IMPOTENCE

Diagnosis and
Management of Erectile
Dysfunction

IMPOTENCE

Diagnosis and Management of Erectile Dysfunction

ALAN H. BENNETT, MD, FACS

Professor of Urological Surgery
Albany Medical College
Albany, New York

W.B. SAUNDERS COMPANY

A Division of Harcourt Brace & Company

Philadelphia   London   Toronto   Montreal   Sydney   Tokyo

W.B. SAUNDERS COMPANY

A Division of Harcourt Brace & Company

The Curtis Center
Independence Square West
Philadelphia, PA 19106-3399

Library of Congress Cataloging-in-Publication Data

Impotence: diagnosis and management of erectile dysfunction / [edited by] Alan
H. Bennett. — 1st ed.
      p.   cm.
   ISBN 0–7216–3768–X
   1. Impotence. I. Bennett, Alan H. (Alan Hugh).
   [DNLM: 1. Impotence.   WJ 709 I348 1994]
RC889.I49   1994
616.6′92—dc20
DNLM/DLC   93–2267

Impotence: Diagnosis and Management of Erectile Dysfunction   ISBN 0–7216–3768–X

Printed in United States of America

Last digit is the print number: 9 8 7 6 5 4 3 2 1

This book is dedicated to Ronald Virag of Paris, France, whose seminal work and innovative ideas in the field of impotence have made much of what is published in these pages possible. His guidance and friendship over the past decade have been an invaluable resource to me and to others who have devoted a significant portion of their careers to improving male sexual health.

Contributors

James H. Barada, MD
Assistant Professor of Surgery, Albany Medical
College; Attending Physician, Albany Medical
Center Hospital and Albany Memorial Hospital,
Albany, New York

Vasoactive Pharmacotherapy

Alan H. Bennett, MD, FACS
Professor of Urological Surgery, Albany Medical
College, Albany, New York

Iatrogenic Causes of Impotence

George S. Benson, MD
Professor of Surgery (Urology), University of
Texas Medical School at Houston; Staff
Urologist, Hermann Hospital; Chief of Urology,
Lyndon Baines Johnson Hospital,
Houston, Texas

Endocrine Factors Related to Impotence

Richard E. Berger, MD
Professor of Urology, University of Washington;
Attending Physician at University of
Washington Affiliated Hospitals,
Seattle, Washington

Nonvascular Causes of Impotence

Jeffrey P. Buch, MD
Assistant Professor of Surgery (Urology),
University of Connecticut Health Center;
Attending Staff, John Dempsey Hospital;
Consulting Staff, Gaylord Rehabilitation
Hospital; Courtesy Staff, Hartford Hospital,
Farmington, Connecticut

Disorders of Ejaculation

Culley C. Carson, MD
Professor and Chief of Urology, University of
North Carolina School of Medicine,
Chapel Hill, North Carolina

Impotence and Chronic Renal Failure

George J. Christ, PhD
Assistant Professor and Director of Basic
Research, Department of Urology, Albert
Einstein College of Medicine, Bronx, New York

Anatomy and Physiology of the Penis

Michael Condra, PhD
Assistant Professor, Department of Psychology,
Queen's University, Kingston, Ontario, Canada

The Pharmacology of Impotence

Charles J. Devine, Jr., MD
Professor, Department of Urology, Eastern
Virginia Medical School; Director, Devine
Center for Genitourinary Reconstructive
Surgery, Sentera Norfolk General Hospital;
Emeritus Staff, Department of Urology,
Children's Hospital of the King's Daughters,
Norfolk, Virginia

*Bends of the Penis, Peyronie's Disease, and Other
Problems*

Craig F. Donatucci, MD
Assistant Professor of Urology and Head, Section
of Male Sexual Dysfunction, Division of
Urology, Department of Surgery, Duke
University Medical Center,
Durham, North Carolina

Dysfunction of the Venoocclusive Mechanism

Irwin Goldstein, MD
Professor of Urology, Boston University School of
Medicine, Boston, Massachusetts

Epidemiology of Impotence
*Pelvic, Perineal, and Penile Trauma-Associated
Arteriogenic Impotence: Pathophysiologic
Mechanisms and the Role of Microvascular
Arterial Bypass Surgery*

Dimitrios G. Hatzichristou, MD
Fellow, Department of Urology, Boston University
School of Medicine, Boston, Massachusetts;
Lecturer, Department of Urology, School of
Medicine, Aristotelian University of
Thessaloniki, Greece

Epidemiology of Impotence
Pelvic, Perineal, and Penile Trauma-Associated
Arteriogenic Impotence: Pathophysiologic
Mechanisms and the Role of Microvascular
Arterial Bypass Surgery

Jeremy W. P. Heaton, MD
Associate Professor, Department of Urology,
Queen's University; Attending Staff, Kingston
General Hospital and Hotel Dieu Hospital,
Kingston, Ontario, Canada

The Pharmacology of Impotence

Mark S. Hirsch, MD
Resident in Urology, Montefiore Medical Center/
Albert Einstein College of Medicine,
Bronx, New York

Anatomy and Physiology of the Penis

Gerald H. Jordan, MD
Professor of Urology, Eastern Virginia Medical
School; Director, Devine Center for
Genitourinary Reconstruction Surgery, Sentera
Norfolk General Hospital; Attending Physician,
Leigh Memorial and Children's Hospital of the
King's Daughters, Norfolk, Virginia

Bends of the Penis, Peyronie's Disease, and Other
Problems

Bernard F. King, MD
Assistant Professor of Radiology, Mayo School of
Medicine; Consultant in Radiology, Mayo
Clinic, Rochester, Minnesota

The Diagnostic Algorithm
Radiologic Evaluation of Impotence

Milton M. Lakin, MD, FACP
Professor and Head, Section of Male Sexual
Medicine, Department of Urology, Cleveland
Clinic Foundation, Cleveland, Ohio

Penile Prostheses

Ronald W. Lewis, MD
Professor of Urology, Mayo School of Medicine;
Consultant in Urology, Mayo Clinic,
Rochester, Minnesota

The Diagnostic Algorithm
Radiologic Evaluation of Impotence

Tom F. Lue, MD
Professor, Department of Urology, University of
California at San Francisco School of Medicine,
San Francisco, California

Dysfunction of the Venoocclusive Mechanism

Eric L. Martin, MD
Instructor of Surgery, Albany Medical College;
Chief Resident, Urology, Albany Medical
Center Hospital, Albany, New York

Iatrogenic Causes of Impotence

Roger M. McKimmy, MD
Chief Resident, Division of Urology, Department
of Surgery, Albany Medical College and Albany
Medical Center Hospital, Albany, New York

Vasoactive Pharmacotherapy

Michael A. McKusick, MD
Assistant Professor of Diagnostic Radiology, Mayo
Medical School; Consultant in Diagnostic
Radiology, Mayo Clinic and Mayo Foundation,
Rochester, Minnesota

Radiologic Evaluation of Impotence

Arnold Melman, MD
Professor and Chairman, Albert Einstein College
of Medicine/Montefiore Medical Center,
Bronx, New York

Anatomy and Physiology of the Penis

Drogo K. Montague, MD
Professor of Surgery (Urology), The Ohio State
University College of Medicine; Head, Section
of Prosthetic Surgery, Department of Urology,
and Director, Center for Sexual Function,
Cleveland Clinic Foundation, Cleveland, Ohio

Penile Prostheses

Alvaro Morales, MD, FRCSC
Professor, Department of Urology, Queen's
    University; Attending Staff and Urologist-in-
    Chief, Kingston General Hospital and Hotel
    Dieu Hospital; Consultant Staff, St. Mary's of
    the Lake Hospital, Kingston, Ontario, Canada

The Pharmacology of Impotence

Perry W. Nadig, MD
Clinical Professor of Urologic Surgery, University
    of Texas Health Science Center, San Antonio;
    Active Staff, Santa Rosa Hospital and
    Metropolitan General Hospital,
    San Antonio, Texas

Vacuum Therapy and Other Devices

Edoardo S. Pescatori, MD
Staff, Institute of Urology, University of Padova,
    Padova, Italy

*Pelvic, Perineal, and Penile Trauma-Associated
    Arteriogenic Impotence: Pathophysiologic
    Mechanisms and the Role of Microvascular
    Arterial Bypass Surgery*

Gilbert Rigaud, MD
Resident in Urology, University of Washington
    Affiliated Hospitals, Seattle, Washington

Nonvascular Causes of Impotence

Ivan Rothman, RN, MN
Research Nurse Clinician, Department of Urology,
    University of Washington Medical Center,
    Seattle, Washington

Nonvascular Causes of Impotence

Mehdi Sarkarati, MD
Instructor in Surgery, Harvard School of
    Medicine, Boston; Chief, SCI Service,
    Brockton/West Roxbury Veterans Affairs
    Medical Center, West Roxbury, Massachusetts

Sexual Dysfunction and Spinal Cord Injury

Kathleen Blindt Segraves, PhD
Assistant Professor of Psychiatry, Case Western
    Reserve School of Medicine; Director of
    Behavioral Medicine, Department of Psychiatry,
    MetroHealth Medical Center, Cleveland, Ohio

Psychogenic Impotence

R. Taylor Segraves, MD, PhD
Professor of Psychiatry, Case Western Reserve
    School of Medicine; Interim Chairperson,
    Department of Psychiatry, MetroHealth Medical
    Center, Cleveland, Ohio

Psychogenic Impotence

Ira D. Sharlip, MD
Assistant Clinical Professor, Department of
    Urology, University of California at San
    Francisco; Vice Chairman, Department of
    Urology, California-Pacific Medical Center,
    San Francisco, California

*Vasculogenic Impotence Secondary to
    Atherosclerosis/Dysplasia*

Maryrose P. Sullivan, PhD
Research Associate, Biomedical Engineer, West
    Roxbury Veterans Affairs Medical Center,
    West Roxbury, Massachusetts

Sexual Dysfunction and Spinal Cord Injury

Martyn A. Vickers, Jr., MD
Assistant Professor of Urology Surgery, Harvard
    Medical School, Boston; Staff Physician in
    Urology, Brigham and Women's Hospital and
    West Roxbury Veterans Affairs Medical Center,
    West Roxbury, Massachusetts

Sexual Dysfunction and Spinal Cord Injury

Subbarao V. Yalla, MD
Associate Professor of Urology, Harvard Medical
    School, Boston; Chief of Urology, West
    Roxbury Veterans Affairs Medical Center,
    West Roxbury, Massachusetts

Sexual Dysfunction and Spinal Cord Injury

Preface

In the past decade and a half, impotence has been the focus of numerous scientific developments. Research into the anatomy, physiology, and biochemistry of erectile function has made it possible to define specific organic disorders that can result in impotence. Now, with a high degree of accuracy, clinicians are able to differentiate between organic and psychogenic causes.

Epidemiologic studies demonstrate that impotence is a common disorder: one in five men over the age of 50, and one in four over the age of 65, suffer from erectile or ejaculatory dysfunction (Gallop Survey, October, 1991). This same survey indicates that only 27% of men with impotence discuss the problem with their physicians. To extrapolate from this small survey conclusions that apply to the entire population is difficult, but it can safely be estimated that 10% of the male population or 10 to 20 million men are impotent in the United States. In 1990, Biomedical Business International estimated that 116,500 men received treatment for impotence in the United States: intracavernosal pharmacotherapy, 42,500; vacuum systems, 44,000; penile implants, 28,500; and vascular or surgical repair, 1,500. To this number should be added patients who are receiving oral agents, testosterone supplementation, or sexual counseling in one form or another. Thus, it is entirely possible that in 1990 one quarter of a million men were actually treated for impotence in the United States.

Impotence: Diagnosis and Management of Erectile Dysfunction brings together experts in the basic science and the clinical management of impotence. The text will cover current methods of diagnosing and treating the impotent male as well as discuss the current research that is ongoing in the various areas of impotence management.

Alan H. Bennett, MD

Contents

CHAPTER 1

Epidemiology of Impotence

Irwin Goldstein

Dimitrios G. Hatzichristou

Impairment of erectile function, although nominally a benign disorder, has a profound impact on the well-being of many men.[1] It has been estimated that 10 million American males have impotence.[2,3] The National Center for Health Statistics data from the National Ambulatory Medical Care Survey showed that in 1985 in the United States, impotence accounted for over 400,000 outpatient physician visits, over 30,000 hospital admissions, and a total cost of 146 million dollars.[4]

Epidemiologic studies on the prevalence of impotence and its possible physical and psychologic correlates have been limited in purpose and scope. The methods for obtaining study populations differed, the criteria for defining impotence varied, the reports of impotence were not stratified by age, and none examined physiologic correlates.[5] Recently, the Massachusetts Male Aging Study (MMAS), the first large epidemiologic study on sexual function in a general population, provided normative data on impotence, defining its prevalence and identifying physiologic and psychologic correlates.[6-9] In this chapter, we review the contemporary knowledge of the epidemiology of impotence and the first results of the MMAS.[6-8]

EPIDEMIOLOGIC STUDIES ON IMPOTENCE: AN OVERVIEW
Prevalence

There have been few epidemiologic studies in the general population on male sexual dysfunction.[5] Kinsey's survey in 1948 represented the first comprehensive study on sexual behavior.[10] It included 12,000 males from representative samples of the general population stratified for age, education, and occupation. Results were based on detailed, structured interviews. Kinsey found that impotence increased with age. It occurred in less than 1% of the male population before the age of 19, in less than 3% of men younger than 45 years, in 6.7% of men between 45 and 55 years, and in 25% by the age of 75 years. In 1979 in a reanalysis of

Kinsey's data, Gebhard and Johnson reported that in a sample of 5460 white males and 177 black males, 42% had erectile problems.[11] The prevalence of ever having had trouble getting or keeping an erection "more than incidentally" was 18.9% in noncollege-educated white males, 5.6% in college-educated white males, and 6.4% in college-educated black males, all between the ages of 15 and 81 + years.

Other studies, investigating the prevalence of impotence in the general population, included small samples. In 1977, Ard reported on the sexual attitudes and behaviors of 161 couples married more than 20 years.[12] Erectile problems were self-reported by 3% of the male sample. A year later, Frank et al. reported on 100 "normal" volunteer couples who were married and sexually active.[13] The mean age of the men was 37 ± 11 years. Forty percent of the men reported erectile or ejaculatory dysfunction. In 1979, Nettelbladt and Uddenberg reported that 40% of 58 randomly selected males, mean age 31, living with their partner, noted some degree of erectile dysfunction, and 7% could not penetrate during coitus.[14] The instrument of the study was not discussed.[14] Schover, in 1988, used a sexual history form and found that 3% of 92 men in stable relationships had erectile dysfunction. The sample was collected through a newspaper advertisement.[5] Ninety-eight presumably normal, white, British male volunteers, aged 20–35 years, representing a range of social classes, were included in a study by Reading and Wiest in 1984.[15] They found that 8.3% of the men reported impotence and 11% described a decreased desire for any interest in sex. Diokno et al. reported 40% impotence in 283 noninstitutionalized men over age 60.[16] The Baltimore Longitudinal Study of Aging reported that by the age of 55, impotence was a problem in 8% of healthy men. For 65, 75, and 80-year-old men, the prevalence of impotence was 25%, 55%, and 75%, respectively.[17] The Charleston Heart Study Cohort reported as sexually inactive 30% of subjects between 66 and 69 years of age and 60%

of those aged 80 or older.[18] In this study, sexual function was self-reported. In general, all these studies shared problems of both nonrepresentative samples due to the method of sampling and the unknown value of the instruments used to assess erectile function in the various populations.[5]

Data concerning the prevalence of impotence have been reported also in restricted groups of men using medical care. These studies were performed primarily in impotent and ill subjects. Schein et al. reported that the prevalence of impotence in 212 family practice patients with a mean age of 35 years was 27%.[19] Pfeifer and Davis observed in 261 males that age negatively correlated with current sexual function.[20] Mulligan et al. reported that middle-aged men with subjective poor health had a 6-fold increase in the likelihood of being sexually dysfunctional, whereas in those over 70 years, there was a 40-fold increase. The authors noticed that although 50% of males over the age of 80 years reported continued interest in sexual function, only 15% were still engaged in sexual intercourse.[21] Morley found a 27% prevalence of impotence in men over age 50 who elected to have a nutritional and general health screening.[22] He concluded that individuals with impotence were more likely to have a medical disorder, to receive medication, or to be depressed. Such an observation— that there is an increased incidence of impotence in men with medical conditions—is in keeping with the finding of Slag et al., who reported that 34% of 1180 men receiving care at a medical outpatient clinic were impotent.[23] Masters and Johnson noted that 50% of those men requesting treatment for erectile dysfunction had "secondary" impotence.[24]

Vascular Disease and Vascular Risk Factors

Chronic illness has been thought to account for the decline in sexual function with aging.[21] The association of impotence with vascular disease is well documented in the literature. Alterations in the inflow (cavernosal artery insufficiency) and outflow (corporal venoocclusive dysfunction) of blood to and from the penis are thought to be the most frequent causes of organic impotence.[25]

Impairments in the arterial hemodynamics of erection have been demonstrated in patients with myocardial infarction, coronary bypass surgery, cerebral vascular accidents, peripheral vascular disease, and hypertension. Wabrek and Burchell reported that 64% of 131 males, aged 31 to 86 years, hospitalized for an acute myocardial infarction were impotent.[26] In 130 impotent men, the incidence of myocardial infarction was found to be 12% and 1.5%, in patients with abnormal and normal penile–brachial index measurements, respectively.[27] In another study, 57% of patients who underwent coronary artery surgery were "mostly" impotent.[28] Forty to fifty percent of men with clinically significant peripheral arterial disease complained of impotence, and in 80% of these, the cause of the erectile dysfunction was primarily organic.[29] Oaks and Moyer reported that 8% to 10% of untreated hypertensive patients were impotent at the time of the hypertension diagnosis.[30]

Vascular disease has been recognized as a leading cause of impotence in diabetic patients. Several investigators have found high rates of vascular abnormalities in patients with diabetes mellitus, particularly in those who were impotent. In diabetics, the prevalence of impotence has been estimated at 35% to 50%, and in some reports, the percentage was as high as 75%.[1] In 12% of diabetics, impotence was the first sign of the disease.[31] The prevalence of impotence in diabetes has been found to be age-dependent, with impotence existing in 15% and 55% at ages 30 to 34 and 60, respectively.[32] Such age dependency was noticed at an earlier age in diabetes than in the general population. Other studies reported that 9% of 88 diabetics, ages 20 to 29, complained of impotence, and 50% of diabetics became impotent within 10 years of the diagnosis of diabetes.[33] Rubin and Babbott reported that 45% of men with diabetes for more than 5 years developed impotence, although there was no statistical correlation between duration of diabetes and impotence.[34] Diabetic hypertensive men have sexual dysfunction in 40% to 80% of cases.[35] Jevtich et al. noted vascular obstructive changes in 95% of impotent diabetic patients.[36] Lehman and Jacobs reported that 83% of the type I diabetics has vascular abnormalities compared to 57% of the type II diabetics, implying that vascular obstruction correlates with the severity and duration of the diabetes rather than the patient's age.[37] Other studies have shown that diabetic patients with impotence have both impaired neurogenic and endothelium-mediated relaxation of penile smooth muscle.[38]

Several studies in impotent men report that the prevalence of organic impotence increased as the number of vascular risk factors identified in their histories increased. Shabsigh et al. reported that smoking, diabetes, and hypertension are risk factors for vasculogenic impotence and the proportion of abnormal penile vascular findings significantly increased as the number of risk factors increased.[39] Virag et al. investigated the distribution of the four main arterial risk factors (diabetes, cigarette smoking, hypertension, and hyperlipidemia) in 440 impotent men.[29] They reported that in 80% of cases, the cause of impotence is a physiologic abnormality, 53% had arterial atherosclerotic lesions, and 34% had hypercholesterolemia. The study concluded that hypertension, smoking (64%), diabetes (30%), and hyperlipidemia (34%) were all significantly more common in the 440 impotent men studied than in the general population.

Hormones and Impotence

Androgens influence the growth and development of the male reproductive tract as well as secondary sexual characteristics.[40] Their effect on libido and sexual behavior is well established, but the effect of androgens on the erectile mechanism remains unclear.[9,40–46] Testosterone, prolactin, and LH have been studied frequently and reported in the literature. Spark et al. suggested that a single determination of serum testosterone in conjunction with history and physical examination is an adequate screening for endocrinologic causes of impotence,[44] as neuroendocrine dysfunction is found in 1% of impotent men.[46] Slag et al., however, reporting on 188 impotent patients with a mean age 60 years, found hypogonadism in 19%, hypothyroidism in 5%, hyperthyroidism in 1%, and hyperprolactinemia in 4%.[23] Murray et al. reported significant correlations between NPT and serum androgens in men with a number of endocrine disorders.[47] A decrease in total and free testosterone and an increase in steroid-binding protein and plasma gonadotropins that parallel the decline in sexual function have been reported.[31]

Gonadal dysfunction also has been proposed as a cause of impotence in diabetics. Murray et al., in a study of 28 impotent diabetic men, aged 24 to 81, found that 83% of the men with impotence and type II diabetes have decreased Leydig cell function.[47] Thirty-nine percent of those patients were identified as having endocrinologic impotence on the basis of high urinary LH excretion and low serum free testosterone levels. Morphologic studies on the testes of impotent diabetic men found increased interstitial collagen, thickening of the seminiferous tubule wall, peritubular and intertubular fibrosis, and tubular sclerosis, suggesting a primary gonadal disorder.[47]

Drug-Induced Impotence

Drug-induced impotence has been proposed as a common pathophysiologic entity. Slag et al. reported a 25% incidence of drug-associated impotence in a medical outpatient population.[23]

Investigations of drug-associated impotence have been based on hospitalized or medical clinic populations. Neri et al. found an increase in the frequency of erectile failure in patients treated with digoxin,[48] and the Coronary Drug Project Research Group reported a decrease of sexual function in 14.1% of patients treated with clofibrate.[49] Sea-

graves et al.[50] and Horowitz and Gobel[51] noted that male sexual dysfunction has been associated with virtually every available antihypertensive agent. Antihypertensive agents reported to cause impotence include sympatholytics (e.g., alpha-methyldopa with an average frequency of erectile dysfunction of 20% to 30%, guanethidine with 24%, clonidine with 4% to 41%, and reserpine with 30% to 40%), beta-adrenoceptor blocking agents (e.g., propranolol in 13.8% of the patients receiving the drug in doses up to 320 mg daily), vasodilators (e.g., hydralazine), and diuretics (e.g., hydrochlorothiazide, bendrofluazide in 36% of patients, spironolactone in 4% to 30% of patients).[48–53]

Ultimately, it is imperative to define a mechanism of action of each suspected drug associated with impotence. Wein and van Arsdalen noted that the diagnosis of drug-induced sexual dysfunction must be restricted to a reproducible dose-related effect that disappears on discontinuation of the drug.[52]

Lifestyle

Paraaging phenomena, such as cigarette smoking, and the cumulative effects of alcohol consumption, obesity, and diminishing physical activity, have been implicated.

In the literature, cigarette smoking and alcoholism have been associated with cardiovascular disease, whereas moderate alcohol consumption has been reported to have the opposite effect.[54] The organic processes that mediate the effect of chronic alcoholism on sexual function are not known but are likely to include neurologic mechanisms.[55] An increased incidence of cigarette smoking among impotent men has been reported by Gray et al.[56] Condra et al. reported a 58.4% incidence of current smokers and an 81% incidence of current and exsmokers combined in a group of 178 patients referred for evaluation of impotence.[57] Similar rates of cigarette smoking (current and exsmokers combined) among impotent men have been reported by Bornman and du Plessis (93%)[58] and Bähren et al. (82%).[59] Rosen et al. found cigarette smoking to be an independent risk factor for atherosclerotic disease in the hypogastric-cavernous arterial bed of impotent men.[60]

Obesity and physical inactivity are not deterrents of sexual function or desire.[61]

Psychologic Correlates

Until the last decade, impotence was thought to be psychogenic in origin in most of the cases. Hengevelt reported that the literature is replete with descriptions of psychologic causes, mainly in the form of case histories.[62] Rust et al. reported that sexual dysfunction in men was able to predict the existence of marital discord in approximately 25% of cases.[63]

Various investigators have found that psychiatric diseases may have a dynamic causative relation to erectile dysfunction. Thase et al. reported impaired nocturnal penile tumescence (NPT) in depressed men.[64] In a highly selected sample, Segraves and Segraves found 47% erectile impairment in 113 men (mean age 51) who had hypoactive sexual desire disorder and participated in a multisite drug study.[65] In depression, the emotions are flat and self-esteem is low. Cognitive-behavioral theory was the first to assign the role of depression as a cause of erectile dysfunction. LoPiccolo noticed that clinicians tended to mislabel symptoms of depression as being caused by erectile failure rather than correctly categorizing erectile failure as a symptom of underlying depression.[66]

WHY EPIDEMIOLOGIC STUDIES ON IMPOTENCE ARE NEEDED

Epidemiologic information is required (1) to answer questions concerning the frequency of various diseases, whether dysfunction rates are increasing, and who is at risk, (2) to examine potential etiologic factors and target prevention programs, and (3) to establish needs for research investigation.[5]

Epidemiologic studies on sexual behavior (including erectile dysfunction) are lacking.[67] The multiple intervening physiologic and psychologic variables that may adversely influence erectile function remain poorly defined. It is possible that impotence is not age dependent (i.e., an inevitable consequence of aging) but rather due to paraaging phenomena (i.e., associated changes, such as illness, medication usage, increased weight, or psychologic phenomena, such as personality change following retirement or change of social status). Although studies conducted in the last decade implied correlation of vascular risk factors with impotence, predictability of these factors in a normal population was lacking.

The nature and determinants of impotence in aging males, therefore, were obscured by lack of scientific information pertinent to a contemporary, healthy population, particularly in the context of physiologic and psychosocial variables. As a result, the Kinsey survey,[10] conducted over 45 years ago in a social and medical context vastly different from that of the present day, remained the most comprehensive population-based source of data on male sexual behavior in the United States. Studies investigating sexual function regretfully concluded that information about the prevalence of impotence in normal populations was too sparse to provide an adequate standard for comparison and that population-based normative data on sexual dysfunction were urgently needed.[5,68]

Studies of normal or apparently healthy individuals are a sine qua non for the identification of populations at risk as new risk factors come under question, as well as for the understanding and clinical management of those at risk.[67] Furthermore, effective clinical management becomes problematic in the absence of baseline data from normal or healthy populations. This lack of scientific information, especially of the prevalence in the general population and the relationship of impotence to intervening variables of physiologic and psychologic concern, has hindered the true health significance of the field.[69]

THE MASSACHUSETTS MALE AGING STUDY
Study Design

The Massachusetts Male Aging Study (MMAS)[6,7] was a cross-sectional, community-based, random-sample, multidisciplinary epidemiologic survey of health and aging in men aged 40 to 70 years. The study was conducted between 1987 and 1989, in 11 randomly selected cities and towns in the area of Boston. Of the 1709 MMAS subjects, 1290 (75.5%) provided complete responses to all the questions of the sexual function instrument and represented the study sample. This sample size is considerably larger than any similar health research in aging to date and is the largest sexual function survey since Kinsey's work in 1948.[10]

The MMAS study was markedly different not only in size but also in content from studies conducted to date. It included four groups of intervening variables (confounders) that can be related systematically to sexual function: health status and medical care use, and sociodemographic, psychosocial, and lifestyle characteristics. The MMAS data were collected at the subject's home by trained interviewers. This theoretical model reflected the multidisciplinary interests represented among the research team: behavioral science, endocrinology, gerontology, sexual dysfunction. Complete hormone profile data, including reliable measurements of 17 hormones, constituted MMAS as the largest male endocrine database available.[9] Such design enabled the MMAS to be the first study permitting precise estimation of key parameters while controlling for potentially important confounders and identification of statistically predictive risk factors. The large random sample of a general, free-living, noninstitutionalized population of the MMAS, only a fraction of which was sick and interacting with the medical care system, afforded the opportunity to address data concerning a generalized population of men.

The MMAS self-administered sexual activity instrument contained 23 questions, of which 9 related most directly to erectile potency. Erectile potency was addressed as a subjective state, as opposed to the more concretely defined phenomenon of erectile dysfunction.[6] The subjects, however, did not assess their potency status directly. A calibration study was conducted to discriminate different potency profiles.[7] To relate the multidimensional MMAS sexual activity instrument to a direct assessment of potency, the 9 MMAS questions most related to potency were answered by all men appearing at the Department of Urology, Boston University Medical Center, during a 6-month period in 1990. One new question was added asking the patients to rate their potency on a scale where the choices were (1) not impotent, (2) minimally impotent, (3) moderately impotent, and (4) completely impotent. A discriminant function combining the 9 sexual activity responses was performed to impute probabilities of nil, minimal, moderate, or complete impotence to each MMAS respondent on the basis of the 9 discriminant variables.[7] Of the 1290 men of the study sample, the discriminant function correctly classified 98% of men who were not impotent and 80% of men who were impotent. All the misclassified men were assigned to an adjacent category.

Research Questions

Based on analysis of the MMAS data, we addressed the following questions[6,8]

1. What is the prevalence of impotence in a population of normal, nominally healthy, aging men, as measured in a community-based random sample?
2. What are the changes of sexual activity and interest with age, and what is the age trend of impotence in this population?
3. What health indices predict impotence over and above the correlated age trend?

All differences noted in the MMAS were statistically significant at $p < 0.01$. The influence of disease, medication, physiologic measures, and lifestyle measures on the pattern of age-adjusted impotence probabilities were assessed by multivariate linear regression and multivariate analysis of variance (MANOVA).

Prevalence of Impotence

More than half of the men (657/1290) had some degree of erectile dysfunction. The largest category comprised 322 moderately impotent (25%), followed by 210 minimally impotent (17%), and 125 completely impotent (10%) men (Fig. 1–1). The prevalence of impotence in the MMAS sample was 52%.[6]

Impotence and Aging[6,8]
How Do Male Sexual Activity and Interest Change Between the Ages 40 and 70 years?[8]

Sexual activity in the MMAS was divided into two broad categories: subjective phenomena and actual events. There was a consistent decline with age in sexual desire, sexual thoughts and dreams, desired level of sexual activity (subjective phenomena), as well as frequency of intercourse, morning erections, difficulties attaining or maintaining an erection or both (actual events).

Subjective phenomena and actual events appeared to occur together. Levels of satisfaction, however, did not show the same age-related changes. Men in their 60s reported the same levels of satisfaction as younger men in their 40s. At least three interpretations of this finding are possible: (1) men simply accommodate to the age-related declines, (2) their expectation from their sexual lives declines also with age, or (3) their sexual expectation accommodates decreased erectile capabilities, adjusting to the current potency status.

What Variables Account for or Are Correlated with Changes in Male Sexual Activity and Interest?[8]

Aging and its social correlates, taken together, were strongly predictive of decreased involvement with sexual activity and a change in attitude. Good health was associated with more involvement and satisfaction. Depression and regression of anger were strongly associated with decreased sexual satisfaction.[8]

What Is the Age Trend of Impotence?[6]

The cross-sectional trend between ages 40 and 70 years for complete impotence was tripled, the probability of moderate as well as overall impotence doubled, and the probability of minimal impotence remained almost constant (Fig. 1–2). Over that age range, the probability of minimal, moderate, and complete impotence was 16.5%, 17.4% and 4.9% at age 40 and 18%, 34%, and 15% at age 70, respectively. The overall probability of impotence at age 40 was 38.9% and at age 70 was 67.1%.

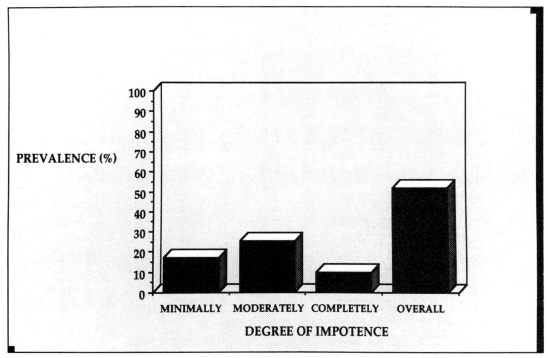

Figure 1–1. Prevalence of minimal, moderate, complete, and overall impotence in the MMAS sample.

Although chronic illness, rather than any intrinsic aspect of age itself, has been suggested as possibly accounting for the decline in sexual function with aging, age was proven to be a predictor of impotence at a statistical significance of $p < 0.0001$.

Disease[6]

Treated diabetes, heart disease, and hypertension as well as untreated ulcer, arthritis, and allergy were the medical conditions associated with impotence. The impotence probability values referenced in succeeding paragraphs have been age-adjusted.

Diabetes

Treated diabetes was associated with probability of impotence (Fig. 1–3). There was a dramatic increase in the probability of complete impotence (tripled, 24.9% to 9.4%), a decrease in the probability of minimal impotence (doubled, 7.7% to 18.2%), and a slight increase in the probability of moderate impotence (30.6% to 24.6%). Overall impotence increased by 11%. These results imply that diabetes exacerbates minimal impotence to complete impotence over and above the higher probability of overall impotence in treated diabetics.

Heart Disease

The probability of minimal, moderate, and complete impotence was 16.1%, 40.7%, and 21.3% among nonsmokers and 16.6%, 21.2%, and 56.4% among current cigarette smokers, respectively, in men being treated for heart disease (Fig. 1–4). The probability of minimal, moderate, and complete impotence for those reporting no heart disease was 18.1%, 24.5%, and 8.5%, respectively, with no difference between smokers and nonsmokers. Although minimal impotence was unchanged, two different patterns were noticed in moderate and complete impotence with respect to cigarette smoking. In the nonsmoking group, both moderate and complete impotence doubled, whereas in the smoking group, moderate impotence decreased slightly and complete impotence increased six times. These data may imply that patients with heart disease and moderate impotence could have complete impotence if they were smokers.

In conclusion, treated heart disease is associated with 78% overall impotence in nonsmokers and 94.3% in smokers.

Hypertension

In nonsmoking men with treated hypertension, no significant differences from the study sample as a whole were noted. Moderate impotence proba-

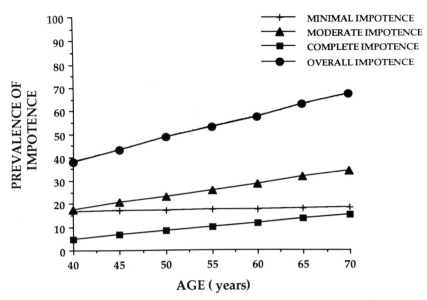

Figure 1–2. The age trend of impotence in the MMAS sample.

bilities were decreased from 23.5% in those without the disease and 31.6% in nonsmokers with treated disease to 19.4%. Complete impotence probabilities were doubled, from 8.6% in those without the disease and 8.5% in nonsmokers with treated hypertension to 19.8% (Fig. 1–5). The overall effect of the disease was characterized by an increase in the probability of complete impotence up to 15%, compared to 8.6% in men without the disease.

Ulcer

Untreated ulcer was associated with 17.6% probability of complete impotence, compared to

9.5% probability in those without the disease. Treated disease was associated with 36.1% moderate impotence, compared to 24.5% and 27% in those without the disease and with untreated disease, respectively.

Arthritis

Among subjects reporting untreated arthritis, the current smokers had a 19.8% probability of complete impotence and the nonsmokers had a 9.4% probability, compared with an 8.7% probability in those without the disease. Treated disease was associated with a significantly increased probability of minimal and mod-

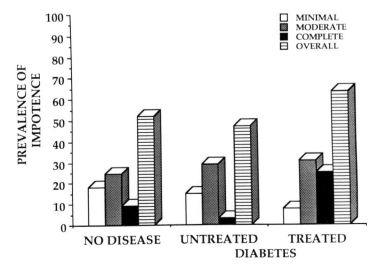

Figure 1–3. Prevalence of minimal, moderate, complete, and overall impotence in untreated and treated diabetics in the MMAS sample.

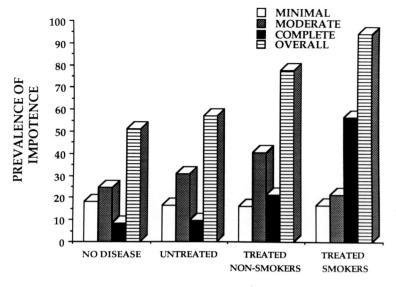

HEART DISEASE

Figure 1—4. Prevalence of impotence in untreated and treated smokers and nonsmokers with heart disease in the MMAS sample.

erate impotence. The overall impotence was 54.5% for nonsmokers and 67% for smokers with untreated disease, 71.7% for those with treated disease, and 49.7% for those without the disease.

Allergy

A similar pattern was found for untreated allergy, although the changes were slighter. Men with untreated allergy had a 12.5% probability of complete impotence (9.8% in those without this condition). The overall impotence was 52% in the

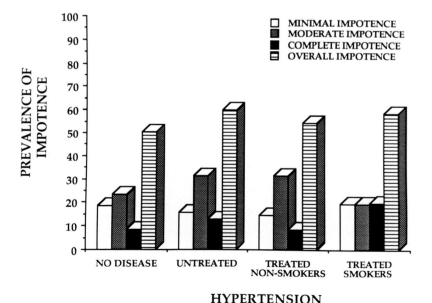

HYPERTENSION

Figure 1—5. Prevalence of impotence in untreated and treated smokers and nonsmokers who are hypertensive in the MMAS sample.

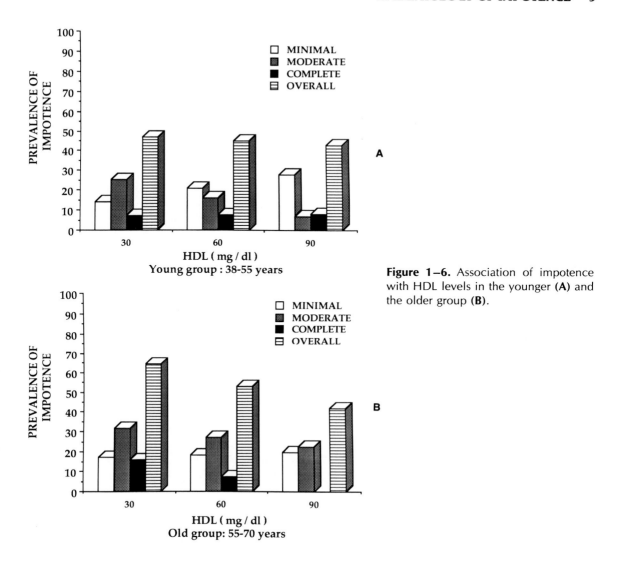

Figure 1–6. Association of impotence with HDL levels in the younger (**A**) and the older group (**B**).

untreated group, 60.6% in the treated group and 52.8% in those without the disease.

Lipids

Raising high-density lipoprotein (HDL) and lowering low-density lipoprotein (LDL) are associated with lack of progression or even regression of coronary disease. In the MMAS, two impotence probability patterns were identified regarding HDL cholesterol. The first represents changes in younger men, age d 38 to 55 years (Fig. 1–6A), and the second represents changes in older men, aged 56 to 70 years (Fig. 1–6B). The probability of moderate impotence in the younger group was 6.7% when the HDL value was 90 mg/dl. The percentage was increased to 16.1% and 25.5% when HDL values decreased to 60 and 30 mg/dl, respectively.

On the other hand, minimal impotence was diminished from 27.7% at an HDL level of 90 mg/dl to 20.9% and 14.1% at HDL levels of 60 and 90 mg/dl, respectively, while the probability of complete and overall impotence remained constant. This implies that men at this age range with minimal impotence may experience moderate impotence if their level of HDL drops from 90 to 30 mg/dl.

Among the older men, no one with complete impotence was identified (0% probability of complete impotence) in those with HDL values more than 90 mg/dl. When the HDL values dropped to 60 or 30 mg/dl, the probability of complete impotence increased to 7.2% and 16.1%, respectively, accompanied by an increase of the overall probability of impotence from 41.9% when the HDL values were 90 mg/dl to 53% and 64.8%

when HDL values decreased to 60 and 30 mg/dl, respectively. These data, added to the finding that total serum cholesterol was not correlated with impotence probability, support HDL levels as a strong determinant of impotence.

Hormones

In the MMAS, one hormone was significantly predictive of the pattern of impotence probability. The adrenal androgen metabolite dehydroepiandrosterone sulfate (DHEAS). DHEAS levels of 0.5 mg/ml were associated with 16% probability of complete impotence, compared to 6.5% and 3.4% probability of complete impotence when the DHEAS levels were 5 and 10 mg/ml, respectively (Fig. 1–7). The probability of minimal impotence decreased as DHEAS levels were decreasing and complete impotence probability was increasing, while the probability of overall and moderate impotence remained unchanged. Therefore, minimally impotent men may become completely impotent if their DHEAS levels decrease from 10 to 0.5 mg/ml. The fact that the serum concentration of DHEAS declines more rapidly with age than many other androgens was not a factor, since the MMAS data were adjusted for age.

Testosterone, either free, albumin-bound, or total, was not statistically significantly correlated with impotence. This may be explained by the metaanalysis of the MMAS data, which suggests that any decline in testosterone with age may be due in large part to ill health rather than being a natural physiologic phenomenon.

No correlation with impotence was found for any other of 17 hormones measured, including prolactin, follicle-stimulating hormone (FSH), luteinizing hormone (LH), sex-hormone binding globulin, androstenedione, androstanediol, and estrogens.

Medications

Impotence was statistically associated with vasodilators and antihypertensive, cardiac, and hypoglycemic medications. No correlation was found between impotence and the use of sympathetic drugs.

In men taking vasodilators, the probability of moderate and complete impotence increased from 24.7% and 9.3% to 41.7% and 36.2%, respectively (Fig. 1–8.). The overall probability of impotence was increased from 51.9% for those not using vasodilators to 91% for those using such agents.

Cardiac drug and antihypertensive users showed two patterns with respect to cigarette smoking. Among subjects using cardiac drugs, the current smokers had a 41.3% probability of complete impotence, compared with 14.3% for the nonsmokers and 8.7% for those not under treatment (Fig. 1–9). Similarly, current smokers taking antihypertensives had a 21.1% probability of complete impotence, compared with 7.5% for the nonsmokers and 9.6% for those not using these medications (Fig. 1–10).

Hypoglycemic agent users had a 25.6% probability of complete impotence, compared with 9.3% for those not in such treatment and 24.9% for treated diabetics.

The impotence probability pattern in users of

Figure 1–7. Association of impotence with DHEAS levels in the MMAS sample.

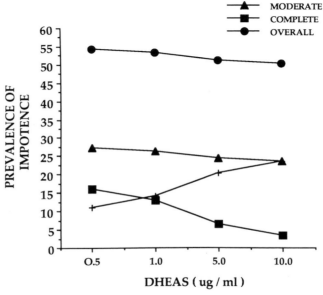

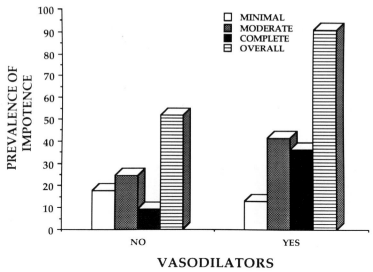

Figure 1–8. Prevalence of impotence in men treated with vasodilators.

these medications, as was expected, closely re-sembled that in subjects reporting treated heart disease, hypertension, or diabetes. Since diabetes, heart disease, and hypertension were associated with impotence in the MMAS sample, it is diffi-cult to indict unequivocally the drugs prescribed to treat those conditions, namely, antiglycemics, antihypertensives, and heart medications, inas-much as virtually all of the men taking the medi-cations had been diagnosed with the corresponding disease.

Cigarette Smoking

Impotence probabilities did not differ signifi-cantly between current smokers and nonsmokers or subjects who reported exposure to cigarette smoke at home or at work and those who reported none. Among current smokers, impotence proba-bilities showed no dependence on dosage (packs per day) or on lifetime pack-years smoked. Ciga-rette smoking, however, had dramatic exacerbating effects in certain subgroups.

The probability of moderate and complete im-

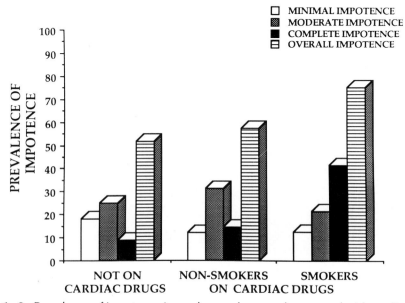

Figure 1–9. Prevalence of impotence in smokers and nonsmokers treated with cardiac drugs.

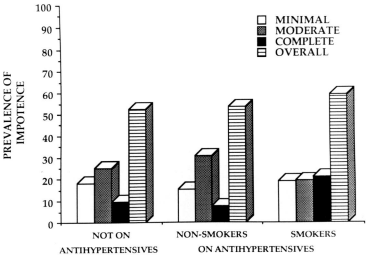

Figure 1–10. Prevalence of impotence in smokers and nonsmokers treated with antihypertensives.

potence in those reported being treated for heart disease were 40.7%, 21.3% among nonsmokers and 21.2% and 56.4% among current cigarette smokers, respectively, as previously reported (Fig. 1–4). Although minimal impotence was unchanged, two different patterns were seen in moderate and complete impotence with respect to cigarette smoking. In the nonsmoking group, both moderate (40.7%) and complete impotence (21.3%) were approximately doubled, and the overall impotence probability approximated 78% whereas in the smoking group, moderate impotence remained constant (21.2%), complete impotence increased six times (56.4%), and the overall probability of impotence reached 94.3%. These data could imply that patients with heart disease and moderate impotence would be completely impotent if they were smokers. The exacerbating effects of smoking were even higher among men with heart disease using cardiac drugs. The current smokers had a 41.3% probability of complete impotence, and the nonsmokers had only a 14.3% probability (Fig. 1–9).

Similar patterns were found in current smokers with treated hypertension and current smokers taking antihypertensive medications (Figs. 1–5 and 1–10). Complete impotence probabilities were doubled, from 8.6% in those without the disease (or 9.6% for those not using these medications) and 8.5% in nonsmokers who were treated with hypertensives (7.5% for nonsmokers taking antihypertensives) to 19.8% in smokers with treated hypertension (21.1% in current smokers taking antihypertensives). Finally, smoking exac-

erbated the probabilities of impotence in one more medical condition. Current smokers with untreated arthritis had a 19.8% probability of complete impotence, and nonsmokers had a 9.4% probability (8.7% in those without the disease).

Lifestyle

Other paraaging phenomena, such as obesity and alcohol consumption, were investigated. No influence on sexual function of such behavior patterns was noticed.

Psychologic Correlates

In the MMAS study, depression, anger either expressed outward or kept inward, and lower levels of dominance were psychologic factors found to be strongly associated with impotence.

Depression

The CES-depression scale[70] data were correlated with impotence. Minimal depression was associated with 4.6% and 42.3% complete and overall impotence, respectively, and major depression was correlated with 40.7% and 100% probability of complete and overall impotence, respectively (Fig. 1–11). Depression, with its highly variable and culture-specific manifestations of persistent sadness, flat affect, and low self-esteem, is seen in a variety of mental and physical disorders and may be diagnosed either as a primary mental disorder or as secondary to an underlying disorder.

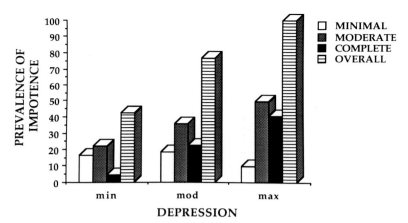

Figure 1–11. Correlation of impotence and depression in the MMAS sample.

Anger

Anger, either suppression or expression (Fig. 1–12), was correlated with 19.2% to 35.4% and 4% to 19% probabilites of moderate and complete impotence, respectively, the range expressing minimal, moderate, and maximal anger, as defined by Spielberger's anger scale.[71] The overall impotence probabilites increased from 37% in those with minimal anger to 74% to 77.4% for the group with maximal anger suppression or expression.

Hostility and expression of anger are associated with many organic diseases, such as peptic ulcer and coronary disease.[72,73] Excessive sympathetic arousal is mediated by chronic anxiety, abnormal personality traits, and problems with expression of emotions, particularly anger. Anger is accompanied by increases in heart rate, mean arterial pressure, and plasma catecholamine levels.[74,75] Excessive sympathetic outflow or elevated blood catecholamine levels or both, in an anxious individual may increase penile smooth muscle tone, opposing the smooth muscle relaxation necesary for erection.[1]

Dominance

The Jackson scale of dominance,[76] used in the MMAS, measures the frequency of attempts to control one's environment and influence others. A higher level of dominance was found to be associated with a 45% probability of overall impotence, and the lower level of dominance was associated with a 64% probability of impotence (Fig. 1–13).

Dominance is a basic personality characteristic, defined as the persistent predisposition to play a prominent or controlling role when interacting with others. Individuals having low levels of dominance

have low self-esteem and may be expected to interact poorly with others in many areas, including sexual interaction. Such characteristics may make them particularly prone to impotence.

CONCLUSIONS

Epidemiologic data on impotence are limited.[5] The MMAS was a methodologically unique effort at examining, in a community-based random sample of noninstitutionalized aging men, a broad and comprehensive set of variables relating to aging and sexual function.[6] The high prevalance of impotence found in the study implies that some degree of erectile dysfunction is present in more than 20 million American men, and impotence, therefore, may be considered a major health concern.

Impotence was strongly associated with age. A consistent decline with age in sexual desire and sexual activity, but not in sexual satisfaction, was reported for the MMAS population.[8] Although these observations may simply mean that subjective and actual events, as well as sexual expectation, follow an age-related decline, they should not rule out the possibility that sexual expectations accommodate decreased erectile capabilities. The importance of these data should be emphasized, since by the year 2030, 20% of the U.S. population will be more than 65 years old,[77] and life expectancy for men has already increased by 3 years.[78]

The multiplicity of potential determinants identified suggests that impotence does not inexorably accompany aging, but it is augmented significantly by modifiable paraaging phenomena. Heart disease and four associated vascular risk factors, diabetes, hypertension, and low serum HDL were signifi-

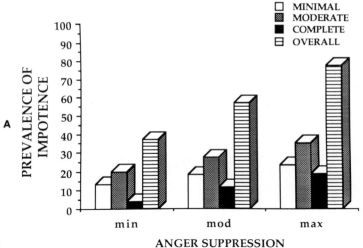

Figure 1–12. Correlation of impotence and anger suppression **(A)** or expression **(B)** in the MMAS sample.

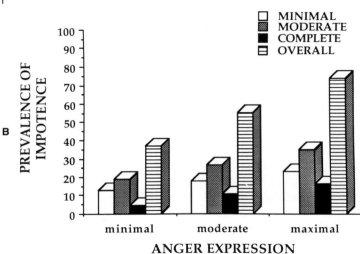

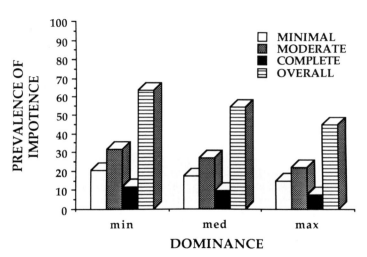

Figure 1–13. Correlation of impotence and dominance in the MMAS sample.

cantly correlated with impotence in the MMAS sample. Cigarette smoking exacerbated the probabilities of impotence, principally in men with cardiovascular disease. It is of interest that DHEAS levels, the only hormone of the 17 measured in the study associated with impotence, have been proposed in the literature as predictors for cardiovascular disease.[79] It may be inferred that vascular compromise, as reflected in cardiovascular or cerebrovascular disease, shares common determinants with vascular impairment of penile erection, the most common cause of organic impotence.

Medications associated with those diseases also were correlated to impotence. In the MMAS observational setting, however, it was not possible to assess if there was a confounding influence of the underlying medical condition causing impotence separate from the medications themselves. A much larger survey or a clinical study focusing on the mechanism of action of each drug suspected of inducing impotence would be required to disentangle the two factors definitively and establish the agent as causative.

All the psychologic factors screened in the study were found to be associated with impotence. Although psychogenic stimuli can facilitate erection, it is clear that cerebral input also can have inhibitory effect on the erectile response. Psychogenic input to the sacral cord may inhibit the reflexogenic erections and, therefore, activation of the parasympathetic dilator nerves to the penis. A man who has been experiencing a pattern of organic erectile dysfunction may be expected to be anxious, depressed, and lacking self-esteem and self-confidence, since performance anxiety and sexual inhibition are among the most common causes of psychogenic impotence.

Limiting our ability to draw conclusions from an observational, cross-sectional study was the fact that biologic, psychologic, and social factors act in concert and influence one another reciprocally. In addition, there have been no previous epidemiologic studies to measure changes in potency status and its intervening variables over time and thus determine the extent to which such changes may account for changes in erectile function in the same subjects over time.

A follow-up longitudinal study, assessing intra-subject changes over a 5–year period interval of the MMAS population, is planned.

ACKNOWLEDGMENT

We acknowledge our indebtedness for their contributions to the Massachusetts Male Aging Study on Impotence to John B. McKinley, Ph.D., Professor of Sociology and Research Professor of Medicine, Boston University and Director, New England Research Institute, Henry Feldman, Ph.D., Associate Professor of Applied Mathematics, Harvard University School of Public Health, and Senior Scientist, New England Research Institute, Robert J.Krane, M.D., Professor and Chairman, Department of Urology, Boston University School of Medicine, and Christopher Longcope, M.D., Professor of Obstetrics, Gynecology and Medicine, University of Massachusetts Medical School. The MMAS was supported by NIH/NIA grant AG04673.

REFERENCES

1. Krane RJ, Goldstein I, Saenz de Tejada I. Impotence. N. Engl J Med 321:1648, 1989.
2. Shabsigh R, Fishman IJ, Scott FB. Evaluation of erectile impotence. Urology 32:83, 1988.
3. Furlow WL. Prevalence of impotence in the United States. Med Aspects Hum Sex 19:13, 1985.
4. National Center for Health Statistics. National Hospital Discharge Survey, 1985. Bethesda, MD: Department of Health and Human Services. DHHS publication No. 87–1751, 1989.
5. Spector IP, Carey MP. Incidence and prevalence of the sexual dysfunctions: a critical review of the empirical literature. Arch Sex Behav 19:389, 1990.
6. Feldman HA, Goldstein I, Hatzichristou DG, et al. Impotence and its medical and psychosocial correlates. (in press)
7. Feldman HA, Goldstein I, Hatzichristou DG, et al. Impotence in Massachusetts males aged 40–70: methods for imputation of uncollected data. (in press)
8. McKinley JB, Feldman HA. Changes in sexual activity and interest in the normally aging male: results from the Massachusetts Male Aging Study. In: Rossi A, ed. Proceedings of the MacArthur Foundation Research Network on Successful Mid-Life Development, 1992.
9. Gray A, Feldman HA, McKinley JB, Longcope C. Age, disease and changing sex hormone levels in middle-aged men: results of the Massachusetts Male Aging Study. J Clin Endocrinol Metab 71:1442, 1990.
10. Kinsey AC, Pomeroy WB, Martin CE. Sexual behavior in the human male. Philadelphia: WB Saunders Co, 1948.
11. Gebhard PH, Johnson AB. The Kinsey data: marginal tabulations of the 1938–1963 interviews conducted by the Institute for Sex Research. Philadelphia: WB Saunders Co, 1979:125.
12. Ard BN Jr. Sex in lasting marriages: a longitudinal study. J Sex Res 13:274, 1977.
13. Frank E, Anderson C, Rubinstein D. Frequency of sexual dysfunction in "normal" couples. N Engl J Med 299:111, 1978.
14. Nettelbladt P, Uddenberg N. Sexual dysfunction and sexual satisfaction in 58 married Swedish men. J Psychosom Res 23:141, 1979.
15. Reading AE, Wiest WM. An analysis of self-reported sexual behavior in a sample of normal males. Arch Sex Behav 13:69, 1984.
16. Diokno AC, Brown MB, Herzog AR. Sexual function in the elderly. Arch Intern Med 150:197, 1990.

17. Morley JE. Impotence. Am J Med 80:897, 1986.
18. Keil JE, Sutherland SE, Knapp RG, et al. Self-reported sexual functioning in elderly blacks and whites. The Charleston Heart Study experience. J Aging Health 4:112, 1992.
19. Schein M, Zyzanski SJ, Levine S, et al. The frequency of sexual problems among family practice patients. Fam Pract Res J 7:122, 1988.
20. Pfeiffer E, Davis GC. Determinants of sexual behavior in middle and old age. J Am Geriatr Soc 20:151, 1972.
21. Mulligan T, Retchin SM, Chinchilli VM, Bettinger CB. The role of aging and chronic disease in sexual dysfunction. J Am Geriatr Soc 36:520, 1988.
22. Morley JE. Impotence in older men. Hosp Pract 4:139, 1988.
23. Slag MF, Morley JE, Elson MK, et al. Impotence in medical clinic outpatients. JAMA 249:1736, 1983.
24. Masters W, Johnson V. Human Sexual Inadequacy. Boston: Little, Brown & Co, 1970.
25. Junemann KP, Persson-Junemann C, Alken P. Pathophysiology of erectile dysfunction. Semin Urol 8:80, 1990.
26. Wabrek AJ, Burchell RC. Male sexual dysfunction associated with coronary heart disease. Arch Sex Behav 9:69, 1980.
27. Morley JE, Korenman SG, Mooradian AD, Kaiser FE. Sexual dysfunction in the elderly male. J Am Geriatr Soc 35:1014, 1987.
28. Gundle GJ, Bozman BR, Tate S, et al. Psychosocial outcome after aortocoronary artery surgery. Am J Psychiatry 137:1591, 1980.
29. Virag R, Bouilly P, Frydman D. Is impotence an arterial disorder? A study of arterial risk factors in 400 impotent men. Lancet 1:181, 1985.
30. Oaks WW, Moyer JH. Sex and hypertension. Med Aspects Hum Sex 6:128, 1972.
31. Whitehead ED, Klyde BJ. Diabetes-related impotence in the elderly. Clin Geriatr Med 6:771, 1990.
32. McCulloch DK, Campbell IW, Wu FC, Prescott RJ, Clarke BF. The prevalence of diabetic impotence. Diabetologia 18:279, 1980.
33. Kaiser FE, Korenman SG. Impotence in diabetic men. Am J Med 85:147, 1988.
34. Rubin A, Babbott D. Impotence and diabetes mellitus. JAMA 168:498, 1958.
35. Zemel P. Sexual dysfunction in the diabetic patient with hypertension. Am J Cardiol 61:27H, 1988.
36. Jevitch MJ, Edson M, Jarman WD, Herrera HH. Vascular factor in erectile failure among diabetics. Urology 19:163, 1982.
37. Lehman TP, Jacobs JA. Etiology of diabetic impotence. J Urol 129:291, 1983.
38. Saenz de Tejada I, Goldstein I, Azadzoi K, et al. Impaired neurogenic and endothelium-mediated relaxation of penile smooth muscle from diabetic men with impotence. N Engl J Med 230:1025, 1989.
39. Shabsigh R, Fishman IJ, Schum C, Dunn JK. Cigarette smoking and other vascular risk factors in vasculogenic impotence. Urology 38:227, 1991.
40. Kwan M, Greenleaf WJ, Mann J, et al. The nature of androgen action on male sexuality: a combined laboratory-self-report study on hypogonadal men. J Clin Endocrinol Metab 57:557, 1983.
41. Maatman TJ, Montague DK. Routine endocrine screening in impotence. Urology 27:499, 1986.
42. Bancroft J, Wu FCW. Changes in erectile responsiveness during androgen replacement therapy. Arch Sex Behav 12:59, 1983.
43. Korenman SG, Morley JE, Mooradian AD, et al. Secondary hypogonadism in older men: its relation to impotence. J Clin Endocrinol Metab 71:963, 1990.
44. Spark RR, White RA, Connolly PB. Impotence is not always psychogenic: newer insights into the hypothalamic-pituitary-gonadal dysfunction. JAMA 243:750, 1980.
45. Nickel JC, Morales A, Condra M, et al. Endocrine dysfunction in impotence: incidence, significance, and cost-effective screening. J Urol 132:40, 1984.
46. Foster RS, Mulcahy N, Callaghan JT, et al. Role of serum prolactin determination in evaluation of impotent patient. Urology 36:499, 1990.
47. Murray FT, Wyss HU, Thomas RG, et al. Gonadal dysfunction in diabetic men with organic impotence. J Clin Endocrinol Metab 65:127, 1987.
48. Neri A, Aygen M, Zuckerman Z, et al. Subjective assessment of sexual dysfunction of patients on long-term administration of digoxin. Arch Sex Behav 9:343, 1980.
49. Coronary Drug Project Research Group. Clofibrate and niacin in coronary heart disease. JAMA 231:360, 1975.
50. Seagraves RT, Madsen R, Carter CS, et al. Erectile dysfunction associated with pharmacological agents. In: Seagraves RT, Schoenberg HW, eds. Diagnosis and Treatment of Erectile Disturbances. New York: Plenum, 1985:22.
51. Horowitz JD, Gobel AJ. Drugs and impaired male sexual function. Drugs 18:206, 1979.
52. Wein AJ, van Arsdalen K. Drug-induced male sexual dysfunction. Urol Clin North Am 15:23, 1988.
53. Goldstein I, Krane RJ. Drug-induced sexual dysfunction. World J Urol 1:239, 1983.
54. Fried LP, Moore RD, Pearson TA. Long-term effects of cigarette smoking and moderate alcohol consumption on coronary artery diameter. Am J Med 80:37, 1986.
55. Schiavi RC. Chronic alcoholism and male sexual dysfunction. J Sex Marital Ther 16:23, 1990.
56. Gray RR, Keresteci AG, StLuis EL, et al. Investigation of impotence by internal pudendal angiography: experiences with 73 cases. Radiology 144:773, 1982.
57. Condra M, Morales A, Owen JA, et al. Prevalence and significance of tobacco smoking in impotence. Urology 27:495, 1986.
58. Bornman MS, du Plessis DJ. Smoking and vascular impotence. S Afr Med 70:329, 1986.
59. Bähren W, Gall H, Scherb W, et al. Arterial anatomy and arteriographic diagnosis of arteriogenic impotence. Cardiovasc Intervent Radiol 11:195, 1988.
60. Rosen MP, Greenfield AJ, Walker TG, et al. Cigarette smoking: an independent risk factor for atherosclerosis in the hypogastric-cavernous arterial

bed of men with arteriogenic impotence. J Urol 145:759, 1991.

61. Renshaw DC. Sex and eating disorders. Med Aspects Hum Sex 4:56, 1990.
62. Hengevelt MW. Erectile disorders: a psychosexological review. In: Jonas U, Thon WF, Stief CG, eds. Erectile dysfunction. Berlin: Springer-Verlag, 1991:207.
63. Rust J, Golombok S, Collier J. Marital problems and sexual dysfunction: how are they related? Br J Psychiatry 152:629, 1988.
64. Thase ME, Reynolds CF III, Jennings JR, et al. Nocturnal penile tumescence is diminished in depressed men. Biol Psychiatry 24:33, 1988.
65. Segraves KB, Segraves RT. Hypoactive sexual desire disorder: prevalence and comorbidity in 906 subjects. J Sex Marital Ther 17:55, 1991.
66. LoPiccolo J. Management of psychogenic erectile failure. In: Tanagho EA, Lue TF, McClure RD, eds. Contemporary Management of Impotence and Infertility. Baltimore: Williams & Wilkins, 1988:133.
67. Booth W. The long-lost survey on sex. Science 239:1084, 1988.
68. Quinn MM, Wegman DH, Greaves IA, et al. Investigation of reports of sexual dysfunction among male chemical workers manufacturing stilbene derivatives. Am J Indust Med 18:55, 1990.
69. National Institutes of Health Consensus Development Conference on Erectile Impotence. Planning Committee Meeting. February 20–21, 1992, Bethesda, MD.
70. Radloff L. The CES-D scale: a self-report depression scale for research in the general population. Appl Psych Meas 1:385, 1977.
71. Spielberger CD, Johnson EH, Russell SF, et al. The experience and expression of anger: construction and validation of an anger expression scale. In: Chesney MA, Rosenman RH, eds. Anger and Hostility in Cardiovascular and Behavioral Disorders. New York: Hemisphere McGraw-Hill, 1985.
72. Langeluddecke P, Gouldston K, Tennant C. Psychological factors in dyspepsia of unknown cause: a comparison with peptic ulcer disease. J Psychosom Res 34:215, 1990.
73. Chesney MA, Rosenman RH. Anger and Hostility in Cardiovascular and Behavioral Disorders. New York: Hemisphere McGraw-Hill, 1985.
74. Verrier RL, Dickerson LW. Autonomic nervous system and coronary blood flow changes related to emotional activation and sleep. Circulation 83(Suppl II):81, 1991.
75. Euler US. Quantification of stress by catecholamine analysis. Clin Pharmacol Ther 5:398, 1964.
76. Jackson DN. Personality Research Form Manual. Port Huron: Research Psychologists Press, 1984.
77. United States Bureau of the Census. Statistical brief. Data from the Census of Population, Vol 1, Chap D, Part 1. Washington, DC: US Department of Commerce Library of Congress Publication PC80-D 1–86, 1984.
78. Metropolitan Life Insurance Company. Trends in longevity after age 65. Statis Bull 68:10, 1987.
79. Barrett-Connor E, Khaw K-T, Yen SSC. A prospective study of dehydroepiandrosterone sulfate. N Engl J Med 315:1519, 1986.

CHAPTER 2

Anatomy and Physiology of the Penis

Arnold Melman

George J. Christ

Mark S. Hirsch

ANATOMY
Corpora Cavernosa

The composition of the penis has been described as three cylindrical erectile bodies bound together and surrounded by connective tissue.[1] Two of the three bodies, the paired corpora cavernosa, are arranged side by side in the dorsal part of the penis. They constitute the dorsal and lateral portions of the organ. The corpora cavernosa, but not the corpus spongiosum, are covered by a thick fascial layer, the tunica albuginea. Recent studies[2] have shown that the tunica is a multilayered structure comprised of alternating bands of circular and longitudinal collagen. We suggest that as the diameter of the cavernous bodies increases, the tunical layers stretch and compress the traversing veins. Immunohistochemical studies have demonstrated the presence of types I and III collagen in the tunica.[3,4] The midline septum consists of vertical strands of collagen that allow free access of blood from one side of the corpora to the other. The tunical surfaces of the corpora cavernosa are fused in the midline except proximally, where they separate to form the tapered crura. The crura are firmly bound on each side to the periosteum of the ischial rami. The crura are covered on their caudad surfaces by variable quantities of striated ischiocavernosi muscles.

Corpus Spongiosum

The unpaired corpus spongiosum, representing the third erectile body, lies ventrally, in a median groove created by the paired cavernous bodies. Unlike the cavernous bodies, it consists of only a thin fascial layer covering sinusoidal tissue, whose center is the urethra. At its distal end, the spongiosum expands into the glans penis. The base of the glans is molded over and attached to the distal rounded ends of the cavernous bodies. The proximal portion

of the glans has a slightly larger diameter than the shaft of the penis and projects posteriorly as the corona. At its proximal end, the spongiosum expands to form the bulb of the penis. The bulbous urethra lies in the superficial perineal space, apposed to the caudal border of the urogenital diaphragm. Its posterior portion projects slightly beyond the urethral entrance. The striated bulbocavernosus muscle covers the bulbous urethra and is responsible for emptying urine and semen from the lumen.

Skin

The skin covering the penis is thin, loosely bound to the shaft, free of adipose tissue, and pigmented on its ventral surface, along the median raphe. Though free of hair for the most part, there are sweat and sebaceous glands. At the distal part of the shaft, the skin folds on itself as the prepuce, then continues as a very thin and adherent layer covering the glans. A small secondary fold of skin, the frenulum, extends just proximal to the external urethral meatus along the median raphe to the deep prepuce.

Fascia

The superficial fascia of the penis is a thin layer of connective tissue with scattered smooth muscle cells and elastic fibers. It is directly contiguous with that of the scrotum. The weak association between the deep and superficial fascial layers allows for remarkable looseness of the penile skin. The deep penile fascia (Buck's fascia) is a thin, strong layer that envelops all three erectile bodies from the base of the glans to the bony attachment at the root. At its proximal portion, it invests the ischiocavernosi and bulbospongiosum as a separate layer, the external perineal fascia. Because of its capsulelike enclosure of the penis, an abscess, hematoma, or leakage of urine from the penile urethra is confined to the penis. A leakage of urine from the membranous urethra, however, can spread between the deep and superficial fascial layers into the penis, scrotum, lower abdomen, and upper thigh.[5]

The cavernous bodies themselves are enveloped by a dense, fibrous envelope, the tunica albuginea. The deeper fibers of the tunica surround each corpus cavernosum individually and converge medially to form the septum of the penis. The septum is largely incomplete in its anterior portion but becomes complete prior to the divergence of the crura. Although the tunica is attached to the deep penile fascia, sufficient space exists for the passage of vessels and nerves (Fig. 2–1). The corpus spongiosum is covered by its own tunica, which is thinner and more elastic than that of the corpora cavernosa. The glans has no fibrous sheath but contains much fibrous connective tissue.

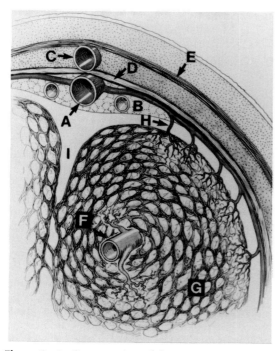

Figure 2–1. Cross-section of the corpora cavernosa, deep dorsal vein (**A**), dorsal artery (**B**), superficial dorsal vein (**C**), Buck's fascia (**D**), Dartos fascia (**E**), cavernous artery (**F**), corporal smooth muscle arranged in a trabecular fashion (**G**), emissary vein (**H**), medial septum of the corporal bodies (**I**). (From Lerner SE, Melman A, Christ GJ. A review of erectile dysfunction: New insights and more questions. J Urol 149:1246, 1993, ©American Urological Association.)

Ligaments

The weight of the penis is supported by two fibrous bands, the fundiform and suspensory ligaments. The more elastic fundiform ligament is a direct continuation of the deep subcutaneous fascia of the anterior abdominal wall. It is firmly attached to the rectus sheath. It splits dorsally to surround the body of the penis and becomes interspersed in the superficial penile fascia. The triangular suspensory ligament lies deep to the fundiform. It arises from the anterior surface of the pubic symphysis and extends to the dorsum of the penis, where it attaches to the deep penile fascia on both sides.[6]

Parenchyma

The corporal parenchyma is a well-vascularized, spongelike network of trabeculae composed of smooth muscle, collagen, and extracellular matrix. The spaces formed by this meshwork, the cavernous spaces or lacunae, are lined by intact endothelium.[7] The predominant type of collagen found in the corpora is type IV.[3] The fact that endothelial cells are known to secrete type IV collagen and that this collagen type forms the basement membranes of most blood vessels supports the theory that the penis is a specialized vascular organ (Fig. 2–2). When appropriately stimulated, the smooth muscle of the trabeculae is capable of marked changes in tone. It is the relaxation of the trabecular smooth muscle that initiates the dilatation of the cavernous spaces and their subsequent filling with blood. One important mediator of this response is the autonomic nervous system (Fig. 2–3).

Parasympathetic Innervation

Although the number of cholinergic nerve fibers within the corpora has been reported as limited,[7] small bundles of them have been identified in the trabecular matrix. The origins of these fibers are the anterior divisions of spinal nerve roots S2 to S4. These preganglionic parasympathetic fibers enter the pelvis as the nervi erigentes (pelvic nerves). The nervi erigentes course laterally in the endopelvic fascia, in close proximity to the hypogastric vessels. They terminate beside the rectum in the pelvic plexus. Branches of the pelvic plexus supply the bladder, lower ureter, seminal vesicles, prostate, rectum, urethra, and corpora cavernosa. The critical branches in erectile physiology, the cavernous nerves, travel along the posterolateral aspects of the prostate to supply the corpora. At the base of the prostate, the cavernous nerves are located relatively lateral to the prostatic capsule. As the cavernous nerves pass distally along the pros-

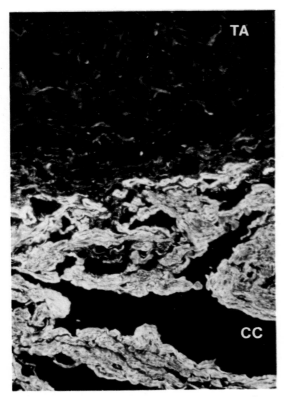

Figure 2–2. Section of tunica albuginea (TA) and corpus cavernosum (CC) of an impotent patient secondary to venous leak. There is intense staining of type IV collagen in the corpus cavernosum as compared to the nonstaining tunica. Collagen type IV 1:320, indirect immunofluorescence (FITC) method. × 200. (From Luangkhot R, Rutchik S, Agarwal V, et al. Collagen alterations in the corpus cavernosum of men with sexual dysfunction. J Urol 148:467, 1992, ©American Urological Association.)

tate, it is important to note their spatial relationship to the gland. It has been helpful to visualize the position of the nerves as the hour positions on the face of a clock. For example, at the prostatic apex, they lie in close proximity to the capsule at the 5 and 7 o'clock positions. At the membranous urethra, they are located at the 3 and 9 o'clock positions, just external to the striated muscles. At the level of the proximal bulbous urethra, they ascend to the 1 and 11 o'clock positions, where they enter the penis at the convergence of the corpora cavernosa.

Sympathetic Innervation

The thoracolumbar portion of the spinal cord, specifically T11 to L2, gives rise to the sympathetic fibers that supply the penis. These fibers course in the retroperitoneal space to reach the major presacral plexus, located anterior and inferior to the aortic bifurcation. They then leave this plexus primarily via the hypogastric nerves. These nerves contribute to the pelvic plexus and the cavernous nerves of the penis.[8]

Somatic Innervation

The dorsal nerve of the penis supplies the corpora cavernosa, the penile skin, and the glans penis. It is a terminal branch of the pudendal nerve. The pudendal nerve is formed from the anterior divisions of S2 to S4. It courses out of the pelvis through the greater sciatic foramen, across the ischial spine, and back into the pelvis via the lesser sciatic foramen. It travels with the internal pudendal vessels along the lateral pelvic wall of the ischiorectal fossa. At the level of the urogenital diaphragm, it divides into three terminal branches: the inferior hemorrhoidal, the perineal, and the dorsal nerves. The dorsal nerve passes medially to the inferior pubic ramus, through the urogenital diaphragm, and along the dorsum of the penis in the space immediately deep to Buck's fascia.

The pudendal nerve supplies both sensory innervation to the penis and motor innervation to the striated perineal musculature. At one time, it was thought that the striated muscles of the penis helped to impede venous outflow during erection. However, it has been demonstrated that animals without bulbocavernosus and ischiocavernosi muscles[9] and humans without function in these muscles[10] demonstrated adequate erections. Therefore, in its somatic efferent role, the pudendal nerve contributes little to erection.

Arterial Supply

The paired internal pudendal arteries are the major branches that supply the penis. They generally arise from the ischiopudendal trunks of the internal iliac arteries. The internal pudendal artery originates at the greater sciatic foramen, crosses the back of the tip of the ischial spine, and enters the perineum through the lesser sciatic foramen. It then passes through Alcock's canal in the ischiorectal fossa to become the penile artery (the perineal portion of the internal pudendal artery). It is at this position that the artery is most vulnerable to external trauma. Here, a pelvic fracture or blunt compressive force to the perineum, such as a straddle injury, can cause total arterial occlusion.[11]

The penile artery passes through the urogenital diaphragm and along the medial margin of the inferior ramus of the pubis. The classic representation of the penile artery is that in the perineum it divides into four terminal branches, the bulbar, ure-

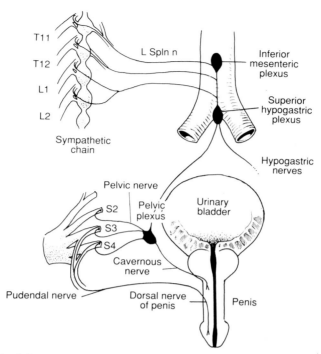

Figure 2–3. Schematic representation of the autonomic innervation of the penis.

thral, dorsal, and cavernous (deep penile) arteries. The bulbar artery supplies the bulb of the urethra. The urethral artery runs in a longitudinal direction within the spongiosal tissue. Along its route, it supplies the corpus spongiosum, urethra, and glans. The dorsal artery of the penis runs deep to Buck's fascia, medial to the paired dorsal nerves and lateral to the single deep dorsal vein. The dorsal artery terminates in short helical branches in the glans penis. Along its route, it divides into a number of circumflex branches that pass around the corpus cavernosum and spongiosum. The cavernosal (deep penile) artery enters the corpus cavernosum at the base of the penis and runs centrally to its tip. Along its course, it gives off two types of branches. One supplies the smooth muscle and nerve fibers of the cavernosal trabecular tissue. The other divides into a series of helicine arteries. Blood flow in the helicine arteries is unique in that it passes directly into the cavernous sinusoidal spaces without first traversing a capillary bed.[12] The shape and length of the helicine arteries allow the penis to elongate and dilate without compromising blood supply to the corpora.

Selective pudendal angiography has shown that there is wide variation in distribution of the penile arteries in normal men. In one study, the classic pattern of the penile arteries was truly representative in only <18% of cases.[13] Frequent variants are found, including dorsal arter-

ies supplying the corporal trabeculae and vessels on one side supplying the contralateral corpus (Fig. 2–4).

Venous Drainage

Three major sets of veins drain the penis: the superficial, intermediate, and deep systems (Fig. 2–5).

The superficial system, which arises in the penile skin and subcutaneous tissues superficial to Buck's fascia, drains via the superficial dorsal vein. This is usually a single vessel but may be multiple or forked. It usually empties into one saphenous vein but may empty into the femoral or inferior epigastric vein.

The intermediate system, deep to Buck's fascia and superficial to the tunica, drains the glans, the distal portion of the corpus spongiosum, and the corpora cavernosa. Many short, straight veins from the glans and ventral corpus spongiosum converge in a retrocoronal plexus. The deep dorsal vein of the penis is formed from this convergence. It runs toward the pubis in the dorsal sulcus between the corpora cavernosa. Small emissary veins, from the dorsal and lateral corpora cavernosa, pierce the tunica, combine as circumflex veins, and empty into the deep dorsal vein. This large vein is usually single and empties into the periprostatic plexus of Santorini.

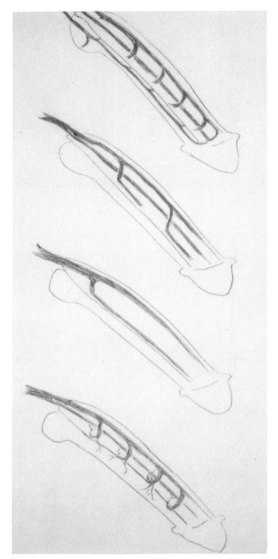

Figure 2–4. Cast studies of cadaver penises by Puech-Leao demonstrate frequent variations of penile arterial anatomy. From top downward: classically described anatomy, single dorsal artery supplying both sides, deep penile artery arising from the dorsal artery, dorsal artery supplying trabecular substance.

The deep system drains the proximal portion of the corpus spongiosum and a large portion of the corpora cavernosa. Small bulbar veins arise in the proximal corpus spongiosum and empty directly into the deep penile (cavernous) veins. Posterior urethral veins either join the bulbar veins or drain directly into the pudendal plexus. Small emissary veins from the corpora cavernosa also empty into the deep veins.

Lue et al. have demonstrated the presence of cavernosal veins lying on the medial cephalad sur-

face of the corpora that drain into the hypogastric system.[14] Crural veins exit from the perineal surface of the crura, course laterally, and drain directly into the internal pudendal veins.

Electron microscopy of the corpora has identified an extensive subtunical venous plexus.[15] These venules drain the corpora cavernosa. They course obliquely in the space deep to the tunica and just superficial to the cavernosal tissue. Their coalescence forms small, tunica-piercing, emissary veins. The passive occlusion of these tiny venules is of critical importance in restricting venous outflow during erection[16] (Fig. 2–6).

PHYSIOLOGY
Mechanism of Erection

When the penis is flaccid, the corporal smooth muscle is in a tonically contracted state, largely under sympathetic modulation. Blood flow to the penis during this period is minimal, sufficient only for nutritional purposes (8 ml/min/100 g).[1] Activation of the parasympathetic nervous system is associated with the release of endogenous vasorelaxants that elicit the relaxation of corporal and arterial smooth muscle. A rapid increase in arterial blood flow occurs, with subsequent engorgement of the corporal trabecular spaces and penile rigidity. To obtain a robust penile erection, a complex series of neurovascular events must occur. In fact, there are four crucial physiologic requirements for penile rigidity: intact neuronal innervation, intact arterial supply, appropriately responsive corporal smooth muscle, and intact venous mechanics. More specifically, corporal smooth muscle relaxation may be elicited as a spinal reflex or as a supraspinal psychogenic impulse. In the so-called reflexogenic erection, direct genital stimulation is transmitted via the dorsal nerve to the pudendal nerve to reach the sacral spinal cord. The response arises in the sacral cord and travels via the pelvic nerve to the cavernosal nerves and into the corporal trabeculae via autonomic nerve fibers. Psychogenic erections are not as clearly defined. In the proper hormonal milieu, various sexual stimuli are processed in the cerebral cortex and transmitted via hypothalamic and thalamic centers to the sympathetic thoracolumbar cord and the parasympathetic sacral cord. From there, autonomic pathways are more well known.

Given an adequate neurohormonal stimulus and appropriately responsive corpora, the next requirement in the creation of a rigid erection is the ability to increase penile arterial flow. Blood flow must increase fivefold to tenfold to obtain a robust erection. Newman and Northrup demonstrated that erections could be created in cadavers by infusing saline into the dorsal penile artery at flow rates

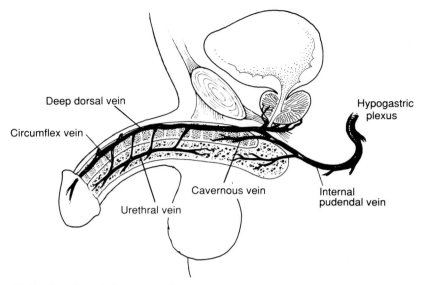

Figure 2–5. Drawing of the intermediate and deep venous drainage systems of the penis.

greater than 25 ml/min.[12] Obviously, these corpora are devoid of smooth muscle activity. If arterial obstruction exists, the reduction in flow can prevent penile erection.[17]

Several putative endogenous vasorelaxants are thought to contribute to the modulation of corporal smooth muscle tone. Among these are norepinephrine, acetylcholine, vasoactive intestinal polypeptide (VIP), prostaglandins, and endothelial-derived factors, including nitric oxide. The exact

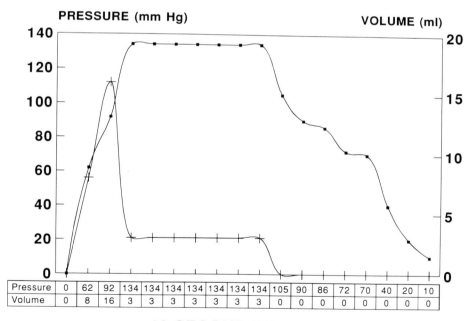

Pressure	0	62	92	134	134	134	134	134	134	134	105	90	86	72	70	40	20	10	
Volume	0	8	16	3	3	3	3	3	3	3	0	0	0	0	0	0	0	0	

10 SECOND INTERVALS

✦ **Pressure** ╋ **Volume**

Figure 2–6. Cavernosometric tracing from a patient with psychogenic impotence. Note that the maintenance of intracorporal pressure at full erection (134 mm Hg) requires relatively little inflow. This demonstrates the adequacy of the venoocclusive mechanism.

mechanism by which this neurohormonal cocktail is able to integrate the rapid and coordinated responses of the corporal smooth muscle is uncertain.

The fourth and final requirement for rigidity is the occlusion of venous outflow. For years, it was thought that venous occlusion was an active constriction, modulated either by pelvic musculature or by intravenous polsters.[18] Now, however, the predominant theory is the passive venoocclusive mechanism of outflow impedance. Briefly, as the sinusoids dilate and arterial flow rushes in under high pressures, the relaxed trabecular walls are forced against the tunica albuginea. The delicate subalbugineal venous plexus lacks muscular walls.[16] The pressure within the bulging sinusoidal spaces is transmitted to these thin venules, causing their compression and the subsequent reduction in venous outflow. It is important to reiterate that the tone of the corporal smooth muscle serves a capacitance function in this tissue[19] and, as such, is the primary determinant of both arterial and venous blood flow.

Although, as mentioned, there is no clear consensus concerning the precise control of corporal smooth muscle tone, numerous putative modulators have been identified.

Adrenergic Contributions

A wealth of clinical and experimental observations implicate a significant role for the sympathetic nervous system in erectile physiology. For example, adrenergic nerve fibers and high concentrations of norepinephrine have been demonstrated in the trabeculae of the corpora and in the tunica of small corporal blood vessels.[7,20] Futhermore, pharmacologic studies of isolated human corporal strips have demonstrated contractile responses to phenylephrine that may be blocked by alpha-adrenergic antagonists[21] (Fig. 2–7). This effect is thought to be mediated directly by postsynaptic alpha$_1$-adrenoceptors and modulated by presynaptic alpha$_2$-adrenoceptors.[22,23] Also of interest is the fact that alpha-adrenoceptors greatly outnumber beta-adrenoceptors in the corpora[24] and that beta blockade has little effect on isolated human corporal strips despite the presence of a significant beta$_2$-adrenergic component.[25] Such observations indicate that relaxation of corporal smooth muscle by hormonal activation of the beta$_2$-adrenergic receptor plays little, if any, role in normal erectile physiology.

Clinically, intracorporal injection of phentolamine (an alpha-blocker) is an accepted and successful method of diagnosing and treating erectile dysfunction.[26] As expected, pharmacologically induced priapism may be treated with intracorporal adrenergic vasoconstrictors.[27] However, it is im-

portant to emphasize that despite the importance of the alpha-adrenergic component, recent studies predictably indicate that in penile flaccidity, and perhaps detumescence as well, other hormonal systems interact to modulate corporal tone.[28–32]

Cholinergic Contribution

For years, it was widely held that the parasympathetic nervous system was the predominant effector of erection.[33–35] Although cholinergic nerves are present in the corpora[36] and probably do play a role in erection, they likely play a less important role than previously thought.

Much evidence exists supporting a more limited involvement of the cholinergic system. First, in vitro testing of human corporal strips with acetylcholine has produced variable results, including tissue contraction[37] and tissue relaxation.[38] Second, cholinergic blockade with atropine during such pharmacologic studies does not fully ablate the effect of electrically induced smooth muscle relaxation.[39] Finally, neither the intravenous, intraarterial, nor intracorporal injection of acetylcholine elicits penile erection, nor has the use of atropine been successful in blocking erection.[40,41] A more likely explanation for the role of the parasympathetic nervous system is that it may contribute to the suppression of adrenergic tone and may enhance the action of some other nonadrenergic, noncholinergic neurotransmitter.

Nonadrenergic, Noncholinergic Contribution
PROSTAGLANDINS

Prostaglandins are known to contribute to the modulation of vascular tone. Human corporal tissue has been shown to be capable of producing prostaglandins.[42] Pharmacologic studies of the effect of prostaglandins on isolated human corporal strips demonstrate that prostaglandin F$_{2\text{-alpha}}$ (PGF$_{2\alpha}$) and prostaglandin I$_2$ (PGI$_2$) promote tissue contraction, whereas prostaglandin E$_1$ (PGE$_1$) and E$_2$ (PGE$_2$) promote tissue relaxation.[43] The physiologic mechanism of action is presumably similar to that of other vascular tissues in which PGF$_{2\alpha}$ is known to elicit contractile responses subsequent to increases in intracellular calcium levels.[44] Conversely, PGE$_1$ acts by raising intracellular cyclic adenosine monophosphate (cAMP) levels and thus relaxes corporal smooth muscle.[45] Clearly, the interplay between intracellular calcium and cAMP levels is an important determinant of corporal smooth muscle tone. Thus, the therapeutic success of intracorporal PGE$_1$ and PGE$_2$ injection in the treatment of erectile dysfunction comes as no surprise.[46]

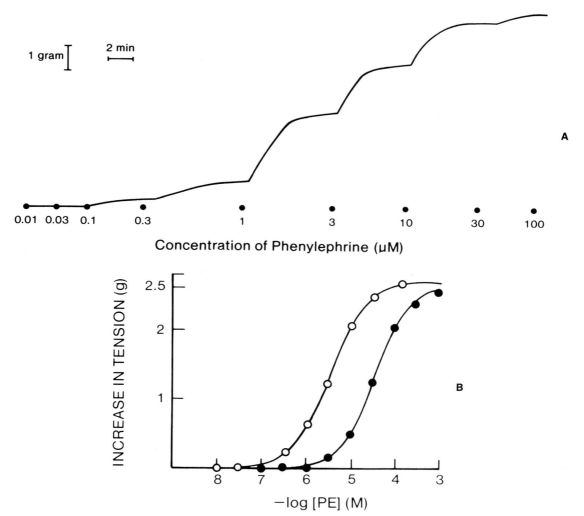

Figure 2–7. A, Representative tracing of the graded contractile response of human isolated erectile tissue to phenylephrine at 32° C. Note the absence of oscillations and the stability of the phenylephrine-induced contractile response. **B,** Representative computer fit curves to observed concentration–response curve data in the absence (*left*) and presence (*right*) of prazosin. Note the complete surmountability and the parallel rightward shift in the phenyl-ephrine concentration–response curve produced by prazosin. (From Christ GJ, Maayani S, Valcic M, and Melman A. Pharmacological studies of human erectile tissue: characteristics of spontaenous contractions and alterations in alpha-adrenoceptor responsivenss with age and disease in isolated tissues. Br J Pharm 101:375, 1990.)

VASOACTIVE INTESTINAL POLYPEPTIDE (VIP)

VIP is a potent vasodilator that has been implicated as a possible neurotransmitter associated with erection. VIP immunoreactive fibers have been demonstrated in the human corpora,[47] and VIP is known to relax corporal strips from humans and monkeys in a dose-dependent manner.[48–51] Clinically, nerves containing VIP have been found in the human corpora, and these have been noted to be reduced in number in impotent men.[52] However, intracorporal injection of VIP has had limited success in the treatment of erectile dysfunction.

ENDOTHELIUM-DERIVED RELAXING FACTOR (EDRF)

The endothelium of many vascular tissues is known to release a variety of vasoactive substances that regulate the tone of the surrounding vascular smooth muscle. Endothelium-derived relaxing factor (EDRF) is such a substance.[53] Studies from a variety of laboratories indicate that EDRF in the corpora may well be nitric oxide or a nitric oxide-like substance.[54,55] The exact source of nitric oxide during physiologic erection is uncertain. However, there is evidence demonstrating that both nonadrenergic, noncholinergic neurons and lacunar endothelial cells are capable of releasing nitric oxide.[56-58]

Regardless of the origin, increased release of nitric oxide is followed by its subsequent diffusion into the vascular smooth muscle cell.[56,58,59] Once inside the smooth muscle cell, nitric oxide is thought to act by activating the soluble guanylate cyclase enzyme, thus increasing intracellular cyclic guanosine monophosphate (cGMP) levels and causing relaxation of corporal smooth muscle (Fig. 2–8).

The preponderance of evidence suggests that nitric oxide is an important modulator of corporal smooth muscle tone. However, its exact role in relation to the plethora of other identifiable vasoactive substances is still to be determined.

ENDOTHELIN

Endothelin is one of the most potent constrictors yet determined. Cultured corporal endothelial cells have been shown to release endothelin.[28] More-over, addition of endothelin to isolated corporal tissue strips elicits a dose-dependent contractile response.[28] It has been postulated that endothelin, along with other endothelium-derived vasoconstrictors (e.g., thromboxane A_2, leukotrienes, $PGF_{2\alpha}$) may act as important modulators of flaccidity and detumescence in the human penis.[28-30]

Role of Gap Junctions in the Corpora

It has been suggested that a mechanism must exist for the efficient intracorporal spread of a local erectile stimulus. That is, given the relatively sparse neuronal innervation of the corpus cavernosum, the limited local action of vasodilators, and the dense collagenous matrix of the corpora, it appears that simple drug diffusion alone cannot be responsible for the rapid and coordinated erectile response characteristic of the penis.[60] The demonstration that gap junctions exist between corporal smooth muscle cells both in vitro and in situ provides a likely intercellular conduit for the amplification of local neural or hormonal stimulation[61-63] (Fig. 2–9).

Several detailed descriptions of gap junctions in this and other publications are available.[64-66]

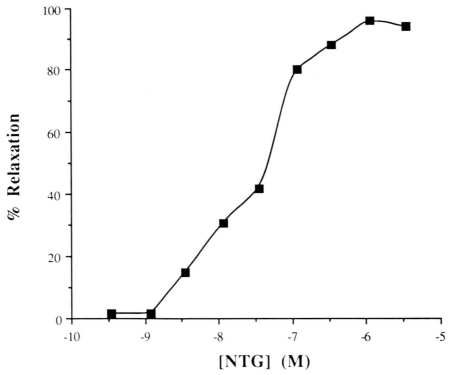

Figure 2–8. Representative computer fit concentration–response curve from isolated human erectile tissue, demonstrating smooth muscle relaxation induced by nitroglycerin. Tissue had been precontracted with 75% of the maximal response dosage of phenylephrine.

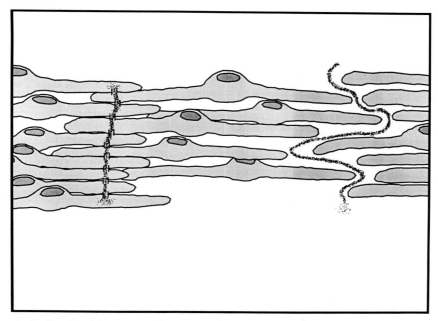

Figure 2–9. Depicted is a group of cavernosal smooth muscle cells connected by a network of small gap junctions that are a hallmark of this tissue. The stippled area to the right outlines the abundance of cavernous spaces in the corpora. Smooth muscle cells in distant areas of the corpora might be coupled with respect to both second messenger exchange and response generation, even though they are not directly activated individually.

Briefly, gap junctions are aggregates of intercellular channels that coalesce to form junctional plaques between apposed cells from a variety of tissues. Individual intercellular channels consist of the union of six homologous membrane-spanning proteins from each cell, known as connexins, that join to provide aqueous intercellular channels between adjacent cells (Fig. 2–10). These intercellular channels facilitate the free passage of current-carrying ions (i.e., calcium) and physiologically relevant intracellular second messengers (i.e., inositol triphosphate, cAMP).[64,65] Thus, intercellular communication at gap junctions has been postulated to contribute to the coordination of cellular responses in tissues as diverse as the myocardium,[67,68] uterus,[69] and ureter.[70] Moreover, as mentioned previously, there is compelling physiologic evidence to support a role for gap junctions in erectile physiology.

More specifically, our recent work has demonstrated the following. (1) Relatively small gap junctions (connexin43,<0.25 μm) are found between corporal smooth muscle cells both in vitro and in situ.[71] (2) Electrophysiologic studies have demonstrated that cultured corporal smooth muscle cells are well coupled electrically, exhibiting the multiple channel sizes characteristic of connexin43.[72] Moreover, the distribution of channel sizes, and thus junctional conductance, is regulated

by alpha$_1$-adrenergic receptor activation, as well as several physiologically relevant second messenger systems.[72] (3) Intracellular injection of fluorescent dyes, such as lucifer yellow and Fura-2, results in rapid intercellular spread of dye through gap junctions (Fig. 2–11). (4) Calcium imaging studies using the calcium-sensitive dye Fura-2 have

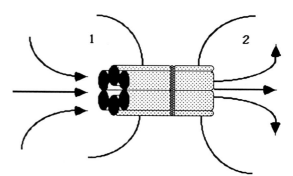

Figure 2–10. Schematic depiction of the architecture of a gap junction channel. Note that each cell of a pair (denoted as **1** and **2**) contributes a hemichannel that is comprised of six homologous membrane-spanning proteins. The intercellular junction is formed by the joining of a hemichannel from each of two cells. These aqueous intercellular channels permit partial cytoplasmic continuity between adjacent cells.

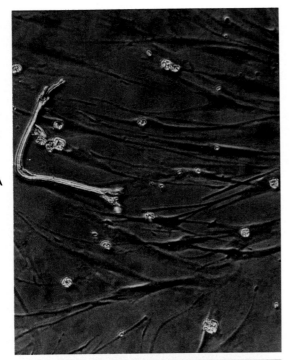

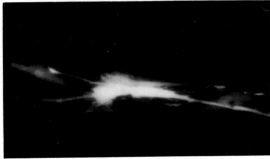

Figure 2–11. Use of fluorescent dye techniques to study intercellular coupling among cultured corporal smooth muscle cells. **A,** Phase contrast image of cultured smooth muscle cells. ×40. **B,** Fluorescence image of the same field of cells at the same magnification. This is a typical example of how a single smooth muscle cell (*center*) can be loaded with fluorescent dye from a microelectrode. In this experiment, the cell is loaded by passive diffusion of the gap junction permeant, fluorescent dye carboxyfluorescein. The dye rapidly diffuses down its chemical gradient: that is, the microelectrode pipette tip contains approximately 20 Mm concentration of carboxyfluorescein. The fluorescence image was taken approximately 3 min after injection of the initial cell and demonstrates the rapid intercellular spread of dye to several other corporal smooth muscle cells in the field.

demonstrated that both calcium ions and IP 3 are freely diffusible through gap junctions between adjacent corporal smooth muscle cells in culture.[73] (5) Electrophysiologic recordings of single corporal smooth muscle cells reveal the absence of action potentials despite the presence of small inward Ca^{2+} currents.[74] (6) Consistent with these observations, pharmacologic studies on isolated corporal tissue strips have indicated that gap junctions contribute significantly to pharmacomechanical coupling and syncytial tissue contraction during activation of the alpha$_1$-adrenergic receptor.[63]

REFERENCES

1. Wagner G. Erection: anatomy. In: Wagner G, Green R, eds. Impotence: Physiological, Psychological, Surgical Diagnosis and Treatment. New York: Plenum Press, 1981:7–24.
2. Hsu LG, Brock G, Martinez-Pinncor L, et al. The three-dimensional structure of the human tunica albuginea: anatomical and ultrastructural levels. Int J Impot Res 4(Suppl 2):P41, 1992.
3. Luangkhot R, Rutchik S, Agarwal V, et al. Collagen alterations in the corpus cavernosum of men with sexual dysfunction. J Urol 148:467, 1992.
4. Padma-Nathan H, Cheung D, Perelman J, et al. The effects of aging, diabetes, and vascular ischemia on the biochemical composition of collagen found in the corpora and tunica of potent and impotent men. Int J Impot Res 2:75, 1990.
5. Clemente CD, ed. Gray's Anatomy, 13th ed. Philadelphia: Lea & Febiger, 1985:1559–1563.
6. Moore KL. Clinically Oriented Anatomy. Baltimore: Williams & Wilkins, 1980:312–324.
7. Benson GS, McConnell JA, Lipschultz LI, et al. Neuromorphology and neuropharmacology of the human penis. J Clin Invest 65:506, 1980.
8. Walsh PC, Donker PJ. Impotence following radical prostatectomy: insight into etiology and prevention. J Urol 128:492, 1982.
9. Semans JH, Langworthy OR. Observations on neurophysiology of sexual function in the male cat. J Urol 40:839, 1939.
10. Kollberg S, Petersen I, Stener I. Preliminary results of an electromyographic study of ejaculation. Acta Chir Scand 123:478, 1962.
11. Krane RJ. Sexual function and dysfunction. In: Walsh PC, Gittes RF, Perlmutter AD, Stamey TA, eds. Campbell's Urology. Philadelphia: WB Saunders Co, 1986; 1:700–735.
12. Newman HF, Northrup JD. Mechanism of human penile erection: an overview. Urology 17:399, 1981.
13. Bookstein JJ, Nad Lang E. Penile magnification phamacoarteriography: details of intrapenile arterial anatomy. Am J Radiol 148:883, 1987.
14. Aboseif S, Breza R, Lue TF, Tanagho EA. Penile venous drainage in erectile dysfunction. Anatomical, radiological and functional considerations. Br J Urol 64:183, 1989.
15. Lue TF, Tanagho EA. Physiology of erection and

pharmacological management of impotence. J Urol 137:829, 1987.

16. Fournier GR Jr, Juenemann KP, Lue TF, Tanagho EA. Mechanisms of venous occlusion during canine penile erection: an anatomic demonstration. J Urol 137:163, 1987.

17. Goldstein I, Krane RJ. Effects of hypotension on the hemodynamics of erection. Surg Forum 34:662, 1983.

18. Conti G. L'erection du penis humain et ses bases morphologic vasculares. Acta Anat 14:217, 1952.

19. Saenz de Tejada I, Moroukian P, Tessier J, et al. Trabecular smooth muscle modulates the capacitor function of the penis: studies on a rabbit model. Am J Physiol 260:H1590, 1991.

20. Melman A, Henry D. The possible role of the cat-echolamines of the corpora in penile erection. J Urol 121:419, 1979.

21. Christ GJ, Maayani S, Valcic M, Melman A. Pharmacological studies of human erectile tissues: characteristics of spontaneous contractions and alterations in alpha-adrenocepter responsiveness with age and disease in isolated tissue. Br J Pharm 101:375, 1990.

22. Hedlund H, Andersson KE, Mattiasson A. Pre- and postjunctional adreno and muscarinic receptor functions in the isolated human corpus spongiosum urethrae. J Auton Pharm 4:241, 1984.

23. Molderings GH, Gothert M, Van Ahlen H, Porst H. Noradrenaline release in human corpus cavernosum and its modulation via presynaptic alpha-2-adrenoceptors. Fund Clin Pharm 3:497, 1989.

24. Levin RM, Wein AJ: Adrenergic alpha-receptors outnumber beta-receptors in human penile corpus cavernosum. Invest Urol 18:225, 1980.

25. Giraldi A, Valcic M, Wagner G, et al. Subthreshold forskolin does potentiate cAMP formation in response to activation of both beta-2-adrenergic and PGE1 receptors in cultured human corpus cavernosum smooth muscle cells. Int J Impot Res 4 (Suppl 2):A41, 1992.

26. Brindley GS. Cavernosal alpha-blockade: a new technique for investigating and treating erectile impotence. Br J Psych 143:332, 1983.

27. Dittriich A, Albrecht K, Bar-Moshe O, Vandendris M. Treatment of pharmacological priapism with phenylephrine. J Urol 146:323, 1991.

28. Saenz de Tejada I, De las Morenas A, Goldstein I, Traish AM. Endothelin: localization, synthesis, activity and receptor types in human penile corpus cavernosum. Am J Physiol 261:H1078, 1991.

29. Lau LC, Adaiken PG, Rarnam SS. Effect of endothelin-1 on the human corpus cavernosum and penile vasculature. Asia Pacific J Pharm 6:287, 1991.

30. Holmquist F, Andersson KE, Hedlund H. Actions of endothelin on isolated corpus cavernosum from rabbit and man. Acta Physiol Scand 139:113, 1990.

31. Hedlund J, Andersson KE, Fovaeus M, et al. Characterization of contraction-mediating prostanoid receptors in human penile erectile tissues. J Urol 141:182, 1989.

32. Hedlund H, Andersson KE, Holmquist F, Uski T. Effects of thromboxane receptor antagonist AH 23848 on human isolated corpus cavernosum. Int J Impot Res 1:19, 1989.

33. Eckhard C. Untersuchungen über die Erection des Penis Beim Hunde: Beitrage zur Anatomie und Physiologie von C. Eckhard, III band, 1863.

34. Brindley GS. Pilot experiments on the actions of drugs injected into the human corpus cavernosum penis. Br J Pharm 87:495, 1986.

35. Wagner G, Brindley GS. The effect of atropine and c-blockers on human penile erection. In: Zorgniotti AW, Rossi G, eds. Vasculogenic Impotence. Springfield, Ill: Charles C Thomas, 1980:77–81.

36. Shirai M, Sasaki K, Kikimaru A. Histochemical investigation on the distribution of adrenergic and cholinergic nerves in the human penis. J Am Med Wom Assoc 27:403, 1972.

37. Adaikan PG, Karin SR, Kottegoda SR, Ratnam SS. Cholinoreceptors in the corpus cavernosum muscle of the human penis. J Auton Pharm 3:107, 1983.

38. Hedlund H, Andersson KE. Comparison of the responses to drugs acting on adrenoceptors and muscarinic receptors in human isolated corpus cavernosum and cavernous artery. J Auton Pharm 5:81, 1985.

39. Saenz de Tejada I, Blanco R, Goldstein I, et al. Cholinergic transmission in human corpus cavernosum. Am J Physiol 254:H459, 1988.

40. Dorr LD, Brody MJ. Hemodynamic mechanisms of erection in the canine penis. Am J Physiol 213:1526, 1967.

41. Wagner G. Erection physiology and endocrinology. In: Wagner G, Green R, eds. Impotence: Physiological, Psychological, Surgical Diagnosis and Treatment. New York: Plenum Press, 1981:25.

42. Roy AC, Tan SN, Kottegada SR. Ability of the human corpus cavernosa muscle to generate prostaglandin and thromboxanes in vivo. Med Sci 12:608, 1984.

43. Hedlund H, Andersson KE. Contraction and relaxation induced by some prostanoids in isolated human penile erectile tissue and cavernous artery. J Urol 134:1245, 1985.

44. Balwierczak JL. The relationship of KCl and prostaglandin F2-alpha mediated increases in tension of the porcine coronary artery with changes in intracellular calcium measured with Fura-2. Br J Pharm 104:373, 1991.

45. Bhargava G, Valcic M, Melman A. Human corpus cavernosa smooth muscle cells in culture: influence of catecholamines and prostaglandins on cAMP formation. Int J Impot Res 2:35, 1990.

46. Gerber GS, Levine LA. Pharmacological erection program using prostaglandin E1. J Urol 146:786, 1991.

47. Gu J, Polak JM, Probert L, et al. Peptidergic innervation of the human male genital tract. J Urol 130:386, 1983.

48. Steers WD, McConnell J, Benson GS. Anatomical localization and some pharmacological effects of

vasoactive intestinal peptide in human and monkey corpus cavernosum. J Urol 132:1048, 1984.

49. Willis E, Ottesen B, Wagner G, et al. Vasoactive intestinal peptide (VIP) as a putative neurotransmitter involved in penile erection. Life Sci 33:383, 1983.

50. Adaiken PG, Kottegoda SR, and Ratnam SS. Is vasoactive intestinal peptide the principal transmitter involved in human penile erection? J Urol 135:638, 1986.

51. Hedlund H, Andersson KE. Effects of some peptides on isolated human penile erectile tissue and cavernous artery. Acta Physiol Scand 124:413, 1985.

52. Gu J, Polak JM, Lazarides M, et al. Decrease of vasoactive intestinal polypeptide (VIP) in the penises from impotent men. Lancet 2:315, 1984.

53. Furchgott RF, Zawadzki JV. The obligatory role of the endothelial cells in the relaxation of arterial smooth muscle by acetylcholine. Nature 288:373, 1980.

54. Ignarro LJ, Bush PA, Wood KS, et al. Endothelium-derived relaxing factor produced and released from the artery and vein is nitric oxide. Proc Natl Acad Sci USA 84:9265, 1987.

55. Palmer RM, Perrige AG, Moncada S. Nitric oxide release accounts for the biological activity of endothelium-derived relaxing factor. Nature 327:524, 1987.

56. Kim N, Azadzoi KM, Goldstein I, Saenz de Tejada I. A nitric oxide-like factor mediates nonadrenergic, non-cholinergic neurogenic relaxation of penile corpus cavernosum smooth muscle. J Clin Invest 88:112, 1991.

57. Azadzoi KM, Kim N, Brown ML, et al. Endothelium-derived nitric oxide and cyclooxygenase products modulate corpus cavernosum smooth muscle tone. J Urol 147:220, 1992.

58. Rajfer J, Aronson WJ, Bush PA, et al. Nitric oxide as a mediator of relaxation of the corpus cavernosum in response to nonadrenergic, noncholinergic neurotransmission. N Engl J Med 326:90, 1992.

59. Ignarro LJ, Bush PA, Buga GM, et al. Nitric oxide and cyclic GMP formation upon electrical field stimulation cause relaxation of corpus cavernosum smooth muscle. Biochem Biophys Res Commun 170:843, 1990.

60. Campos de Carvalho AC, Moreno AP, Christ GJ, et al. Junctional communication between vascular smooth muscle cells (human corpus cavernosum) in culture. Soc Cell Biol XX:XXX, 1990.

61. Moreno AP, Campos de Carvalho AC, Christ GJ, et al. Gap junctions between human corpus cavernosum smooth muscle cells in primary culture: electrophysiological and biochemical characteristics. Int J Impot Res 2(Suppl 2):55, 1990.

62. Spray DC, Moreno AP, Campos de Carvalho AC, et al. Junctional communication between corpus cavernosum smooth muscle cells. Proc Fifth World Cong Microcirc 104, 1991.

63. Christ GJ, Moreno AP, Spray DC. Intercellular communication through gap junctions: a potential role in pharmacomechanical coupling and syncytial tissue contraction in vascular smooth muscle isolated from the human corpus cavernosum. Life Sci 49:PL-195, 1991.

64. Bennett MVL, Spray DC. Gap Junctions. Cold Spring, NY: Cold Spring Harbor Laboratory, 1985.

65. Bennett MVL, Barrio L, Bargiello TA, et al. Gap junctions: new tools, new answers, new questions. Neuron 6:305, 1991.

66. Hertzberg EL, Johnson R, eds. Gap Junctions. New York: Alan R. Liss, 1988.

67. Barr L, Dewey MM, Berger W. Propagation of action potentials and the structure of the nexus in cardiac muscle. J Gen Physiol 48:797, 1965.

68. Spray DC, Burt JM. Structure–activity relations of the cardiac gap junction channel. Am J Physiol 27:C195, 1990.

69. Garfield RE, Cole WC, Blennerhassett MG. Gap Junctions in Uterine Smooth Muscle. Boca Raton, Fla: CRC Press, 1989.

70. McDougal WS. Kidney and ureter. In: Gillenwater JY, Grayhack JT, Howards SS, Duckett JW, eds. Adult and Pediatric Urology. St. Louis: Mosby–Year Book, 1991:545–570.

71. Campos de Carvalho AC, Roy C, Moreno AP, et al. Gap junctions formed of connexin43 are found between smooth muscle cells of human corpus cavernosum. J Urol 149:1568, 1993.

72. Moreno AP, Campos de Carvalho AC, Christ GJ, et al. Gap junctions between human corpus cavernosum cells: gating properties and unitary conductance. Am J Physiol 264:C80, 1993.

73. Christ GJ, Moreno AP, Melman A, Spray DC. Gap junction-mediated intercellular diffusion of Ca^{2+} in cultured human corporal smooth muscle cells. Am J Physiol 263:C373, 1992.

74. Christ GJ, Spray DC, Melman A, Brink P. Electrophysiological studies of ion channels in cultured human corporal smooth muscle cells. Int J Impot Res 4(Suppl 2):A40, 1992.

CHAPTER 3

Endocrine Factors Related to Impotence

George S. Benson

ENDOCRINE FACTORS IN MALE SEXUAL DYSFUNCTION

The role of androgens in penile erection in man is not known. The incidence of endocrinopathy in the impotent population has ranged from 1.7% to 35%.[1] The value of hormonal screening and which studies to obtain in the evaluation of the impotent patient remain controversial. Despite these uncertainties, decisions about endocrine evaluation and management of patients with erectile dysfunction must be made frequently.

THE EFFECT OF HORMONES ON MALE SEXUAL FUNCTION

Significant data concerning the effects of androgens on sexual function have been accumulated from studies in animals, particularly the rat. In this animal model, castration produces a rapid disappearance of serum testosterone. Castrated animals exhibit diminished ejaculatory behavior, decrease in number of intromissions, and loss of mounting behavior. Administration of testosterone to previously castrated rats restores normal sexual activity.[2] Although testosterone is known to affect spinal reflex activity,[3] the primary site of testosterone action on the control of sexual function is probably the brain. The implantation of small amounts of testosterone into the hypothalamic preoptic area, but not into other parts of the brain, restores normal sexual behavior to castrated rats.[2]

Rats are not people, and the relationship between androgens and sexual function in man is not as clear. The difficulties encountered in separating libido from erectile activity when performing clinical studies are well known. Studies on the effects of castration and studies using testosterone replacement in hypogonadal patients have been conducted. In 1963, Ellis and Grayhack reported that a significant number of patients (16 of 82) retained their potency following castration for the treatment of prostate cancer.[4] In these patients, castration plus estrogen therapy resulted in more erectile problems than did castration alone. Retained potency also has been described following bilateral orchiectomy by other authors.[5,6] These studies have been criticized because all the data were generated by questioning patients and are, therefore, subjective. No objective studies were performed. Although it can be argued that no reliable studies exist to determine a patient's ability to achieve penile erection in a sexual setting, the necessity for androgens for penile erection in man remains in doubt.

Several well-designed placebo-controlled studies on the effect of androgen replacement in hypogonadal men have been performed.[2,7,8] In this group of patients, testosterone replacement does increase sexual interest and activity. The beneficial effects of testosterone replacement on erectile capability are less clear. Hypogonadal men report fewer spontaneous daytime penile erections and experience abnormal nocturnal penile tumescence (NPT) when objectively studied in sleep laboratories. The abnormal NPT studies revert to normal when these hypogonadal men are treated with testosterone.[9,10] When hypogonadal men view erotic films or engage in fantasy, however, their erectile responses are normal. In summary, therefore, although nocturnal erections appear to be testosterone dependent, attaining penile erection in sexual settings may not be related to circulating androgen levels. These observations support the hypothesis that, in man, testosterone enhances libido but does not directly control penile erection in a sexual setting. Certain stimuli, therefore, appear to be androgen sensitive, and others do not. Although a threshold level of serum testosterone for normal sexual activity probably exists, changes in serum testosterone levels within the normal range do not correlate with sexual interest or activity.[2] In impotent men without androgen deficiency, testosterone is no more effective than placebo in restoring sexual potency. In a well-controlled study of impotent patients without testosterone deficiency, more than one half of the patients reported marked improvement in potency regardless of whether they received testosterone or placebo.[11]

Male sexual function is probably also influenced by hormones other than androgens. Most men with hyperprolactinemia experience both loss of libido and impotence.[12] A very small number of patients with hyperprolactinemia and normal serum testosterone levels have been reported, but the vast majority of patients with hyperprolactinemia have markedly depressed serum testosterone levels.[13] The interactions between prolactin and testosterone are not clear. Increased prolactin may inhibit the action of luteinizing hormone (LH) on Leydig cell function. Alternatively, prolactin may decrease the secretion of LH either by inhibiting the response of the pituitary to LHRH or by decreasing the secretion of LHRH from the hypothalamus.[13] Impotence in patients with hyperprolactinemia is not solely related to low testosterone levels. In these patients, testosterone therapy does not correct erectile dysfunction. Sexual function does improve, however, when prolactin levels are lowered by treatment with bromocriptine. This finding has led to speculation that the hyperprolactinemia per se may be the cause of erectile dysfunction.[13] Other evidence has been presented supporting the hypothesis that the primary effect of increased prolactin levels is to diminish libido and that impotence seen in this syndrome is secondary or psychogenic.[14,15]

HYPOTHALAMIC-PITUITARY-GONADAL AXIS

Regulation of serum testosterone levels is controlled by the hypothalamic-pituitary-gonadal axis (Fig. 3–1). Normally, 1% to 3% of the total testosterone is in the free fraction, and the remaining 97% to 99% is transported in plasma bound to albumin and testosterone-binding globulin (TeBG). Only a small fraction of the total testosterone is, therefore, biologically available to target organs. Blood levels of TeBG are influenced by both hormonal factors and disease states. Estrogens and thyroid hormone increase plasma TeBG levels and, therefore, reduce the free testosterone fraction. Conversely, TeBG levels are decreased by androgens, growth hormone, glucocorticoids, and obesity. When TeBG levels fall, more biologically active free testosterone is available.[16]

Most serum testosterone is produced by testicular Leydig cells, and a small amount of androgen is synthesized in the adrenal cortex. Leydig cell secretion of testosterone is controlled by LH. LH is secreted by cells located in the anterior pituitary and is a glycoprotein hormone that consists of two noncovalently linked subunits, termed α and β. LH shares a common α subunit with thyroid-stim-

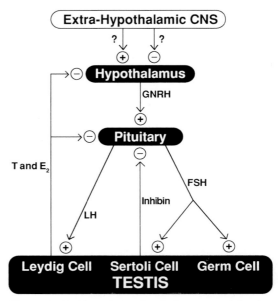

Figure 3–1. Hypothalamic-pituitary-gonadal axis.

ulating hormone (TSH), follicle-stimulating hormone (FSH), and human chorionic gonadotropin (HCG), but each hormone has a unique β subunit that confers biologic specificity. The isolated β subunits themselves are biologically inactive.[17] LH is secreted in episodic bursts, which in man are estimated to occur at a frequency of 4.4 pulses per hour.[18] LH secretion is, in turn, stimulated by the pulsatile release of gonadotropin-releasing hormone (GnRH), a decapeptide produced in the medial basal hypothalamus. GnRH released by the hypothalamus reaches the pituitary via the hypophyseal-portal system. GnRH release is influenced by a variety of neurotransmitters or peptides or both. Animal data demonstrate that norepinephrine, when administered intraventricularly, stimulates LH secretion in vivo and GnRH production by hypothalamic tissue in vitro.[19] Naloxone, an opiate antagonist, increases the frequency and amplitude of LH pulsatile secretion in normal men.[20] Dopamine, histamine, and other putative neurotransmitters also have been shown to affect GnRH and LH release.[21]

LH secretion is regulated by circulating levels of both androgen and estrogen through negative feedback. The relative importance of androgens and estrogens in controlling LH release is difficult to ascertain because testosterone is metabolized to both dihydrotestosterone (DHT) and estradiol. Furthermore, the exact site of action of androgens and estrogens in suppressing LH release is not clear and may include activity at both hypothalamic and pituitary levels.

FSH is also released from the pituitary in response to pulsatile GnRH stimulation. Like LH, FSH is a glycoprotein that is composed of two subunits. The α subunit of FSH is identical to the α subunit of LH. The unique β subunit of FSH is, therefore, responsible for stimulating spermatogenesis, the primary physiologic effect of FSH. Neither LH nor FSH is bound to plasma proteins to any significant degree. FSH secretion is controlled, at least in part, by GnRH, and like LH, FSH is secreted in a pulsatile manner. FSH levels are also controlled by inhibin, a polypeptide produced by Sertoli cells, via a negative feedback mechanism. Although LH and FSH appear to be secreted by the same pituitary cell type and release of both hormones is stimulated in a pulsatile manner by GnRH stimulation, differences in FSH and LH release do exist. A greater LH release than FSH release from the pituitary is seen following GnRH stimulation.[22] Testosterone administration markedly suppresses LH, but not FSH, levels.[23]

ENDOCRINE EVALUATION

The mechanism considered responsible for erectile dysfunction in most endocrine causes of impotence is hypogonadism or low levels of circulating androgens. As previously discussed, however, circulating androgen levels in man do not always correlate with erectile ability, and to view decreased serum testosterone levels as the only cause of impotence is probably too simplistic. The classification of endocrinopathies associated with erectile dysfunction based on serum levels of testosterone and gonadotropins is, however, clinically useful. Hypogonadism may be secondary to any abnormality of the hypothalamic-pituitary-gonadal axis. Because this axis functions primarily as a negative feedback system, the site of pathology usually can be determined by measurement of serum testosterone and gonadotropins. Low testosterone levels may be associated with either low, normal, or high levels of gonadotropins. Low testosterone levels associated with low gonadotropins (LH and FSH) imply disease at the level of the hypothalamus or pituitary and is termed hypogonadotropic hypogonadism. When low testosterone levels are associated with increased (or normal) levels of gonadotropins, the site of pathology is presumed to be the testis and is termed hypergonadotropic hypogonadism, or primary testicular failure.

The history and physical examination may be of some help, but a firm diagnosis of hypogonadism is almost always made by laboratory testing. In general, the two most helpful findings during the history and physical examination in suggesting the diagnosis of hypogonadism in the adult are decreased libido and decreased testicular size and consistency.[1] Small testes, however, are not necessarily diagnostic of low circulating testosterone levels. Significant seminiferous tubular damage can occur with traumatic, chemical, or viral insult, with relative preservation of Leydig cell function. Other historical and physical findings consistent with hypothalamic, pituitary, or testicular disease, such as headaches, visual symptoms, and hypogonadal facies, are generally nonspecific.

The diagnosis of hypogonadism (either hypogonadotropic or hypergonadotropic) is established by hormonal evaluation. Measurement of serum testosterone by radioimmunoassay (RIA) is the initial study of choice. Normal values vary somewhat between different laboratories but are generally in the 300 to 1200 ng/dl range. Testosterone levels do vary and exhibit diurnal variation, with morning peaks. For this reason, a diagnosis of hypogonadism should not be made from a single testosterone determination, particularly if the blood is drawn in the afternoon. Since most of the action of testosterone is mediated by the free (nonprotein bound) fraction, measurement of free testosterone and TeBG levels has been advocated as being preferable to measurement of total testosterone. If serum testosterone levels are normal, hypogonadism is ruled out, and no further evaluation is necessary. When a low testosterone is identified, further evaluation is necessary to differentiate hypogonadotropic from hypergonadotropic states and to exclude hyperprolactinemia. Measurement of LH and FSH usually differentiates whether the hypogonadism is secondary to testicular or to pituitary-hypothalamic disease. Increased levels of LH and FSH are seen with primary testicular failure. With pituitary or hypothalamic disorders, LH and FSH levels are either normal or decreased.

The differentiation of hypothalamic from pituitary disease requires stimulation studies by agents that act selectively on either the hypothalamus or the pituitary. Clomiphene citrate has been used to determine hypothalamic dysfunction. Clomiphene blocks the negative feedback by estradiol on the hypothalamus and thus increases secretion of GnRH.[24] LH and FSH are determined before and after clomiphene administration, and an increase in gonadotropins (doubling of LH levels) in response to clomiphene implies a functioning hypothalamic-pituitary axis. The GnRH stimulation test also may help to differentiate pituitary from hypothalamic disease. Since GnRH acts directly on the pituitary, patients with pituitary disease should not demonstrate increases in LH and FSH with GnRH stimulation.[25] In patients with low testosterone levels, stimulation with HCG may aid in separating hypothalamic-pituitary disease from primary testicular pathology. The biologic action of HCG is similar to that of LH. A rise (doubling) in serum testosterone following HCG administration implies normal Leydig cell function. Finally, most patients with hyperprolactinemia secondary to pituitary tumors also demonstrate decreased serum testosterone levels.[13,26] If a low testosterone level is found in the evaluation of a man with erectile dysfunction, serum prolactin should be determined.

SPECIFIC ENDOCRINOPATHIES ASSOCIATED WITH ERECTILE DYSFUNCTION

Specific diseases that lead to hypogonadism and erectile dysfunction are conveniently classified as being either hypergonadotropic (testicular failure) or hypogonadotropic (pituitary-hypothalamic) disorders. In addition, a miscellaneous group of diseases thought to exert at least some deleterious effect on sexual function through endocrinologic effects is described (Fig. 3–2).

Hypergonadotropic Hypogonadism (Testicular Failure)
Testicular Absence (Anorchia and Castration)

The absence of palpable testes on physical examination is obvious in patients experiencing erectile dysfunction with anorchia or after surgical castration. Anorchia, or vanishing testes syndrome, is seen uncommonly in children and is thought to be the result of prenatal torsion or vascular compromise. The regression of mullerian structures and the development of male external genitalia argue for the presence of a functional testis during fetal

development. Diagnosis consists of the findings of elevated LH and FSH levels, low testosterone levels, and lack of elevation of testosterone levels with HCG stimulation.[27] Lifelong therapy with testosterone beginning at the time of expected puberty is indicated. The effects of postpubertal castration on sexual function have been discussed previously. Following castration, testosterone levels generally fall to less than 50 ng/dl.[28,29] This level corresponds to testosterone values seen in normal, nonpregnant females. Even with this low level of testosterone, however, some men report adequate sexual functioning. Men who have undergone castration clearly need no laboratory investigation before proceeding to androgen replacement therapy. In most men, however, bilateral orchiectomy is performed for the treatment of prostate cancer. Testosterone replacement in these patients is contraindicated, and therapy of erectile dysfunction with either a vacuum constriction device, intracavernosal drug injection, or penile prosthesis should be considered.

Congenital and Chromosomal Abnormalities

Hypoplastic testes associated with hypogonadism occur in Noonan's syndrome and Klinefelter's syndrome. The clinical features in Noonan's syndrome in the male are similar to those seen in Turner's syndrome (XO) in the female. This autosomal dominant inherited disease is characterized by short stature, webbed neck, and cardiovascular abnormalities.[30] Hypoplastic, often cryptorchid, testes are commonly seen, and testosterone levels are characteristically low to normal. After puberty,

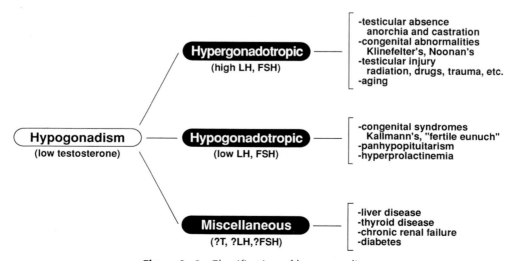

Figure 3–2. Classification of hypogonadism.

LH and FSH levels are elevated, and therapy consists of testosterone replacement. Klinefelter's syndrome is karyotypically defined as the presence of two or more X chromosomes and at least one Y chromosome. Patients with Klinefelter's syndrome typically are tall and have gynecomastia, small, firm testes, and azoospermia. Many of these patients are diagnosed during an infertility evaluation, although motile spermatozoa in the ejaculate have been observed in some patients with Klinefelter's syndrome.[31] Testosterone levels are low to normal, and LH and particularly FSH levels are elevated. Although infertility in these patients is rarely reversible, testosterone replacement is indicated for clinical signs of androgen deficiency.

Testicular Injury and Drug Effects

Although testicular damage from radiation, chemicals, trauma, viral illness, or cancer chemotherapy usually results in a more profound effect on the seminiferous tubules than on Leydig cell function, clinical symptoms of androgen deprivation also may result. Leydig cell function is relatively resistant to radiation, although doses of greater than 2000 rad directed at the testes have been associated with decreased testosterone production.[32] Evidence has been presented that not only seminiferous tubule damage but also Leydig cell damage occurs both during the acute phase of mumps orchitis and following recovery.[33] Serum testosterone levels are usually normal in men who have received cancer chemotherapy.[34] Drug use and drug therapy may be a common cause of androgen deficiency states. Cannabis, cocaine, and opiates have been implicated in sexual dysfunction,[35] and the use of marijuana and heroin has been associated with low testosterone levels.[36] Alcohol abuse has been associated with impotence, and decreased serum testosterone levels have been demonstrated in intoxicated male alcoholics and in nonalcoholic men given large amounts of alcohol for several days.[37] Spironolactone may depress libido, and adverse side effects of this agent, including gynecomastia and impotence, have been attributed to endocrine effects.[38] Cimetidine, an H_2 receptor blocker, is in widespread use for treatment of peptic ulcer disease. This agent is known to have antiandrogen effects, and erectile dysfunction has been reported in approximately 50% of patients taking this drug.[39] It is difficult to define the exact mechanism of action of cimetidine that is responsible for the reported erectile dysfunction because this agent also increases prolactin levels[40,41] and theoretically can block peripheral H_2 receptors in corporal smooth muscle.

Effects of Aging

Although decline in gonadal function with aging is not as significant in men as in women, changes do occur. A decrease in both total and free testosterone levels has been documented to occur with aging, although concentrations of these hormones usually are maintained within the normal range.[42] This decrease in testosterone levels has been attributed to both testicular and pituitary-hypothalamic changes. Since an increase in LH and FSH levels as well as a decreased response to HCG have been demonstrated, a decline in testicular Leydig cell function is thought to occur.[43] In addition, a decrease in pituitary response to GnRH stimulation also occurs.[44] These endocrine changes occurring at multiple sites may be secondary to concomitant diseases or simply to the effects of aging itself. Nevertheless, there is no evidence that treating erectile dysfunction in older men who have testosterone levels in the normal range with parenteral testosterone is more efficacious than placebo. In addition, testosterone therapy possesses inherent risks.

Hypogonadotropic Hypogonadism (Pituitary-Hypothalamic Disease)
Congenital Syndromes

Kallmann's syndrome is the most common form of hypogonadotropic hypogonadism. Classically, this syndrome consists of low testosterone and LH and FSH levels and anosmia, although patients with Kallmann's syndrome with normal olfactory function have been described. Other abnormalities, including mental retardation, deafness, color blindness, and craniofacial defects, are associated with this syndrome. Patients often have delayed puberty. Since the administration of GnRH results in elevated levels of LH and FSH, the primary pathology is thought to be in the hypothalamus.[45] Autopsy studies reveal no pituitary pathology, and anterior pituitary function is normal except as judged by low LH and FSH levels. Testosterone may be administered to induce masculinization and for improvement in libido and potency, recognizing the deleterious effects of testosterone on spermatogenesis.

In contrast to Kallmann's syndrome in which both LH and FSH levels are depressed, a syndrome of isolated LH deficiency (fertile eunuch) is recognized. Spermatogenesis is seen on testicular biopsy, and FSH levels are normal.[46] Serum LH and testosterone levels are, however, markedly depressed. These patients have a eunuchoid appearance but usually normal-sized testicles. Probably because of markedly low testosterone levels, spermatogenesis usually is impaired. HCG therapy is indicated for both the androgen deficiency and the infertility.

Two other congenital hypogonadotropic syndromes are recognized primarily by their associated anomalies. The Prader-Labhart-Willi syndrome consists of hypotonia, hypomentia, hypogonadism, and obesity.[47] A hypothalamic disorder is thought to be responsible because chronic GnRH treatment increases LH and FSH levels.[48] The Laurence-Moon-Biedl syndrome is an autosomal recessive inherited syndrome characterized by hypogonadism associated with mental retardation, retinitis pigmentosa, polydactyly, renal anomalies, and cryptorchidism. Erectile dysfunction in patients with these syndromes is rarely of clinical concern.

Acquired Syndromes

Hypogonadism secondary to gonadotropin deficiency can occur in panhypopituitarism from a variety of causes. Pituitary ablation by surgery or irradiation, infarction, infiltrative or granulomatous disease, or from any mass lesion involving the hypothalamus or pituitary may result in panhypopituitarism. Hormonal abnormalities consist not only of hypogonadism but also of adrenal and thyroid dysfunction. Symptoms of decreased libido and erectile dysfunction may occur before symptoms referable to other organ systems. In postpubertal patients, in fact, symptoms of hypogonadism are often the earliest signs of panhypopituitarism secondary to a pituitary tumor.[49] Finding of a low testosterone and subsequently low LH and FSH levels should lead to the diagnosis of pituitary disease. Magnetic resonance imaging (MRI) or computed tomography (CT) of the head is usually indicated in these patients.

Hyperprolactinemia is classically associated with a pituitary tumor. In this clinical setting, decreased libido and erectile dysfunction are reported by the majority of patients.[1,13] In addition, hyperprolactinemia is associated with a myriad of conditions, including other central nervous system diseases, endocrinopathies, liver disease, renal disease, and a variety of drugs.[49] In addition to complaints of sexual dysfunction, patients may exhibit gynecomastia, although galactorrhea is uncommon. Testosterone levels are almost always low, as are LH levels. Because serum testosterone levels are almost always decreased, many investigators believe that a serum prolactin test does not need to be performed as a screening test in otherwise asymptomatic men complaining of erectile dysfunction.[1] Only if the testosterone is low is the serum prolactin determined. Prolactin probably exerts its effect at the level of the hypothalamus by diminishing GnRH secretion.[13]

Although there is a clear relationship among hyperprolactinemia, low serum testosterone levels, and impotence, the mechanisms responsible for erectile dysfunction with hyperprolactinemia are not solely secondary to decreased testosterone levels. Administration of testosterone does not restore sexual function to these patients as long as prolactin levels are elevated.[13] Prolactin clearly exerts detrimental effects on erectile function that are not mediated through lowering of testosterone levels, but these effects are not well understood. The use of bromocriptine has revolutionized the treatment of hyperprolactinemia secondary to pituitary tumors.[13,50] Prolactin release by the pituitary is inhibited by dopamine. Bromocriptine is a dopamine agonist that lowers prolactin levels and restores testosterone levels to normal. Potency may be restored, and tumor size may be reduced. In some patients, however, surgical ablation of the pituitary tumor is necessary. The use of bromocriptine in hyperprolactinemic states not associated with a pituitary tumor is not well defined.

Miscellaneous Diseases

A variety of systemic diseases associated with erectile dysfunction may exert some of their effects through endocrinologic mechanisms. The reasons why patients with diabetes mellitus, thyroid dysfunction, liver disease, adrenal disease, and chronic renal failure complain of erectile dysfunction are not well understood. Sexual dysfunction in diabetics is probably primarily related to vascular or neurologic changes or both. Although prior studies have shown no differences in hormonal levels between impotent and potent diabetics,[51] more recent studies have suggested that impotent diabetics do have lower testosterone and higher LH levels than controls.[52] Erectile dysfunction has been associated with both hyperthyroidism and hypothyroidism. In patients with thyrotoxicosis, serum levels of total testosterone often are elevated, whereas free testosterone levels are normal. This finding is attributed to an elevated level of TeBG in these patients.[53] In addition, LH levels and estradiol are elevated, and a decreased Leydig cell response to HCG has been observed.[53,54] This latter finding is compatible with Leydig cell dysfunction in hyperthyroid states. Whether the erectile dysfunction is caused by hormonal abnormalities or the overall impact of thyrotoxicosis is not known.

Hypothyroidism also has been associated with sexual dysfunction. Total testosterone levels are decreased, but probably as a result of decrease of TeBG levels, as free testosterone levels are normal. Hypothyroidism is also associated with increased prolactin levels, and hyperprolactinemia may be, at least in part, responsible for erectile dysfunction in these patients.[55] Hypogonadism is frequently seen in patients with chronic liver disease. Particularly in patients with alcoholic liver disease, plasma testosterone levels may be reduced and LH levels elevated.[56] Diminished response to HCG stimulation has been observed. In addition, estradiol levels are elevated. For this reason, gynecomastia may occur in addition to testicular atrophy. Since high LH levels respond inadequately to GnRH or clomiphene citrate, a hypothalamic-pituitary defect probably coexists with testicular dysfunction.[57] Prolactin levels are elevated also in men with hepatic cirrhosis.[58]

Patients with adrenal disease, particularly Cushing's disease, complain of decreased libido and impotence. As with many systemic diseases, these symptoms are thought to be related to both testicular and hypothalamic-pituitary factors.[59] A poor LH and FSH response to GnRH is thought to be secondary either to the space-occupying effect of the pituitary tumor or to the deleterious effects of high cortisol levels on gonadotrope function. Increased cortisol levels may directly adversely affect testicular function.[60] Endocrine changes related to chronic renal failure are discussed in Chapter 8. Although all of these systemic diseases often are associated with demonstrable hormonal changes, the relationship between these changes and erectile dysfunction remains largely speculative. Although low testosterone levels may be documented, it is naive to expect that testosterone replacement will restore potency in all of these patients.

ANDROGEN THERAPY AND ITS COMPLICATIONS

Although some hypogonadal states can be treated with HCG and the treatment of choice for hyperprolactinemia is bromocriptine, testosterone is the mainstay of therapy for the vast majority of hypogonadal men with erectile dysfunction. Although the goal of therapy is to keep serum testosterone levels in the normal range, there are few data to indicate that tight control of serum testosterone levels is of benefit. Most dose and injection interval regimens are based on pharmacokinetic studies and not on observed clinical benefit.

Unmodified testosterone is rapidly metabolized, whether given orally or parenterally, and therapeutic blood levels are difficult to attain or maintain. Successful androgen replacement therapy has relied on modification of testosterone by either esterification of the 17 beta-hydroxyl group or alkylation at the 17 alpha-position.[61] The alkylated testosterone drugs methyltestosterone and fluoxymesterone have been used widely primarily because they can be given orally. Both agents have the significant disadvantage of poor gastrointestinal absorption

and liver toxicity.[62] For these reasons, their use has been replaced by the parenteral use of esterified testosterone.

Testosterone cypionate and testosterone enanthate, both esterified testosterone, are recommended as the drugs of choice for androgen replacement. Both drugs are administered by intramuscular injection. Dosage and interval of administration are based on pharmacokinetic studies in hypogonadal males.[63,64] If the goal of therapy is to keep serum testosterone levels constantly within the normal range, 200 mg of testosterone enanthate given every 2 weeks or 300 mg every 3 weeks appears reasonable. Serum levels peak at supraphysiologic levels at 24 h and then gradually decline. Most patients treated with testosterone will experience an increase in libido, but beneficial effects on penile erection are less predictable.

Significant side effects can and do occur with treatment with testosterone. Informed consent should be given before initiating therapy, and the need for follow-up examination and studies must be stressed. The relationship of testosterone therapy to prostate cancer, hepatotoxicity, and cardiovascular complications should be discussed. Because of these side effects, testosterone should be administered only for the indication of hypogonadism.

No evidence exists implicating testosterone therapy as a cause of prostate cancer, but testosterone is contraindicated in the presence of prostate cancer. Before initiating therapy, a digital rectal examination and a prostate-specific antigen (PSA) test should be performed. Particularly in our litigious society and with the widespread use of PSA for prostate cancer screening, older patients on testosterone therapy should be followed by their treating physician for the development of prostate cancer. Despite the fact that hepatotoxicity has been markedly reduced when esterified rather than alkylated testosterone is used, evaluation of liver function studies before and periodically during therapy is prudent.

Androgen therapy has been demonstrated to increase hematocrit and red blood cell volume.[65] In a recent study, 2 of 15 patients who had significant increases in whole body hematocrit suffered strokes, and 1 had a transient ischemic attack (TIA) while on testosterone therapy. Testosterone causes elevation of hematocrit values most likely by stimulating erythropoietin production, and patients with hematocrit values greater than 48% appear to be at risk from cardiovascular complications.[66] Testosterone administration also leads to sodium retention and may adversely contribute to preexisting congestive heart failure.[62] Hyperlipidemia has been reported to occur following androgen administration.

In summary, a number of significant complications can occur during testosterone therapy. Patients should be evaluated regularly with at least a history and physical examination, PSA, serum multiple analysis (SMAC), and hematocrit.

CONCLUSION

The relationship between hypogonadism and erectile dysfunction is poorly understood. Specifically, what is the role of serum testosterone in the production of penile erection? Does testosterone replacement in hypogonadal states restore potency through an endocrinologic mechanism, or are responses secondary to placebo effect? What is a reasonable laboratory endocrine evaluation for the patient who has erectile dysfunction?

In a recent (December 1992) "Consensus Development Conference Statement" on impotence sponsored by the National Institutes of Health, several very reasonable assessments and recommendations were made. In addition to a history and physical examination, the conference concluded that

Endocrine evaluation consisting of a morning serum testosterone is generally indicated. Measurement of serum prolactin may be indicated. A low testosterone level merits repeat measurement together with the assessment of LH, FSH, and prolactin levels. Other tests may be helpful in excluding unrecognized systemic disease and include a complete blood count, urinalysis, creatinine, lipid profile, fasting blood sugar, and thyroid function studies.

In my opinion, a testosterone and SMAC constitute reasonable, cost-effective laboratory screening studies if the history and physical examination do not indicate other specific pathology. Evidence has been presented, however, that determination of testosterone is necessary only when patients have decreased libido or atrophic testes.[1]

The NIH consensus conference's recommendations for endocrine therapy are as follows.

For some patients with an established diagnosis of testicular failure (hypogonadism), androgen replacement therapy may sometimes be effective in improving erectile dysfunction. A trial of androgen replacement may be worthwhile in men with low serum testosterone levels if there are no other contraindications. In contrast, for men who have normal testosterone levels, androgen therapy is inappropriate and may carry significant health risks, especially in the situation of unrecognized prostate cancer. If androgen therapy is indicated, it should be given in the form of intramuscular injections of testosterone enanthate or cypionate. Oral androgens, as currently available, are not indicated. For men with hyperprolactinemia, bromocriptine therapy often is efficacious in normalizing the prolactin level and improving sexual function.

These guidelines are current, sound, and cost effective.

When evaluating a patient with complaints of erectile dysfunction, endocrine causes should be

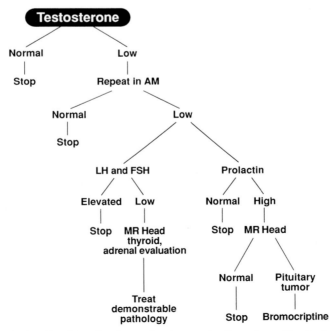

Figure 3–3. Algorithm for the endocrine evaluation of erectile dysfunction.

screened with a careful history and physical examination. The history should be directed at excluding liver, thyroid, adrenal, and renal disease and diabetes. The level of libido should be ascertained. Physical examination should be directed at determining the presence of systemic disease. The size and consistency of the testes should be determined. The endocrine laboratory evaluation should consist of determination of serum testosterone (and prolactin if decreased libido or atrophic testes are found). If low serum testosterone is identified, determination of serum prolactin, LH, and FSH is indicated. High prolactin levels or low LH and FSH levels require further endocrine evaluation, to include radiologic investigation of the head (Fig. 3–3). When androgen replacement therapy is deemed necessary, testosterone enanthate or cypionate is indicated, and careful follow-up for complications of androgen therapy is required. Most men who experience erectile dysfunction and who have low testosterone levels do not have the Laurence-Moon-Biedl or the Prader-Labhart-Willi syndrome. In many patients, no definitive diagnosis can be made. When prescribing testosterone therapy, we should remember that a significant number of men with no testicles are reported to have erections.[67] A primary objective of future research should be to determine the direct effects of serum testosterone levels on erectile function in man.

REFERENCES

1. Johnson AR, Jarow JP. Is routine endocrine testing of impotent men necessary? J Urol 147:1542, 1992.
2. Davidson JM. Hormones and sexual behavior in the male. Hosp Pract 10:126, 1975.
3. Hart BL. Physiology of sexual function. Vet Clin North Am 4:557, 1974.
4. Ellis WJ, Grayhack JT. Sexual function in aging males after orchiectomy and estrogen therapy. J Urol 89:895, 1963.
5. McCullagh EP, Renshaw JF. The effects of castration in the adult male. JAMA 103:1140, 1934.
6. Roen PR. Impotence: a concise review. NY State J Med 65:2576, 1965.
7. Skakkeback NE, Bancroft J, Davidson DW, et al. Androgen replacement with oral testosterone undecanoate in hypogonadal men: a double-blind controlled study. Clin Endocrinol 14:49, 1981.
8. Luisi M, Franchi F. Double-blind group comparative study of testosterone undecanoate and mesterolone in hypogonadal male patients. J Endocrinol Invest 3:305, 1980.
9. Cunningham GR, Karacan I, Ware JC, et al. The relationships between serum testosterone and prolactin levels and nocturnal penile tumescence (NPT) in impotent men. J Androl 3:241, 1982.
10. Kwan M, Greenleaf WJ, Mann J, et al. The nature of androgen action on male sexuality: a combined laboratory self-report study on hypogonadal men. J Clin Endocrinol Metab 57:557, 1983.
11. Benkert O, Witt W, Adam W, et al. Effect of testosterone undecanoate on sexual potency and the hypothalamic-pituitary-gonadal axis of impotent males. Arch Sex Behav 8:471, 1979.
12. Perryman RL, Thorner MO. The effects of hyperprolactinemia on sexual and reproductive function in men. J Androl 5:233, 1981.
13. Carter JN, Tyson JE, Tolis G, et al. Prolactin-secreting tumors and hypogonadism in 22 men. N Engl J Med 299:847, 1978.
14. Bancroft J, O'Carroll R, McNeilly A, et al. The effects of bromocriptine on the sexual behavior of hyperprolactinemic man: a controlled case study. Clin Endocrinol 21:131, 1984.
15. Schwartz MF, Bauman JE, Master WH, et al. Hyperprolactinemia and sexual disorders in men. Biol Psychiatry 17:861, 1982.
16. Glass AR, Swerdloff RS, Bray GA, et al. Low serum testosterone and sex-hormone-binding globulin in massively obese men. J Clin Endocrinol Metab 45:1211, 1977.
17. Catt KD, Dufau ML, Tsuruhara T. Absence of intrinsic biological activity in LH and hCG subunits. J Clin Endocrinol Metab 36:73, 1973.
18. Veldhuis JD, Evans WS, Rogol AD, et al. Intensified rates of venous sampling unmask the presence of spontaneous, high-frequency pulsations of luteinizing hormone in man. J Clin Endocrinol Metab 59:96, 1984.
19. Negro-Vilar A, Ojeda SR, McCann SM. Catecholaminergic modulation of luteinizing hormone-releasing hormone release by median eminence terminals in vitro. Endocrinology 104:1749, 1979.
20. Ellingboe J, Veldhuis JD, Mendelson JH, et al. Effect of endogenous opioid blockade on the amplitude and frequency of pulsatile luteinizing hormone secretion in normal men. J Clin Endocrinol Metab 54:854, 1982.
21. Glass AR, Vigersky RA. Pituitary-testicular axis. In: Lipshultz LI, Howards SS, eds. Infertility in the Male, 2nd ed. St. Louis: Mosby–Year Book, 1991:21.
22. Mortimer CH, Besser GM, Hook J, et al. Intravenous, intramuscular, subcutaneous and intranasal administration of LH/FSH-RH: the duration of effect and occurrence of asynchronous pulsatile release of LH and FSH. Clin Endocrinol 3:19, 1974.
23. Stewart-Bentley M, Odell W, Horton R. The feedback control of luteinizing hormone in normal adult men. J Clin Endocrinol Metab 38:545, 1974.
24. Winters SJ, Janick JJ, Loriaux DL, et al. Studies on the role of sex steroids in the feedback control of gonadotropin concentrations in men. II. Use of the estrogen antagonist, clomiphene citrate. J Clin Endocrinol Metab 48:222, 1979.
25. Marshall JC. Investigative procedures. Clin Endocrinol Metab 4:545, 1975.
26. Miller JB, Howards SS, McLeod RM. Serum prolactin in organic and psychogenic impotence. J Urol 123:862, 1980.
27. Levitt SB, Kogan SJ, Schneider KM, et al. Endo-

crine tests in phenotypic children with bilateral impalpable testes can reliably predict "congenital" anorchism. Urology 11:11, 1978.

28. Sciarra F, Soreini G, DiSilverio F, et al. Plasma testosterone and androstenedione after orchiectomy in prostatic adenocarcinoma. Clin Endocrinol 2:110, 1973.

29. Shearer RJ, Hendry WF, Sommerville IF, et al. Plasma testosterone: an accurate monitor of hormone treatment in prostatic cancer. Br J Urol 45:668, 1973.

30. Nora JJ, Nora AH, Sinha AK, et al. The Ullrich-Noonan syndrome (Turner phenotype). Am J Dis Child 127:48, 1974.

31. Foss GL, Lewis FJW. A study of four cases with Klinefelter's syndrome, showing motile spermatozoa in their ejaculates. J Reprod Fertil 25:401, 1971.

32. Brauner R, Czernichow P, Cramer P, et al. Leydig cell function in children after direct testicular irradiation for acute lymphoblastic leukemia. N Engl J Med 309:25, 1983.

33. Adamopoulous DA, Lawrence DM, Vassilopoulous P, et al. Pituitary-testicular interrelationships in mumps orchitis and other viral infections. Br Med J 1:1177, 1978.

34. Chapman RM, Sutcliffe SB, Rees LH, et al. Cyclical combination chemotherapy and gonadal function. Lancet 1:285, 1979.

35. Seagraves RT, Madsen R, Carter CS, et al. Erectile dysfunction associated with pharmacological agents. In: Seagraves RT, Schoenberg HW, eds. Diagnosis and Treatment of Erectile Disturbances. New York: Plenum Press, 1985:23.

36. Mendelson JH, Mendelson JE, Patch VD. Plasma testosterone levels in heroin addiction and during methadone maintenance. J Pharmacol Exp Ther 192:211, 1975.

37. Rubin HB, Henson DE. Effects of drugs on male sexual function. In: Thompson T, Daws PB, eds. Advances in Behavioral Pharmacology. New York: Academic Press, 1979;2:65.

38. Loriaux DL, Menard R, Taylor A, et al. Spironolactone and endocrine dysfunction. Ann Intern Med 85:630, 1976.

39. Jensen RT, Collen MJ, Pandol SJ, et al. Cimetidine-induced impotence and breast changes in patients with gastric hypersecretory states. N Engl J Med 308:883, 1983.

40. Hall WW. Breast changes in males on cimetidine. N Engl J Med 295:841, 1976.

41. Carlson HE, Ippoliti AF. Cimetidine, an H_2 antihistamine, stimulates prolactin secretion in man. J Clin Endocrinol Metab 45:367, 1977.

42. Vermeulen A, Rubens R, Verdonch L. Testosterone secretion and metabolism in male senescence. J Clin Endocrinol Metab 34:730, 1972.

43. Rubens R, Dhont M, Vermeulen A. Further studies on Leydig cell function in old age. J Clin Endocrinol Metab 39:40, 1974.

44. Harman SM, Tsitouras PD, Costa PT, et al. Reproductive hormones with aging. II. Basal pituitary gonadotropins and gonadotropin responses to LHRH. J Clin Endocrinol Metab 54:547, 1982.

45. Hoffman AR, Crowley WF. Induction of puberty in men by long-term pulsatile administration of low-dose gonadotropin releasing hormone. N Engl J Med 397:1237, 1982.

46. Faimen C, Hoffman DL, Dyan RJ, et al. The fertile eunuch syndrome: demonstration of isolated luteinizing hormone deficiency by radioimmunoassay techniques. Mayo Clin Proc 43:661, 1968.

47. Bray GA, Dahms WT, Swerdloff RS, et al. The Prader-Willi syndrome: a study of 40 patients and a review of the literature. Medicine 62:59, 1983.

48. Tolis G, Verdy IM, Friesen HG, et al. Anterior pituitary function in the Prader-Labhart-Willi (PLW) syndrome. J Clin Endocrinol Metab 39:1061, 1974.

49. Streem SB. The endocrinology of impotence. In Bennett AH, ed. Management of Male Impotence. Baltimore: Williams & Wilkins, 1982:26.

50. Franks S, Jacobs HS, Martin N, et al. Hyperprolactinaemia and impotence. Clin Endocrinol 8:277, 1978.

51. Wright AD, London DR, Holder G, et al. Luteinizing release hormone tests in impotent diabetic males. Diabetes 25:975, 1976.

52. Murray FT, Wyss HU, Thomas RG, et al. Gonadal dysfunction in diabetic men with organic impotence. J Clin Endocrinol Metab 65:127, 1987.

53. Chopra IJ, Tulchinsky D. Status of estrogen-androgen balance in hyperthyroid men with Grave's disease. J Clin Endocrinol Metab 38:269, 1974.

54. Kidd GS, Glass AR, Vigersky RA. The hypothalamic-pituitary-testicular axis in thyrotoxicosis. J Clin Endocrinol Metab 48:798, 1979.

55. Snyder PJ, Jacobs LS, Utiger RD, et al. Thyroid hormone inhibition of the prolactin response to thyrotropin-releasing hormone. J Clin Invest 52:2324, 1973.

56. Chopra IJ, Tulchinsky D, Greenway FL. Estrogen-androgen imbalance in hepatic cirrhosis. Ann Intern Med 79:198, 1973.

57. Van Thiel DH, Lester R, Sherins RJ. Hypogonadism in alcoholic liver disease: evidence for a double defect. Gastroenterology 67:1188, 1974.

58. Van Thiel DH, McClain CJ, Elson MM, et al. Evidence for autonomous secretion of prolactin in some alcoholic men with cirrhosis and gynecomastia. Metabolism 27:1778, 1978.

59. Luton J-P, Theiblot P, Valcke J-C, et al. Reversible gonadotropin deficiency in male Cushing's disease. J Clin Endocrinol Metab 45:488, 1977.

60. Glass AR, Smith CE, Kidd GS, et al. The response of the hypothalamic-pituitary-testicular axis to surgery. Fertil Steril 30:560, 1978.

61. McClure RD. Endocrine evaluation and therapy. In: Tanagho EA, Lue TF, McClure RD, eds. Contemporary Management of Impotence and Infertility. Baltimore: Williams & Wilkins, 1988:84.

62. Wilson JD, Griffin JE. The use and misuse of androgens. Metabolism 29:1278, 1982.

63. Snyder PJ, Lawrence DA. Treatment of male hypogonadism with testosterone enanthate. J Clin Endocrinol Metab 51:1335, 1980.

64. Sokol RZ, Palacios A, Campfield LA, et al. Comparison of the kinetics of injectable testosterone in

eugonadal and hypogonadal men. Fertil Steril 37:425, 1982.

65. Palacious A, Campfield LA, McClure RD, et al. Effect of testosterone enanthate on hematopoiesis in normal men. Fertil Steril 40:100, 1983.

66. Krauss DJ, Taub HA, Lantinga LJ, et al. Risks of blood volume changes in hypogonadal men treated with testosterone enanthate for erectile impotence. J Urol 146:1566, 1991.

67. Heim N. Sexual behavior of castrated sex offenders. Arch Sex Behav 10:11, 1981.

CHAPTER 4

The Diagnostic Algorithm

Ronald W. Lewis

Bernard F. King

No one particular diagnostic plan is the only correct way to evaluate the impotent patient. An approach that works at a multidisciplinary tertiary medical center is presented as a framework on which to build a point of departure for a discussion of timing and need for each of the diagnostic steps (Fig. 4–1). This algorithm is very pragmatic and one that will work for the small office as well as the largest referral center. It is also a system of workup that lends itself to cost containment, which must be considered in the context of the present and future economic realities of available health care dollars. Finally, this system of diagnostic steps has to be placed into the greater context of goal-directed therapy, a term first used by Lue.[1]

The goal-directed approach is established at the first encounter with the patient. The goals for the patient and partner, when available (and every effort should be made to have the partner present),[2] to solve the erectile dysfunction problem facing them is paramount in planning the next necessary diagnostic steps. At the first information-gathering encounter with the patient in which medical history is taken and physical examination is performed, it is also as important to find out what the couple knows about the various therapeutic choices for this disorder (conceptions and misconceptions) and what solutions have been tried. Age and medical condition of the patient will often limit his therapeutic choices. Some colleagues have criticized goal-directed therapy as loss of control of their role as physician; on the contrary, it only further strengthens this role. An unbiased presentation to the patient and his partner of all options available to treat their particular erectile dysfunction will allow clearer diagnostic step planning as the patient responds to this information.

HISTORY AND PHYSICAL EXAMINATION

The single most important step in the diagnosis of male erectile dysfunction is the history and physical examination (Fig. 4–1). Key elements in the history taking are outlined in Table 4–1. A sexual function questionnaire often will increase the efficacy of the initial evaluation. An example of such a questionnaire used at the Cleveland Clinic is shown in Figure 4–2. All areas of disorders of sexual dysfunction, including lack of or decreased desire, erectile dysfunction, ejaculatory dysfunction, and orgasmic difficulties, should be explored with the patient. The exact nature of the erectile dysfunction should be documented, whether it is complete or partial, whether it is intermittent or situational, the time and situation of onset, how long the problem has been present, whether there is an abnormal curvature of the penis associated with the dysfunction, and whether there is a loss of penile sensation or pain with erection. The history also should document the patient's previous workup and treatment. The possibility of neurogenic impotence is probably best determined at the initial fact-finding session if a history of neurologic disease or injury (by trauma or surgery) to the nerves responsible for erection is present. Occasionally, a diagnosis of diabetes mellitus will be made initially in the patient with erectile dysfunction, particularly if the patient has not had routine health care or if there is a strong family history of the disorder. A careful endocrine history will aid the physician in the selection of the laboratory diagnostic steps. The cardiac and peripheral vascular history is important for establishing etiology of the impotence and also aids in diagnostic planning. The psychologic history is extremely important, particularly for signs or symptoms of depression, a disorder seen in men at the same ages that most erectile dysfunction occurs. Often this plays a major etiologic role. We prefer the patient to give the marital and sexual history without the partner present, otherwise he may be inhibited in presenting all the facts. Later, obtaining the partner's views of the same historical information often will provide helpful insights for etiology and management. An accurate assessment of any use and the degree of use of tobacco, alcohol, illicit or prescribed

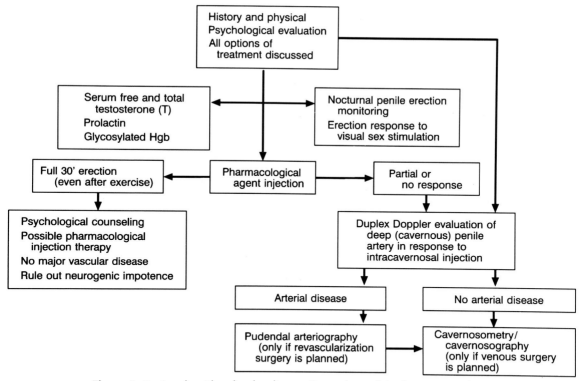

Figure 4–1. An algorithm for the diagnostic workup of the impotent patient.

drugs, and all medications is necessary at the time of the initial history, since there may prove to be a causal relationship that may have implications for therapeutic choices.[3,4] Sleep disorders are suggested by excessive snoring or restlessness at night or daytime somnolence or both.

A psychologic evaluation of the impotent patient by a trained professional is optimal, and this person often is part of the initial evaluation team at aca-demic centers.[5–7] A self-administered mental status or sexual inventory questionnaire may be of value, although the validity of existing tests has been questioned.[8] However, even in the most simple office setting, some evaluation of the mental status of the erectile dysfunction patient must be made.

The physical evaluation of the impotent patient is usually a limited, specialized examination (Table 4–2). The examination is concentrated on an evaluation of the penis, particularly corporeal palpation, the rest of the genitalia, the perineum, and the rectum. At the time of the rectal evaluation, the presence of the bulbocavernosal reflex can be determined by appreciation of rectal sphincter tightening on squeezing of the glans penis. In addition, the prostate is assessed. Determination of penile and perineal sensation is made at this initial physical evaluation.

TABLE 4–1
Evaluation of Impotency

History
Genitourinary disease or surgery
Symptoms of vascular or endocrine disease
Systemic debilitating disease
Neurologic disease
Vascular, neurologic, spinal, or inguinal surgery
Genital, pelvic, or spinal trauma
Sleep disorders
Psychologic history
Marital and sexual history
Nocturnal, early morning, nonintercourse erections
Medications
Tobacco or alcohol use
Other drug use or abuse

LABORATORY TESTS

There are three serum tests that are basic in almost all patients with erectile dysfunction: free (nonprotein-bound) and total testosterone and prolactin. Some have questioned the need for routine prolactin screening.[9] Serum testosterone is particularly important when the erectile dysfunction is only partial, that is, when the patient is able to get

THE CLEVELAND CLINIC FOUNDATION/THE CENTER FOR SEXUAL FOUNDATION
SEXUAL FUNCTION QUESTIONNAIRE

PLEASE ANSWER THESE QUESTIONS IN WRITING AND BRING THEM WITH YOU TO YOUR APPOINT-
MENT WITH DR. _____ ON _____.

The following questionnaire is designed to help your physician evaluate your sexual problem and its impact on your life. Some of the questions will be reviewed with you at the time of your interview. Please circle the appropriate answers. If you have any questions or additional comments please list them at the end of your questionnaire. Of course, this information is confidential.

Name _____   Age _____

Clinic Number _____   Date _____
(LEAVE CLINIC NUMBER BLANK IF UNKNOWN)

1. **Education**
   - a. completed high school   yes   no
   - b. completed college   yes   no
     degree:
   - c. completed postgraduate school yes   no
     degree:
   - d. skilled trade   yes   no
   - e. other

2. **Employment**
   - a. Are you currently employed?   yes   no   retired   disabeled
   - b. What is (or was) your job or profession?

3. **Marital Status**

   Single   Married   Divorced   Widower
   - a. If you are married (if not married, please go to 3.c. below)
     1. How many years have you been married?
     2. How would you describe the quality of your marriage?
        good   fair   poor
     3. How would you describe the quality of your sexual relationship?
        good   fair   poor
     4. Do you believe that your wife contributes to your sexual problem?
        yes   no
        If so, please describe briefly.
        _____
        _____
        _____

     5. Is your wife interested in having your sexual problem treated?
        yes   no   doesn't care
   - c. If you are not married, do you have a regular or steady sexual partner?
     yes   no

4. **Past Medical History**
   - a. Do you have any medical illnesses or conditions?
     yes   no
     If so, please list
     _____
     _____

     - b. Have you taken any medication in the past year)?
       yes   no
       If so, please list
       _____
       _____

     - c. List any operations you have had and their dates.
       _____
       _____

     - d. Have you ever received radiation, x-ray, or Cobalt treatments? Do not include x-rays for diagnostic purposes?
       yes   no
       If so, please state why, the date and the number of treatments given.
       _____
       _____

     - e. Have you ever had a serious injury or accident resulting in permanent damage?
       yes   no
       If so, please describe briefly.
       _____
       _____

     - f. How much alcohol (beer, wine, whiskey, etc.) do you drink?
       per day   per week   (circle one, then list type and amount)
       _____
       _____

5. **Psychological**
   - a. Have you ever seen a psychiatrist or a psychologist?
     yes   no
     If so, please describe the reason and the date(s).
     _____
     _____

   - b. Do you have any important personal problems that may be interfering with your sexual or job performance?
     yes   no
     If so, please describe.
     _____
     _____

   - c. Would you describe yourself as being an anxious or depressed person?
     yes   no
     If so, please describe what you mean.
     _____
     _____

6. Have you ever seen another physician regarding your sexual problem?
   yes   no
   If so, please give the dates, the doctor's opinion, and treatment offered or received.
   _____
   _____

7. Describe in your own words your sexual problem and how it is currently affecting your life.
   _____
   _____

8. **Erections** (Hard-ons)
    a. When was the last time you had a normal erection?
    b. Do you have erections now?
        yes   no

    c. If you answered yes to 8b how would you describe the quality?
        good   fair   poor
    d. Are your erections straight or curved? If they are curved, please describe them or draw a picture.

    e. Do you ever have erections at night?
        yes   no
    f. Do you ever awaken with erections in the morning?
        yes   no
    g. If the answer to e and/or f is yes, how do they compare with your sexually induced erections?
        Please describe this. _____
        _____

    h. When was the last time you had sexual intercourse?

    i. Does the quality or duration of your erection vary at times?
        yes   no
    j. Does your ability to have erections vary with different sexual partners?
        yes   no   I don't know
    k. Do you have any concern regarding the size of your penis?
        yes   no

9. **Climax or Orgasm**
    a. Are you able to have a climax or an orgasm?   yes   no
        If so, how was this achieved?
        vaginal penetration   manual   oral   anal
    b. Does semen (fluid) come out the end of your penis when you have an orgasm?
        yes   no
    c. Can you masturbate to climax?
        yes   no   I don't know
        If so, does your penis get hard at this time?   yes   no
    d. Do you now have or have you ever had premature ejaculations?
        (unintentional ejaculation or climax prior to vaginal penetration or shortly afterwards)
        yes   no
    e. Does reaching a climax seem to take a long time?
        rarely or never   occasionally   frequently
    f. Is your climax or orgasm ever painful?
        yes   no
    g. Is sensation (feeling) in your penis normal?
        yes   no

10. **Desire**
    a. Do you think that your level of interest in sexual relations (how often you feel "horny")
        is (circle one):
        about right for my age   less than it should be   more than it should be
    b. Do you avoid having sexual relations even though desire (a "horny" feeling) is present?
        rarely or never   occasionally   frequently   a partner has not been available
    c. Does your wife or primary sex partner provide you with the amount and quality of
        sexual stimulation you would like?
        rarely or never does   occasionally does   usually does
        a partner has not been available
    d. Does your wife or primary sex partner seem to have a level of interest in sex that is:
        low   about right   excessive   a partner has not been available
    e. Does your wife or primary sex partner get a climax or orgasm during intercourse?
        rarely or never   ocassionally   usually or frequently   don't know
        a partner has not been available
    f. Which of the following best describes the attitude of your wife or primary sex partner towards
        your sexual problem?
        doesn't care   upset   disappointed   accepting and understanding
        a partner has not been available

11. Would you like a report sent to your doctor?
    yes   no
    If yes, please provide the following information:
    Doctor's Name _____
    Address (please include zip code) _____
    _____

    Type of doctor (circle)
    Family Doctor   Internist   Urologist   Psychiatrist or Psychologist
    Other _____

12. Any remarks you wish to add?
_____
_____
_____

Figure 4–2. Example of a sexual function questionnaire. This one, which is used at the Cleveland Clinic, consists of a four-page evaluation (presented here on two pages).

TABLE 4–2
Evaluation of Impotency

Physical Examination
Secondary sexual characteristics
  Gynecomastia
Genitalia
Rectal evaluation
Neurologic
  Perineal and penis sensation
  Bulbocavernosal reflex
Pulses
  Femoral
  Distal extremities

Evaluation of the Man with Impotence in the Era of Vacuum Devices and Intracavernous Therapy—What Is Being Done or Should Be Done?
I. Goal-directed therapy
  A. Patient's age and health status
  B. Inform the patient (and partner) of therapeutic choices
  C. Awareness of patient's (and partner's) goals of therapy
  D. Tailor diagnostic evaluation and therapy in face of steps A–C
II. Minimal workup in context of goal-directed therapy
  A. History and physical examination are always necessary
  B. If vacuum device (V/D) chosen, diagnostic evaluation is minimal
    1. Free and total testosterone if erectile dysfunction is partial
    2. Prolactin
    3. Glycosylated hemoglobin in patients with no previous medical evaluation for diabetes mellitus (DM) or with family or personal history of DM
    4. Careful use in patients with bleeding disorders and contraindicators in patients with priapism history without permanent fibrosis
  C. If penile implant initially chosen, diagnostic evaluation is minimal
    1. Ensure patient understands options of treatment available
    2. Some insurance coverage requires proof of organic cause of impotency
      a. Nocturnal penile tumescence (NPT) (measure tumescent events with rigidity)
      b. Color duplex Doppler evaluation of penile arteries
    3. Explain consequences and complications of penile implant
      a. Infection
      b. Mechanical failure requiring reoperation
  D. If pharmacologic injection chosen
    1. Endocrine evaluation as in V/C device (steps 1–3)
    2. Need for office testing or intercourse trial or both
    3. Multiple agents and combinations available
      a. Papaverine alone
      b. Papaverine with phentolamine
      c. Prostaglandin E_1 (PGE_1)
      d. All three preferred at Mayo Clinic
        Papaverine 75 mg, phentolamine 2.5 mg, 5 PGE_1 25 μg-4.25 ml
        Dose 0.25 ml (4.4 mg papaverine, 0.15 mg phentolamine, 1.5 μg PGE_1)
  E. If vascular surgery or if patient or insurer desires to know, etiology workup becomes more comprehensive
    1. ± NPT
    2. Endocrine workup as in A, (steps 1–3)
    3. Office pharmacologic agent injection—if positive response (i.e., full erection by 10–15 min lasting 30 min) no significant vascular disease present—negative test inconclusive
    4. Color duplex Doppler evaluation of cavernosal arteries
      a. Abnormal (peak systolic arterial velocity >30 cm/sec and diameter of artery >0.7 mm after injection)—pelvic arteriography if patient a surgical candidate
      b. Normal with good erection—no significant vascular disease

TABLE 4–2
Evaluation of Impotency *Continued*

---

     c. Normal with poor or no erection, either another office injection or home test or cavernosometry/cavernosography if patient wishes to be considered for venous surgery

     d. High end diastolic velocity (>3–5 cm/sec) with poor or no erection—cavernosometry/cavernosography if patient candidate for venous surgery

  F. If psychologic basis is considered main etiology

     1. NPT

     2. Office injection testing—usually positive

  G. Do not forget that some patients are not interested in any of current therapeutic options; thus, none of the above may be this patient's choice

---

some rigidity or tumescence with sexual activity. When this clinical condition exists and the free testosterone is abnormally low, the patient will usually improve with parenteral testosterone. Multiple serum values for testosterone or pooled samples will correct for the daily fluctuations in serum levels of this hormone, but one sample obtained in the morning is usually adequate. If the result is normal for free and total testosterone, there is no need for further testing. Repeating the study on another day is reasonable if there is discordance between the free and total values or if the levels are low, before starting any intramuscular therapy. Although serum testosterone usually is decreased in the presence of significantly elevated prolactin,[10] there have been a number of reported incidences of elevated prolactin values with normal serum testosterone to warrant including this test in the essential hormone screen.[11] If serum prolactin is elevated, a CT scan of the head is needed to determine the presence of a large prolactin-secreting tumor in the pituitary. Serum luteinizing hormone (LH) and follicle-stimulating hormone (FSH) can be determined later if serum testosterone is low and prolactin is normal to determine if the condition is hypergonadotrophic or hypogonadotrophic hypogonadism, for there is a possibility that this information may affect treatment choice. An initial complete hormone screen for pituitary, adrenal, and thyroid hormones is not cost effective but should be ordered if the history and physical examination suggest an endocrine disorder. If the patient is a diabetic, has a family history of diabetes mellitus, or has a history of or physical evaluation that shows balanoposthitis, a glycosylated hemoglobin test is ordered as part of the initial essential laboratory blood work. This is a much better indication of consistent blood sugar levels than is a single fasting blood sugar. Newly diagnosed or poorly managed patients with diabetes mellitus or disorders of endocrine organs should be referred to the appropriate specialist. Urine, prostatic, or urethral cultures can be obtained in the presence of a history of urinary infection or signs and symptoms of a urinary infection. A complete blood count, serum chemical profile including a fasting blood sugar, or specific serum tests, such as blood urea nitrogen or creatinine, can be ordered if the patient has not had routine health screening. A serum lipid panel is necessary if there is a suspicion of vascular disease, particularly if any vascular intervention is planned, since there is a contraindication to such treatment until serum lipids are controlled.

Nocturnal Penile Tumescent Monitoring

There is some controversy among experts in the field of impotency about the need for and timing of nocturnal penile tumescent (NPT) monitoring in the impotent patient.[12–15] It is problematic that nocturnal penile rigidity (NPR) was not the original abbreviation used to designate this study, since it is imperative to know the degree of rigidity, not of tumescence, to determine the intactness of physiologic parameters for erections. NPT testing in a formal sleep laboratory with evaluation of rigidity is definitely indicated when a major sleep disorder is suspected from the history. This is also the preference at our institution when psychogenic impotence is highly suspected from the history, when there is a strong sense of secondary gain for the patient, such as workmen's compensation or other insurance cases, and when the patient shows an excellent response to an intracavernous injected agent but gives a definitive history of total erectile dysfunction in the absence of neurogenic disease or trauma. Under the last three circumstances, NPT testing with an instrument that can monitor tumescence and rigidity without formal sleep laboratory evaluations is also acceptable. There is only one instrument available for this testing, the Rigiscan (Dacomed Corporation, Minnetonka, MN).[16] Rigiscan monitoring cannot detect a sleep disorder or lack of REM sleep, but it is a much more economical test. If normal erections occur with good circumference changes and good rigidity, a psychologic etiology for the erectile dysfunction can be highly suspected, although NPT alone cannot unequivocally distinguish organic from psychogenic impotence. Visual sex stimulation erectile response may prove to be a more efficient and accurate test to differentiate psychogenic and organic impotence, but this remains to be tested.[14]

Pharmacologic Agent Injection Testing

The office injection of a vasoactive agent or agents has become a very efficient and convenient diagnostic step in evaluation of the impotent patient.[17] A full rigid erection occurring within 10 to 15 min of the injection that lasts for at least 30 min is indicative of no major vascular disorder. If no significant erection occurs by 15 min, the patient adds manual stimulation, the combined injection and stimulation test of Lue (CIS test).[1] A slow erectile response taking 30 min or longer is suggestive of arterial disease. A rapid full erection by 10 min that quickly dissipates over the next 10 min suggests venoocclusive dysfunction. The lack of response to this test is not definitely indicative of vascular disease. There can be a different response to the same agent in the same patient on different occasions. Distress from the needle injection can produce a sympathetic response with norepinephrine release, leading to no or partial response. A lack of response to the agent or agents in an office setting does not mean that a patient motivated for this type of therapy might not have success with injection therapy with his sex partner at home. Patients with neurogenic impotence are extremely sensitive to these agents, and if there is a history of neurologic disease or trauma, the first testing dose should be lowered. At our institution, 10 μg of prostaglandin E_1 (PGE_1) or 0.25 ml of a triple mixture (4.4 mg of papaverine, 0.15 mg of phentolamine, and 1.5 μg of PGE_1) is the preferred agent for office testing. A consistent failure to respond to a vasoactive agent is highly suspicious for a vascular or sinus smooth muscle disease, and color duplex Doppler sonographic evaluation of the penile arteries and the cavernosal tissue is the next diagnostic step. Priapism (any painful prolonged erection or an erection lasting over 3 to 4 h) occurs on the initial office injection 5% to 10% of the time. The patient should not leave the office with an erection that has not resolved. Priapism associated with injection testing or therapy is best treated with insertion of a 19-gauge needle into the corpora tissue at the base of the penis and withdrawal of 20 to 30 ml of blood. If the penis remains soft after this for 10 to 15 min, no further therapy is indicated. However, if the erection returns, another 20 to 30 ml of blood is aspirated, followed by instillation of 200 to 400 μg of phenylephrine for flushing. (We keep a stock solution of phenylephrine at a concentration of 500 μg/ml refrigerated in our clinic for such emergencies.)

Other Neurologic Testing

Decreased tactile sensation on the penis or perineum on physical examination, a history of an inability to sustain an erection with a sense of decreased feeling of contact or penile sensation during sexual intercourse, or a weak or absent bulbocavernous reflex suggests sensory deficit neurogenic impotence. Other more sophisticated neurologic tests, such as biothesiometry, bulbocavernosus reflex latency, or somatosensory evoked potentials from the tibial nerve and from the dorsal penile nerve, may increase the diagnostic accuracy of a sensory disorder.[18,19] Although there are no proven tests to evaluate for autonomic nerve defects, an afferent autonomic pathway disorder may be diagnosed by measuring the urethroanal reflex latency.[19,20] Measurement of intracavernous nerve activity via needle electrodes has been proposed as a possible direct evaluation tool for determination of autonomic nerve function, but this has to be evaluated further.[21-23]

Color Duplex Doppler Sonographic Evaluation

After a failed office injection test or after the initial interview with the patient who is motivated to know the etiology of his erectile dysfunction, we prefer the color duplex Doppler sonography evaluation of the cavernous tissue and the penile artery after injection of a vasoactive agent.[24] We originally used 60 mg of papaverine as the agent for this test, but after learning of the triple agent (A. Bennett, personal communication, 1989), we started using 0.25 mg of the triple agent. Since September 1991, we have used 10 μg of PGE_1 for this test. We do not believe that the arterial response varies among these agents, although others disagree.[25] We modified Lue's original technique of duplex Doppler ultrasonography by adding the use of color imaging, which greatly enhanced the ease of location of the penile artery and, hence, the rapidity of performance of the test.[24,26]

If the patient has bilateral peak systolic velocities of ≥30 cm/sec, dilation of the cavernosal arteries to a diameter of 0.7 mm or more, and a good erection secondarily from the injection, there is no significant arterial disease. If the clinical response is poor, i.e., erection is not strong, the 15 to 20 min end-diastolic velocity is greater than 3 cm/sec, and there are good peak systolic velocities, a venoocclusive disorder is highly suspected.

If the end-diastolic velocity is 0 or a minus value indicating retrograde flow in the artery (because of greater intracavernous pressure than diastolic pressure), no venoocclusive disorder is present. Under these circumstances, we do no other diagnostic test to determine venoocclusive function. If arterial disease or venoocclusive disorder is suspected from color duplex Doppler sonography testing, more definitive and more invasive diagnostic testing is performed, such as arteriography or cavernosometry and pharmacocavernosography, but only if the patient is a candidate for vascular surgery and is aware that long-term success from vascular procedures varies greatly. In addition, a thorough gray scale examination with and without color Doppler ultrasonography is performed on the cavernosal tissue looking for arterial–sinusoidal fistulas or Peyronie's plaque or both.

Vascular Disease Invasive Testing

We perform pelvic and pudendal arteriography only on those patients who have positive findings for vascular disease or disorder on the color duplex Doppler ultrasonography evaluation and who accept a potentially high failure rate. These patients should be carefully counseled in the other options of management, such as injection therapy, vacuum constriction devices, and penile prostheses. The preferred test for diagnosis of a venoocclusive disorder is pump infusion or gravity cavernosometry.[27,28] We believe that a functional test of the penile arteries, such as color duplex Doppler, and the anatomic test of pelvic arteriography are both necessary for diagnosis of arterial disease. The patient who is to have arterial surgery should also have an evaluation for venoocclusive dysfunction (by cavernosometry and pharmacocavernosography), since this disorder also can be present, and venous ablation surgery should be performed at the same time as the deep dorsal vein arterialization or revascularization surgery.

DIAGNOSTIC ALGORITHM USE WITH GOAL-DIRECTED THERAPY

In summary, all patients with a diagnosis of erectile failure undergo an initial history and physical evaluation, as outlined, with input from the partner if possible. Some mental status evaluation is preferable at this initial encounter. A careful presentation of the options of treatment for erectile failure is made to the couple. The physician then determines, based on the patient and his partner's goals and desires to know the exact etiology of the erectile difficulty, what the next step is to be. If the patient has not had routine health care monitoring, some basic laboratory tests should be performed, especially checking for diabetes in the face of a strong family history or history of infection disorders, such as balanoposthitis. Whether to screen all patients for testosterone and prolactin depends mostly on the philosophy of the physician. As a general cost-effective screening test, it is not reasonable, but it is preferred if the patient still has some moderate degree of rigidity with sexual activity and notices as a major part of his complaint a marked decrease in desire, sexual energy, or libido. There may be no need for further testing. For example, a patient in good general health in his 70s with total erectile failure with good libido who, after carefully having the vacuum constriction device presented (this is done at our institution by having the couple view a composite video of four different devices), chooses this therapy usually is given instructions and a prescription for one of the devices. This same approach is used for any patient regardless of age or circumstances who chooses the vacuum constriction device.

Nocturnal penile erection testing is performed in patients in whom a primary psychologic etiology is thought to be present, in patients suspected, from their history, of having a major sleep disorder, and in patients in whom major invasive vascular surgery is planned.

In patients who choose injection therapy after the initial goal-directed therapy information session, an injection is given at the first office visit as well. The preference at our clinic is the triple mixture of papaverine, phentolamine, and PGE_1 (0.25 ml) or PGE_1 alone (10 μg). This initial dose is decreased in those patients suspected of having a neurologic cause of impotency. If a rigid erection does not occur 10 min after the injection, manual self-stimulation is encouraged. If the patient does not respond to this initial office injection, he either returns for a higher dose in the office, receives another injection on another day for intercourse trial at home or a nearby hotel room with his partner, or is scheduled for evaluation of the cavernosal arteries with color duplex Doppler ultrasonography. If a patient has a full rigid erection by 10 min or with manual stimulation at 20 min and the erection lasts for 20 to 30 min, he is instructed in home pharmacologic injection therapy or a pharmacologic erection program (PEP). If the erection persists for more than 2 h or is painful after 1 h, it is pharmacologically reversed with 200 to 400 μg of phenylephrine after placing a 19-gauge needle in one side of the cavernous tissue at the lateral base of the penis and aspirating 10 to 20 ml of blood. If priapism or a prolonged erection occurs, the patient returns for another lower dosing session. An example of the patient who often follows this immediate office injection trial pathway is the patient who is impotent after radical pelvic surgery, such as radical retropubic prostatectomy, who had normal erections before his cancer surgery.

Many times, patients want to know the exact etiology of their erectile dysfunction and to know all possible options of treatment for their erectile dysfunction, including possible vascular surgery, particularly if they are under age 50 or are required by their insurance plans to clearly establish the organic etiology. In these cases, color duplex Doppler ultrasonography is the next evaluation scheduled after the initial office visit (Fig. 4–1). If this shows bilateral arterial disease and the patient is a candidate for vascular surgery, the next step is pelvic arteriography. If the patient gets a good clinical response to the injected agent at the time of the test and wishes to pursue home injection therapy, even in the presence of arterial disease, he is instructed in the home injection technique. If he is motivated for injection therapy with a poor or no response at the time of this testing, he is further tested in the clinic or home setting with a higher dose or a different agent or agents. In patients with good arterial peak systolic velocity and diameter dilation who do not have 0 or negative end-diastolic velocities, who have poor or no clinical response to the injected agent(s), and who wish to consider venous surgery, the next evaluation is cavernosometry and pharmacocavernosography. These evaluations are performed also before surgery on any patient who is to have arterial surgery. We do not perform the more invasive vascular studies in any patient who has a usable response to the vasoactive agents unless he is totally unable to choose home injection therapy. There is no need to perform these more invasive tests if the patient does not wish it or is a suitable candidate for vascular surgery.

In patients who have an excellent erectile response to the office injection agent(s) or show no vascular disease on the color duplex Doppler sonogram, have an excellent erection at the time of testing, and do not have a history or physical evidence of neurologic disease, a psychologic basis must be suspected, even in the absence of suspected psychologic impotence at the initial history-taking session. A more intense psychologic evaluation is recommended. A negative clinical erection at the time of intracavernosal injection does not rule out psychologic impotence, however, and this is an example of when the history, the NPT data, and psychologic testing must be integrated to establish a diagnosis.

If the patient and partner are motivated to choose the penile prosthesis as a first therapeutic choice, it is important for the treating physician to ensure that they know the exact alternative choices and the possible risks and complications of the penile prosthesis. The exact workup beyond the initial history and physical examination and psychologic screening depends on the need for the medical insurer to have an established diagnosis. It is extremely important to make sure that there is no active infection and that the patient with diabetes mellitus is under good control.

REFERENCES

1. Lue TF. Impotence—a patient's goal-directed approach to treatment. World J Urol 8:67–74, 1990.
2. Leiblum SR, Rosen RC. Couples therapy for erectile disorder: conceptual and clinical consideration. J Sex Med Ther 17:147–159, 1991.
3. Segraves RT, Madsen R, Carter CS, Davis JM. Erectile dysfunction associated with pharmacological agents. In: Segraves RT, Schoenberg HW, eds. Diagnosis and Treatment of Erectile Disturbances—A Guide for Clinicians. New York: Plenum Medical Book Co, 1985:23–63.
4. Wein AJ, Van Arsdalen KN. Drug-induced male sexual dysfunction. Urol Clin North Am 15:23–31, 1988.
5. Williams DE. Impotence: psychological contributions to etiology of management. In: Lewis RW, Barrett DM, eds. Problems in Urology—The Impotent Man. Philadelphia: JB Lippincott Co, 1991:510–518.
6. LoPiccolo J, Daiss S. Psychologic issues in the evaluation erectile failure. In: Tanagho EA, Lue TF, McClure RD, eds. Contemporary Management of Impotence and Fertility. Baltimore: Williams & Wilkins, 1988:104–120.
7. Kaplan HS. Psychiatric evaluation and therapy: what's new? In: Lue TF, ed. World Book of Impotence. London: Smith-Gordon, 1992:59–64.
8. Segraves RT, Schoenberg HW, Segraves KAB. Evaluation of the etiology of erectile failure. In: Segraves RT, Schoenberg HW, eds. Diagnosis and Treatment of Erectile Disturbances—A Guide for Clinicians. New York: Plenum Medical Book Co, 1985:165–195.
9. Nickel JC, Morales A, Condra M, et al. Endocrine dysfunction in impotence: incidence, significance, and cost-effective screening. J Urol 132:40–43, 1984.
10. Leonard MP, Nickel CJ, Morales A. Hyperprolactinemia and impotence: why, when, and how to investigate. J Urol 142:992–994, 1989.
11. Canning JR, Renshaw DC, Flanigan RC, Young MJ. Prolactin and impotence. Int J Impot Res 4 (Suppl 2):P47, 1992.
12. Karacan I, Howell JW. Use of nocturnal penile tumescence in diagnosis of male erectile dysfunction. In: Tanagho EA, Lue TF, McClure RD, eds. Contemporary Management of Impotence and Fertility. Baltimore: Williams & Wilkins, 1988:95–103.
13. Morales A, Condra M, Reid K. The role of nocturnal penile tumescence monitoring in the diagnosis of impotence: a review. J Urol 143:441–446, 1990.

14. Morales A, Condra M, Surridge DH, Heaton JP. Nocturnal penile tumescence monitoring: is it necessary? In: Lue TF, ed. World Book of Impotence. London: Smith-Gordon, 1992:67–73.

15. Allen RP, Brendler CB. Comment—nocturnal penile tumescence with polysomnography (NPT-PSG) remains the only objectively validated procedure for differential diagnosis of organic versus psychogenic erectile impotence. In: Lue TF, ed. World Book of Impotence. London: Smith-Gordon, 1992: 67–73.

16. Kessler WD. Nocturnal penile tumescence. Urol Clin North Am 15:81–86, 1988.

17. Lewis RW. Pharmacologic erection. In: Lewis RW, Barrett DM, eds. Problems in Urology—The Impotent Man. Philadelphia: JB Lippincott Co, 1991:541–558.

18. Padma-Nathan H, Gerstenberg TC. Neurogenic erectile dysfunction—diagnosis and management. In: Lewis RW, Barrett DM, eds. Problems in Urology—The Impotent Man. Philadelphia: JB Lippincott Co, 1991:527–540.

19. Bemelmans BLH, Meuleman EJ, Anten BWN, et al. Penile sensory disorders in erectile dysfunction: results of a comprehensive neuro-urophysiological diagnostic evaluation in 123 patients. J Urol 146:777–782, 1991.

20. Sarica Y, Karacan I. Electrophysiological correlates of sensory intervation of the vesico-urethral junction and urethra in man. Neurol Urodyn 6:477–484, 1988.

21. Wagner G, Gerstenberg T, Levin RJ. Electrical activity of corpus cavernosum during flaccidity and erection of the human penis: a new diagnostic method? J Urol 142:723–725, 1989.

22. Stief CG, Djamilian M, Schaebstaud F, et al. Single potential analysis of cavernous and electric activity: a possible diagnosis of autonomic impotence? World J Urol 8:75–79, 1990.

23. Stief CG. Single potential analysis of cavernous electric activity (SPACE)—does this interpretation of cavernous electric activity allow the diagnosis of cavernous autonomic dysfunction? In: Lue TF, ed. World Book of Impotence. London: Smith-Gordon, 1992:95–100.

24. Hattery RR, King BF, Lewis RW, et al. Vasculogenic impotence: duplex and color Doppler imaging. Radiol Clin North Am 29:629–645, 1991.

25. Meuleman EJH, Bemelmans BLH, Doesburg WH, et al. Penile pharmacological duplex ultrasonography: a dose–effect study comparing papaverine/phentolamine and prostaglandin E1. J Urol 148: 63–66, 1992.

26. Lue TF, Hricak H, Marich KW, et al. Vasculogenic impotence evaluated by high-resolution ultrasonography and pulsed Doppler spectrum analysis. Radiology 155:777–781, 1985.

27. Lewis RW. Venogenic impotence: diagnosis, management, and results. In: Lewis RW, Barrett DM, eds. Problems in Urology—The Impotent Man. Philadelphia: JB Lippincott Co, 1991:567–576.

28. Meuleman EHJ, Wijkstra H, Doesburg WH, Debruyne FMJ. Comparison of the diagnostic value of pump and gravity cavernosometry and evaluation of the cavernous veno-occlusive mechanism. J Urol 146:1266–1270, 1991.

CHAPTER 5

Radiologic Evaluation of Impotence

Bernard F. King

Ronald W. Lewis

Michael A. McKusick

The use of imaging tools in the diagnosis of impotence has become quite complex. The radiologic diagnosis of impotence consists of various evaluations of the corpora cavernosal tissue itself, the arterial supply to the corpora cavernosa, and the venous drainage system of the corpora cavernosa. In this chapter, we discuss in detail color duplex sonography, pelvic arteriography, cavernosometry, cavernosography, and radiologic diagnostic problems with penile prostheses.

DUPLEX SONOGRAPHY

Since 1982, many patients with impotence have been evaluated initially with an intracavernosal injection of a vasodilating pharmacologic agent. In theory, in pharmacologically induced erections, there should be little influence from psychologic factors or neurologic pathways.[1] Therefore, arterial inflow and venoocclusive mechanisms should be intact if a patient develops an erection after intracavernosal injection of a pharmacologic agent. Evidence suggests that this technique can miss some patients with a vasculogenic component to their impotence. In addition, as a screening test, it fails to differentiate arteriogenic from venogenic impotence. Duplex sonography of the penis was introduced by Lue et al. in 1985, and the technique has been refined by several investigators.[2-12] This technique allows for estimation of velocity of blood flow and change in the diameter of the cavernosal artery in patients with possible arteriogenic impotence. In addition, evaluation of the arterial waveform and evaluation of the draining veins of the penis can provide a means of evaluating venogenic impotence.

Duplex Sonography Technique

When impotent patients are referred for duplex sonography of the penis, no special preparation is necessary. The examination should be done in a quiet room with minimal distractions or interruptions. The examination is performed with the patient in the supine position, with the penis on the anterior abdominal wall. High-frequency (7.5–10 MHz), linear-array, ultrasound transducers should be used to image the penis in the longitudinal and transverse planes.

Duplex sonography of the cavernosal arteries is best accomplished in a longitudinal, parasagittal plane from a ventral approach (Fig. 5–1). In the flaccid state, the cavernosal arteries may follow a tortuous course and can be seen only intermittently on a single longitudinal plane. In the erect state, the cavernosal artery assumes a straighter course.

The first step is to obtain cavernosal artery diameter measurement before injection of a vasodilating agent. This baseline measurement of each cavernosal artery diameter is necessary to determine the degree of change following the intracavernosal artery injection of the vasodilating agent. Magnified views of the cavernosal arteries are used for measurement purposes, and internal lumen diameter measurements are obtained. Because of the wide variability within each artery, multiple measurements on each side can be obtained and averaged.

After cavernosal artery diameter measurements are made, a vasodilating agent is injected into the penis. The types and doses of vasodilating agents that are used vary widely (Table 5–1). Initially, many investigators injected 60 mg of papaverine (2 ml) into either the left or right corpus cavernosum. Some have used papaverine (40 mg) and phentolamine (2.5 mg), whereas others have used a triple agent consisting of papaverine (4.4 mg), phentolamine (0.15 mg), and prostaglandin E_1 (PGE_1, 1.5 μg) in 0.25 ml or PGE_1 alone (10–20 μg).[13] The incidence of priapism varies from 3% to 10% of patients and may be related to dose and combination of agents. It was thought that small doses of these vasodilating agents used together resulted in an additive effect that allowed one to

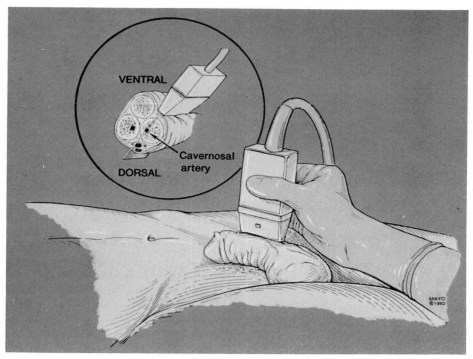

Figure 5–1. Technique drawing depicting the penis and the anatomic position on the anterior abdominal wall. The transducer is placed along the ventral aspect of the penis, and imaging is obtained in the longitudinal, parasagittal plane directed at the cavernosal artery. (Mayo Foundation, used with permission.)

use minimal doses of these agents with optimal response and minimal discomfort. However, early experience in our practice suggested that the incidence of priapism approached 8% to 10% using a triple agent. Therefore, we now use PGE_1 (10 µg) alone in an attempt to minimize the risk of priapism. PGE_1 used alone can result in a minor degree of pain and discomfort that may affect the patient's psychologic status during the examina-

TABLE 5–1
Vasodilating Agents for Impotence Evaluations

Agents	Mode of Action
Papaverine	Direct smooth muscle relaxant via interference with calcium flow during muscle contraction
Phentolamine	Induces smooth muscle relaxation by blocking alpha-adrenergic receptors; potentiates the action of papaverine
Prostaglandin E_1	Involved in the production of nitric oxide—a potent smooth muscle relaxant

tion. The optimal dose of vasodilating agent or combination of agents is uncertain.[14]

After injection, the vasodilating agent diffuses readily from one corpus cavernosum to the other because of the fenestrations within the septum of the penis. It is, however, important to inject the vasodilating agent accurately into the dorsal two thirds of the proximal portion of the penile shaft so that the agent does not enter the corpus spongiosum, the urethra, or the glans (Fig. 5–2). All patients should be instructed to contact their referring physician or go directly to an emergency room for evaluation and treatment of possible priapism if a painful erection occurs or if an erection does not subside after 1 to 2 h. Pharmacologically induced priapism is defined as persistent painful erection of the penis 1 to 3 hs after intracavernosal injection of a vasodilating agent. Persistent priapism (greater than 4–6 h) can result in ischemic necrosis and fibrosis of cavernosal tissue. Patients who are prone to priapism include those with a history of neurogenic impotence or sickle cell disease or trait and patients on heparin therapy. The use of smaller doses of vasodilating agents or performance of the examination without pharmacologic agents may be warranted in these patients.[15]

Treatment of priapism should be carried out by

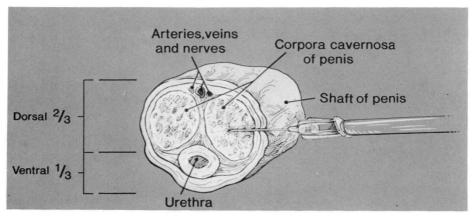

Figure 5–2. Cross-sectional drawing of the penis depicting the correct injection method of vasodilating agents into the dorsal two thirds of the penile shaft. Care must be taken not to inject into the ventral one third of the penis to avoid injecting the vasodilating agents into the urethra or corpus spongiosum. (Mayo Foundation, used with permission.)

a trained urologist and usually consists of aspirating approximately 20 ml of blood from a corpus cavernosum. If this fails to relieve the priapism, a small dose of a vasoconstricting agent (i.e., phenylephrine HCl, 200–400 µg) diluted in 1 ml of normal saline (500 µg/ml) can be injected intracavernosally to facilitate vasoconstriction and cessation of the erection.[13]

Following the intracavernosal injection of a vasodilating agent, the postinjection diameters of the cavernosal arteries are measured (Fig. 5–3), and dynamic velocity measurements are obtained up to 20 min postinjection. Doppler analysis of the cavernosal artery is optimally obtained near the base of the penis, where the Doppler angle is the smallest. A Doppler angle of less than 60 degrees should be achieved. Spectral analysis of the Doppler wave-

form in the cavernosal arteries enables measurement of peak systolic (PSV) and end diastolic velocities (EDV) (Fig. 5–4).

There continues to be debate about the optimal time after pharmacologic enhancement to record cavernosal artery PSV and EDV measurements. In our experience, peak systolic velocities vary in quartiles between 5 and 20 min postinjection.[16] Because of this time variation, we obtain velocity measurements at 5 min intervals in both cavernosal arteries for at least 20 min after injection of a vasodilating agent.

The dynamic duplex sonographic evaluation of the cavernosal arteries after the intracavernosal injection of a vasodilating agent reveals a progression of normal phases in the spectral waveform (Fig. 5–5).[11] These dynamic changes in the Doppler

Figure 5–3. Longitudinal ultrasound study of the right cavernosal artery (arrows) following the injection of a vasodilating agent. Note that the internal lumen diameter measures 1.1 mm.

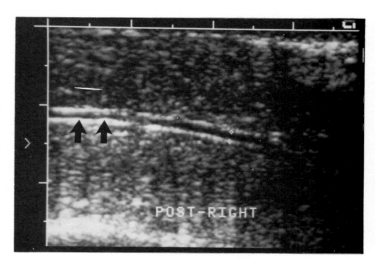

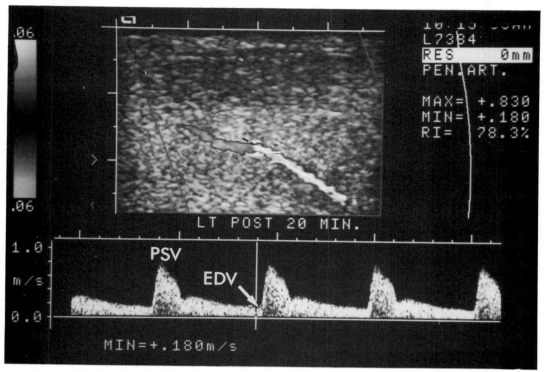

Figure 5–4. Longitudinal Doppler ultrasound study of the left cavernosal artery 20 min post-injection of a vasodilating agent. From the Doppler waveform, one can estimate the peak systolic velocity (PSV) and the end diastolic velocity (EDV).

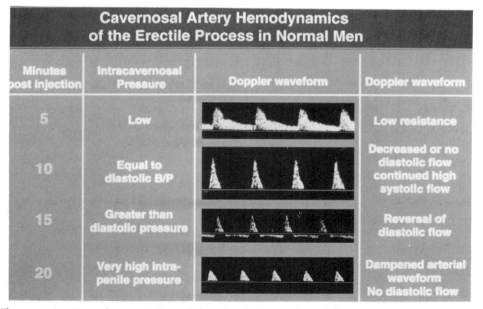

Figure 5–5. Normal progression of the Doppler waveform following the intracavernosal injection of a vasodilating agent. These changes in Doppler waveform correspond to changes in intracavernosal pressure as an erection develops.

waveform tend to occur within 20 min after the intracavernosal injection of a vasodilating agent and reflect the changes in intrapenile pressure during a normal erection. Dynamic evaluation of this waveform along with measurements of PSV, EDV, and diameter changes allows for the most accurate assessment of each patient for possible arteriogenic or venogenic impotence.

Arteriogenic Impotence

According to most investigators, PSV following the intracavernosal injection of a vasodilating agent appears to be the most promising parameter when evaluating patients for possible arteriogenic impotence. In a study of normal male volunteers, it was found that the normal average peak systolic velocity following intracavernosal injection of a vasodilating agent is approximately 30 to 40 cm/sec.[11] Lue et al. found that the majority of patients who have a moderate to good response to papaverine clinically have peak systolic velocities of 25 cm/sec or greater.[2] In addition, no patients in their study who had a poor response to papaverine injection had peak systolic velocities exceeding 25 cm/sec. Collins and Lewandowski found that patients who responded sonographically to papaverine had average peak systolic velocities of 26.8 cm/sec.[4] Early in our experience, we reported a series of 12 patients with suspected arteriogenic impotence who underwent pelvic arteriography.[9] All 5 patients with abnormal findings on arteriography in this early study also had peak systolic velocities of less than 25 cm/sec. Six of seven patients with normal arteriograms had peak systolic velocities in their cavernosal arteries of 25 cm/sec or greater. Thus, these early studies indicated that a peak systolic velocity of 25 cm/sec or less suggests inadequate arterial inflow to permit clinically moderate to good erections.

Benson and Vickers grouped impotent patients into three subgroups based on cavernosal artery peak systolic velocities.[10] The first subgroup was considered normal and found to have average peak systolic velocities of 47 cm/sec. The second group of patients were thought to have mild to moderate arterial insufficiency, with average peak systolic velocities of 35 cm/sec. A third group with severe arterial insufficiency was found to have average peak systolic velocities of 7 cm/sec. From these data, other authors have concluded that peak systolic velocity of 30 cm/sec could correctly distinguish patients with adequate arterial inflow from those with severe arterial disease.[8]

Our recent experience revealed that a dynamic study up to 20 min postinjection and a 30 cm/sec cutoff value yielded an 83% sensitivity for detection of bilateral, hemodynamically significant arterial stenoses when compared to conventional angiography.[16] Thus, velocity measurements alone may not detect all patients with arteriogenic impotence. This may be explained by the fact that arterial blood flow is not only a function of velocity in a particular vessel but also a function of the cross-sectional area of the lumen of the vessel. However, the initial size of the artery is probably not a good indicator of arterial disease, and the arterial compliance and ability to dilate may be more important. Therefore, a 75% increase in vessel diameter appears to be the best indicator of normal arterial compliance and vessel dilatation.[2] Assessment of cavernosal blood flow should include PSVs as well as the degree of arterial dilatation to provide the most sensitive means of detecting arteriogenic impotence.

From these studies, it seems logical to assume that PSVs in the cavernosal arteries of less than 25 cm/sec after administration of a vasodilating agent should suggest arterial inflow disease and should lead to a more definitive evaluation with selective internal pudendal arteriography if clinically warranted (Fig. 5–6). PSV values between 25 and 30 cm/sec and a 75% increase in vessel diameter should be considered borderline. PSV measurements greater than 30 cm/sec accompanied by a 75% increase in vessel diameter should be considered normal.

Several circumstances warrant special consideration. If there is a marked discrepancy between the velocities of the two cavernosal arteries (greater than 10 cm/sec difference), unilateral arterial disease of the penis may be present. Adequate blood flow through one cavernosal artery may be all that is needed for adequate erection. However, unilateral disease of the penis may be significant in certain individuals, and appropriate arteriography may need to be pursued.[17] Another exception occurs when the PSV is greatly elevated (i.e., over 100 cm/sec). This high velocity has been seen in patients with diffuse vascular spasm or small vessel disease (i.e., diabetes mellitus) or both. Such patients demonstrate little or no change in cavernosal arterial diameter measurements before and after injection of a vasodilating agent. Therefore, if normal or high velocities in the cavernosal arteries are detected, one should closely evaluate the caliber of the cavernosal arteries. If the caliber does not significantly increase following the vasodilating agent, the patient may have diffuse small vessel disease (i.e., diabetes) or diffuse vasospasm (nicotine abuse, medications), with artificially high velocities because of a small vessel lumen.

Recent evidence suggests that the sensitivity and accuracy of cavernosal artery duplex sonography may be increased by evaluation of additional parameters, such as systolic acceleration. Acceleration (PSV-EDV/pulse rise time) values less than 400 cm/sec² in the cavernosal arteries also may be an indicator of arteriogenic impotence.[18] Arteriolar dysfunction within the cavernosal tissue of the penis and sinusoidal dysfunction are potentially important factors in vasculogenic impotence.[19] It is clear that more work is needed in evaluation of the cavernosal artery Doppler waveform as it relates to arterial inflow disease to the penis.

The direction of blood flow in the cavernosal artery can be reversed. It has been shown that reversal of flow in diastole is a normal phenomenon in later stages of erection (Fig. 5–7). However, systolic flow reversal may indicate proximal penile artery occlusion with collateral flow in a retrograde fashion into the affected cavernosal artery.[17] Reversal of systolic flow in the cavernosal artery may warrant further evaluation with conventional angiography. Proximal penile artery occlusion can result from trauma, corporal fibrosis, or atherosclerotic vessel disease.

Collateral vessels from the contralateral cavernosal artery, dorsal penile artery, or spongiosal artery often can be seen with color Doppler sonography. These collateral vessels may be normal or

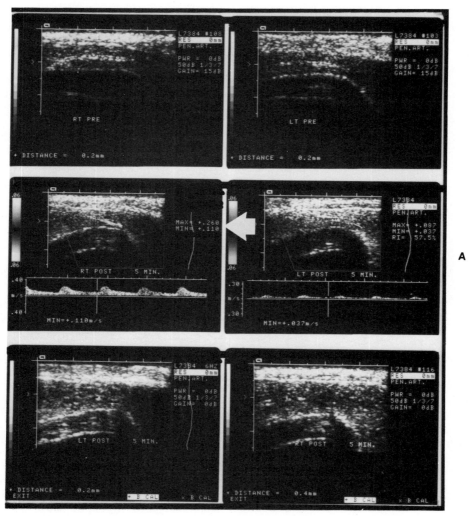

Figure 5–6. **A** and **B,** Abnormal duplex Doppler sonogram in a patient with arteriogenic impotence. The precavernosal artery measurements revealed the internal lumen diameter of the cavernosal arteries to measure 0.2 mm. Following injection of a vasodilating agent, there was suboptimal (less than 75%) arterial dilatation. In addition, suboptimal peak systolic velocities (less than 25 cm/sec) in both cavernosal arteries were noted throughout the examination. Note that peak systolic velocities are listed in the right upper corner of each image (MAX) *(arrow)*. End diastolic velocities are listed as MIN.

Continued on following page

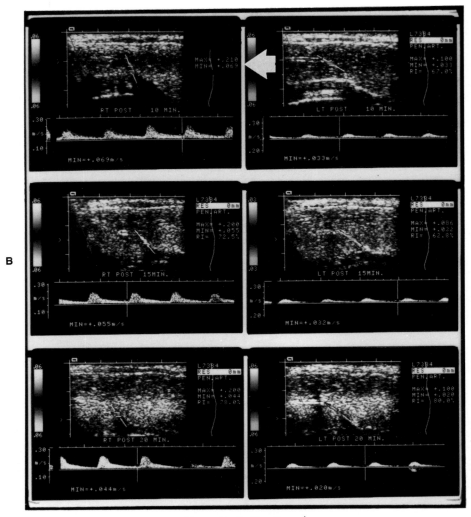

Figure 5–6. *Continued*

may indicate proximal disease in the affected artery.

Particular attention should be given to the presence of arterial sinusoidal fistulas or arterial venous fistulas within the corporal tissue of the penis in patients who have developed erectile dysfunction following trauma. These lesions often are very amenable to surgical repair. Partial priapism can be an accompanying sign in arterial sinusoidal fistulas, and color Doppler evaluation often can locate the fistula in question (Fig. 5–8).[20]

Venogenic Impotence

Venogenic impotence may be due to poor venoocclusion of the corporal bodies. Although the exact cause of venous leakage is unknown, it may be secondary to stretching or thinning of the thick tunica albuginea. Inadequate compression of the

emissary veins draining the sinusoids between the expanding corpora cavernosa tissue and the tunica albuginea during tumescence and rigidity is the paramount reason for venous leak. When these emissary veins are not adequately compressed, venous outflow from the cavernosa continues to occur. Tumescence may be achieved, but rigidity is never accomplished.

Traditionally, venogenic impotence has been evaluated with cavernosometry and cavernosography. However, these examinations are invasive and not optimal for screening purposes. Therefore, many have advocated duplex sonography as a screening examination for venogenic impotence.

During the duplex Doppler examination of the cavernosal arteries in the normal patient, there is an initial increase in diastolic and systolic velocities immediately after intracavernosal injection of vasodilating agents. This corresponds to the physiologic dilatation of the cavernosal artery, helicine arteries, and sinusoidal spaces. As the sinusoidal spaces are dilating and filling, resistance in the cavernosal artery is low, and forward diastolic flow is prominent (Fig. 5–7). However, when the venoocclusive mechanism engages, the sinusoids become maximally distended and intracavernosal pressure dramatically increases. At this point, vascular resistance increases and diastolic flow ceases or even reverses. If a patient's venoocclusive mechanism is not intact, excessive venous leakage will persist, and intracavernosal pressure will remain low. The Doppler spectral waveform in this instance will continue to exhibit the prominent for-

ward diastolic flow of a low-resistance vascular bed throughout the examination. Therefore, patients who continue to have high EDVs (over 3 cm/sec) throughout the examination (up to 15–20 min) despite normal arterial inflow (peak systolic velocities of 30 cm/sec or greater) may have venogenic impotence (Fig. 5–9). Cavernosometry and cavernosography should be considered in these patients. Patients who demonstrate reversal of diastolic flow in both cavernosal arteries should have an intact venoocclusive mechanism and should not have venogenic impotence.[16]

The majority of venous efflux from the corpora cavernosa occurs via the deep dorsal vein. Some

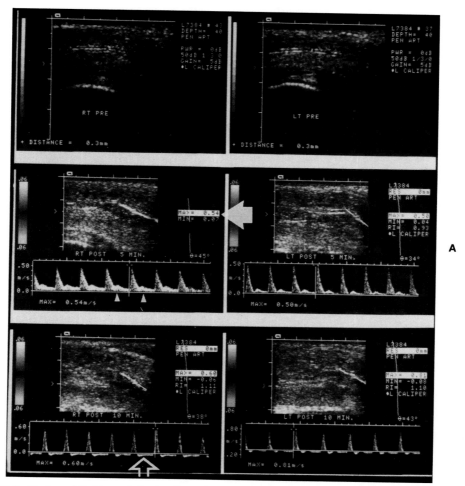

Figure 5–7. **A** and **B,** Normal duplex Doppler sonogram of the cavernosal arteries. Note that there is normal arterial dilatation (greater than 75% increase in artery diameter) in the cavernosal arteries after injection of a vasodilating agent. (Peak systolic velocities are listed as MAX in the right upper corner of each image. End diastolic velocities are listed as MIN, *large arrow.*) Note the normal increase in forward diastolic flow at 5 min postinjection *(arrow heads).* Also note the normal reversal of diastolic flow at the 10, 15, and 20 min measurements *(open arrows).* This reversal of diastolic flow is normal and correlates well with the increasing intracavernosal pressure needed to initiate and maintain an erection.

Continued on following page

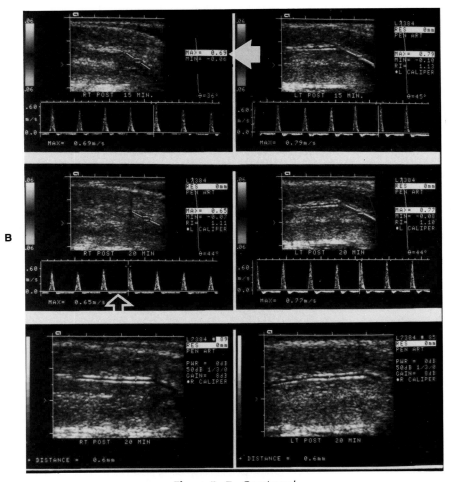

Figure 5-7. *Continued*

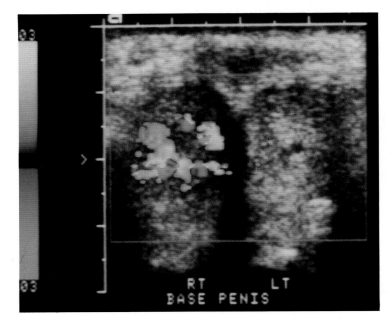

Figure 5-8. Transverse color Doppler sonogram of the right (RT) and left (LT) corpora cavernosa. Notice that within the right corpus cavernosum there is a large area of confluent color flow indicating an arterial cavernosal fistula that was confirmed at angiography and surgery.

Receiver Operator Characteristic Curve (ROC)
Correlating EDV With Cavernosometry For Detection of Venous Leak

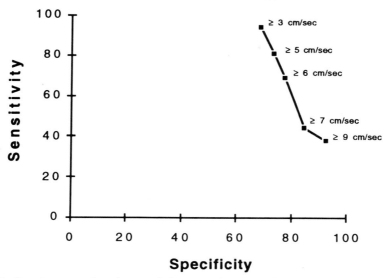

Figure 5–9. Receiver operator-characteristic curve demonstrating sensitivities and specificities of various end diastolic velocities (EDV) (obtained at 15–20 min postinjection) in the detection of venogenic impotence using cavernosometry as the gold standard. An EDV of >3 cm/sec at 15 to 20 min postinjection yields the best sensitivity with fair specificity in the detection of venogenic impotence.

investigators have recommended measurements of velocity in the deep dorsal penile vein as a means of detecting excessive venous leakage.[21] It appears that transient early dorsal vein flow is normal in many patients. However, persistent dorsal vein flow at 20 min postinjection may indicate excessive venous leakage, although our experience suggests that both normal patients and patients with excessive venous leakage may have high deep dorsal vein velocities up to 20 min postinjection.[22] In addition, some patients who have excessive venous leakage on cavernosometry and cavernosography may leak primarily via the crural veins near the base of the penis and not via the deep dorsal penile vein. These crural veins are not accessible to duplex sonographic evaluation. For these reasons, deep dorsal vein flow analysis does not appear to be a consistently reliable method for evaluation of a patient with possible venogenic impotence.

Pitfalls and Duplex Doppler Sonography for Impotence

Although intracavernosal injection of vasodilating agents is supposed to bypass the psychologic stimulus needed for an erection, excessive psychologic overlay may result in an impaired response to vasodilating agents. Suboptimal PSVs (less than 25 cm/sec) can occur as a result of excessive alpha-adrenergic tone in normal patients with excessive anxiety. Therefore, patients should be studied in an appropriate setting with the least amount of distractions.

Early investigators recommended that velocity measurements should be obtained at 5 to 10 min after injection. Recent studies have indicated that the response to intracavernosal vasodilating agents varies among individuals, and PSV in normal males can occur at any time from 5 to 30 min postinjection.[16,21] Therefore, to detect maximum velocities, the PSV should be measured at least at 5, 10, 15, and 20 min after injection and longer if necessary.

Because normal individuals may have high EDVs early in the examination (5–10 min after injection), abnormal EDV measurements should be assessed only at the later time periods (15–20 min). Persistent low resistant spectral waveforms at these later times in association with normal cavernosal artery PSVs should indicate persistent and excessive venous leakage as a possible cause of the patient's impotence. If measurements are only made at 5 or 10 min postinjection, a false interpretation of excessive venous leakage could be made. Therefore, high EDVs can indicate excessive venous leakage only when obtained at 15 to 20 min post-injection and if there is adequate arterial inflow (PSV >30 cm/sec).

Proper injection of the vasodilating agents is paramount in obtaining accurate results. If the vasodilating agent is injected into the corpus spongiosum, erection may not occur. In addition, the vasodilating agent may enter the urethra inadvertently and not have an effect on the cavernosa.

PELVIC ARTERIOGRAPHY

More invasive arteriographic evaluation is reserved for patients who are candidates for percutaneous balloon angioplasty or surgery. A history of severe pelvic trauma usually is present in young patients who have arterial disease as a major cause of their impotence. Older patients often report symptoms and signs of small vessel diseases, such as angina or claudication. Many of the patients with arteriogenic impotence have a history of tobacco use. In general, only patients who are candidates for surgery should undergo angiographic evaluation of impotence. We do not perform this surgery in patients over the age of 60. Before angiography at our institution, all patients undergo a screening evaluation with color duplex Doppler ultrasonography of the deep penile (cavernous) arteries.

Anatomy

The internal pudendal artery (IPA) is the major artery of erection, supplying also the perineum and external genitalia (Fig. 5-10). The IPA originates as a branch of the anterior division of the hypogastric (internal iliac) artery, where several variations can occur. According to Huguet et al., in 65% of cases, the IPA shares a common trunk with the inferior gluteal artery.[23] In 30% of cases, the IPA will be seen as the terminal anterior division branch of the hypogastric artery. In less than 5% of cases, the IPA will arise as an isolated branch of the hypogastric artery, and rarely, it will arise as a branch of either the obturator or hemorrhoidal artery. The IPA is normally about 3 mm in diameter.

Huguet et al. have suggested dividing the course of the internal pudendal artery into three distinct segments (Figs. 5-10B and 5-11).[23,24] Segment I begins with the origin of the IPA and ends where this vessel penetrates Alcock's (pudendal) canal. This segment includes what has also been referred to as the intrapelvic and gluteal sections of the IPA. Radiographically, segment I is seen from the origin of the IPA, usually from the inferior margin of the sacroiliac joint, to the inferior line of the superior pelvic ramus. This portion of the IPA gives off branches to the sacral plexus, muscle groups, urinary bladder, and occasionally the middle hemorrhoidal artery.

Segment II of the IPA lies within Alcock's canal. Radiographically, this portion of the IPA is seen to project within the obturator foramen on the ipsilateral anterior oblique view of the pelvis. This corresponds to the posterior perineal section of the IPA, where it gives off branches to the inferior hemorrhoidal artery and the superficial perineal artery. The superficial perineal artery is a constant branch of the IPA and, hence, can be used as a landmark (Fig. 5-11B). There are three types of origin of the superficial perineal artery depending on its relationship to the superior line of the inferior pubic ramus.[23] In general, type I branching indicates that the superficial perineal artery originates within the confines of the obturator foramen. This type is seen in 70% of cases. Type II originates below the obturator foramen, and type III originates above. Beyond the origin of the superficial perineal artery, the IPA is commonly referred to as the common penile artery.

Segment III of the IPA corresponds to the anterior perineal section passing through the urogenital diaphragm. Angiographically, in the anterior oblique view of the pelvis, this segment of the IPA is seen beginning at the anterior-inferior margin of the obturator foramen just before the artery projects under the ischiopubic ramus and ends with the origin of the cavernosal (deep) artery of the penis. This segment of the artery gives rise to the artery to the bulb of the penis, the urethral branch, and finally the dorsal and cavernosal branches.

The branches of the common penile artery must be opacified and identified during angiographic evaluation of impotence. The single best projection for evaluation of the common penile artery branches is the ipsilateral anterior oblique projection, usually from 25 to 45 degrees off axis, with the penis stretched out on the medial surface of the opposite thigh. Bookstein has suggested 23 degrees of caudal angulation of the x-ray tube to help prevent vessel overlap (personal communication). With this projection, all the common penile artery branches can be easily accounted for.

The first significant penile branch artery, the artery to the bulb, arises from the common penile artery, where it is projected over the ischiopubic ramus. This branch passes just slightly cephalad, then courses inferior to the common penile artery. A dense contrast blush of the bulb of the urethra usually makes this artery very easy to distinguish. The next branch, not often visualized, is the urethral artery, a small-caliber branch projected along

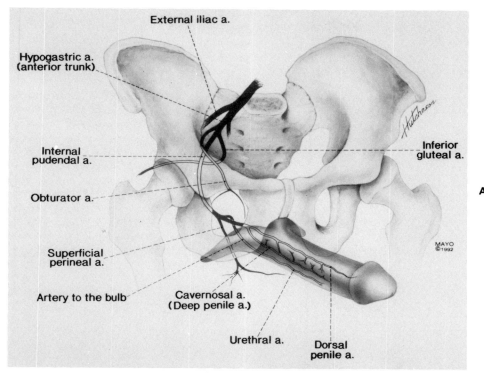

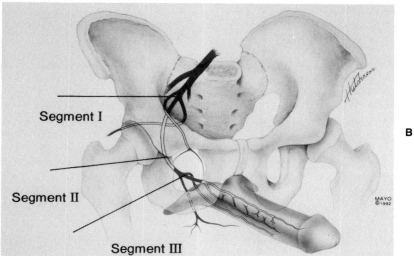

Figure 5–10. A, Diagrammatic representation of the arterial blood flow to the penis projected over the bony landmarks. These can be visualized best if the patient is placed in the appropriate oblique position with the penis in the semierect state (due to the intracavernous vasoactive agent), draped over the contralateral thigh, opposite the artery that has been injected. The internal pudendal artery usually supplies the cavernosal tissue with one of its terminal branches, the cavernosal artery. Other landmark vessels are identified on the diagram. **B,** Three segments of internal pudendal artery. Segment I, from origin to where artery enters Alcock's (pudendal) canal. Segment II lies within Alcock's canal. Segment III begins with the origin of the artery to the bulb of penis until the cavernosal artery branches off. (Mayo Foundation, used with permission.)

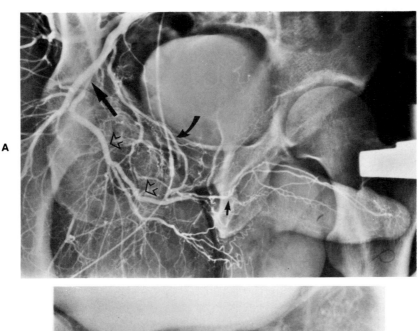

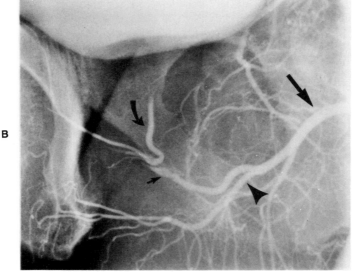

Figure 5–11. A, Right internal pudendal artery (IPA) in ipsilateral anterior oblique projection. Catheter-induced spasm is seen in the proximal aspect of the segment I portion of the IPA *(large arrow). Open arrowheads* denote segment II of the IPA in Alcock's canal. Segment III of the IPA ends at the origin of the cavernosal artery *(small arrow)*. Note accessory IPA *(curved arrow).* **B,** Left internal pudendal artery (IPA) *(large arrow)* in the anterior oblique projection with 23 degree caudal tube angulation. Type I branching of superficial perineal artery *(arrowhead)*. Artery to the bulb *(small arrow)*. Retrograde filling of an accessory IPA *(curved arrow)*. Note how this projection avoids vessel overlap at the base of the penis.

the lower surface of the penis. The urethral artery can arise as a branch of the artery to the bulb or from one of the penile arteries. The continuing common penile artery then divides into the deep penile or cavernosal artery and the dorsal artery of the penis.

The most important artery to visualize in angiography for impotence is the deep penile artery or the cavernosal artery. Very rarely, this artery may be bifid in one cavernous space. It is not uncommon for both cavernous arteries to arise from one of the common penile arteries. It is necessary to use intracavernous pharmacologic agents to visualize the cavernosal arteries, since this system is such a high-resistance system due to sinus smooth muscle contraction. If these arteries are normal and

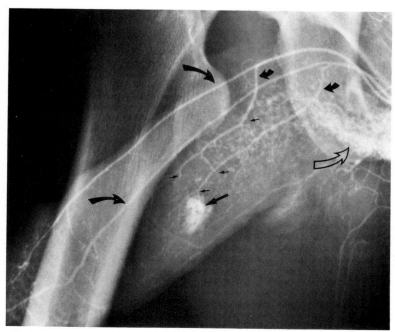

Figure 5–12. Intrapenile vascular anatomy. Dorsal arteries *(large curved arrows)* give rise to the distal cavernosal arteries *(small curved arrows)*. Note helicine branches *(small straight arrows)* and contrast staining of the cavernosal tissue *(curved open arrow)*. The dense blush in the cavernosal tissue *(large straight arrow)* at the vasodilator injection site is normally seen only in patients with adequate arterial inflow.

intracavernous pressure has been decreased with intracavernous agents, multiple helicine branches can be seen with contrast staining of the corpus cavernosum in the later films (Fig. 5–12). The deep penile artery is usually 0.5 mm in diameter.

Depending on the rotation and orientation of the penis as it is projected over the downward contralateral inner thigh, the dorsal artery may be projected either superiorly or inferiorly to the cavernous artery as it courses along the penile shaft. It is usually more superior in position and larger, 0.5 to 0.8 mm in diameter. Near the glans, it is not uncommon for the dorsal artery to anastomose in a circular fashion with the opposite artery. As a normal variation, there can be multiple branches from the dorsal artery to the cavernous tissue along the shaft of the penis (Fig. 5–12).

Not uncommonly, an accessory internal pudendal artery arises from the anterior division of the internal iliac (hypogastric) artery, a remnant of the umbilical, ischial, or obturator artery (Fig. 5–13).[23,25,26] On internal pudendal arteriograms performed in patients with varicoceles who were not impotent, Curet et al. found an accessory internal pudendal artery in 3 of 9 cases.[27] Rosen et al. found an accessory pudendal artery in 13 of 195 men undergoing angiographic evaluation of impotence.[28] The accessory pudendal artery is more

common on the right. It usually takes its origin as either a terminal branch of the anterior division of the hypogastric artery or as a very early branch of the main IPA. The accessory pudendal artery projects above the obturator foramen and has a more superior and medial course toward the penis. It most often gives origin to the dorsal and cavernosal arteries but sometimes also the bulbous branch and, occasionally, only to the dorsal artery. An accessory branch should be searched for if the main IPA gives rise only to the superficial perineal and bulbar branch arteries.

It is not uncommon for both deep and both dorsal arteries to arise from one pudendal artery (Fig. 5–14). In addition, anastomotic bridges between IPAs or bulbar arteries can be appreciated at the base of the penis near the crura of the erectile bodies in the infrapubic region. Variations and collateral branches are numerous, and the reader is referred to other detailed publications discussing these.[23–25,28,29]

Angiographic Technique

Many angiographic techniques have been advocated over the years for evaluating the impotent patient. We review several of these as a historical perspective to what is properly called

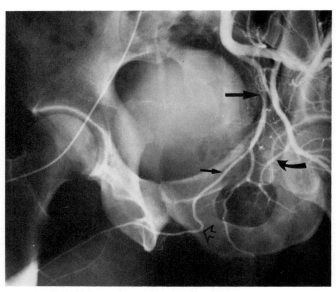

Figure 5–13. Left hypogastric artery injection. An accessory internal pudendal artery (IPA) *small arrow)* arising from the obturator *(large arrow).* Note characteristic vertical descent to base of penis with continuation as common penile artery *(open arrowhead).* The IPA shows slow filling *(curved arrow).*

the pharmacoangiographic evaluation of impotence.

Pelvic arteriography performed for the diagnosis of arteriogenic impotence should include a nonselective pelvic angiogram with a catheter in the aorta above the bifurcation as well as bilateral selective pudendal arteriography (Fig. 5–15). The aortic flush study may demonstrate abnormalities of large vessel that may be amenable to balloon dilatation or definitive pelvic vascular surgery (Fig. 5–16).[30,31] These narrow segments amenable to balloon dilatation or definitive pelvic vascular surgery usually involve the distal aorta and common iliacs or the origins of the internal iliacs or hypogastric arteries. The inferior epigastric arteries, branches of the external iliac arteries that are most often used as donor vessels for revascularization, also are visualized with aortography, particularly in the late phases of the injection (Fig. 5–15).

Ginestie and Romieu were the first to describe in detail techniques of selective internal pudendal arteriography in evaluation of the impotent patient.[25] Many of their original technical recommendations have not changed, and they include (1) a transfemoral percutaneous approach, (2) an anterior oblique view for ipsilateral artery study, (3) an indwelling urethral catheter to aid in distinguishing small penile vessels from scrotal and other small pelvic vessels, (4) the use of low-viscosity contrast warmed to body temperature, (5) slow injection of contrast (3 ml/sec) to aid in preventing arterial spasm, and (6) films taken every second from 10 to 20 sec after injection. They suggested unilateral puncture of the axillary artery or, preferably, bilateral puncture of the femoral artery for

study of the pelvic arteries in the impotent patient. Others prefer the axillary approach, although this is required only if there is occlusive disease of both iliac vessels.[27] However, with the development of specialized angiographic catheters, unilateral femoral puncture allowed for visualization of arteries supplying both sides of the penis.[32,33] Originally, Ginestie and Romieu suggested placing a sack of flour on the penis and dependent contralateral thigh to equalize densities for better imaging of the penile arteries. This was continued to be recommended by others up to 1986 with a description of the use of 2 kg of flour in a sterile plastic bag to act as a photon absorber and to allow for better visualization of the small penile arteries.[33,34] Today, selection of the proper radiographic technique and collimation will give the same result. In 1978, Michal and Pospichal described better visualization of the penile arteries when arteriography was performed at the time of simultaneous infusion of the corpora cavernosa with heparinized saline.[35] With these techniques, selective pudendal arteriography was shown to visualize the terminal branches of the internal pudendal/common penile artery, including the artery to the bulb, the urethral artery, the dorsal penile artery, and the deep cavernous or central penile artery.

Although Ginestie and Romieu had suggested a preheated, hydrosoluble, low-viscosity contrast material injected at 3 ml/sec, with 60 ml used for each internal pudendal artery study, others later suggested 30 to 50 ml of contrast injected at 2 to 4 ml/sec.[24,25,32–35] Low-osmolar or nonionic high-concentration contrast agents have been used for superselective studies in a volume of 30 to 60 ml injected at a rate of 3 to 6 ml/sec.[26,29]

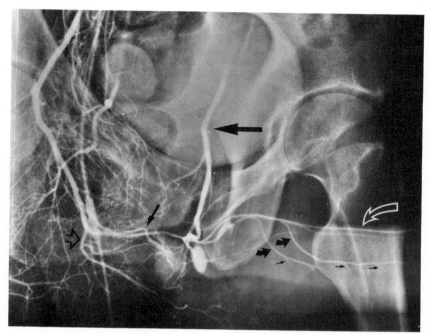

Figure 5–14. Right internal pudendal (IPA) injection. Type II superficial perineal artery *(open arrowhead).* Artery to the bulb *(straight arrow)* with contrast staining. Retrograde filling of opposite IPA *(large arrow)* via cross-filling at base of penis. Note how both dorsal *(white curved arrow)* and cavernosal arteries *(small curved arrows)* fill from the right IPA injection. Helicine branches *(tiny arrows).*

Film sequence was described originally by Ginestie and Romieu to begin at 10 sec of injection and consist of one film per second for 20 sec.[25] Other studies began at the end of injection and were comprised of either one film per second for 20 sec,[33] one film per second from 8 to 22 sec or 30 sec after starting the injection,[32,36] or one film every 2 sec beginning with the injection and lasting for 25 films.[24] Brühlmann et al. suggest 15 films in the following sequence: one film per second for 5 sec, one film every 2 sec for 10 sec, and one film every 3 sec for 15 sec.[26] Bookstein and Lang suggest filming at two films per second for 3 sec, one film per second for 6 sec, and one additional film after another 3 sec.[29]

Michal and Pospichal were the first to suggest using 1 mg of acetylcholine in 20 ml of saline as a vasodilator before injecting contrast.[35] When combined with infusion of the corpora with heparinized saline at 30 ml/min, the technique was called phalloarteriography, and it greatly enhanced visualization of the penile arteries. Curet et al. have suggested that hyperosmolar contrast media has a vasodilatory effect.[27] Bookstein et al. have suggested pharmacoarteriography using nitroglycerin (Nitrobid) 300 mg diluted in 10 ml of isotonic saline, infused in 2-ml bursts over a period of 30 secs, 1 min before arteriography, alone or with 30

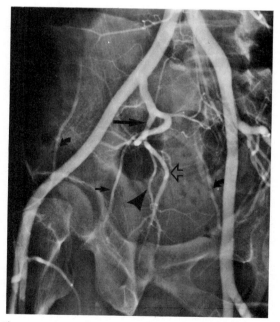

Figure 5–15. Pelvic flush aortogram in right posterior oblique projection. Anterior division of hypogastric artery *(large arrow).* Internal pudendal artery *(arrowhead).* Inferior gluteal artery *(open arrowhead).* Obturator artery *(small arrow).* Inferior epigastric arteries *(curved arrows).*

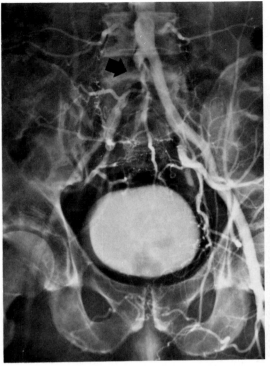

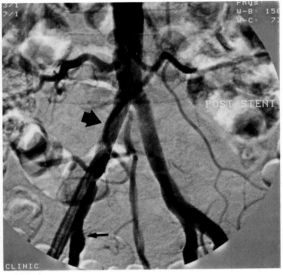

Figure 5–16. A, A 48-year-old man with long smoking history who has three block right buttock claudication and difficulty sustaining an erection during sexual intercourse. Low pelvic flush aortogram shows a right common iliac occlusion *(large arrow)* with delayed filling of the iliac system. **B,** Digital subtraction angiogram after common iliac stent placement. Note the intravascular stent in place and smooth and the normal caliber of the common iliac artery *(large arrow)*. Normal blood flow is seen in the internal iliac artery *(small arrow)*. Following treatment, the patient's claudication and impotence disappeared.

to 50 mg of papaverine.[37] They stated that tolazoline 20 mg, acetylcholine 240 mg over 3 min, and phentolamine 1 mg were less effective dilating agents. In a later publication, Bookstein and Lang advocated using 150 to 200 μg of nitroglycerin mixed with 30 mg of papaverine (diluted in 10 ml of isotonic saline), infused over 30 sec, 1 min before arteriography.[29] St. Louis et al. used 15 mg of papaverine diluted in 10 ml of saline intraarterially immediately before injection of the contrast media.[34] Kunnen et al. saw no advantage using intraarterial papaverine (40 mg).[38]

Intracavernous injection of smooth muscle relaxants, papaverine in particular (40–60 mg), before selective internal pudendal arteriography was described as early as 1986 and was found necessary to visualize the deep (cavernous) penile artery.[29,36,38–40] Gall et al. suggested using intracavernous papaverine (15 mg) and phentolamine (0.5 mg).[41] Bookstein and Lang suggest that this can be an effective alternative to their recommendation of intraarterial injection of vasodilators.[29] Schwartz et al. suggested that with the use of intracavernous

papaverine, nonselective angiography alone is adequate to demonstrate the penile arterial blood supply.[42]

Magnification views were first suggested by Ginestie and Romieu in 1978 and subsequently have been recommended by others.[25,29,34,37,40,43] The necessity for magnification varies with the degree of opacification of the penile arteries and the resolution of the imaging system. Digital subtraction angiography has been reported to produce excellent imaging of the penile arteries with either intraarterial or intravenous injection of the contrast agents, particularly when intracavernous papaverine has been used before contrast.[34,43–45]

Originally, general or epidural anesthesia was thought to be necessary because of the intolerable pain associated with the bolus of contrast, which could cause a reflex contraction of the penile arteries or patient movement during the study.[24,25,32] Mueller and Lue suggested that spinal anesthesia was preferable because blockage of the sympathetic influences would cause relaxation of the cavernous smooth muscle tissue.[39] Later, combination neuroleptic-induced anesthesia or a combination of local anesthesia and intravenous morphine or a sedative, such as diazepam, was described as adequate.[27,28,34,46] St. Louis et al. suggested adding lidocaine (Xylocaine) to the contrast agent in a ratio of 200 mg/100 ml as an analgesic agent.[34]

Our angiographic evaluation of the impotent patient has evolved over the years as experience with the technique has increased. All patients receive IV anesthesia using a combination of fentanyl citrate and madazolam (Versed, Roche Laboratories, Nutley, NJ) to achieve a suitable level of relaxation. Following administration of local and IV anesthesia, a 6-0 French angiographic sheath is introduced into the right common femoral artery. The sheath allows for easy catheter exchange when needed. A 65 cm 5-0 French pigtail catheter is placed in the low abdominal aorta, and bilateral oblique flush pelvic arteriograms are obtained with filming at one per second using either cut film or digital techniques. The patient is centered to include both the aortic bifurcation and the ischial tuberosities. Hexabrix (ioxaglate meglumine 39.3% and ioxaglate sodium 19.6%) (Mallinckrodt Medical Inc., St. Louis, MO) is the contrast of choice with injection rates of 30 ml at 12 ml/sec.

After the pelvic flush angiograms have been performed, we administer 0.25 ml of a mixture of papaverine (4.4 mg), phentolamine (0.15 mg), and PGE_1 (1.5 μg) intracavernosally using a 25-gauge needle.

Using the pigtail catheter with the tip uncoiled and draped over the iliac bifurcation, a guidewire is negotiated into the opposite external iliac artery. A Terumo wire (Meditech Corporation, Watertown, MA) works very well for this purpose. We employ a 5.2F reverse curve Bookstein shape catheter (Cordis Corporation, Miami, FL) for selective study of the internal pudendal artery.[29] This catheter comes with arm lengths of 10, 15, or 20 cm and is reformed easily by advancing it over the wire into the opposite iliac artery. When the knee of the catheter reaches the iliac bifurcation, the wire is withdrawn to that point. With a twist and advancement, the catheter will configure into its preformed shape and, with some practice, allow for easy selection of the IPAs on both sides. If the IPAs cannot be engaged easily, proximal stenosis should be suspected and the anterior division injected instead. We prefer using the IPA because it allows for better opacification of the penile branches. Spasm, however, is common with superselective catheter placement, and care should be taken not to advance the tip too far into the IPA. We normally inject 100 mg of coronary nitroglycerine into the IPA before contrast injection. This seems to decrease the amount of spasm. Excellent opacification of the IPA and its branches will occur with injection of

24 ml of Hexabrix at 4 ml/sec. For smaller vessels, 21 ml at 3 ml/sec works fine. A gentle test injection under fluoroscopy will help determine the needed amount. We use contact cut film technique in the ipsilateral anterior oblique projection. Magnification films are no longer used routinely due to the smaller field of view. Care is taken to position the penis properly so that it is as stretched out as possible on the contralateral thigh. Filming of the selective pudendal artery study is usually performed in the ipsilateral anterior oblique projection at a slant 25 to 45 degrees off axis. A caudal tube angulation of 23 degrees helps to avoid vessel overlap at the base of the penis. Careful attention to penile positioning can avoid problems during later film interpretation. An indwelling Foley catheter has not proven necessary. Patients are centered so that the field of view will include the penile tip in the lower right corner. This is important to enable distinguishing the deep from the dorsal artery in some patients. In most patients, this positioning also will include visualization of the IPA. We use a film series of two per second for 3 sec, one per second for 6 sec, and one per 3 sec for 9 sec for a total of 15 films.

Films are evaluated carefully during the course of the examination to ensure proper demonstration of the intrapenile branches. If a normal appearing IPA ends either in a superficial perineal or bulbar branch, a less selective injection of the anterior division is performed to avoid missing an accessory pudendal artery. Also, in the presence of arterial occlusive disease (whether on the basis of arteriosclerosis or previous trauma) selective injection of other anterior division branches can turn up collateral supply to the penile arteries. Alternatively, less selective angiography is helpful, but vessel overlap can lead to some confusion during film interpretation.

When all of the films have been reviewed and the examination has been determined to be of good quality, the catheter is removed, hemostasis is achieved, and the patient is taken to the postanesthesia room for 30 to 45 min of observation. Our patients routinely are studied as outpatients and go home if there are no complications after 6 h of careful postcatheterization observation.

In summary, almost all modern techniques of angiography have been applied to improve visualization of the penile arteries in the impotent patient being investigated for arteriogenic impotence. Intracavernous smooth muscle relaxants have particularly improved visualization of the deep penile arteries. This relaxation of the corpora tissue allows for a more rapid infusion of small amounts of contrast. Bookstein et al. have suggested that if normal penile arterial architecture is seen on the first selective study, the opposite side need not be investigated.[37] Until angiographic data are evaluated in the same patient in correlation with functional arterial studies, such as the duplex Doppler evaluation of the central penile arteries, we prefer bilateral selective arteriography in the angiographic study of the impotent patient.

The Abnormal Pelvic Arteriogram

In the landmark publication of Ginestie and Romieu, 25% of 250 patients were found to have arterial stenosis, occlusions, or, more rarely, dysplasia.[25] Michal and Pospichal, in their description of phalloarteriography, suggested that the overwhelming majority of patients with impotence have abnormal pelvic arteries.[35] Historically, others have reported significant obstructive disease in 23% to 92% of their patients.[26,36,41-43,45] Struyven et al. suggested dividing abnormal vessels seen on internal pudendal arteriography into three categories: obstructive, traumatic, or dysplastic.[33] Huguet et al. suggested that atheromatous lesions usually affect the ischiorectal segment of the internal pudendal artery in patients 50 to 60 years of age.[23] They also described localized compressive lesions of the third arterial segment (the perineal) affecting patients between the ages of 50 and 55 years, which other authors had classified as dysplasias. They found that these occur in the region where the pudendal artery crosses the urogenital diaphragm, and they refer to this disorder as "perineal outlet syndrome."[24]

Brühlman et al. have suggested that vascular abnormalities in impotent patients almost always indicate obstructive changes in the common or deep penile arteries, with disease of the IPA as well, in about one fourth of these patients.[26] Gray et al. classified abnormalities in arteries with respect to the most proximal lesion in 57 selective arteriographic studies.[32] They found 4 normal studies (7%), 3 that showed iliac artery stenosis (5%), 18 that showed IPA disease (31%), and 32 that showed more distal small penile artery disease (56%). Schwartz et al. found arteriosclerosis at the base of the penis in 21 patients and in the ischiorectal segment or Alcock's canal in 11 patients on nonselective studies following cavernosal injections with papaverine in 32 of 36 abnormal angiograms.[42] Bilateral arterial disease is said to be present in 47% to 77% of studied patients.[26,32] Juhan et al., agreeing with the earlier opinions of Ginestie and Romieu, state that more proximal lesions are almost always bilateral.[24,25] Vascular abnormalities due to injury associated with pelvic trauma have been reported in 5% to 7% of arteriograms performed for impotence.[24,26,29] Zorgniotti et al. and other investigators have reported examples of ar-

teriovenous malformations associated with trauma.[47-51] These traumatic injuries to intracavernosal arteries can result in direct arterial communication with cavernosal tissues. Preliminary evaluation with color Doppler sonography is helpful to determine the site of injury and further direct angiographic investigation (Fig. 5-8). An arteriogram is important to confirm the diagnosis. Selective embolization of the feeding artery at the site of injury should be attempted before surgical intervention (Fig. 5-17).

Figures 5-18, 5-19, and 5-20 show various manifestations of the arteriogram in patients with arteriogenic impotence.

CAVERNOSOMETRY AND CAVERNOSOGRAPHY

Earlier publications have described cavernosography as useful for the evaluation of Peyronie's disease, penile trauma, priapism, and infilrative diseases of the penis.[52-58] In fact, in one of these reports, Datta described corpus cavernosography as not useful in the evaluation of impotence.[55] Veterinarians were the first to describe the usefulness of corpus cavernosography in the 1970s for evaluating impotence in the bull.[59-61] In a landmark series of three publications from 1974 to 1975, Fitzpatrick described first direct dorsal vein puncture and then corpus cavernosography to diagnose valvular incompetence of the dorsal vein and intercommunicating venous drainage.[62-64] In 1976, Ney et al. described a timed fixed contrast disappearance cavernosography study.[65] The contrast drained rapidly and completely by 75 min in the impotent patients compared to 90 min in the two normal men. In 1979, Ebbehøj and Wagner were the first to report a diagnostic dynamic cavernosography study, presenting four cases of abnormal drainage of the cavernous bodies that were successfully treated surgically.[66] Wagner subsequently showed that venoocclusion was a necessary part of erection in a xenon washout study performed during visual sex stimulation.[67] Two reports in 1981 and 1982 described cavernosography as a method of evaluating impotency.[68,69] However, both studies concentrated on the diagnosis of structural abnormalities within the cavernous tissue or the suspensory ligament. Virag described a group of patients as having venous incompetence based on initiation and maintenance infusion flow rates of more than 200 ml/min and 100 ml/min, respectively.[70]

Puyau and Lewis, aware of Virag and Wagner's studies, developed a dynamic cavernosography technique in 1981 that was reported in 1983 and 1984.[71,72] These investigators concentrated on initiation flow studies and simultaneous intracavernosal pressure measurements on infusion cavenosometry and cavernosography with a controlled volume of contrast, until both corpora filled completely or a total of 50 ml of 30% diatrizoate meglumine was injected at a rate of 2 ml/sec. On cavernosography, there was a significantly greater number of draining veins and incomplete filling of the corpora in those patients who did not obtain an erection even at the low flow rates. In a series of articles in 1984, Delcour and Wespes and associates from Brussels, Belgium, reported a similar infusion pump technique for cavernosometry, but they aptly stressed maintenance flow rates.[73-75] In 1985, Porst et al. reported very high flow rates in two patients with venous insufficiency.[76] In 1986, the Brussels group and Lue in San Francisco in-

troduced the use of papaverine intracavernosally as a more physiologic way to perform cavernosometry.[77-79] In 1987, Puyau et al. published a study showing differences between cavernosometry and cavernosography in the same patient on the same study before and after papaverine.[80] In 1987, Bookstein et al. further stressed the accuracy of and coined the phrase "pharmacocavernosography and pharmacocavernosometry" using 60 ml of papaverine and 1 mg of phentolamine.[81] Four earlier studies had advised that cavernosography should be performed after obtaining erection by infusion of saline, a much more complicated procedure requiring a much larger volume of fluid in those with a large venous leak.[82-85]

Other methods to diagnose a venoocclusive dis-

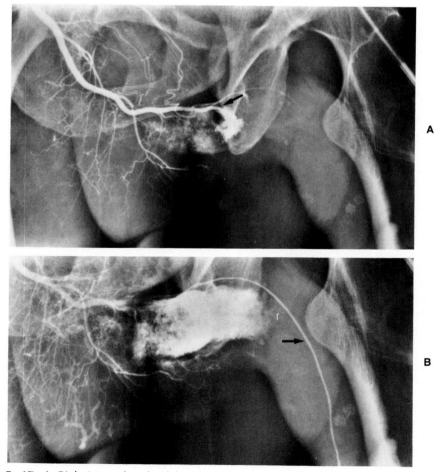

Figure 5–17. A, Right internal pudendal artery injection. Early film shows abrupt termination of the cavernosal artery *(arrow)* with immediate contrast filling of the cavernosal tissue. Intense cavernosal staining is due to a posttraumatic cavernosal artery–sinusoidal fistula. Large caliber of the cavernosal artery compared to the normal-sized dorsal artery results from the marked increase in blood flow. **B,** Late arterial phase film shows extensive cavernosal staining from arterial injury. Normal dorsal artery *(arrow).*

Continued on following page

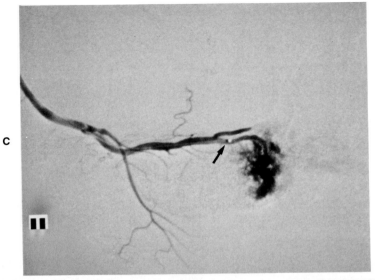

C

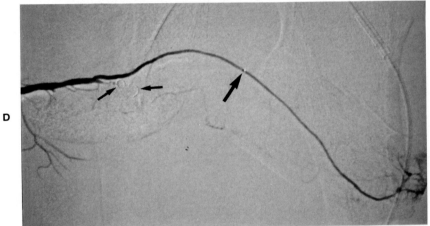

D

Figure 5–17, cont. C, Digital subtraction angiogram. Closeup view before embolization shows the catheter tip in the cavernosal artery *(arrow)*. **D,** Postembolization digital subtraction angiogram. Two 3 mm coils occlude the cavernosal artery *(small arrows)*. Note lack of cavernosal staining. Angiogram shows the catheter tip *(large arrow)* in the dorsal artery, which remains completely patent posttreatment.

order besides pump infusion initiation or maintenance flow rates (pump cavernosometry or pharmacocavernosometry) include the pressure/volume ratio (PVR) and pharmacologic maintenance erectile flow method of Bookstein,[81,86] outflow resistant measurement from the University of Washington group,[87,88] pressure decay measurements from the Boston University group's dynamic infusion cavernosometry and cavernosography (DICC),[89] and gravity cavernosometry from the San Paulo, Brazil, group.[90]

A comparison of various cavernosometric criteria for venogenic impotence and pharmacocavernosography was made in 60 patients at the Mayo Clinic to determine which test would be the most accurate to diagnose venogenic impotence. Cavernosometry was performed concurrently before and after injection of a pharmacologic agent. The pharmacologic agents used in the study were 60 mg of papaverine or a mixture of 45 mg of papaverine and 2.5 mg of phentolamine. After the postpharmacologic maintenance flow rate was determined, the pressure was brought to a steady state of 150 mm Hg, the infusion was stopped, and the rate of fall was measured over a 30-sec period (phase II of DICC). After obtaining the two maintenance flow rates (both before and after infusion of pharmacologic agents) and measuring the drop

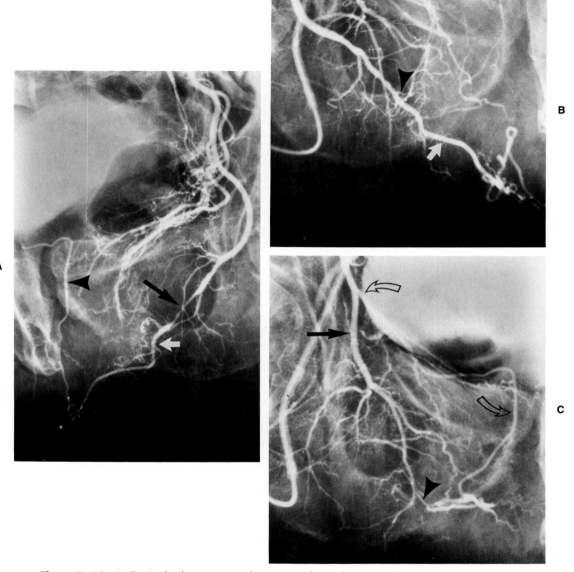

Figure 5–18. A, Typical atheromatous disease involving the internal pudendal artery in Alcock's canal *(large arrow)* with occlusion of common penile artery in a 54-year-old with arteriogenic impotence. Also shown are the superficial perineal artery *(white arrow)* and crossfilling of the contralateral accessory internal pudendal artery *(arrowhead)*. **B,** Same patient as in **A.** Right IPA injection shows moderate atheromatous disease in Alcock's canal plus occlusion of segment III *(arrowhead)*. Superficial perineal artery *(white arrow)*. **C,** Obturator artery *(large arrow)* injection in this same patient shows origin of the accessory internal pudendal artery *(curved arrows)*. Note how segment III of the IPA fills in a retrograde fashion back to the level of occlusion *(arrowhead)*.

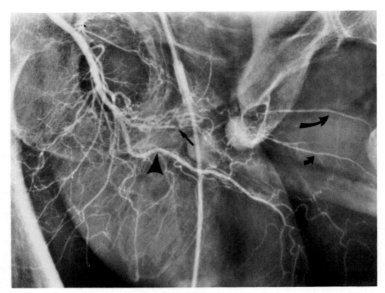

Figure 5–19. A 44-year-old man with a history of pelvic trauma. Right common penile artery occlusion *(small arrow)* with multiple collateral vessels at base of penis. Dorsal and cavernosal filling *(large and small curved arrows, respectively).* Superficial perineal artery *(arrowhead).*

in pressure from 150 mm Hg steady state, a cavernosographic film was obtained with diluted contrast injected in an attempt to obtain a pressure of at least 90 mm Hg at the time the film was taken. All 60 patients were being evaluated for impotence, and their average age was 52 years. Thirty-five of 60 patients (58%) showed a significant venous leak during the cavernosography phase of the study. The cavernosometry tests were considered positive for venous leak if the maintenance flow rate without pharmacologic agents was greater than 100 ml/min and the maintenance flow rate after pharmacologic agents was greater than 50 ml/min. Any pressure drop of over 50 mm Hg, that is, from 150 mm Hg to 100 mm Hg over the 30 sec, was considered positive for a venous leak. All of the patients showed a drop to more than 50 mm Hg after the steady state of 150 mm Hg had been reached, and the infusion was discontinued except for 1 patient in whom both maintenance cavernosometry and pharmacocavernosography did not indicate a venous leak. However, only 58% of the patients were found to have a significant venous leak by maintenance cavernosometry and pharmacocavernosography. Therefore, we believe that the second phase of DICC results in an overdiagnosis of venous leak.

In 1991, Mueleman et al. compared various diagnostic criteria using infusion pump and gravity cavernosometry in two groups of patients, those obtaining an erection after 50 mg of papaverine and those who did not obtain erection after injection on two occasions.[91] A sophisticated statistical analysis of the results shows that the two tests found to be most significant for diagnosis of venooclusive dysfunction were infusion pump maintenance flow rate and steady-state intracavernous pressure in millimeters of mercury by gravity cavernosometry.

Pump infusion maintenance flow rates in healthy or normal subjects were reported in four studies.[77,87,88,92] All subjects had maintenance flow rates less than 50 ml/min, and 45% of the 37 subjects had flow rates less than 14 ml/min.

Based on our data, the data in the literature, and the previous discussion, we have developed a technique of cavernosometry/pharmacocavernosometry/pharmacocavernosography that will collect data about the various best diagnostic tests for venooclusive dysfunction at Mayo Clinic (Table 5–2). We consider a maintenance flow rate of greater than 100 ml/min on cavernosometry as diagnostic of venooclusive dysfunction before a pharmacologic agent is given. We consider 75 to 100 ml/min a questionable area of evaluation on this cavernosometry study. After the pharmacologic agent is given, we consider a maintenance flow rate of greater than 50 ml/min diagnostic of venooclusive disorder and a flow rate of 30 to 50 ml/min in the borderline area. In patients who have had a flow less than 30 ml/min to maintain an erection after a pharmacologic agent, we have not seen significant venous runoff on pharmacocavernosography when injected at a rate to produce an intracavernosal pressure of 90 mm Hg. Therefore,

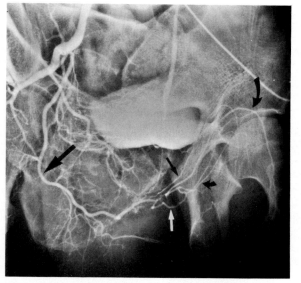

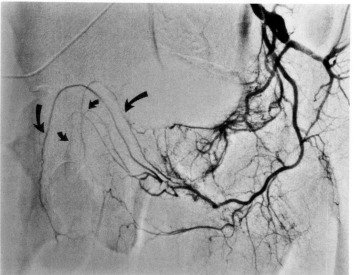

Figure 5–20. A 50-year-old man with a 5-year history of erectile dysfunction. **A,** Abrupt occlusion of the common penile artery. Left internal pudendal artery *(large straight arrow).* Well-developed collateral *(white arrow)* fills the right dorsal artery *(large curved arrow)* and both cavernosal arteries *(small curved arrow).* The left dorsal artery *(small straight arrow)* arises proximal to the occlusion. **B,** Subtraction film on same patient as in **A.** Note how this film technique reveals more details of the intrapenile vessels. Dorsal arteries *(large curved arrows).* Cavernosal arteries *(small curved arrows).*

we no longer obtain pharmacocavernosometry for such patients.

Radiologic Anatomic Orientation for Cavernosography

Veins draining the corpora cavernosa can be classified into three systems: superficial, interme-diate, and deep (Fig. 5–21). The superficial system primarily drains the skin of the penis, but it also can drain through communicators some of the deeper systems of the penis, including some vessels from the corpora cavernosa. The primary vein co-alescing to drain the system is the superficial dorsal penile vein, which drains into the external pudendal vein at the base of the penis. The external pudendal

TABLE 5−2
Technique of Cavernosometry/Pharmacocavernosometry/Pharmacocavernosography

Two 19-gauge needles placed into each corpus cavernosum (obliquely, toward patient's head), without anesthesia, laterally along shaft of penis under sterile conditions

One needle connected for pressure measurement via a transducer connected to a physiologic recorder or monitor

Other needle connected to an infusion roller pump for infusion of heparinized saline solution (1000 U/100 ml) prewarmed to body temperature

Record baseline pressure

Infuse fluid at 50 ml/min increments until full erection occurs (90−100 mm Hg), then decrease flow to obtain flow rate needed to maintain erection (do not infuse above 300 ml/min)

Inject pharmacologic agent (usually 45 mg of papaverine and 2.5 mg of phentolamine) through the needle

Record baseline pressure 10 min later

Obtain steady state intracavernous pressure using gravity flow

Repeat infusion pump flow study obtaining flow rate to maintain erection (do not infuse above 150 ml/min)

Inject 30% diatrozoate or iothalamate meglumine (60 ml full strength or 120 ml 50% dilution with saline at same rate as last maintenance flow rate and obtain cinefluoroscopic images, or spot static x-ray images (AP and oblique) for pharmacocavernosography

vein subsequently drains into the saphenous vein in a subcutaneous course. The saphenous vein drains into the femoral veins. Occasionally, the superficial system receives tributaries from the corpora cavernosa on the lateral surface of the base of the penis. In addition, the corpus spongiosum veins drain into the superficial system. Rarely, there may be small tributaries from the glans to the superficial dorsal vein. It is rare that abnormal drainage from the corpora cavernosa occurs only in the superficial system in patients with venoocclusive disorder. The main vessel draining the in-

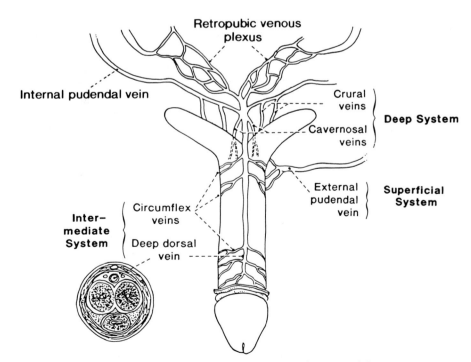

Figure 5−21. Diagrammatic representation of the venous drainage of the corpora cavernosal tissue. There can be communicators from the intermediate system to the superficial system at the distal end of the penis and near the base of the penis. The primary drainage is through the intermediate system, whose main trunk is the deep dorsal vein. The deep system is at the base of the penis and consists of crural and cavernosal veins.

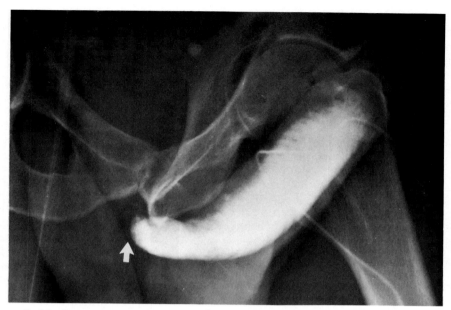

Figure 5–22. Cavernosogram in a normal patient who obtained a rigid erection with the infusion of contrast, at which time the intracavernosal pressure was 100 mm Hg. Notice that the contrast does not efflux from the contained space of the corpora cavernosa through any veins. There is poor filling of the contrast into the crural portion, beyond the white arrow, of the corpora cavernosa because of the complete venous occlusion obtained with the high pressure.

termediate system is the deep dorsal vein, which can consist of more than one trunk along the shaft of the penis, but these usually coalesce at the base of the penis in the infrapubic region as one single trunk. This deep dorsal vein drains into the preprostatic or retropubic venous plexus and occasionally into the internal pudendal veins. It receives drainage from the corpora cavernosa by the circumflex veins or from direct emissary veins of the dorsal midline on the shaft of the penis. Along its course on the dorsal surface and at its base in the infrapubic region, the deep dorsal vein also may receive contributories from superficial veins that will penetrate Buck's fascia. It is constituted initially by several trunks draining the glans approximately 1 cm from the glans sulcus. Two sets of veins make up the deep system, the crural veins and the cavernosal veins. The crural veins can drain directly into the retropubic venous plexus or, as is more usual, into the internal pudendal veins. They arise from the lateral and posterior surface of the corpora cavernosal bilaterally. The cavernosal veins are extensions of direct emissary veins from the medial portion of each of the corpora cavernosa before they diverge to attach to the ischial tuberosity. They can drain into an infrapubic plexus. The communicating drainage is a common drainage with the deep dorsal vein or into the internal pudendal veins. The retropubic venous plexus and the

internal pudendal veins eventually join and drain into the internal iliac veins.

Cavernosography in the Normal Male

Reports of cavernous venous drainage from pharmacocavernosography in potent patients is limited. Wespes et al. reported no significant venous leakage in 5 psychogenically impotent patients.[77] A similar report came from Bookstein.[86] Steif et al. reported only slight cavernosal venous drainage on cavernosography (in 4 patients) or pharmacocavernosography (in 8 patients) in patients with congenital penile deviation.[93] Lue et al. showed minimal (trace visualization of the cavernous deep dorsal vein) or no venous drainage at all in 11 patients who had a full rigid erection after 60 mg of papaverine.[79] Fuchs et al. had similar findings in 10 potent volunteers after 60 mg of papaverine, except in 1 patient, who showed significant venous opacification, but the photograph in this article shows that this study was performed with the penis in a flaccid state.[94] Vickers et al. did find runoff into cavernous veins (and also the external pudendal vein in 1 patient) in 3 of 6 patients with erectile dysfunction that subsequently spontaneously resolved.[92] (See Fig. 5–22 for an example of a cavernosogram in a subject without a venoocclusive disorder.)

Pharmacocavernosography in Patients with Venoocclusive Disorders

Courtheoux et al. classified venous drainage on cavernosography into three types: (1) by deep dorsal vein, (2) by the superficial network, and (3) a combination of both.[95] Hartnell et al. included six types by adding drainage into the deep crural veins if present in types 1–3 (now classified as 1a, 2a, 3a) as subtypes 1b, 2b, or 3b.[96] The breakdown of the site of venous leakage in patients with venoocclusive dysfunction has been reported in several publications[94,97,98] (Table 5–3).

See Figures 5–23 through 5–29 for examples of the various types of abnormal venous drainage that can be seen on corpus cavernosography or pharmacocavernosography in the patient with venoocclusive dysfunction. These are examples of drainage by the patterns described in Table 5–3.

In summary, carvernosography cannot be discussed without the accompanying cavernosometry data. The performance of cavernosometry after injection of a pharmacologic agent is certainly more physiologic, since the smooth muscles of the sinus spaces are relaxed by these agents. The method requires less infusion of saline, a very important consideration in patients in whom a fluid load is a limiting factor. However, two sets of maintenance flow rates have been verified consistently by cavernosography to be diagnostic for significant venous leakage. If a maintenance flow rate of greater than 100 ml/min is necessary to obtain an intracavernous pressure of 90 to 100 mm Hg in a patient in the performance of cavernosometry without pharmacologic agents, a significant venous leak can be diagnosed. If the infusion required is from 75 to 100 ml/min, the cavernosometry data should be correlated with the degree of venous leakage seen on cavernosography, the patient's clinical history, and the response to pharmacologic agent. The high maintenance flow rates and high volume of fluid probably overcome the smooth muscle resistance of the sinus spaces to produce conditions more like physiologic erection in those patients who have not had pharmacologic agents. If the maintenance flow rate is greater than 40 to 50 ml/min after pharmacologic agents in the cavernosometry study, a significant venous leakage is almost always seen on the pharmacocavernosography films.

There is no doubt that because of the low volumes of dilute contrast used, the cavernosography phase of the study should always be performed after the infusion of pharmacologic agents. Numerous studies have shown consistently that unless there has been sinus dilatation by the intracavernous

TABLE 5–3
Site of Venous Leakage in Venoocclusive Dysfunction

	Study 1[a] No. of Patients (%)	Study 2[b] No. of Patients (%)	Study 3[c] No. of Patients (%)
Site of Leakage			
Superficial system only	6 (6)	—	—
Intermediate system only	9 (9)	8 (18)	6 (17)
Deep system only	16 (17)	—	9 (25)
Cavernous veins only	15 (16)		
Crural veins only	1 (1)		
Superficial and intermediate systems	11 (12)	6 (13)	8 (22)
Intermediate and deep systems	23 (24)	14 (30)	9 (25)
Deep dorsal vein and cavernous veins	7 (7)	—	—
Deep dorsal vein, cavernosal veins, and glans/spongiosum	—	17 (37)	—
Deep system and spongiosum	—	—	2 (5.5)
All three systems	24 (25)	1 (2)	2 (5.5)
Total patients	96	46	36

[a] = Data from Aboseif SR, et al. Br J Urol 64:183, 1989.
[b] = Data from Shabsigh R, et al. J Urol 146:1260, 1991.
[c] = Data from Fuchs et al. J Urol 141:1353, 1989.
[d] = Leakage through deep dorsal vein and glans/spongiosum.

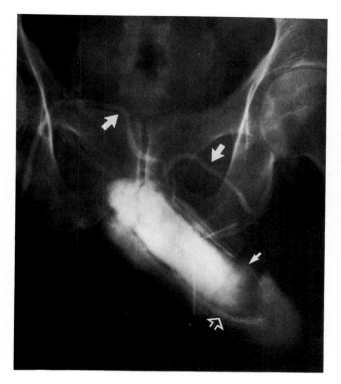

Figure 5–23. Drainage primarily through the superficial system on a cavernosogram in an impotent patient. Note that this patient's drainage is through both external pudendal veins *(large arrows)*. There is good demonstration of drainage from a glans vessel *(small arrow)* into the superficial system and drainage from the glans into spongiosal veins *(open arrow)* as well.

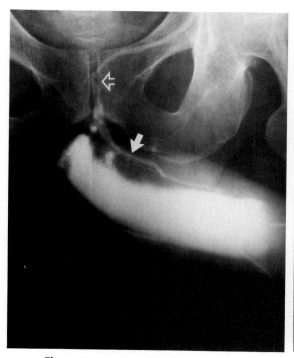

A

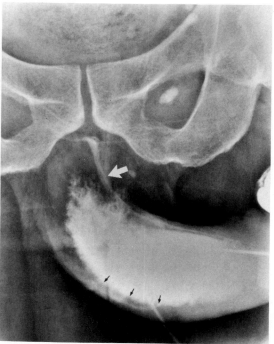

B

Figure 5–24. A and **B,** Cavernosograms performed at a flow rate necessary to produce an intracavernous pressure of 100 mm Hg in two patients that show drainage primarily through the intermediate system deep dorsal vein *(closed white arrows)* draining into the retropubic venous plexus *(open arrow)* in the infrapubic region. There seem to be communications also between the corpora cavernosum and the spongiosum in **B** *(small black arrows).*

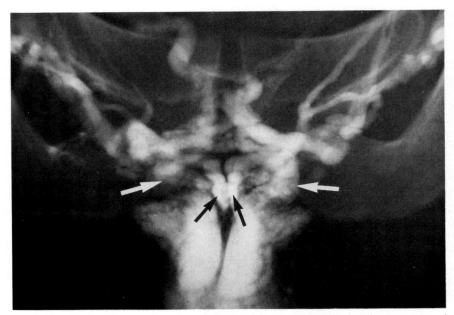

Figure 5–25. Cavernosogram showing drainage primarily through the deep system of the penis of a patient who has massive venous drainage into a complex retropubic plexus from both crural *(black arrows)* and cavernosal veins *(white arrows).*

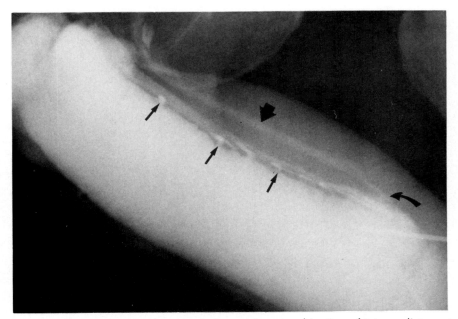

Figure 5–26. Cavernosogram showing drainage into a combination of intermediate system deep dorsal vein into which circumflex veins *(black arrows)* can be seen draining along the shaft of the penis and superficial penile vein *(large black arrow).* There is a direct communication between the superficial and the intermediate systems near the glans *(curved arrows).*

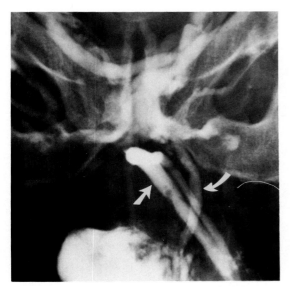

Figure 5–27. This cavernosogram shows drainage into a combination of the intermediate and deep systems at the base of the penis of a patient with moderate venous leakage. Drainage into a complex dorsal vein *(straight arrow)* and a large left cavernosal vein *(curved arrow)* into a complex retropubic plexus is shown.

agents, many effluxing veins will be seen on the cavernosography film. Cavernosography films should be taken at a time when the pressure in the intracavernous body is 90 to 100 mm Hg or a full rigid erection has been produced. This may be a valid criterion for a study in the normal male, but it often is not possible to attain these pressures in the patient with a venous leak. Sometimes in a patient with a severe venous leak, this pressure cannot be achieved with the infusion of 60 to 120 ml of contrast agent.

PENILE PROSTHESES

The treatment of impotence varies. However, a common treatment is placement of a penile prosthesis. Because impotence is a common problem and because these devices are becoming more and more popular, it is important that one understands pelvic radiographs of patients with mechanical malfunctions of their prostheses. Because of potential malfunction, it is important to be familiar with the appearance of normal, noninflatable and inflatable prostheses and to be able to recognize the radiographic appearance of the more common causes of malfunction in inflatable penile prostheses.

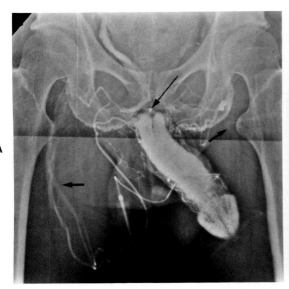
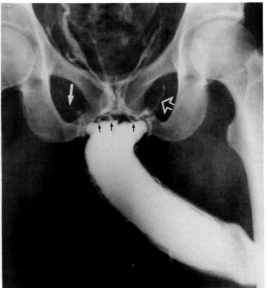

Figure 5–28. These cavernosograms show drainage into a combination of the superficial and deep systems. **A,** Drainage into the saphenous system bilaterally *(short black arrows)* and a cavernosal vein *(long black arrow)* from the right corpus cavernosum. **B,** Drainage through crural and cavernosal deep veins *(small black arrows)* into the retropubic venous plexus. There is also drainage from the superficial system at the base of the penis into the right external pudendal *(white arrows)*. Although there is a small vein seen draining the lateral aspect of the left crura, this, in fact, is a deep vein and drains into the internal pudendal vein *(open arrow)*.

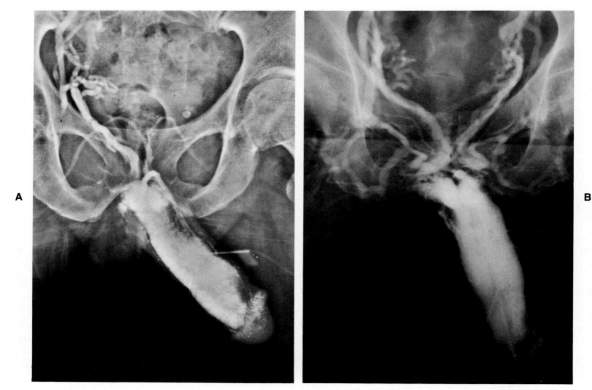

Figure 5–29. A and **B,** These cavernosograms show massive drainage in patients in whom intracavernosal pressure could not be increased to 100 mm Hg because of the severe venous runoff. Both patients show massive drainage from a combination of the superficial, intermediate, and deep systems into very complex retropubic and saphenous venous systems.

TABLE 5–4
Classification of Penile Prostheses

Noninflatable and Semirigid
Nonmalleable
    1. Small Carrion prostheses (Heyer-Schulte Corp., Minneapolis, MN)
    2. Finney-Flexirod I, II (Surgitek, Inc., Racine, WI)[a]
Malleable
    1. AMS600 (American Medical Systems, Minnetonka, MN)
    2. JONAS (Dacomed Corp., Minneapolis, MN)
    3. Mentor malleable (Mentor Corp., Goleta, CA)

Self-Contained Inflatable and Mechanical Prostheses
Inflatable
    1. Hydroflex and Dynaflex (American Medical Systems)
    2. Flexi-flate 1 and 2 (Surgitek, Inc.)[a]
Mechanical
    1. Omni or Duriphase (Dacomed Corp.)

Inflatable: Multicomponent
    1. AMS700 series and 700Cx, or? (American Medical Systems)
    2. Mentor IPP (Mentor Corp.)
    3. Uniflate[b] (Surgitek Inc.)[a]
    4. Mentor GFS[b] Mark II (Mentor Corp.)

[a]No longer marketed.
[b]These models have combined the pump and reservoir into one unit and, therefore, have fewer components.

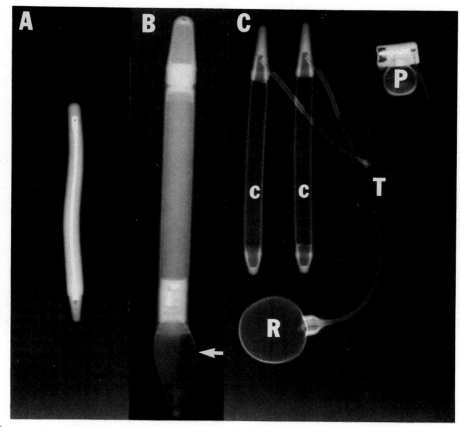

Figure 5–30. Plain radiograph of the three basic types of penile prostheses. **A,** Plain radiograph of a single semirigid malleable penile prosthesis cylinder (AMS600, American Medical Systems, Minnetonka, MN). **B,** Plain radiograph of a self-contained, inflatable penile prosthesis cylinder (Dynaflex, American Medical Systems). The self-contained pump *(arrow)* is near the tip of the prosthesis. **C,** Plain radiograph of a multicomponent inflatable penile prosthesis (AMS700 Series, American Medical Systems). The pump (P), reservoir (R), tubing (T), and cylinders (C) are all filled with radioopaque contrast solutions at the time of surgery. (Mayo Foundation, used with permission.)

Classification

There are three major types of penile prostheses (Table 5–4) (Fig. 5–30). The first penile prostheses introduced consisted of a single semirigid acrylic or silicone rod placed into the penis. These were quickly followed by paired intracavernosal devices.[99-101] Subsequently, paired malleable rods were developed for placement into each corpus cavernosum. Then, hydraulic prostheses were developed. The hydraulic penile prostheses (IPP) either can be self-contained in one single unit or can be made up of many components. Finally, nonhydraulic self-contained devices have been developed that consist of a number of plastic segments connected by a spring-action cable. All three types of penile prostheses are in use.

Radiographic Manifestations of Malfunctioning Penile Prostheses

Mechanical malfunctions of penile prostheses occur most commonly with IPPs. However, noninflatable, semirigid and malleable prostheses can develop mechanical complications. Rarely, patients may experience complete breaks through the semirigid silicone prostheses. Reports of erosion of a semirigid or malleable prostheses through the skin or end of the urethra have been noted. This later complication is usually obvious on physical examination. In addition, small breaks or fraying of the braided silver wire core in some malleable prostheses have been found. Despite the excellent radiopacity of the silver core, many of the breaks or small areas of

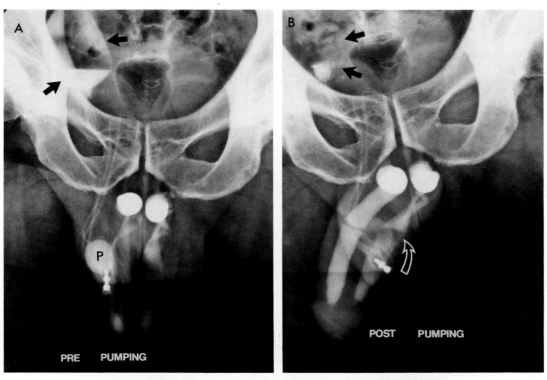

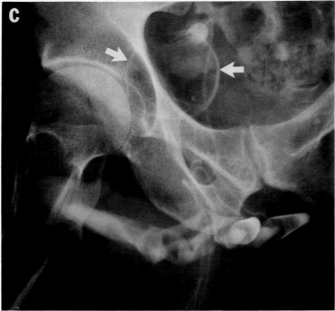

Figure 5–31. A, Plain radiograph of a patient with a multicomponent, inflatable prosthesis before pumping and inflating the prosthesis. Note that the reservoir *(large arrows)* is abnormally collapsed in the resting state. **B,** Same patient after pumping and inflating the prosthesis. Note that the reservoir *(large black arrows)* is abnormally completely empty and the penile prosthesis cylinders are not fully distended *(open curved arrow)*. This lack of adequate distention of the penile cylinders is due to the inadequate fluid present in the reservoir before pumping. **C,** A different patient, in whom the reservoir *(white arrows)* is completely empty because of leaking of the iodinated contrast material out of the reservoir into the surrounding tissues and subsequently being absorbed. Also note the collapsed penile cylinders, which along with the empty reservoir, indicate prior leakage of the contrast media out of the system.

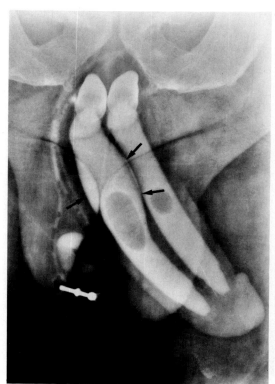
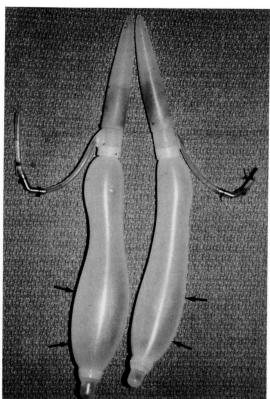

Figure 5–32. A, Radiograph of a multicomponent inflatable penile prosthesis, demonstrating aneurysmal dilatation *(arrows)* of the penile cylinders. **B,** Image of the penile cylinders after surgical removal, demonstrating aneurysmal dilatation *(arrows)* of both penile cylinders.

fraying have been underestimated on plain film radiography.

Why an inflatable multicomponent prostheses malfunctions is often difficult to evaluate with physical examination. Most malfunctions of multicomponent IPPs can be assessed adequately with a single oblique pelvic radiographic with the prostheses inflated. One of the more common malfunctions of mechanical IPPs is inadequate inflation of the prostheses to achieve a satisfactory erection. Pelvic radiography often reveals a marked decrease in the amount of fluid in the reservoir. The penile cylinders often are underinflated. The water-soluble iodinated contrast material that leaks out of the reservoir of cylinders is rapidly absorbed and excreted by the kidneys and is, therefore, not visible on plain radiographs (Fig. 5–31). Another complication of inflatable multicomponent prostheses is aneurysmal dilatation or buckling of the cylinder. This often is due to a structural deficiency within the cylinder or possibly to preexisting weakness in the tunica albuginea. These cylinder aneurysms are seen easily on plain radiographs (Fig. 5–32).

Patients often experience gradual loss of penile rigidity, or patients may have erections that become angulated or asymmetric. Rupture of the outer layers of the cylinder also can occur (Fig. 5–33). This may result in dramatic focal ballooning of the cylinder. Malposition of the cylinder can appear as kinking on the radiograph (Fig. 5–34).

Kinks or separation of the tubing of these multicomponent inflatable prostheses can occur and usually develop within the first few months after surgery. Kinking or separation of the tubing can be seen easily on plain radiographs. Often a patient can function with just one cylinder if the other cylinder has to be removed (Fig. 5–35).

Pump migration or malfunction should be considered in any patient with a nonfunctioning prosthesis who has an apparently normal pelvic radiograph (Fig. 5–36).

Erosions of the pump or reservoir have been known to occur. Reservoirs usually erode into the bladder. Close scrutiny of the radiograph can reveal an abnormal location of the pump (Fig. 5–37).

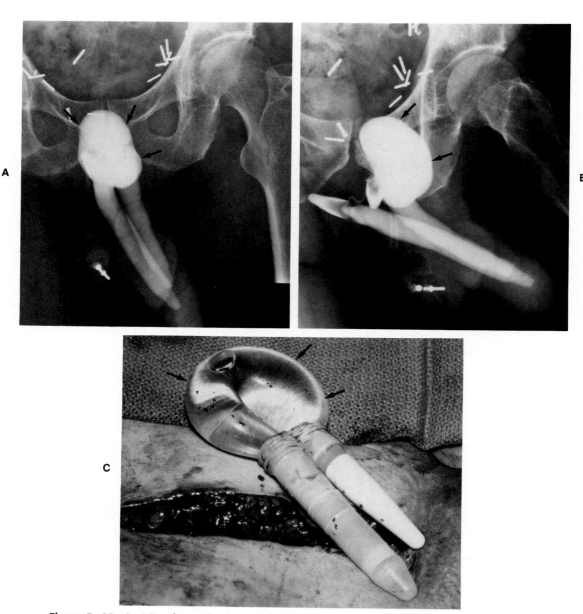

Figure 5–33. A, AP radiograph of a multicomponent inflatable penile prosthesis. Note the large well-defined collection of contrast media *(arrows)* near the base of the penile cylinders. Also note the apparent shortening of the left penile cylinder relative to the right. **B,** Oblique radiograph of the same patient, demonstrating a dramatic ballooning of the base of the left penile cylinder *(arrows)*. **C,** Image of the left penile cylinder after surgical removal, demonstratng rupture of the outer supportive layer of the penile cylinder and ballooning of the inner layer containing the contrast media *(arrows)*.

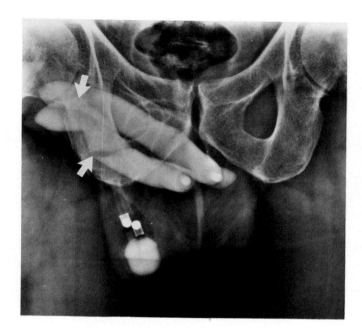

Figure 5–34. AP radiograph of a multicomponent inflatable penile prosthesis, demonstrating malposition of the right penile cylinder *(arrows)*. Malposition of the right penile cylinder is demonstrated by kinking and bending on the radiograph.

Figure 5–35. An oblique radiograph of a multicomponent inflatable penile prosthesis, in which there is only one penile cylinder. The left penile cylinder has been surgically removed, and the tubing previously connected to the left penile cylinder has been capped *(arrow)*.

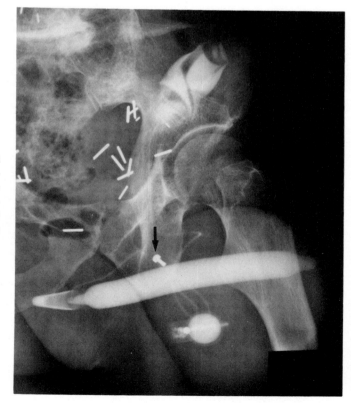

Figure 5–36. AP radiograph of a multicomponent inflatable penile prosthesis. Note that the small metallic ball *(arrow)* in the pump has been dislodged from the valve mechanism (V). This type of three-way ball valve mechanism is no longer used. The new two-way ball valve mechanisms (see Fig. 5–34) appear to have fewer ball valve malfunctions.

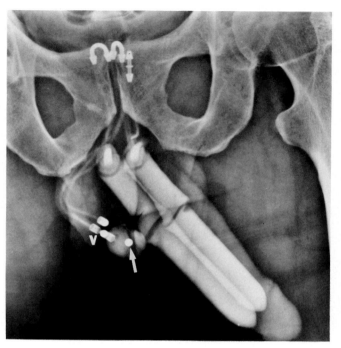

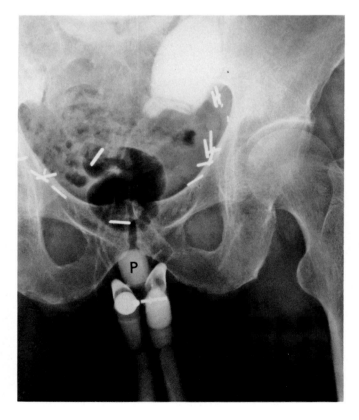

Figure 5–37. AP radiograph of a multicomponent inflatable penile prosthesis, demonstrating malposition of the pump (P) proximal to the penile cylinders. The pump should be in the scrotum distal to the penile cylinders (see Fig. 5–34).

Pump erosions usually are easily detected on physical examination. Detection of reservoir erosion into the bowel or the bladder is often difficult on a plain radiograph and often requires endoscopy or surgery for diagnosis.

Inflatable self-contained prostheses also may malfunction. Fracture of the reservoir or mechanical malfunction of the spring-action cable (Omniphase) may occur. In some cases, there is no mechanical dysfunction, and the patient has had difficulty in using the pump.

The wide variety of prostheses available and the constant change and improvement in many of these prostheses make it difficult to identify clearly the exact type of prosthesis on plain film radiography. However, plain film radiography can aid in solving problems in patients with malfunctioning penile prostheses.

ACKNOWLEDGMENT

We would like to express special thanks to Sonja Schleusner for the preparation of this manuscript.

REFERENCES

1. Buvat J, Bervat-Hertaut M, Dehaene JL, et al. Is intravenous injection of papaverine a reliable screening test for vasculogenic impotence? J Urol 135:476, 1986.
2. Lue TF, Hricak H, Marich KW, et al. Vasculogenic impotence evaluated by high-resolution ultrasonography and pulsed Doppler spectrum analysis. Radiology 155:777, 1985.
3. Mueller SC, Lue TF. Evaluation of vasculogenic impotence. Urol Clin North Am 15:65, 1988.
4. Collins JP, Lewandowski BJ. Experience with intracorporeal injection of papaverine and duplex ultrasound scanning for assessment of arteriogenic impotence. Br J Urol 59:84, 1987.
5. Desai DM, Gingell JC, Skidmore R, et al. Application of computerized penile arterial waveform analysis in the diagnosis of arteriogenic impotence: an initial study of potent and impotent men. Br J Urol 60:450, 1987.
6. Gall H, Barhren W, Scherb W, et al. Diagnostic accuracy of Doppler ultrasound technique of the penile arteries in correlation to selective arteriography. Cardiovasc Intervent Radiol 11:225, 1988.
7. Robinson LQ, Woodcock JP, Stephenson TP. Duplex scanning in suspected vasculogenic impotence: a worthwhile exercise? Br J Urol 63:432, 1989.
8. Krysiewicz S, Mellinger BC. The role of imaging in the diagnostic evaluation of impotence. AJR 153:1133, 1989.
9. Quam JP, King BF, James EM, et al. Duplex and color Doppler sonographic evaluation of vasculogenic impotence. AJR 153:1141, 1989.
10. Benson CB, Vickers MA. Sexual impotence caused by vascular disease: diagnosis with duplex sonography. AJR 153:1149, 1989.
11. Schwartz AN, Wang KY, Mack LA, et al. Evaluation of normal erectile function with color flow Doppler sonography. AJR 153:1155, 1989.
12. Paushter DM. Role of duplex sonography in the evaluation of sexual impotence. AJR 153:1161, 1989.
13. King BF, Hattery RR, James EM, et al. Duplex sonography in the evaluation of impotence: current techniques. Semin Intervent Radiol 7:215, 1990.
14. Meuleman EJ, Bemelmaus BLH, Doesburg WH, et al. Penile pharmacological duplex ultrasonography: a dose–effect study comparing papaverine, papaverine/phentolamine, and prostaglandin E$_1$. J Urol 148:63, 1992.
15. Sidi AA. Vasoactive intracavernous pharmacotherapy. Urol Clin North Am 15:95, 1988.
16. Roth JC., King BF, Hattery RR, et al. Vasculogenic impotence: dynamic duplex and color Doppler penile sonography. (Submitted for publication)
17. Hattery RR, King BF, Lewis RW, et al. Vasculogenic impotence: duplex and color Doppler imaging. Radiol Clin North Am 29:629, 1991.
18. Valji K, Bookstein JJ. Diagnosis of arteriogenic impotence: efficacy of duplex sonography as a screening tool. AJR 160:65, 1993.
19. Bookstein JJ, Valji K. The arteriolar component of impotence: a possible paradigm shift. AJR 157:932, 1991.
20. Kleer E, Lewis RW, King BF, et al. The use of color duplex Doppler and pelvic arteriography for the diagnosis of unusual penile abnormalities. Int J Impot Res 4(Suppl 2):A75, 1992.
21. Fitzgerald SW, Erickson SJ, Foley WD, et al. Color Doppler sonography in the evaluation of erectile dysfunction: patterns of temporal response to papaverine. AJR 157:331, 1991.
22. King BF. Color Doppler flow imaging evaluation of the deep dorsal penile vein in vascular impotence. Radiol Soc North Am 1989:371. Abstract—scientific program.
23. Huguet JF, Clerissi J, Juhan C. Radiological anatomy of pudendal artery. Eur J Radiol 1:278, 1981.
24. Juhan CM, Padula G, Huguet JF. Angiography in male impotence. In: Bennett AH, ed. Management of Male Impotence. Baltimore: Williams & Wilkins, 1982:73.
25. Ginestie JF, Romieu A. Radiologic Exploration of Impotence. Boston: Martinus Nijhoff, 1978.
26. Brühlmann W, Pouliadis G, Zollikofer CH, et al. Arteriography of the penis in secondary impotence. Urol Radiol 4:243, 1982.
27. Curet P, Grellet J, Perrin D, et al. Technical and anatomic factors in filling of distal portion of internal pudendal artery during arteriography. Urology 29:333, 1987.
28. Rosen MP, Greenfield AJ, Walker TG, et al. Arteriogenic impotence: findings in 195 impotent men examined with selective internal pudendal angiography. Radiology 174:1043, 1990.
29. Bookstein JJ, Lang E. Penile magnification phar-

macoarteriography: details of intrapenile artery anatomy. AJR 148:883, 1987.

30. Castaneda-Zuniga WR, Smith A, Kaye K, et al. Transluminal angiography for treatment of vasculogenic impotence. AJR 139:371, 1982.
31. Bookstein JJ, Valji K. Transluminal therapeutic interventions in vasculogenic impotence. In: Papanicolaou N, ed. Radiology of Impotence and Infertility. Lippincott's Reviews—Radiology. Philadelphia: JB Lippincott, 1992:631.
32. Gray RR, Keresteci AG, St. Louis EL, et al. Investigation of impotence by internal pudendal angiography. Experience with 73 cases. Radiology 144:773, 1982.
33. Struyven J, Gregior W, Giannakopoulos X, et al. Selective pudendal arteriography. Eur Urol 5:233, 1979.
34. St. Louis EL, Gray RR, Grosman H. Simplified technique of internal pudendal angiography in the investigation of impotence. Cardiovasc Intervent Radiol 9:22, 1986.
35. Michal V, Pospichal J. Phalloarteriography in the diagnosis of erectile impotence. World J Surg 2:239, 1978.
36. Delcour C, Vandenbosch G, Delatte P, et al. Technical advances in penile arteriography. AJR 150:803, 1988.
37. Bookstein JJ, Valji K, Parsons L, et al. Pharmacoarteriography in the evaluation of impotence. J Urol 137:333, 1987.
38. Kunnen M, DeMeyer JM, DeSy WA. Pudendal arteriography, without penile vasodilation: practically worthless! Acta Urol Belg 56:315, 1988.
39. Mueller SC, Lue TF. Evaluation of vasculogenic impotence. Urol Clin North Am 15:65, 1988.
40. Goldstein I. Arterial revascularization procedures. Semin Urol 4:252, 1986.
41. Gall H, Bahren W, Steif CG, et al. Diagnosis of vasculogenic impotence—comparing investigation by Doppler sonography and arteriography. Acta Urol Belg 56:246, 1988.
42. Schwartz AN, Freidenberg D, Harley JD. Nonselective angiography after intracorporeal papaverine injections: an alternative technique for evaluating penile artery integrity. Radiology 167:249, 1988.
43. Delcour C, Vandenbosch G, Wespes E, et al. Pudendal arteriography. Acta Urol Belg 56:308, 1988.
44. Leipner Von N, Porst H, Koster O, et al. DSA und konventionelle angiographie im vergleich bei der angiographischen diagnostik der impotentia coeundi. Fortschr Roengenstr 144:516, 1986.
45. Nessi R, De Flaviis L, Bellinzoni G, et al. Digital angiography of erectile failure. Br J Urol 59:584, 1987.
46. Lue TF, Tanagho EM. Physiology of erection and pharmacological management of impotence. J Urol 137:829, 1987.
47. Zorgniotti AW, Shaw WW, Padula G, et al. Impotence associated with pudendal arteriovenous malformations. J Urol 132:128, 1984.
48. Witt MA, Goldstein I, Saenz de Tejada I, et al. Traumatic laceration of intracavernosal arteries: the pathophysiology of nonischemic, high flow, arterial priapism. J Urol 143:129, 1990.
49. Walker TG, Grant PW, Goldstein I, et al. "High-flow" priapism: treatment with superselective transcatheter embolization. Radiology 174:1053, 1990.
50. Visvanathan K, Burrows PE, Shillinger JF, et al. Posttraumatic arterial priapism in a 7-year-old boy: successful management by percutaneous transcatheter embolization. J Urol 148:382, 1992.
51. Gudinchet F, Fournier D, Jichlinski P, et al. Traumatic priapism in a child: evaluation with color flow Doppler sonography. J Urol 148:380, 1992.
52. Fetter TR, Yunen JR, Dodd G. Application of cavernosography in the diagnosis of lesions of the penis. AJR 90:169, 1963.
53. Hamilton RW, Swann JC. Corpus cavernosography in Peyronie's disease. Br J Urol 39:409, 1967.
54. Fitzpatrick TJ. Spongiosograms and cavernosograms: a study of their value in priapism. J Urol 109:843, 1973.
55. Datta NS. Corpus cavernosography in conditions other than Peyronie's disease. J Urol 118:588, 1977.
56. Pliskow RJ, Ohme RK. Corpus cavernosography in acute "fracture" of the penis. AJR 133:331, 1979.
57. Raghavaiah NV. Corpus cavernosogram in the evaluation of carcinoma of the penis. J Urol 120:423, 1978.
58. Grosman H, Gray RR, St. Louis EL, et al. The role of cavernosography in acute "fracture" of the penis. Radiology 144:787, 1982.
59. Ashdown RR, Gilanpour H. Venous drainage of the corpus cavernosum in impotent and normal bulls. J Anat 117:159, 1974.
60. Young SL, Hudson RS, Walker DF. Impotence in bulls due to vascular shunts from the corpus cavernosum penis. J Am Vet Med Assoc 171:643, 1977.
61. Ashdown RR, David JSE, Gibbs C. Impotence in the bull: abnormal drainage of the corpus cavernosum penis. Vet Rec 104:423, 1979.
62. Fitzpatrick TJ. Venography of the deep dorsal venous and valvular systems. J Urol 111:518, 1974.
63. Fitzpatrick TJ. The corpus cavernosum intercommunicating venous drainage system. J Urol 113:494, 1975.
64. Fitzpatrick TJ, Cooper JF. A cavernosogram study on the valvular competence of the human deep dorsal vein. J Urol 113:497, 1975.
65. Ney C, Miller HL, Friedenberg RM. Various applications of corpus cavernosography. Radiology 119:69, 1976.
66. Ebbehøj J, Wagner G. Insufficient penile erections due to abnormal drainage of cavernous bodies. Urology 13:507, 1979.
67. Wagner G. Erection: physiology and endocrinology. In: Wagner G, Green R, eds. Impotence: Physiological, Psychological, Surgical Diagnosis and Treatment. New York: Plenum, 1981:25.

68. Velcek D, Evans JA. Cavernosography. Radiology 144:781, 1982.

69. Herzberg Z, Kellett MJ, Morgan RJ, et al. Method, indications and results of corpus cavernosography. Br J Urol 53:641, 1981.

70. Virag R. Arterial and venous hemodynamics in male impotence. In: Bennett AH, ed. Management of Male Impotence. Baltimore: Williams & Wilkins, 1982:108.

71. Puyau FA, Lewis RW. Corpus cavernosography: pressure flow and radiography. Invest Radiol 18:517, 1983.

72. Lewis RW, Puyau FA, Kerstein, et al. Corpora cavernosa outflow as defined by dynamic cavernosography: implications in the evaluation and treatment of impotence. In: Virag R, Virag-Lappas H, eds. Proceedings of the First World Meeting on Impotence. Paris: Les Editions du CERI, 6:190, 1984.

73. Delcour C, Wespes E, Schulman CC, et al. Investigation of the venous system in impotence of vascular origin. Urol Radiol 6:172, 1984.

74. Wespes E, Schulman CC. Parameters of erection. Br J Urol 56:416, 1984.

75. Wespes E, Delcour C, Struyven J, et al. Cavernometry–cavernography: its role in organic impotence. Eur Urol 10:229, 1984.

76. Porst A, Altwein JE, Bach D, et al. Dynamic cavernosography: venous outflow studies of cavernous bodies. J Urol 134:276, 1985.

77. Wespes E, Delcour C, Struyven J, et al. Pharmacocavernometry: cavernography in impotence. Br J Urol 58:429, 1986.

78. Delcour C, Wespes E, Vandenbosch G. Impotence: evaluation with cavernosography. Radiology 161:803, 1986.

79. Lue TF, Hricak H, Schmidt RA, et al. Functional evaluation of penile veins by cavernosography in papaverine-induced erection. J Urol 135:479, 1986.

80. Puyau FA, Lewis RW, Balkin P, et al. Dynamic corpus cavernosography: effect of papaverine injection. Radiology 164:179, 1987.

81. Bookstein JJ, Valji K, Parsons L, et al. Penile pharmacocavernosography and cavernometry in the evaluation of impotence. J Urol 137:772, 1987.

82. Delcour C, Wespes E, Schulman CC, et al. Investigation of the venous system in impotence of vascular origin. Urol Radiol 6:190, 1984.

83. Virag R, Spence PP, Frydman D. Artificial erection in diagnosis and treatment of impotence. Urology 24:157, 1984.

84. Malhotra CM, Balko A, Wincze JP, et al. Cavernosography in conjunction with artificial erection for evaluation of venous leakage in impotent men. Radiology 161:799, 1986.

85. Porst H, vanAhlen H, Vahlensieck W. Relevance of dynamic cavernosography in the diagnosis of venous incompetence in erectile dysfunction. J Urol 137:1163, 1987.

86. Bookstein JJ. Cavernosal veno-occlusive insufficiency in male impotence: evaluation of degree and location. Radiology 164:175, 1987.

87. Freidenberg DH, Berger RE, Chew DE, et al. Quantitation of corporeal venous outflow resistance in man by corporeal pressure flow evaluation. J Urol 138:533, 1987.

88. Lowe MA, Schwartz AN, Berger RE. Controlled trial of infusion cavernosometry in impotent and potent men. J Urol 146:783, 1991.

89. Goldstein I. Vasculogenic impotence: its diagnosis and treatment. In: deVere White R, ed. Sexual Dysfunction Problems in Urology. Philadelphia: JB Lippincott, 1987:547.

90. Puech-Leao, Chao S, Glina S, et al. Gravity cavernosometry: a simple diagnostic test for cavernosal incompetence. Br J Urol 4:93, 1989.

91. Mueleman EJH, Wijkstra H, Doesburg WH, et al. Comparison of the diagnostic value of pump and gravity cavernosometry in the evaluation of the cavernous veno-occlusive mechanism. J Urol 146:1266, 1991.

92. Vickers MA, Benson C, Dluhy R, et al. The current cavernosometric criteria for corporovenous dysfunction are too strict. J Urol 147:614, 1992.

93. Stief CG, Wetterauer U, Sommerkamp H. Intraindividual comparative study of dynamic and pharmacocavernosography. Br J Urol 4:93, 1989.

94. Fuchs AM, Mehringer CM, Rajfer J. Anatomy of penile venous drainage in potent and impotent men during cavernosography. J Urol 141:1353, 1989.

95. Cortheoux P, Maiza D, Henriet JP, et al. Erectile dysfunction caused by venous leakage: treatment with detachable balloons and coils. Radiology 161:807, 1986.

96. Hartnell GG, Mulcahy MJ, Kaiely EA, et al. Digital subtraction dynamic cavernosography. Br J Radiol 61:679, 1978.

97. Aboseif SR, Breza J, Lue TF, et al. Penile venous drainage in erectile dysfunction: anatomical, radiological and functional considerations. Br J Urol 64:183, 1989.

98. Shabsigh R, Fishman IJ, Toombs BD, et al. Venous leaks: anatomical and physiological observations. J Urol 146:1260, 1991.

99. Houspian DM, Amis ES. Penile prosthetic implants: a radiographic atlas. Radiographics 9:707, 1989.

100. Cohan RH, Dunnick NR, Carson CC. Radiology of penile prosthesis. AJR 152:925, 1989.

101. Parker MS, Cohan RH. Radiology of penile prosthesis. In: Papanicolaou N, ed. Radiology of Impotence and Infertility. Lippincott's Reviews— Radiology. Philadelphia: JB Lippincott Co, 1992.

CHAPTER 6

Psychogenic Impotence

Kathleen Blindt Segraves

R. Taylor Segraves

In this chapter, we address some of the methods and issues regarding assessment and treatment of psychogenic erectile dysfunction. The available research data are reviewed, and we attempt to summarize what appears to be current clinical wisdom.

Historically, it was assumed generally that the majority of cases of erectile dysfunction were psychogenic.[1-4] More recently, research has suggested that organic causes may be more common than previously realized.[5-9] In the past 10 years, there has been a proliferation of diagnostic procedures for evaluating the medical aspects of erectile functioning. Procedures are available to evaluate vascular, hormonal, and neurogenic factors involved in erectile problems. The proliferation of new technologies has resulted in identifying organic anomalies that may relate to erectile dysfunction. Melman et al. suggest that organic factors can be identified in about 50% of the patients with erectile disorders.[10,11] Advancement in effective treatment options has increased the interest and importance of differentiating organic from psychogenic erectile disorders.

A multitude of functions determine normal erectile functioning. A variety of biologic, psychologic, and interpersonal influences bear on sexual functioning. Because there are no firmly established guidelines, diagnostic evaluation of this complaint varies considerably from practitioner to practitioner and from center to center. However, there appears to be some uniformity in that most centers begin the process of assessment with a review of the patient's medical, sexual, and psychosocial history.

A presumptive diagnosis of psychogenic erectile disorder first requires an adequate medical assessment. The necessary physical evaluation to ascertain a working hypothesis of psychogenic etiology is reviewed in other chapters of this text. Unfortunately, not all cases can be divided into either organic or psychogenic etiology. Many patients have a mixed etiology and require a multitherapeutic approach. For example, a diabetic male who has an episodic problem of erectile failure may, over time, develop erectile problems associated with his fear of failure. This performance anxiety in response to the fear of failure may result in a psychogenic erectile disorder in a man with some organic impairment. Hence, identification of both organic and psychogenic factors would have separate treatment ramifications. Identifying treatable organic factors is important, as it would clearly be a disservice to the patient to treat an organically based erectile disorder exclusively with psychotherapy.

PSYCHOSOCIAL ASSESSMENT

The major purpose of a complete psychosocial assessment is to gather sufficient information concerning the patient's life situation and sexual behavior to be able to hypothesize psychologic influences that may be contributing to or maintaining the erectile problem. This assessment first examines the context in which the erectile problem occurs (Table 6-1). The information gained may offer important insights into possible contributing factors. The clinician might begin the assessment by asking the patient general questions about his sexual functioning, followed by more direct and explicit questions. One of the first tasks of the assessment is to determine if the patient has an erectile disorder. Some men will complain of erectile dysfunction when further assessment reveals that they have unrealistic expectations. For example, a man in his 60s may want to perform at the same frequency as when he was in his 20s or may expect a full erection every time he engages in any form of sexual activity. Some men will complain of erectile failure when the primary problem is premature ejaculation. The man may ejaculate before penetration and is unable to immediately regain his erection. A careful assessment becomes necessary to determine if the erectile dysfunction predated and contributed to the development of premature ejaculation, or if the reverse is true.

The clinician might find a number of different questions useful when eliciting important diagnostic information. During this evaluation process, it is helpful to ask the patient for a detailed description of the sexual problem, including the circumstances surrounding its onset and any events af-

TABLE 6–1
Psychiatric Assessment

I. Is the presenting complaint an erectile disorder?
    A. Rule out unrealistic expectations
        1. Expectations of unchanged sexual frequency in older men
        2. Full erection at will
    B. Rule out premature ejaculation
        1. Loss of erection before penetration
II. Is the problem secondary to another problem?
    A. Rule out affective disorder
        1. Major depressive disorder
    B. Rule out substance abuse
        1. Alcohol and recreational drug abuse
    C. Rule out other sexual disorders
        1. Desire disorder (hypoactive desire disorder)
        2. Sexual aversion disorder
III. Identify contributing psychosocial factors
    A. Rule out stress prior to onset
    B. Rule out ongoing stress
    C. Rule out marital discord
    D. Rule out partner emotional or physical unavailability
IV. Identify contributing psychosexual factors
    A. Rule out sexual adjustment problems
        1. Drive discrepancies
        2. Discrepancies in sexual preference (intercourse AM vs PM, position preference)
    B. Rule out performance anxiety
    C. Rule out partner sabotage
    D. Rule out sexual dysfunction in partner
    E. Rule out sexual misinformation
    F. Rule out poor sexual skills or techniques
        1. Lack of adequate penile stimulation
        2. Excessive stimulation resulting in premature ejaculation

fecting its course. Reports of sudden onset not associated with change in medical status or medication would raise questions about concurrent stressors that may be associated with the problem's onset. Questions concerning environmental stress, such as major life changes, acute or chronic illness of partner or self, death of a loved one, loss of work, financial concerns, and infidelity of spouse or self, may help to identify psychogenic etiologic factors (Table 6–2).

The clinician would also attempt to determine what are the man's thoughts relating to his presenting complaint and attempt to identify his automatic self-statements, fantasies, or self-explanations concerning the erectile dysfunction. Identifying what a man thinks has bearing on treatment planning. For example, if a man believes his erectile disorder is a symptom of an undiagnosed pros-

tate cancer, he may not want talking therapy, which may result in his dropping out of treatment or not following a psychiatric referral. Repeated erectile failure may result in a self-statement suggesting poor self-esteem and a state of demoralization. For example, the man may be haunted by negative self-statements, such as "I will always be a failure," "I am no good," or "There is no hope for my problem." Such a man might benefit from a direct intervention, which would provide a reliable erection along with psychotherapy.

Questions concerning why the patient is seeking treatment at this time may identify sources of stress that may be maintaining the problem. For example, one may discover that the patient is seeking treatment because of an escalating marital discord. One needs to identify the relationship factors impinging on the sexual relationship. The attitudes and expectations of the sexual partner may provide useful information about the pressure the patient feels to perform adequately. For example, the man's sexual history might indicate that his erectile problem has developed gradually over the past 3 or 4 years but has suddenly become quite severe in the last 2 years. The relationship assessment reveals that the couple has been attempting to conceive a child for the past 2 years. The partner informs the patient when intercourse must take place. Hence, the patient is expected to engage in intercourse on scheduled days dictated by basal temperature charts or medical interventions unrelated to his sexual drive. The woman may implicitly or overtly blame the man for their infertility, since he is not able to perform at critical times of her cycle. The problem is made worse when the man knows that the infertility specialist as well as auxiliary staff are aware of his problem.

The clinician would need to rule out other psychiatric disorders that may be associated with erectile impairment, such as affective disorder and substance abuse. Decreased libido and erectile dysfunction may be symptoms of a major depressive disorder. Depression can affect nocturnal penile tumescence (NPT) evaluations. The NPT of a man who is clinically depressed may demonstrate an absence of or minimal nocturnal erections. Without identifying the depressive episode, the NPT might suggest an organic erectile disorder. Effectively treating the depression may result in a reversal of the erectile disorder. The differential assessment would include identifying sexual problems in other phases of the sexual response cycle, such as the desire phase, which might result in the primary diagnosis of hypoactive sexual desire disorder. It is not unusual for a man to have a primary diagnosis of hypoactive sexual desire with a secondary diagnosis of erectile disorder.[12,13] If it appears that the man is having arousal problems because he is

TABLE 6–2
Sexual History Data Predictive of a Psychogenic Erectile Disorder

Highly Suggestive*
1. Adequate morning erection ($\geq$ 2 per week)
2. Adequate erection during foreplay
3. Adequate spontaneous erections
4. Adequate masturbatory erections
5. Adequate erections induced through fantasy
6. Adequate erections with someone other than partner

Possibly Suggestive
1. Abrupt onset associated with psychosocial stress (divorce, illness in family, loss of job, affair, etc.)
2. Abrupt onset not related to change in medical status or medication
3. Problem maintaining an erection to intromission

*Adequate is defined as sufficient for penetration if it were to occur during a sexual encounter.

attempting intercourse when his libido or drive is low, treatment would focus on what appears to be the primary problem, hypoactive desire, rather than the erectile complaint. Assuming that hormone studies are normal, one approach would be to help the man identify his level of desire and suggest that he attempt intercourse only when his level of desire or drive is high.

The use of sexual symptomatology to differentiate psychogenic from organic erectile disorders is an important step in the psychosexual assessment.[14–18] One of the primary indications of a psychogenic etiology is when the man reports experiencing an adequate (sufficient for penetration if intercourse were to take place) erection on awakening or in other noncoital situations.[18] Some men report being able to achieve an erection during various sexual activities, such as sexual foreplay or masturbation or with a new or different partner.[14–18] The ability to experience an erection under any noncoital condition is a simple predictive screen for psychogenicity (Table 6–2). Sexual symptomatology is clinically useful, although it might not be accurate in all situations and is dependent on the accuracy of the patient's self-report. Generally, the ability to have an erection during a noncoital activity suggests that the sexual problem has a psychogenic component.

THEORIES OF ETIOLOGY

Assumptions regarding the etiology of psychogenic erectile disorder are associated with a variety of theoretical orientations. These theoretical assumptions are related to different treatment approaches. The most enduring schools of thought are primarily psychodynamic, cognitive-behavioral, and systems theory. The models are rarely applied in pure form. For example, behavioral approaches usually include identifying thoughts as well as observable behaviors, and systems theory often includes cognitive-behavioral assessment and treatment approaches. The Masters and Johnson approach is an amalgam of behavioral and systems theory.

Traditional psychoanalytic theory views erectile disorders as a symptom of unresolved conflicts generated during early psychosexual development. Psychoanalytic theory suggests that the unresolved Oedipal complex leads to an arrested psychosexual development, which is the genesis of erectile problems.[1] Failure to obtain or maintain an erection sufficient for intercourse was thought to be due to guilt because of the unconscious forbidden wish to have sex with the mother.[1,19] The erectile problem suggests the patient's inability to differentiate between mother and other women. The anxiety associated with erectile problems is related to castration anxiety, the unconscious fear that the father, or the perceived powerful person, will punish the man for engaging in sex with the woman (mother figure). Levine and Althof proposed an updated "psychodynamic model for conceptualizing the pathogenesis of arousal problems that involves the resonation of forces that derive from three spheres of causality: (1) performance anxiety, (2) antecedent life changes and (3) developmental vulnerabilities."[20]

Beginning in the late 1950s, a behavioral approach to sexual problems was developed based on learning theory. A behavioral assessment was conducted to find the discrete components of sexual activity. The patient would keep a structured diary recording behaviors that surround and include all sexual behaviors (identifying the antecedents, sexual attempt, and consequences). This method focused on the current sexual problem. Reversing the sexual complaint is facilitated by changing the antecedent (stimulus) or consequence (positive or negative reinforcers) of the attempt at sexual intercourse. The conditioned anxiety response and the use of systematic desensitization as proposed by Wolpe in the late 1950s was a major force in this method of treatment. Erectile disorders were conceptualized as being the result of a conditioned anxiety response to a particular set of sexual stimuli.[21] Treatment was to recondition the person's reaction to the anxiety-producing stimulus. The field of behavioral therapy has expanded to include cognitive factors.

Cognitive-behavioral therapists apply social

learning theory to sexual complaints. This approach "emphasizes the role of incorrect information, skill deficits, and dysfunctional anxieties concerning sexual performance, or concerning what is considered proper sexual behavior."[22] The therapist begins by identifying the patient's internal thoughts and affect as well as the external behaviors or cues that precede or follow the failed sexual encounter.[21,23–26] The cognitive-behavioral approach views sexual problems as a set of discrete internal and external behaviors that can be changed using the principles of behavioral analysis and social learning theory.

Over the years, therapists treating sexual problems found that interventions based on social learning theory and anxiety reduction methods proposed by Masters and Johnson did not reverse many of the sexual problems. There was a heterogeneous group of patients with very complex sexual problems that were resistant to change. The field began to shift to a systems approach for the most resistant situations. Therapists began to use systemic interventions. There are various definitions for systems theory. One definition is that the primary focus is on the dyad and the reciprocal interactions within the couple. Communication problems and power struggles, according to this approach, could result in erectile problems.[3,27–29] Another definition of systems theory includes an expanded concept of the interactional scheme. Cultural and religious differences and family of origin alliances all have an impact on the couple's equilibrium that can secondarily affect the couple's sexual relationship. Often, unresolved family of origin issues and alliances may be contributing to the problem.[30] For example, the erectile disorder may be related to the man's unconscious anger that his wife is more attached to her father than to him. The systems approach would include an analysis of how the erectile disorder might serve as an adaptive process to maintain homeostasis within the couple. For example, his erectile problem protects the wife from confronting her fears about adult sexual relationships, or the problem may help the couple regulate their mutual discomfort with the level of closeness and other intimacy issues (e.g., fear of engulfment, boundaries, personal space).

TREATMENT APPROACHES
Direct and Indirect Methods

A number of methods are available for the treatment of psychogenic erectile disorders. Matching the hypothesized contributing factors with appropriate interventions is the key to efficient and efficacious treatment. Treatment can logically be grouped into interventions that approach the erectile difficulty somewhat indirectly, such as behavioral and marital therapy, and other methods, which can be classified as direct. The direct methods include oral medications such as yohimbine, intracavernosal injections, vacuum device with constriction rings, and the use of surgical prosthetic devices. The decision of which approach to take can prove far more involved than one might expect. Clearly, most of the direct methods are capable of restoring the capacity to obtain and maintain an erection sufficient for coitus. However, these methods cannot ensure that the patient wants to use his restored erectile ability or that his partner is receptive to renewed sexual activity. On the other hand, severe psychologic sequelae of direct interventions appear to be relatively uncommon. Although not frequent, it is possible that a patient who experienced a reversal of his problem through a direct approach may continue to be dissatisfied with the treatment result because his initial discomfort may relate to issues other than erectile failure. He may experience marital discord following the intervention or bring legal action to remedy what he perceives as an unsatisfactory result. Precise information about the frequency of patients' negative responses to a direct method is not available.

Unfortunately, there often is a polarization toward the treatment of erectile disorders between urologic surgeons and mental health professionals. The latter group advocates indirect treatment approaches and frequently is suspicious of the motives of physicians who use direct approaches to treat impotence. A certain degree of mistrust of the alternative treatment camp and subspecialists is common. Part of this can be understood by reflecting on the type of patients seen by each specialist. Physicians treating impotence rarely see the successful outcomes of psychotherapy for erectile problems and may have only a few patients who have benefited when referred to psychotherapists. Previous research has suggested that most referrals to psychiatry are not consummated, primarily because the patient does not keep the original or return appointments.[31,32] On the other hand, the typical psychiatrist does not have reason to see the typical patient who has been successfully treated. Instead, the psychiatrist may be referred patients who are discontent with the treatment they received from their primary physician or surgical specialist. The selection bias in patients, plus current financial pressures in medicine, can contribute to considerable subspecialty mistrust and misperception. Fortunately, in a number of hospital settings, surgeons and mental health professionals have begun to work together to assess the feasibility of direct methods of treatment for psychogenic erectile problems.

PSYCHOTHERAPY
Treatment Outcome

The outcome reported for psychotherapy of psychogenic erectile problems varies considerably from clinical series to clinical series. This variability probably relates to various factors, including differences in therapist skill and technique as well as differences in patient populations. It is probable that some patients with organic contributions to their erectile failure have been included in some psychotherapeutic trials, obviously lowering success rates.[33] It is being recognized that lifelong and acquired psychogenic erectile disorders represent two discrete groups of patients, each with its own response to therapy. Acquired or secondary erectile failure is far more common than lifelong erectile dysfunction and generally is easier to treat.

The available data clearly indicate that secondary impotence with acute onset and of brief duration in patients with good previous sexual functioning is more likely to respond favorably to psychotherapy.[20,34–37] Often, the precipitant is clearly identifiable and easily ameliorated with reassurance or brief behavioral therapy. A 50-year-old man who has never been able to have coitus is quite different from the same aged man who has been sexually potent in all but the last 6 months, when he was unemployed as a result of downsizing within his corporate office. Erectile dysfunction of brief duration with an obvious stressor preceding onset is responsive to a variety of interventions. On the other hand, erectile disorders of insidious onset and long duration often are extremely resistant to indirect interventions (psychotherapy).[37]

Another factor shown to influence prognosis in response to psychologic intervention is the patient's entry point into the medical system. Men who self-refer themselves to a urologist are unlikely to follow through with psychiatric referral.[31] Men who view their problem as biologic and not in the head may require a different type of psychologic intervention.

Men who seek treatment for erectile problems from various medical specialties may have concurrent medical problems resulting in erectile problems with a mixed etiology. Often, patients with organic etiologies may develop a psychogenic overlay. Patients with mixed etiologies may benefit from brief psychotherapy. However, a man who believes that erectile difficulties are the exclusive result of a physical problem is less likely to engage in formal psychotherapy.

Due to the heterogeneity of the population and the variability within the treatment approaches, comparative analysis of efficacy is problematic. Within the field, there is a lack of agreement regarding standard criteria for successful treatment. Effectiveness varies when evaluating short-term vs long-term improvements. Also, the effectiveness of sex therapy is difficult to determine because many patients report positive changes in many aspects of their lives following sex therapy. Patients often report a reduction in sexual anxiety, increased intimacy, better communication, and increased self-esteem even if the sexual complaint continues.[23]

Psychotherapy Approaches
Psychoanalytic Treatment

Classic psychoanalytic treatment is a process in which the patient engages in intensive long-term (multiple times a week) therapy. The unresolved conflicts, over time, get played out repeatedly within the therapeutic relationship. For example, the patient may express thoughts that indicate unprovoked hostility toward the analyst. Such feelings or expectations that are not directly related to the current situation are called transference. The analyst interprets the transference interactions to promote less dysfunctional ways of relating. Simply defined, the transference process, which is central to all important relationships, is what we expect from another person or situation. "Hope, wish, and fear are names for patterns of expectation that either develop directly through experience or are taught by example. Once established, these anticipatory configurations are mobilized in response to situations that resemble, or seem to resemble, the original conditions that gave rise to the pattern."[38] The erectile disorder may have served as a defense that may no longer be adaptive for the patient during a specific developmental phase.[20] Through the therapeutic alliance, "a patient learns to perceive himself differently; or, to say it another way, a transference pattern—an expectational set is altered through therapy."[39] This psychoanalytic approach has some drawbacks for the resolution of a sexual complaint. Treatment may take years before the erectile problem is resolved. Second, the stringent attribution of unconscious conflicts as the only causal explanation for sexual problems in the traditional analytic approach may limit the usefulness of this method, since it denies the relationship of overt reality factors in problem development. There are no sound empirical data demonstrating the effectiveness of analytic treatment for erectile disorders.[19,40–42]

Cognitive-Behavioral Treatment

Proponents of behavioral therapy see sexual activity as a discrete set of behaviors that can be changed by direct behavioral interventions. The behavior therapist might not work on the dyadic issues unless the relationship issues directly relate to the current erectile problem. Cognitive-behavioral therapy includes analysis of thoughts or internal dialogue associated with the sexual behaviors. This model would include interventions aimed at changing overt and covert behaviors simultaneously. The purpose of identifying the specific overt and covert determinants of sexual behavior is to design treatment approaches based on the patient's unique situation.

Individualized treatment approaches are more likely to be effective in reversing the problem than is a programmed treatment approach to all patients and every sexual complaint. Few therapists simply prescribe rote behavioral exercises. Interventions vary across therapist and the individual's unique set of variables associated with the disorder. The efficacy of behavioral and cognitive behavioral sex therapy is fairly well established for erectile difficulties.[23,25,43,44]

Over the years, the behavioral exercises first introduced by Masters and Johnson have seen a variety of shifts and modifications. Today, the behavioral approaches might include some combination of the following: skills training, basic sex education, cognitive restructuring, relaxation training, assertiveness training, individual therapy, marital or couple's therapy, communication training, and structured home practice assignments.

The goal of cognitive behavioral therapy, which usually occurs in a couples context, is to engender a sense of trust and safety between the couple, to decrease the fear of failure, and to shift attention away from performance or the fear of failure to the experience of sensory and sexual pleasure. This is usually accomplished by the prohibition of coitus and the prescription of home-based, graduated sexual learning experiences (exercises). Depending on the particular case, sexual education and couples therapy may play an important role.[45]

For a male patient who is erroneously convinced that his difficulty is physical and who cannot fathom the possibility of erectile problems having an interpersonal etiology, a different strategy may be effective. The clinician may choose not to confront the patient but to state that no organic etiology can be identified with current technology. The therapist might suggest that erectile problems are often worsened by stress. He or she may then try to relieve some of the self-imposed stress (performance anxiety) through reassurance, stating that this problem often resolves with time. The therapist might suggest that the patient refrain from coitus but continue with sexual foreplay and return in a month. In many cases, the removal of performance anxiety plus the continued stimulation of foreplay may lead the patient to disobey his therapist's recommendation and cure himself.

Proscription of intercourse is an example of a win–win intervention. Simply stated, the patient wins no matter what he does or does not do. If he adheres to the suggestion, he is complying with treatment, but if the patient engages in the forbidden behavior and is successful, he has experienced a positive sexual experience that will help in planning future interventions. If, on the other hand, he attempts unsuccessfully to engage in intercourse, the therapist can instruct the patient that he attempted intercourse too soon. This form of intervention reduces the likelihood of the patient's becoming more discouraged by his erectile problem. Such a negative outcome provides the therapeutic process information about what is going on so that new interventions can be designed.[46]

The proscription, or banning, of sexual intercourse is a component that was emphasized in Masters and Johnson's 2-week residential therapy program.[25,36] Some therapists routinely prohibit sexual intercourse during the initial phase of sex therapy. Tuthill succinctly describes the rationale.[47]

> When intercourse has failed, the patient must stop trying, and retrace the steps of courtship, which in some cases he may never have trod at all. . . . Often the first problem is to persuade them to spend enough time in bed together for spontaneous contact to take place. After a time the search for pleasure becomes his objective, and he forgets that he is trying to achieve intercourse. . . . The essence of treatment is the simple lesson that intercourse is a sensual pleasure or nothing.

Banning coitus may not work or be appropriate for everybody. Some authors suggest that coital prohibition may have a negative impact on the couple's sexual spontaneity and sexual activity, which may lead to a loss of sexual desire.[48] Lipsius suggests that the home practice sensate focus exercises be practiced primarily for pleasure and not intentionally as a prelude to intercourse. This reduces the goal-oriented sexual performance without interfering with spontaneity.[48]

Education is an important part of this model. Often, patients lack sexual skills to enhance arousal. Instructing the couple on skills that facilitate intercourse with a less than turgid erection can be helpful. For example, teaching the couple the stuffing method for intercourse, in which the man or woman manually stuffs the less rigid penis into the vagina, is sometimes helpful. The couple may need to be instructed on basic physiology and arousal strategies. For example, some women assume the man will become aroused with little direct stimulation from her. This situation may result in the man's having difficulty maintaining his erection. The couple might benefit from a discussion about what types of stimulation would be acceptable and arousing for each. If the woman is opposed to oral or manual stimulation of the penis, it may be helpful to suggest that the couple try a vibrator for more intense direct penile stimulation to enhance his erection.

Under the umbrella term of behavioral therapy, a variety of interventions can be found, such as cognitive restructuring, relaxation training, stress management, communication training, and general sex education. However, the behavioral literature is replete with such terms as "home assignments," sometimes called "pleasuring exercises," "sensate focus," and "behavioral tasks." These exercises serve many functions. The exercises provide a safe environment for the couple to learn a new way of relating to one another sexually. Generally, each partner takes turns in the exploration of each other's body, excluding breasts and genitals (alternating giving and receiving sensual pleasure). The focus is not on achieving an erection but rather on personal pleasure. The tasks provide an opportunity to communicate to one's partner what is arousing and what is a turnoff. Over the years, some couples get into set patterns of relating sexually, and often, therapy reveals that sexual repertoires that worked quite well when they were in their 20s are no longer very arousing. Trying to get the couple to build on their sexual repertoire and communicate directly what each finds arousing may result in a shift in emphasis from performance to increased sensual pleasures. This shift in focus may result in enhanced sexual arousal.

During the treatment sessions, the couples talk about their home exercises and reactions to them. Problems and experiences are explored, and alternative strategies are suggested. Over the course of treatment, the amount and type of genital exploration escalates. Intermittent penile caressing resulting in repeated tumescence and detumescence of the penis encourages the couple to experience the penis in various stages of turgidity without pressure to perform. The woman usually is instructed to stimulate the penis until the penis becomes firm. Once firm, she is to stop stimulation until detumescence occurs and then to begin stimulation again. This exercise demonstrates to the couple that if an erection is lost, it can be regained. This experience helps some men learn that without the stress of performance, they can become aware of sensual pleasure associated with erections. However, when the man tries to will an erection, he may have problems succeeding. The couple over time might move to vaginal containment with minimal thrusting with the woman in the superior position. This allows the man time to focus on sensations, and the woman can move gently to help to maintain the erection without speeding to orgasm. The sexual position then alternates, and the man controls his thrusting to orgasm.

Cognitive factors that may affect erectile disorders include persistent erroneous beliefs and assumptions about sexual performance.[38,45,49] A cognitive framework allows the therapist insight into irrational beliefs and expectations that may be reducing the ability to obtain and maintain erections. The cognitive framework provides a method of identifying thoughts, beliefs, worries, or the patient's internal dialogue (thoughts we verbalize to ourselves or self-statements) that are interfering with erectile capacity. The patient learns to identify dysfunctional cognitions, and therapy helps the man to change his internal self-statements or beliefs. For example, the patient might equate love, happiness, and self-esteem with his ability to obtain and maintain an erection. Helping such a patient broaden his definition of sex from intercourse exclusively to a wider range of behaviors that encompass relating intimately may facilitate his ability to experience erections sufficient for intercourse. The cognitive-behavioral framework aims to identify conditions that are interfering with the patient's ability to achieve an erection. For example, the patient might be attempting intercourse when stressed or fatigued. He might be attempting to perform in an environment not conducive to sexual arousal. Some men tune out all sexual thoughts or playfulness until they enter the bed and then expect to be able to perform at will with little foreplay or sexual priming, often resulting in erectile disappointments.

Self-observation often inhibits sexual arousal. Often the man is rating or judging his erection and thinking (cognitive self-statements) "I am not getting hard. . . . She is probably thinking there is something wrong with me. . . . I will not be able to keep my erection. . . . I can tell it's getting soft. . . . I won't be able to please her. . . ." "Regardless of the precipitating factors, most cases of male erectile disorder are maintained by interfering thoughts that may precede and occur during sexual relations."[50] Once the cognitive impediments are identified, the therapist can design interventions that will restructure or reframe the man's self-statements or cognitions. Such restructuring may help to increase arousal and facilitate the ability to obtain and maintain the erection (see Spence,[23] and Beck et al.[51] for reviews of cognitive restructuring). Ideally, the man would change his self-statements to "this feels good. . . . I know that my penis will become hard again. . . . This is exciting having her rub my penis this way. . . ." One goal of this type of intervention is to help the man expand on his ideas of what is sex. Most men with erectile problems equate sex with a hard-as-a-rock erection rather than a wide range of sensual experiences and behaviors.

Some couples have dysfunctional ways of communicating their needs or wishes. Other couples have an impoverished view of what constitutes adult sexual activities. Each member may be unable to self-generate sexually arousing interactions or positive erotic thoughts. Patients who are entrenched in dysfunctional thought processes and are unable to recall positive sexual cognitions or who have a very limited repertoire of sexual behaviors might benefit from the use of audiovisual aids. Some therapists suggest that, when appropriate, the patient or couple view or read erotic material as a means of exposure to sexual fantasies or examples of more arousing sexual thoughts.[52] A book or video may offer examples of sexual behavior that the couple finds arousing and would like to try but are too shy to state orally. After watching the video or reading erotic literature, the couple may be able to verbalize what they would like to try or what they found to be a turnoff. Given the reluctance of some couples to seek out videos or erotic literature, it is very helpful if the therapist has a prepared list of books and videos that can be found easily in public libraries and general video rental stores. The material, listed in a nonjudgmental and sensitive manner, would range from the romantic with no explicit sex scenes to more erotic stories with very explicit sexual activity. A couple may have to sample several different stories to find what is mutually arousing because of the personal nature and wide variation in what people find arousing.

Systemic Interventions

Systems theory embodies many of the earlier approaches (behavioral, cognitive, couples, and family) while encouraging analysis of broader interactional situations. Therapists using this approach do not ascribe blame to a single behavior or person. Instead, the therapist views the circular aspect of the couple's interaction of which the sexual problem is only one component. The therapist makes an assessment of this complicated situation by paying attention to the unspoken and elusive motivation that reinforces the problem. Often, the problem is not as simple as it may appear, and unilateral interventions may have negative interactional consequences. For example, a couple comes to the initial session holding hands, each showing concern for the other. The patient states that he cannot maintain his erections to complete sexual intercourse. This problem has developed over the past 3 years. Both the patient and his partner deny any stress or marital problems. They report seeing a variety of sex therapists. Multiple behavior interventions to restore his ability to maintain his erection were tried with no success. His wife supports the patient's current request to try the vacuum erectile device (VED). Because the

patient has experienced so many failures at sex therapy, the VED is a reasonable next step. The patient returns to the clinic alone, stating that although the VED worked he and his wife are very dissatisfied with treatment. This suggests that the problem is more complex than restoring the patient's erection. The couple is stuck in a self-perpetuating system of circular causality. The circular forces of this couple's system will defeat any intervention designed to restore his erections. A closer look at this system identifies where the couple is stuck. To be sexually functional, this man needs to feel desired by his partner and reassured of his masculine attractiveness. The woman believes that a good wife is always sexually available regardless of her level of sexual desire. He feels that she is never in the mood, and she feels righteous because she is always sexually available. Within this complicated system, the intervention would be to help each member be cognizant of what they want from each other and how they can stop sabotaging the other's needs. Interventions are needed to change the system.

Men with a complaint of erectile dysfunction often have a variety of more complicated dyadic issues that have an impact on sexual behaviors. However, even with the most sophisticated systematic approaches, not all sexual interactional problems are resolvable. For example, a man may no longer be sexually attracted to his partner. Although enhancing the general relationship may lead to a more pleasant situation, the erectile problem may continue. At times, the erectile disorder may serve as a positive adaptation for the couple, and attempting to remove the symptom may result in a patient leaving therapy. For example, the erectile dysfunction may serve to impose a comfortable distance for a couple who are ambivalent about or fear intimacy. The sexual dysfunction becomes the unspoken excuse that allows the couple to reduce anxiety-producing interactions and continue to develop other mutually agreeable aspects of the relationship, or the sexual dysfunction may provide the excuse to leave a relationship when it becomes too intense or engulfing.

The interactional aspect of systems theory provides multiple ways of identifying convoluted relationship situations. The clinician would attempt to identify unspoken beliefs or fears by concentrating on the couple's patterns of sexual interaction, general communication, independence and attachment needs, different needs for sharing and intimacy, attitudes regarding child rearing, sex role and role expectations, jealousy, outside interests, and power struggles in an attempt to restore sexual homeostasis. For example, a man with a long history of erectile disorders may have an unspoken concern about his sense of masculinity. He may

begin to expect rejection or ridicule from his partner because of the emphasis he places on his ability
to obtain and maintain an erection. This can result
in a circle of anxiety or fear of failure that results
in the man mentally removing himself from the
interaction by mentally observing his level of
arousal and the strength of his erection. This observation often results in loss of the erection, which
increases his performance anxiety and inhibits further arousal. Such a man may begin to avoid all
potential sexual encounters because of repeated
failures. The partner may begin to doubt her desirability when her partner no longer pursues her
or ignores all of her sexual overtures. Her sense
of femininity may be threatened, or she may suffer
a loss in self-esteem as she finds she is unable to
arouse her partner. Often, there is discord in non-
sexual activities, and communications are quite disturbed at this phase of the sexual problem. Couples
will often use the words "should" and "ought" to
describe expectations. For example, the man might
think "she should know what I find arousing" or
"she ought to give me more direct stimulation when
my penis becomes soft." Since most of us are not
clairvoyant, there is a need to learn how to communicate our wishes clearly and not depend on the
other partner's ability to read our mind.

Psychotherapy Summary

Psychotherapy for psychogenic erectile dysfunction consists of many approaches and formats.
Successful treatment often relates to a comprehensive biopsychosexual assessment of the problem and appropriate individualized interventions.
Treatment often is facilitated by involving the partner whenever possible. Treatment goals include
changing dysfunctional thoughts, behaviors, and
interactions that are found to inhibit sexual arousal.
The goal of treatment planning is to provide the
minimal interventions necessary to reverse the
problem.

DIRECT METHODS OF INTERVENTION

Invasive and noninvasive medical approaches to
psychogenic impotence have been proposed by
some clinicians under certain circumstances. The
direct methods can be an appropriate intervention
for men who continue to have erectile problems
after an adequate trial of psychotherapy. One ca-
veat of providing a medical approach exclusively
is the covert message given to the patient that his
problem is organic. One might better serve the
patient if the medical intervention is one component within a comprehensive biopsychosocial treatment approach. Because of prevailing financial

constraints, comprehensive programs are not always an option.

Patient satisfaction and compliance may be enhanced by identifying patients who might be dissatisfied with a direct method of producing an erection. Recognizing unrealistic expectations or beliefs of the patient or partner helps to identify
patients who might be at high risk for postinter-
ventional dissatisfaction. Asking the patient what
he expects from the vacuum pump or vasoactive
penile injections will help to determine the appro-
priateness of the proposed intervention. For example, if the man believes that all of his sexual
problems will be ameliorated with the vacuum
pump, he ultimately may be disappointed with
treatment. Patients who believe that their orgasms
will improve or their libido will increase often find
fault with the intervention. Having a reliable means
of obtaining an erection is no guarantee that the
partner will want to engage in sexual activity with
any greater frequency.

Ideally, the direct medical approach should help
with the restoration of self-confidence and reduce
performance anxiety. A man who has stopped attempting to have intercourse and is avoiding potential sexual encounters because of his fear of
failure may, theoretically, benefit from a direct and
reliable method of intervention. Helping the patient
understand how erectile problems develop and the
limitations of the proposed intervention may reduce
treatment disappointments. With a direct method,
he will know that he will have an erection. Such
knowledge may help him focus on the sensual experience of intercourse and away from his status
of erection. The goal would be to shift his attention
from "Will I get erect?" to "I am feeling good, this
is very arousing." A man who values a good-
enough erection (sufficient for penetration) rather
than one who is in search of the rock-hard erection
would have a better prognostic outlook from a medical intervention. A man whose focus is completely
on his penis and not on sensual pleasure or sexual
intimacy is very difficult to treat with a direct
method of intervention. Such a man is often dissatisfied with an erection that is judged to be 90%
full during a vasoactive diagnostic injection examination. However, a man who currently enjoys
sexual intimacy but lacks an erection sufficient for
successful intercourse would most likely be pleased
with direct medical intervention.

Vacuum Erection Device (VED)

The VED was approved by the FDA in 1982 as
a mechanical method of producing an erection.
This is an intervention that appears to be effective
in producing an erection for men with organic,
mixed, and psychogenic etiologies.[53-55] An inter-

esting report by Turner et al. suggests that spontaneous erections significantly improved in men who used the VED for longer than a year.[55] Koreman et al.[56] reported a significant improvement in penile–brachial pressure indexes in men using the vacuum device regularly for 6 months. Some of the men in the sample were able, on occasion, to have intercourse without using the device. High percentages (80% to 95%) of patient satisfaction have been reported in the literature.[54,55] However, more studies are needed to determine long-term satisfaction with the VED.[55,57,58]

Altof and Turner "suggest that prior to deciding on this option and/or purchasing the device a man and his partner should come in for a demonstration and teaching session. This meeting provides a better sense of whether and how the system will work."[59] The couple might first view a video before working with a clinician who would answer questions and educate the couple by recommending methods to circumvent the technical nuances of the VED. The erection produced by the VED differs from a spontaneous erection in several ways. The surface temperature of the penis is somewhat cooler than normal body temperature. Also, because the tumescence begins at the constricting band, the penis pivots at the base, which may require manual insertion of the penis for intercourse.[50,59]

There have been no reports of adverse psychologic sequelae when the VED was used by men who have a psychogenic etiology to their erectile disorder. Altof and Turner report "vacuum tumescence therapy with psychogenically dysfunctional patients (most of whom were in concomitant psychotherapy) indicated that these devices helped restore sexual confidence and moderate performance anxiety in approximately one-third of the sample."[59]

The recommended maximum time limit for the VED of 30 min may have an added therapeutic benefit for men with psychogenic erectile disorders. Many men delay using the device until they are closer to the time of penetration. When the main contributing factor is performance anxiety, the VED provides the man with erectile insurance. Hence, the man may engage in sexual foreplay knowing that if he does not have a spontaneous erection, he has the VED. The goal is to regain confidence and in time reduce the need for the VED. Unfortunately, if a man engages in foreplay and stops to use the VED, it may have a negative impact on the spontaneity of the couple's lovemaking, which eventually may result in a decreased sex drive. Single males without a steady partner often are reluctant to use the VED because it is cumbersome and is difficult to conceal from a new partner.

The VED offers a reliable temporary reversal of erectile difficulties. This device appears to be relatively safe and is noninvasive. From a systems perspective, ascertaining the man and his partner's expectations may reduce disappointment with this intervention. For example, a couple who expect that using the device will result in the resolution of marital discord may find that the psychosocial problems remain the same or worsen with the VED. Wincze and Carey suggest[50]

> The vacuum device may be used as a good diagnostic tool for implant candidates about whom there is some doubt. Because the vacuum device is noninvasive, there are fewer problems that may occur if the device does not work out. If a man and his partner have difficulty with or complaints about the use of the vacuum device, it is likely that they would also have difficulty with the implant.

Vasoactive Therapy

The preceding section on the VED addressed some of the basic issues regarding direct methods of intervention. Men who do not have a steady partner often opt for vasoactive therapy, since it is easier to conceal than the VED with constriction band. There is little evidence regarding the long-term negative psychologic sequelae from intracorporeal injections. Clinicians present strong arguments in favor of and against the therapeutic benefit derived from vasoactive injections for psychogenic erectile problems.

Wincze and Carey's clinical observations[50] suggest that loss of desire and ability to reach orgasm occur in some men using injection therapy. They also report a concern about the partner's diminished level of arousal and desire when the man uses the self-injection method of treatment. Suggesting the possibility of a negative impact on the partner, "for most individuals, it is very arousing and affirming to watch their partner's arousal grow as a result of their own sexual attraction or skills. If erections are caused by injection rather than foreplay, then a primary source of psychological feedback may be lost."[50] Continued reliance on the direct method of intervention may result in a decrease in sexual desire and arousal in some partners.[50,58–60]

The potential for psychologic or intrapersonal problems is increased when such interventions are given without adequate counseling or patient education. The man has the means to induce a reliable erection when he is not fully sexually aroused, and this might result in a less than optimal sexual experience.[60] If this becomes a regular pattern, the man might experience a decline in sexual desire and begin to avoid all forms of sexual behavior. Clinicians who anticipate such a problem can work with the patient before implementing the intervention by teaching the patient to be aware of his true level of desire. Such a patient might benefit from prohibition of intercourse when his internal dialogue contains "ought" or "should" regarding initiating sexual intercourse. He should be instructed not to initiate sexual intercourse until his sexual desire or drive is quite high. This is often difficult for many men, who believe that a man should be able to become fully aroused at will and with little foreplay.[38,45,50,60] Patients whose history suggests a good premorbid sexual relationship would probably benefit and have fewer problems with a more direct approach to psychogenic erectile problems.

Penile Implants

Patient selection for the various direct methods of treating psychogenic erectile disorders is not based on empirical studies but rather on clinical wisdom. Within the field of sexual treatment, one can find a spectrum of attitudes and biases. Many of the direct methods lack long-term follow-up to suggest set guidelines for determining who is a good candidate.

Most urologists would be hesitant to suggest a surgical procedure, such as the penile implant, as a first intervention for a man with a presumptive psychogenic etiology. Some surgeons require a psychiatric evaluation before implantation of a penile prosthesis. There is little agreement on what should be included in the evaluation. The range of psychosexual evaluations within the field is quite broad. Some evaluations include only a brief mental status examination. Another approach might be so comprehensive as to create a time barrier based on arbitrary paternalistic biases. For example, the evaluation may require that a man receive an extensive psychologic assessment, participate in some prescribed psychotherapy, or participate in a fair trial of yohimbine, followed by the VED or injection therapy before a surgical intervention is considered. These treatment protocols are determined by clinical wisdom, since there are no empirical studies to support the choice or order of interventions for psychogenic erectile disorder. Generally, most centers require some psychologic assessment to determine who might be poor candidates for surgery.[60-62] A poor candidate is a man who because of lack of interpersonal and communication skills, avoidance behavior, low sexual desire, ejaculatory problems, poor self-image, marital discord, unrealistic expectations, or a combination of these factors may be dissatisfied with the implant.[60,62] Determining the individual's risk factor and treating each aspect of the potential problem before direct surgical intervention might reduce patient dissatisfaction (Table 6–3).[60]

Pharmacotherapy

The major drug used to treat psychogenic impotence in the United States is yohimbine. A number of controlled studies[63,64] have indicated moderate efficacy in the treatment of psychogenic impotence. To date, no psychiatric contraindication or adverse psychiatric consequence has been iden-

TABLE 6–3
Common Risk Factors for Postimplantation Sexual Dissatisfaction

Risk Factor	*Impact After Surgery*
Belief that size of penis is crucial in sex	Disappointment with penile length, girth, or rigidity
Belief that foreplay is a nuisance	Inability of either partner to reach orgasm because intercourse is begun without high sexual arousal
Poor sexual communication	Inability to modify sexual caressing or intercourse techniques to compensate for differences between penile prosthesis and a natural erection
Premature ejaculation	Intercourse still is too brief for satisfaction, or man feels compelled to continue thrusting without arousal
Decreased orgasmic intensity	Orgasms remain disappointing to the man
Male low sexual desire	Frequency of sex remains very low
Female low sexual desire	Bickering about the frequency of sex increases, and the husband may initiate an affair
Untreated postmenopausal vaginal atrophy	The woman has severe dyspareunia
Erectile dysfunction was psychogenic	Because psychogenic problems often serve a function, a technical cure destabilizes the relationship or leads to a new sexual problem, such as psychogenic pain or inability to reach orgasm

From Shover LR. Sex therapy for the penile prosthesis recipient. Urol Clin North Am 16:91–98, 1989.

tified. Thus, many centers use this as a first-line intervention for patients who are resistant to the concept of psychotherapy.

SUMMARY

Men seek treatment for erectile disorders from a variety of medical specialists. The man will often ask specifically for a means to ensure an erection, which does not include psychotherapy. Pharmacotherapy may be a reasonable intervention, but it is of moderate efficacy for reversing erectile disorders.[63-65] Technology is available to provide a reliable erection. However, men who use one of the new technologies to induce an erection (vasoactive injections, vacuum devices, penile implant) may continue to return to the treating physician to voice his dissatisfaction with his erections and treatment. Because men with a primary diagnosis of psychogenic erectile disorder seldom accept a good-enough erection and are looking for a rock-hard erection, it is very important to screen patients for their expectations before treatment.[60,61] There are potentially many reasons why such a man might be disappointed with his ability to induce an erection at will. Some men may be engaging in sex when they are not mentally aroused or when experiencing low sexual desire and, therefore, may report the sexual encounter as being unfulfilling. Some men see foreplay as unnecessary given their ability to induce an erection using the VED or vasoactive injections. A technologically induced erection may result in a loss in sexual desire and arousal in either the patient or partner, and this may increase marital discord. With some men, the new technology does not reduce performance anxiety. Such men may never attempt intercourse without the vacuum device or self-injections. However, other men find that the new technologies enhance their sense of self-esteem and reduce performance anxiety, which in time may decrease their reliance on the intervention.[50,59]

There are few data regarding psychologic harm from the new technologies. However, it makes clinical sense to begin treatment with the most noninvasive methods and, after a fair trial, continue to the next level of intervention. Assessing the patient's and partner's expectations before the intervention may help to reduce posttreatment dissatisfaction. Telling the patient and partner the advantages and disadvantages of the intervention may reduce some of the postprocedure problems. One consideration that comes into play is cost. Psychotherapy may require many visits that may not be covered by the patient's insurance. The vacuum device initially is a considerable expense when compared to self-injections, but eventually, the VED becomes more cost efficient.

SPECIAL SITUATIONS

Some men who experience erectile disorders may be in situations that require some modification of standard treatment approaches. While the basic treatment principles are maintained, slightly different strategies and knowledge may be required when working with special populations. For example, a man without a steady partner may avoid relationships because he fears rejection, or he may not know how to conceal the vasoactive injection vials or VED from a new partner. A gay couple may be experiencing problems maintaining an erection because they find safe sex less arousing. A physically disadvantaged man may require additional help circumventing obstacles relating to a lack of dexterity or prosthetic devices. These are important treatment issues that are beyond the scope of this text. Texts that provide comprehensive information regarding special treatment issues are available.[50,66-70]

CONCLUSION

No matter what intervention is implemented to reverse erectile problems, the difficulty may persist. Although the chief complaint suggests that the man is sufficiently bothered by the problem to use help, many men will not be compliant. Men who are referred to sex counselors fail to make any appointments. Some men who have received a reliable method of obtaining an erection (VED, vasoactive injections, penile implant) may return to complain about their erections or may drop out of treatment without explanation. When all interventions fail, it may be useful to reexamine the psychosocial conditions to identify the potential function being served by this symptom. One might question whether the problem protects the man from becoming involved. One might hypothesize that the erectile problem is a way of expressing anger or dominance over his partner. However, as therapists and surgeons, we need to accept the humbling reality that our best intentions and our most efficient technologic advancements will not reverse all complaints of psychogenic erectile failure.

REFERENCES

1. Freud S. A child is being beaten: a contribution to the study of the origin of sexual perversions. In: Strachey J ed and trans. The Standard Edition of the Complete Psychological Works of Sigmund Freud. London: Hogarth Press. 1955; 17:175–204.
2. Tyler EA. Sexual-incapacity therapy. In: Freedman DX, Dyrud JE, eds. American Handbook of Psychiatric Treatment. New York: Basic Books, 1975.
3. Kaplan HS. The New Sex Therapy. New York: Brunner/Mazel, 1974.
4. Wagner G, Green R. Impotence, Physiological, Psy-

chological, Surgical Diagnosis and Treatment. New York: Plenum Press, 1981.

5. Strauss EB. Impotence from a psychiatric standpoint. Br Med J 1:697, 1950.
6. Martin LM. Erectile impotence: it can be highly treatable. Geriatrics 35:79, 1980.
7. Spark RF, White RA, Connolly PB. Impotence is not always psychogenic. JAMA 243:750, 1980.
8. Segraves RT, Schoenberg HW, Zarins CK, et al. Characteristics of erectile dysfunction as a function of medical care system entry point. Psychosom Med 43:227, 1981.
9. Karacan I, Salis PJ, Williams RL. The role of the sleep laboratory in diagnosis and treatment of impotence. In: Williams RL, Karacan I, eds. Sleep Disorders, Diagnosis and Treatment. New York: John Wiley, 1982.
10. Melman A, Kaplan D, Redfield J. Evaluation of the first 70 patients in the Center for Male Sexual Dysfunction of Beth Israel Medical Center. J Urol 131:53, 1984.
11. Melman A, Tiefer L, Pedersen R. Evaluation of the first 406 patients in urology department-based center for male sexual dysfunction. Urology 32:6, 1988.
12. Segraves KB, Segraves RT. Multiple phase sexual dysfunction. J Sex Educ Ther 17:153, 1991.
13. Segraves KB, Segraves RT. Hypoactive sexual desire disorder: prevalence and co-morbidity in 906 subjects. J Sex Marital Ther 17:55, 1991.
14. Derogatis LR, Melisaratos N. The DSFI: a multidimensional measure of sexual functioning, J Sex Marital Ther 5:244, 1979.
15. Derogatis LR, Meyer JK. A psychological profile of the sexual dysfunctions. Arch Sex Behav 8:201, 1979.
16. Kockott G, Feil W, Revenstorf D, et al. Symptomatology and psychological aspects of male sexual inadequacy: results of an experimental study. Arch Sex Behav 9:457, 1980.
17. Abel GG, Becker JU, Cunningham-Rathner J, et al. Differential diagnosis of impotence in diabetics. Neurol Urodynamics 1:57, 1982.
18. Segraves KA, Segraves RT, Schoenberg HW. Use of sexual history to differentiate organic from psychogenic impotence. Arch Sex Behav 16:125, 1987.
19. Reynolds BS. Psychological treatment models and outcome results for erectile dysfunction: a critical review. Psychol Bull 84:1218, 1977.
20. Levine SB, Altof SE. The pathogenesis of psychogenic erectile dysfunction. J Sex Educ Ther 17:251, 1991.
21. Wolpe J. Psychotherapy by Reciprocal Inhibition. Stanford, Calif: Stanford University Press, 1958.
22. Gambrill ED. Behavior Modification: Handbook of Assessment, Intervention, and Evaluation. San Francisco: Jossey-Bass Publishers, 1978:923.
23. Spence SH. Psychosexual Therapy: A Cognitive-Behavioral Approach. Psychology and Health Series 6. Marcer C, series ed. New York: Chapman & Hall, 1991.
24. Dengrove E. Therapeutic approaches of impotence in the male. III: Behavior therapy of impotence. J Sex Res 7:177, 1971.

25. Masters WH, Johnson VE. Human Sexual Inadequacy. Boston: Little, Brown, and Co, 1970.
26. Murphy CV, Mikulas WL. Behavior features and deficiencies of the Masters and Johnson program. Psychol Rec 24:221, 1974.
27. Segraves RT. Marital Therapy: A Combined Psychodynamic Behavioral Approach. New York: Plenum Press, 1982.
28. Bowen M. Family Therapy in Clinical Practice. New York: Jason Aronson, 1978.
29. Verhulst J, Heinman J. An interactional approach to sexual dysfunction. Am J Fam Ther 7:19, 1979.
30. LoPiccolo J. Management of psychogenic erectile failure. In: Tanagho E, Lue T, McClure R, eds. Contemporary Management of Impotence and Infertility. Baltimore, Williams & Wilkins, 1988.
31. Segraves R, Schoenberg HW, Zarins CK. Referral of impotent patients to a sexual dysfunction clinic. Arch Sex Behav 11:521, 1982.
32. Tiefer L, Melman A. Adherence to recommendations and improvement over time in men with erectile dysfunction evaluated in a urology department. Arch Sex Behav 16:301, 1987.
33. Heiman JR, LoPiccolo J. Clinical outcome of sex therapy. Arch Gen Psychiatry 40:443, 1983.
34. Annon JS. The behavioral treatment of sexual problems. In: Brief Therapy. Honolulu: Enabling Systems, 1974, vol 1.
35. Ellis A. Treatment of erectile dysfunction. In: Leiblum SR, Pervin LA, eds. Principles and Practices of Sex Therapy. New York: Guilford Press, 1980.
36. Kolodny RC, Masters WH, Johnson VE. Textbook of Sexual Medicine. Boston, Little, Brown, and Co, 1979.
37. Kolodny RC. Evaluating sex therapy: process and outcome at the Masters and Johnson Institute. J Sex Res 17:301, 1981.
38. Zilbergeld B. The New Male Sexuality. New York: Bantam, 1992.
39. Basch FB. Doing Psychotherapy. New York: Basic Books, 1980:35–36.
40. Cooper AJ. Treatment of male potency disorders: the present status. Psychosomatics 12:335, 1971.
41. LoPiccolo J, Hogan D. Multidimensional behavioral treatment of sexual dysfunction. In: Pomerleau OF, Brady JP, eds. Behavioral Medicine. Baltimore: Williams & Wilkins, 1979.
42. Wright S, Perreault R, Mathieu M. Treatment of sexual dysfunction: a review. Arch Gen Psychiatry 34:881, 1977.
43. Marks IM. Review of behavioral psychotherapy 2: sexual disorders. Am J Psychiatry 138:750, 1981.
44. Meyer JK. Training for the treatment of sexual disorders. In: Meyer JK, Schmidt CW, Wise TN (eds): Management of Sexual Disorders. Baltimore: Williams & Wilkins, 1983:368–379.
45. McCarthy BW: Erectile dysfunction and inhibited sexual desire: cognitive-behavioral strategies. J Sex Educ Ther 18:22, 1992.
46. Fennell MJV. Depression. In: Hawton K, Salkovskis PM, Kirk J, Clark DM, eds. Cognitive Behavior Therapy for Psychiatric Problems: A Practical Guide. Oxford: Oxford University Press, 1989.

47. Tuthill JF. Impotence. Lamcet 128:124, 1955.
48. Lipsius SH. Prescribing sensate focus without proscribing intercourse. J Sex Marital Ther 13:106, 1987.
49. Zilbergeld B. Male Sexuality. New York: Dell, 1978.
50. Wincze JP, Carey MP. Sexual Dysfunction: A Guide for Assessment and Treatment. New York: Guilford Press, 1991:114–131.
51. Beck AT, Rush AJ, Shaw BG, Emery G. Cognitive Therapy of Depression. London: Wiley, 1979.
52. Bjorksten OJW. Sexually graphic material in the treatment of sexual disorders. In: Meyer JK, ed. Clinical Management of Sexual Disorders. Baltimore: Williams & Wilkens, 1976.
53. Cooper AJ. Preliminary experience with a vacuum tumescence device (VCD) as a treatment for impotence. J Psychosom Res 31:413, 1987.
54. Nadig P. Six years experience with the vacuum tumescence device. Int J Impot Res 1:55, 1989.
55. Turner LA, Altof SE, Levine SB, et al. Treating erectile dysfunction with external vacuum device: impact upon sexual psychological and marital functioning. J Urol 144:79, 1990.
56. Koreman S, Viosca S, Kaiser F, el al. Use of a vacuum tumescence device in the management of impotence. J Am Geriatr Soc 38:217, 1990.
57. Tiefer L, Pedersen B, Melman A. Psychosocial follow-up of penile prosthesis implant patients and partners. J Sex Marital Ther 14:184, 1988.
58. Pederson B, Tiefer L, Ruiz M, Melman A. Evaluation of patients and partners one to four years following penile prosthesis surgery. J Urol 139:956, 1988.
59. Altof SE, Turner LA. Self-injection therapy and external vacuum devices in the treatment of erectile dysfunction: methods and outcomes. In: Rosen RC, Leiblum SR, eds. Erectile Disorders: Assessment and Treatment. New York: Guilford Press, 1992:229.
60. Shover LR. Sex therapy for the penile prosthesis recipient. Urol Clin North Am 16:91, 1989.
61. Tiefer L, Moss S, Melman A. Follow-up of patients and partners experiencing penile prosthesis malfunction and corrective surgery. J Sex Marital Ther 17:113, 1991.
62. Tiefer L. In pursuit of the perfect penis: the medicalization of male sexuality. Am Behav Sci 29:579, 1986.
63. Riley AJ, Goodman RE, Kellett JM, Orr R. Double-blind trial of yohimbine hydrochloride in the treatment of erection inadequacy. J Sex Marital Ther 4:17, 1989.
64. Sussett JG, Tessier CD, Wincze J, et al. Effect of yohimbine hydrochloride on erectile impotence: a double-blind study. J Urol 141:1360, 1989.
65. Reid K, Morales A, Harris C, et al. Double-blind trial of yohimbine in treatment of psychogenic impotence. Lancet 2:421, 1987.
66. Shover LR, Jensen SB. Sexuality and Chronic Illness: A Comprehensive Approach. New York: Guilford Press, 1988.
67. Rosen RC, Leiblum SR, eds. Erectile Disorders: Assessment and Treatment. New York: Guilford Press, 1992.
68. McCarthy BW. Treatment of erectile dysfunction with single men. In: Rosen RC, Leiblum SR, eds. Erectile Disorders: Assessment and Treatment. New York: Guilford Press, 1992:313–340.
69. Reynolds B. An audio tape adjunct in the treatment of sexual dysfunction in men without partners. J Sex Educ Ther 18:35, 1992.
70. Schover LR. Erectile failure and chronic illness. In: Rosen RC, Leiblum SR, eds. Erectile Disorders: Assessment and Treatment. New York: Guilford Press, 1992:341–367.

CHAPTER 7

Nonvascular Causes of Impotence

Richard E. Berger

Ivan Rothman

Gilbert Rigaud

Penile erection is produced by a complex series of events involving cognition, peripheral sensory input, central and peripheral autonomic nervous events, and hormonal and vascular events. Many of the vascular factors are discussed in other chapters of this book. In this chapter, we discuss some of the possible nonvascular causes of erectile dysfunction. These include chronic disease, diabetes mellitus, central nervous system diseases, and the effects of aging. We also discuss the tests available to assess neurologic function as it relates to erectile physiology.

NEUROPHYSIOLOGY OF ERECTION

The neural mechanisms responsible for erection in man are poorly understood. This is especially true in the understanding of the central processing of sexual stimuli. Peripherally, the penis is innervated by both divisions of the autonomic nervous system as well as by somatic sensory nerves (Fig. 7–1). Sensory innervation to the penis is provided primarily by the pudendal nerve. The pudendal nerve arises from the S2–S4 segments of the spinal cord in Onuf's nucleus. It passes between the coccygeus and pyriformis muscles and leaves the pelvis through the greater sciatic foramen. It then crosses the ischial spine and reenters the pelvis through the lesser sciatic foramen. The pudendal nerve leaves the pelvis again via Alcock's canal and splits into a sensory branch to the penis (dorsal nerve of the penis) and motor branches to the rectum and bulbocavernosus and isciocavernosus muscles (perineal nerve).[1] The dorsal nerve of the penis runs on the dorsum of the penis laterally to the glans. It supplies the skin of the dorsal and lateral aspects of the shaft and the glans penis. This nerve makes an important contribution to sexual function, and its interruption in animal studies produces significant sexual dysfunction[2] (Fig. 7–2).

The perineal nerve also provides sensory afferents to the penis. It is said to terminate in the urethral mucous membrane and has been shown to innervate the skin of the urethral aspect of the penile shaft, the ventral glans, and perimeatal tissue.[3] Other sensory fibers come from the ilioinguinal nerve and provide innervation to the skin of the ventral base of the penis along with the anterior half of the scrotum.

Motor innervation is provided by both parts of the autonomic system. Stimulation of parasympathetics in animal studies invariably result in erection, whereas stimulation of sympathetics causes detumescence.[4] Parasympathetic innervation originates in the intermediolateral gray matter of the spinal cord at the S2–S4 levels. These fibers exit through the anterior foramina of S2–S4 (nervi erigenti) and join the fibers from the hypogastric nerve (sympathetics) to form the pelvic plexus. The pelvic plexus lies over the lateral aspect of the rectum and innervates the rectum, bladder, prostate, seminal vesicles, and penis. The most caudal fibers travel along the posterolateral aspect of the prostate to innervate the corpora of the penis (cavernous nerves). At the level of the prostatic urethra, the cavernous nerves are quite distant from the prostatic capsule. However, they travel toward the apex of the prostate and lie only a few millimeters away at the 5 and 7 o'clock positions.[5] The cavernous nerves form several bundles on each side of the urethra between the 3 and 9 o'clock positions just external to the striated muscles. From the membranous urethra, fibers of the cavernous nerves penetrate the tunica albuginea of the corpus spongiosum to innervate the vasculature and erectile tissue of the corpus spongiosum and glans penis. The remaining fibers from the cavernous nerves ascend gradually toward the 1 and 11 o'clock positions, where the crura of the corpora cavernosa converge to the midline. These nerves then penetrate the corpora cavernosa to supply the cavernous

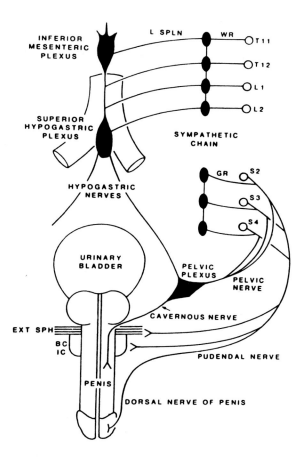

Figure 7–1. Diagram showing the sympathetic, parasympathetic, and somatic efferent pathways to the penis. L SPLN, lumbar splanchnic nerves; GR, gray rami; WR, white rami; BC, bulbocavernosus muscle; IC, ischiocavernosus muscle; EXT SPH, external urinary sphincter. (From DeGroat W, Steers WW. Neuroanatomy and neurophysiology of penile erection. In: Tanago EA, Lue TF, McClure RD, eds. Contemporary Management of Impotence and Infertility. © 1988, the Williams & Wilkins Co., Baltimore.)

vein and terminal branches of the urethral, dorsal, and deep dorsal penile arteries.[6]

Sympathetic innervation of the penis originates in the intermediolateral gray matter of the spinal cord at the T10–L2 levels. These fibers course retroperitoneally and condense into the superior hypogastric plexus (presacral nerve) located just inferior to the aortic bifurcation. Fibers leave the superior hypogastric plexus as the paired hypogastric nerves, which fuse distally and then enter the pelvic plexus (inferior hypogastric plexus). There,

sympathetic fibers mix with parasympathetic fibers and exit as part of the cavernous nerve.

Two kinds of penile erection have been recognized: reflexogenic and psychogenic. Trauma to the spinal cord below the thoracolumbar region results in loss of reflex erection but preservation of psychogenic erections. With higher cord lesions, reflex erection is maintained but psychogenic erection is lost, suggesting the presence of a reflex center for erections located in the sacral cord.[7] This was first demonstrated by the classic experiment of Roos

Figure 7–2. Innervation of the glans of the penis. (From Kaneko S, Bradley WE. Penile electrodiagnosis: penile peripheral innervation. Urology 30:210–212, © Williams & Wilkins, 1987.)

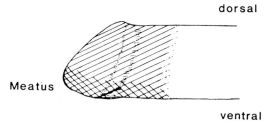

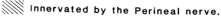

Innervated by the Dorsal nerve of the Penis.

Innervated by the Perineal nerve.

and Bard in cats.[8] Although psychogenic erection seems to be mediated via autonomic pathways, the center for psychogenic erection remains unclear. Several cerebrocortical and subcortical areas have been demonstrated to affect erections and sexual function in general. In man, temporal lobe seizures have been associated with hyposexual and hypersexual behavior.[9] Klüver and Bucy demonstrated the role of the temporal lobe in sexual function. Monkeys demonstrated increased heterosexual, homosexual, and autosexual behavior following bilateral temporal lobectomy.[10] McLean et al. demonstrated positive loci for erection in the gyrus rectus of the cerebral cortex, the cyngulate gyrus, paraventricular nucleus of the hypothalamus, and mammilary bodies.[11,12]

DIAGNOSTIC TESTS FOR NEUROLOGIC FUNCTION IN IMPOTENT MEN

Although great advances have been made in electrodiagnosis and imaging of the nervous system, history and neurologic examination remain the mainstays of the neurologic diagnosis of impotence. Since erection is a complex process involving multiple parts of the nervous system, the sensory, motor, and autonomic systems must all be addressed in the physical examination.[13] From the findings on history and physical examination, sophisticated neurophysiologic and anatomic studies may be performed to further objectify and delineate lesions in the nervous system. The reader is referred to textbooks on neurologic examination.[13]

The association of a neurologic finding with impotence does not mean that it is the decisive or even important factor in the impotence. Many men with neurologic findings also have vascular abnormalities responsible for or contributing to erectile difficulties. Men with physical disorders known to be causally linked to the development of impotence may develop psychogenic impotence. The symptoms the patient describes should prove consistent with diagnosed physiologic abnormalities to be considered significant. Furthermore, therapy does not necessarily follow from diagnosis. Treatments should be found that are compatible with the patient's outlook and lifestyle.

SOMATIC TESTS OF NEUROLOGIC FUNCTION
Vibratory Testing

Rowland[14] tested vibrotactile and electrical stimulation thresholds in the fingertips and ventral surface of the penis. He found that these thresholds were lowest in youngest subjects and higher for aging and diabetic subjects. Others have noted,

however, that vibration fibers are generally of large diameter, whereas autonomic fibers are very small in diameter. Abnormalities of vibration would, therefore, imply coexistence of a large fiber neuropathy as well as a small fiber neuropathy. DeTejada and Goldstein have found vibratory testing useful in predicting abnormal evoked potentials.[15]

Nerve Conduction of the Dorsal Nerve of the Penis

Nerve conduction velocity can be measured in somatic nerves throughout the body. The penis has its somatic innervation via the dorsal nerve of the penis, the perineal nerve, and the ilioinguinal nerve. The dorsal nerve of the penis runs from the base of the penis to the glans and supplies both the dorsal and lateral aspect of the glans penis (Fig. 7–2). This nerve has been shown to be important in sexual behavior in animals.[16] Sensation to the glans penis may be adversely affected by trauma, peripheral neuropathy, or aging. Abnormalities in dorsal nerve conduction would reflect clinical loss of sensation in the penis. This may result in loss of ability to maintain an erection during waking hours while having normal nocturnal erections.

The function of the dorsal nerve may be determined by measuring conduction velocity. Metal electrodes are placed on the dorsum of the penis at the base and the tip or glans in pairs 15 to 20 mm apart. The referential electrodes of the glans are placed distal to the active ones, and those at the base are placed proximally. The ground wire, which is approximately 5 mm wide, is wrapped around the middle of the penile shaft. Gentle stretching of the penis is necessary during this procedure. Square wave impulses with a duration of 0.1 msec with a frequency of 1 Hz are applied to one set of electrodes. The amplitude should be 1.5 to 2 times sensory threshold and up to 200 V. The potential of the electrode is recorded after an average of 30 sweeps. The average value of nerve conduction using such testing is 38 ± 5 m/sec.[17]

Somatosensory Evoked Pudendal Potentials

Somatosensory pudendal-evoked potentials (pudendal SSEPs) evaluate the ability of the nerves in the penis, pelvis, spinal cord, and brain to conduct impulses (Fig. 7–3). Stimulation is supplied to the penis at a rate of 1.5 to 4.7 Hz.[18,19] Intensities should be 2.5 times the threshold. Recordings can be made from a single channel that can be placed 2 cm posterior to the C_z electroencephalogram position in the midline site. Recording electrodes also

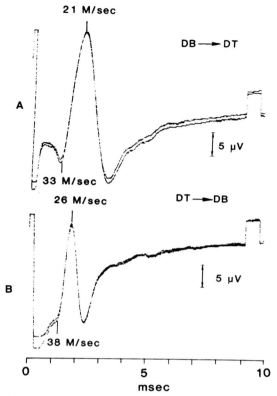

Figure 7–3. Orthodromic and antidromic evoked action potentials of dorsal nerve of penis in an 86-year-old man with hypertension. **A,** Antidromic measurement. NCV-DNP-takeoff: 33 m/sec, NCV-DNP-N1: 12 m/sec. **B,** Orthodromic measurement. NCV-DNP-takeoff: 38 m/sec, NCV-DNP-N1: 26 m/sec. (From Kaneko S, Bradley WE. Penile electrodiagnosis: penile peripheral innervation. Urology 30:210–212, © Williams & Wilkins, 1987.)

can be placed on either side of the center, but maximum response is in the midline.[20] The dorsal nerve SSEP probably has at least three relay sites in the sacral cord, thalamus, and sensory cortex. This test is usually not used for screening but to provide objective evidence for confirmation of an abnormal physical examination. The average conduction time is 23.5 m/sec, with a range of 21 to 29.1.[21] These latencies are about the same as tibial SSEPs.[22] This test is often delayed in spinal diseases, such as multiple sclerosis.[23–26] Most men with abnormal SSEPs also have abnormalities on physical examination. Parys et al. suggested that autonomic fibers also are commonly involved in patients with abnormal penile SSEPs. This is because the pudendal plexus[27] is mixed autonomic and somatic, and patients with lesions of one system often have lesions of the other.

Bulbocavernosus Reflex

The bulbocavernosus reflex is performed by stimulating the penis and recording over the bulbocavernosus muscle. This reflex can measure abnormalities in the sensory somatic peripheral systems as well as the spinal cord. After its first description in 1967,[28] for many years the bulbocavernosus reflex was considered valuable in the investigation of erectile failure. The reflex is thought to be polysynaptic.[29–31] The test is performed by stimulating the penis with ring electrodes around the shaft or by using a hand-held bipolar stimulator.[24,30,32–34] Recording from the bulbocavernosus muscle may be by needle electrodes or skin electrodes.[30,32,33,35–37] Early studies showed that this reflex was prolonged in men with peripheral neuropathy.[32,38] However, response was normal in other patients who were known to have neurogenic impotence. The response can be abnormally prolonged in men with normal erections.[35,39] Lavoisier et al.[35] measured bulbocavernosus reflex in 90 men and cast doubt on the usefulness of this reflex. Nineteen had abnormal bulbocavernosus latencies of greater than 45 msec. Of these 19, 8 had abnormal NPT tests. The neurophysiologic pathways of the bulbocavernosus reflex are not those thought to be of erection. Penile erection results from increased sinusoidal relaxation resulting from sympathetic and parasympathetic nervous systems.[40,41] The bulbocavernosus reflex tests somatic sensation. The minimal latencies of the bulbocavernosus reflex result from impulses in the largest myelinated fibers, both afferent and efferent. These have conduction losses 10 to 15 times faster than those of autonomic fibers. An abnormal bulbocavernosus reflex, therefore, probably represents a coexisting large fiber disorder and not a small fiber neuropathy of the autonomic nervous system affecting penile erection.

Sphincter Electromyography

Sphincter electromyography occasionally may be useful in patients suspected of having multiple system atrophy. Many men with this disease have a long history of impotence.[42] Onuf's nucleus and the anterior horn cells of the spinal cord innervate the striated sphincter. In multiple system atrophy, these cells are selectively lost.[18,43] Prolongation of motor units in the urethral and anal sphincters usually can be demonstrated.[25,44] These units are not lost in Parkinson's disease, which is common in the differential diagnosis.[42] Normal duration of the motor units is 8 msec. In multiple system atrophy, these are in excess of 20 msec. This test is most useful in patients with bladder symptoms, postural hypertension, and possibly mild parkinsonism.

AUTONOMIC NERVOUS SYSTEM TESTS

The autonomic nervous system reacts to many diseases that affect small nerves, the most commonly known of which is diabetes mellitus.[45] Risk factors for the development of diabetic neuropathy and impotence include symptomatic neuropathy, claudication, retinopathy, poor diabetes control, age, and alcohol intake. Most autonomic function tests are aimed at determining general autonomic function. Abnormalities are taken to represent generalized dysfunction, including the autonomic nerves going to the penis, but this has seldom been proven. These autonomic function tests include heart rate changes with Valsalva maneuver and deep breathing and postural change in blood pressure on standing. A summary of some autonomic tests is given in Table 7–1.

R-R Interval Testing

R-R interval testing measures variation in heart rate with inspiration, expiration, and Valsalva. This variation is due to both the sympathetic nervous system (SNS) and the parasympathetic nervous system (PNS). Studies should be performed in the morning after an overnight 8-h fast in a quiet, relaxed atmosphere. The patient should avoid tobacco products for 8 h, alcohol for 12 h, and over-the-counter medicines for 8 h. The patient should not have experienced vigorous exercise or severe emotional upset in the last 24 h. Diabetics should not have taken insulin for at least 8 h and should not have had a hypoglycemic episode in the last 8 h.[46] Beta blockage with propanolol is used to block effects of the SNS when the PNS needs to be studied. Heart rate variation with breathing is due to autonomic reflexes. Tidal volume expands lungs, which activate stretch receptors in the lung, chest wall, and heart chambers and stimulate afferent nerves (the vagus) to the brainstem and the nucleus solitarius. Efferent signals then decrease PNS tone and increase SNS tone by sending impulse down the efferent vagus and cervicothoracic sympathetic nerves, respectfully. These nerves terminate in the heart. The variation in heart rate with inspiration and expiration is measured by (1) standard deviation, (2) mean circular resultant, (3) maximum minus minimum heart rate for each breath, (4) expiration/inspiration ratio (E:I), and (5) Holter monitoring. The mean circular resultant method is not linked to intrinsic heart rate, is affected minimally by premature ventricular contractions (PVCs), and is not affected by change in average heart rate during the study and, therefore, may be the best method. The PNS contributes the major effect on R-R variation in the resting state. R-R variation is age-dependent and dependent somewhat on ideal weight, as PNS activity is reduced in obese individuals.[47]

Orthostatic Hypotension

Orthostatic hypotension is one of the hallmarks of severe autonomic dysfunction. This probably stems from a defect in the SNS. Normally, heart rate response to standing consists of tachycardia at 3 and 12 sec, followed by bradycardia at 20 sec. The initial increase in heart rate is an exercise reflex, whereas subsequent bradycardia is baroreflex mediated. The test commonly is performed on a tilt table. On becoming upright, there is normally a transient rise in blood pressure precipitated by increased intrathoracic and intraabdominal pressures that mechanically compress the aorta. This reduces venous return and reduces stroke volume, leading to a fall in cardiac output in spite of tachycardia due to withdrawal of vagal influence. The total peripheral resistance increases as a result of sympathetic discharge. Within 4 sec after increase, the fall in blood pressure is arrested in normal people and does not fall below 5 mm of mercury of the original pressure. In patients with autonomic dysfunction, there is typically a loss of both blood pressure overshoot and reflex bradycardia.[48]

Cystometry, Uroflorometry, and Urodynamics

Since the bladder is innervated by the PNS and the SNS, study of its function is used to access the autonomic nervous system. Diminished urinary flow rate may result from detrusor dysfunction from parasympathetic autonomic neuropathy but must be differentiated from poor flow rate from urinary obstruction. This can be done by measuring intravesical pressures and relating them to flow rate.

EMG of Corpus Cavernosum

Electromyogram (EMG) of the smooth muscles of the corpora cavernosum has been described by Wagner et al.[49] These recordings are made with a bipolar concentric needle electrode. Recordings are made in the flaccid and erect state. Decreased activity occurs with erections, suggesting that contractions of cavernous smooth muscles are synchronized by sympathetic tone. During erection, the sympathetic tone is reduced, resulting in nonsynchronization of the contractions.[50] Single potential analysis of cavernous electrical activity (SPACE) has also been used.[51] Eleven of 14 impotent men with diabetes over 20 years had clinical findings of cavernous myopathy. Stief et al. found

TABLE 7–1
Clinical Tests of Autonomic Function

Test	Normal Response	Part of Reflex Arc Tested
Noninvasive Bedside Tests		
Blood pressure response to standing or vertical tilt	Fall in BP ≤30/15 mm Hg	Afferent and efferent limbs
Heart rate response to standing	Increase 11–29 bpm/30:15 ratio ≥1.04	Afferent and efferent limbs
Isometric exercise	Increase in diastolic BP, 15 mm Hg	Sympathetic efferent limb
Heart rate variation with respiration	Maximum-minimum heart rate ≥ 15 bpm; E:I ratio ≥ 1.2*	Vagal afferent and efferent limbs
Valsalva ratio	≥ 1.4*	Afferent and efferent limbs
Sweat tests	Sweating all body and limbs	Sympathetic efferent limb
Axon reflex	Local piloerection, sweating	Postganglionic sympathetic efferent fibers
Plasma norepinephrine level	Rise on tilting from horizontal to vertical	Sympathetic efferent limb
Plasma vasopressin level	Rise with induced hypotension	Afferent limb
Invasive Tests		
Valsalva maneuver	Phase I: Rise in BP Phase II: Gradual reduction of BP to plateau; tachycardia Phase III: Fall in BP Phase IV: Overshoot of BP, bradycardia*	Afferent and efferent limbs
Baroreflex sensitivity	(1) Slowing of heart rate with induced rise of BP* (2) Steady-state responses to induced rise and fall of BP	(1) Parasympathetic afferent and efferent limbs (2) Afferent and efferent limbs
Infusion of pressor drugs	(1) Rise in BP (2) Slowing of heart rate	(1) Adrenergic receptors (2) Afferent and efferent parasympathetic limbs
Other Tests of Vasomotor Control		
Radiant heating of trunk	Increased hand blood flow	Sympathetic efferent limb
Immersion of hand in hot water	Increased blood flow of opposite hand	Sympathetic efferent limb
Cold pressor test	Reduced blood flow	Sympathetic efferent limb
Emotional stress	Increased BP	Sympathetic efferent limb
Inspiratory gasp	Reduced hand blood flow	Sympathetic efferent limb
Tests of Pupillary Innervation		
4% Cocaine	Pupil dilates	Sympathetic innervation
0.1% Adrenaline	No response	Postganglionic sympathetic innervation
1% Hydroxyamphetamine hydrobromide	Pupil dilates	Postganglionic sympathetic innervation
2.5% Methacholine, 0.125% pilocarpine	No response	Parasympathetic innervation

*Age-dependent response.
BP, blood pressure; E:I, expiration/inspiration.
From McLeod JG, Tuck RR. Disorders of the autonomic nervous system: Part 2 investigation and treatment. Reprinted with permission from Ann Neurol 21:520, 1987.

51 abnormal recordings in 154 consecutive patients and suggested that damage to the autonomic system may occur much earlier than to the somatic system.[51] These tests remain controversial, however, and have not gained wide acceptance in the diagnosis of nervous system lesions affecting erection.

SPECIFIC DISEASES
Diabetes

Sexual dysfunction is common in diabetic men and women. Ellenberg found the prevalence of impotence in diabetic men to be 50% to 60%.[52] McCulloch et al. studied the natural history of diabetic impotence in a 5-year prospective study of 466 men.[53] Two hundred seventy-five were originally impotent, and 78 (28%) became impotent after 5 years of follow-up. Features found predictive of subsequent impotence were age, amount of alcohol intake, initial diabetic control, intermittent claudication and retinopathy, and the appearance of neuropathy. Only 11 of 129 (8.5%) regained potency who were impotent initially. They also noted that men with impotence but with no clinically apparent vascular or neural damage subsequently developed retinopathy and neuropathy significantly more frequently than did their potent counterparts. The most significant associations with initial impotence were age, treatment with insulin vs oral medication, retinopathy, symptomatic somatic neuropathy, and symptomatic autonomic neuropathy. Braunstein found impotence in 40% of diabetic men.[54] In a review of the literature, he found that impotence ranged from 27% to 75%. He compared this to Kinsey's values and found that at age 60, 20% of the general population had erectile dysfunction, whereas in diabetics, 40% had dysfunction. Jensen et al. compared 80 diabetic men whose mean age was 36 years with healthy age-matched controls.[55,56] Diabetics had a significantly higher rate of erectile dysfunction (34% vs 12%). Jenson et al. noted that 31% also had low sexual desire. Newman and Marcus found the incidence of impotence in men over age 60 who had had diabetes longer than 5 years to be 42.7%.[57]

The pathophysiology of erectile dysfunction in diabetic men is related to both vascular and neurogenic factors. Zuckerman et al. showed that dysfunctional diabetic patients demonstrated weaker nocturnal penile tumescence (NPT) responses than did nondiabetic dysfunctionals or control potent patients, suggesting that this was of an organic nature.[17] Robinson et al. found that in 27 men with diabetes, vascular disease was present in almost all.[58] They also found by thermosensitivity testing that small nerve or fiber dysfunction was present in 17 of 33 diabetics. Hirshkowitz et al. found both neurologic and vascular mechanisms to be involved

in most diabetics.[59] They showed that NPT was not due to disturbed sleep but was related to organic dysfunction. Lipson found that diabetic men had increased susceptibility to side effects from vascular medications, particularly antihypertensives.[60] Bancroft et al. showed that the changes in penile diameter and penile arterial pulse to erotic stimulation in diabetic patients was of less amplitude than in potent diabetic patients and normals.[61] Faerman et al. did not find hormonal differences in diabetics and other impotent patients.[62]

Diabetics are more subject to develop both somatic and autonomic neuropathy than are nondiabetics. DeTejada and Goldstein found the prevalence of peripheral and autonomic neuropathy to be significantly higher in impotent than potent men with diabetes.[15] They found that the neuropathic bladder was often associated with impotence because innervation of these two organs has common origins in the hypogastric sympathetic and pelvic parasympathetic nerves. Since there is no widely accepted test for autonomic innervation of the penis, decreased autonomic function of the bladder was taken to mean that impotence is due to autonomic neuropathy. They found decreased tissue content of norepinephrine acetylcholinesterase and vasoactive intestinal peptide (VIP) in patients with diabetes. Symptoms of neuropathy may be present in diabetic patients or may be subclinical. When present, these include glove and stocking hypoesthesia, decreased urinary flow, disturbances in gastrointestinal motility with constipation, nocturnal diarrhea, nausea and vomiting from gastroparesis, anhydrosis of lower limbs, gustatory sweating, hypoglycemic unawareness, resting tachycardia, and slow pupillary reflexes.

Numerous tests of both somatic and autonomic dysfunction have been used to document neuropathy in diabetics. As mentioned earlier, the bulbocavernosus reflex (BCR) is performed by stimulating the glans penis and measuring the evoked potential in the bulbocavernosus muscle. Latency in a healthy population has varied widely, and, therefore, abnormalities can be difficult to demonstrate.[63] Devathasan et al. found this reflex useful in differentiation in diabetic and nondiabetic impotence due to neuropathy.[64] Sarica and Karacan stimulated the vesicourethral junction and glans penis in 14 normals and 24 diabetic impotent men.[65] Sixty-seven percent of diabetics had absent or delayed BCR to stimulation of vesicourethral junction, and 12.5% had delayed response to the glans penis. Seventy-four percent of men with abnormal BCRs to stimulation at the bladder base had peripheral neuropathy, and the authors suggested that stimulation of the bladder base was preferable to stimulation of the penis. Other investigators have found the BCR not to be a valuable test to determine the cause of diabetic impotence.[63,66,67] Desai et al. believed that the poor reliability of the BCR was probably due to the fact that this reflex incorporates fast conducting myelinated fibers belonging to the A-beta and A-delta groups.[68] These tend to be affected relatively late in the context of diabetic neuropathy, whereas the autonomic nerves are affected early. Autonomic nerves are small diameter myelinated and unmyelinated fibers. Desai et al. suggested that urethral anal responses, such as Sarica and Karacan reported, would be a better test because they incorporate autonomics.[65] They suggested that the BCR test would add a little to the standard peripheral nerve conduction studies, which were at a 94% correct prediction rate.[68]

Some authors advocate dorsal nerve conduction of the penis as a simple and accurate test to diagnose neuropathy in diabetic men. Kaneko and Bradley measured nerve conduction velocity in impotent men with and without diabetes.[69] Average nerve conduction velocity was 37 ± 7 msec in impotent diabetics and 44 ± 7 msec in nondi-

abetics ($p < 0.003$). In the same group of men, they found no difference in BCR (Table 7–2). Pudendal SSEPs also record differences in patients with peripheral neuropathy, as well as CNS lesions (Fig. 7–4).

Since the bladder and the penis are both parasympathetically and sympathetically innervated by the sacral nerves, nerve dysfunction may affect both organs. In diabetics, the correlation with diabetic cystopathy and peripheral neuropathy has ranged from 75% to 100%.[70] Ellenberg studied 45 impotent diabetics. Of these, 37 had neurogenic bladders and 38 had neuropathy. Of 30 potent diabetics, only 3 had neuropathy, and 3 had cystopathy. Buvat et al. found that urinary flow rates were significantly ($p < 0.05$) lower in impotent diabetics (12.5 $\pm$ 3.7 msec) vs nonimpotent diabetics (22.5 $\pm$ 3.6 msec).[71]

Ertekin et al. measured skin potentials from peripheral nerves in the hands, feet, and penis of 41 men.[72] Skin potentials were easily obtained from the hands, feet, and penis of all normal subjects. In diabetic impotent men, the incidence or abnor-

TABLE 7–2
Results of Physiologic Studies

	Nondiabetic	Diabetes Mellitus	Statistical Difference (p value)
No. of patients	29	28	—
Age (years)	59 $\pm$ 10	57 $\pm$ 9	Not significant
Nerve conduction velocity (m/sec)*			
Posterior tibial nerve	44 $\pm$ 7	37 $\pm$ 7	<0.005
Sural nerve	46 $\pm$ 7	41 $\pm$ 8	<0.025
Dorsal nerve of penis			
Takeoff	45 $\pm$ 6	37 $\pm$ 6	<0.0005
N1	34 $\pm$ 4	28 $\pm$ 5	<0.0005
Bulbocavernosus reflex (msec)*	38 $\pm$ 5	39 $\pm$ 6	Not significant
Penile brachial index*	0.95 $\pm$ 0.09	0.83 $\pm$ 0.14	$p < 0.0005$

Effect of Age on Physiologic Studies

Age Versus	Nondiabetic	Diabetes Mellitus
Nerve conduction velocity		
Posterior tibial nerve	$p < 0.01$	Not significant
Sural nerve	Not significant	Not significant
Dorsal nerve of penis		
Takeoff	Not significant	Not significant
N1	$p < 0.05$	Not significant
Bulbocavernosus reflex	Not significant	Not significant
Penile brachial index	$p < 0.005$	Not significant

*Mean $\pm$ standard deviation.
Adapted from Kaneko S, Bradley WE. Penile electrodiagnosis. Reflex latency versus nerve conduction velocity of the dorsal nerve of the penis in diagnosis of diabetic impotence. J Urol 137:933–935 © Williams & Wilkins, 1987.

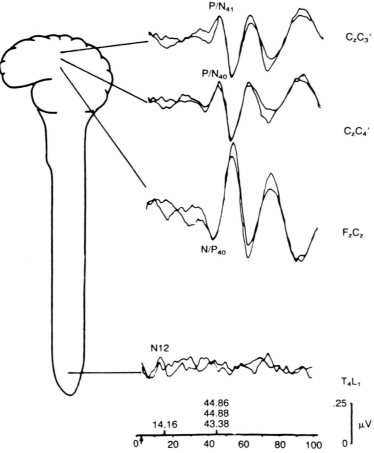

Figure 7–4. Cerebral and sacral waveforms in a dorsal nerve somatosensory evoked potential test. (From Padma-Nathan H, Goldstein I. Neurologic assessment of the impotent patient. In: Montague DK, ed. Disorders of Male Sexual Dysfunction. Chicago: Year Book Medical Publishers, 1988:86–94.)

malities encountered in hand or foot recordings was 28%. They believed this to be the incidence of abnormalities in the sympathetic autonomic nervous system. Fowler et al. did plantar thermal testing in 15 men with erectile dysfunction considered to be neuropathic and diabetics with nonneuropathic erectile dysfunction.[66] They found BCRs to be normal in 5 of 9 men thought to have typical diabetic impotence. Thermal thresholds were absent in all of those tested who had neuropathy. Since heat sensation tests predominantly small myelinated and unmyelinated fibers, thermal testing is a useful test in determining diabetic impotence.

Lack of variation of heart rate is thought to be due to abnormalities of the autonomic nervous system. Some investigators believe that if these cardiac heart rate reflexes are absent, this indicates the likelihood of an abnormality in the nerves sup-

plying the penis. Rothschild et al. compared R-R variation during inspiration/expiration and Valsalva ratio.[73] They found that R-R variation but not Valsalva ratio was decreased in diabetic subjects and in otherwise asymptomatic impotent men. Quadri et al. studied 38 diabetics with erectile dysfunction (ED) and 35 without ED.[74] R-R interval was abnormal in 21 patients with ED (55.3%) and 9 patients without ED (25.7%) ($p < 0.05$). Most investigators consider changes in the R-R interval with respiration to be one of the most sensitive indicators of autonomic dysfunction. Yet these tests have been shown by some to be normal in many diabetic men with impotence,[75] suggesting either a lack of sensitivity or a nonneurologic cause of impotence. One study showed that 6 of 14 men followed for 5 years with impotence as their only symptom had normal autonomic function tests at the beginning and end of the study. Eight other

TABLE 7–3
Diseases Associated with Peripheral Neuropathies

1. Diabetes mellitus	11. Polyarteritis nodosa
a. Polyneurophy	12. Sarcoidosis
b. Uncontrolled diabetic neuropathy	13. Lymphomas
c. Mononeuropathy	a. Systemic
d. Amyotrophy	b. Focal
e. Thorocoabdominal neuropathy	14. Cryoglobulinemia
f. Painful neuropathy	15. Chronic liver disease
g. Hypoglycemic neuropathy	16. Thermal burns
h. Autonomic neuropathy	17. Diphtheria
2. Chronic renal insufficiency	18. Leprosy
3. Carcinoma	19. Herpes zoster
4. Plasma cell dyscrasias	20. Thiamine (vitamin B_1) deficiency
a. Multiple myeloma	21. Riboflavin (vitamin B_2) deficiency
b. Waldenstrom macroglobulinemia	22. Pyridoxine anemia (vitamin B_6) deficiency
c. Other monoclonal gammopathies	23. Pernicious anemia (vitamin deficiency)
d. Primary nonfamilial amyloidosis	24. Malnutrition
e. Osteosclerotic myeloma	25. Postgastrectomy state
5. Rheumatoid arthritis	26. Tropical (nutritional) ataxia
6. Sjögren syndrome	27. Chronic obstructive pulmonary disease (COPD)
7. Scleroderma	28. Polycythemia vera
8. Systemic lupus erythematosus	29. Gout
9. Cranial arteritis	30. AIDS
10. Hypothyroidism	

From Kraft GH. Peripheral neuropathies. In: Johnson EW, ed. Practical Electromyography, 2nd ed. Baltimore: Williams & Wilkins, 1988:246–318. © 1988.

men who developed symptoms of autonomic dysfunction were not impotent. They concluded that impotence in diabetes could occur in the absence of autonomic neuropathy, whereas in others, it appeared to be the earliest symptom of autonomic damage.[75]

Other Neuropathy

Numerous diseases and disorders are associated with both somatic and autonomic peripheral neuropathy, and all of these disorders have been associated with impotence. A summary is presented in Tables 7–3, 7–4, 7–5, 7–6, 7–7.

TABLE 7–4
Hereditary Neuropathies

1. Charcot-Marie-Tooth disease (HMSN I*)	10. Spinocerebellar degenerations of adulthood
2. Hereditary motor-sensory neuropathy II (neuronal form of peroneal muscular atrophy)	11. Familial spastic paraplegia (HSMN V)
3. Dejerine-Sottas disease (HMSN III)	12. Pelizaeus-Merzbacher disease
4. Roussy-Levy syndrome	13. Refsum disease (HMSN IV)
5. Prednisone-responsive hereditary motor sensory neuropathy	14. Fabry disease
6. Hereditary compression neuropathy	15. Metachromatic leukodystrophy
a. Autosomal dominant	16. Krabbe leukodystrophy
b. Autosomal recessive	17. Tangier disease
7. Hereditary compression neuropathy	18. Abeta-lipoproteinemia
8. Riley-Day syndrome	19. Primary amyloidosis
9. Friedreich's ataxia	20. Acute intermittent porphyria
	21. Giant axonal neuropathy

*Hereditary peripheral neuropathies affecting motor and sensory nerves have been classified as hereditary motor sensory neuropathy (HMSN) types I, II, III, IV, and V by the laboratory of P.J. Dyck at the Mayo Clinic. Additional, less common HMSNs also have been described.
From Kraft GH. Peripheral neuropathies. In: Johnson EW, ed. Practical Electromyography, 2nd ed. Baltimore: Williams & Wilkins, 1988:246–318. © 1988.

TABLE 7–5
Toxic Neuropathies

Heavy Metals	Drugs	Organic Compounds
1. Lead	1. Nitrofurantoin (Furadantin)	1. Ethyl alcohol
2. Arsenic	2. Diphenylhydantoin (Dilantin)	2. N-Hexane
3. Thallium	3. Vincristine	3. Acrylamide
4. Mercury	4. Isonizide	4. Triorthocresyl phosphate
5. Antimony	5. Dapsone	5. Methylbutylketone
6. Gold	6. Corticosteroids	6. Carbon disulfide
	7. Sodium cyanate	7. Dichlorophenoxyacetic acid
	8. Halogenated hydroxyquinolines	8. Ethylene oxide
	9. Thalidome	
	10. Hydralazine	
	11. Chloramphenical	
	12. Disulfiram (Antabuse)	
	13. Heroin	
	14. LSD	
	15. Pyridoxine	
	16. Misonidazob	
	17. Amiodarone	
	18. Tetanus toxoid	
	19. Cisplatin	
	20. Amiodorone	
	21. Vacor	

From Kraft GH. Peripheral neuropathies. In: Johnson EW, ed. *Practical Electromyography*, 2nd ed. Baltimore: Williams & Wilkins, 1988:246–318. © 1988.

Multiple Sclerosis

Victims of multiple sclerosis (MS) commonly experience sexual dysfunction. Goldstein et al. found that in a sample of 45 women and 41 men, sexual dysfunction was present in 84 (97%).[76] Erectile dysfunction was present in 29 of 41 (71%) men. Most of these men (76%) also had detrusor hyperreflexia. Vas studied 37 patients with MS, of whom 43.2% complained of impotence.[23] Impotent men with MS more often complained of urgency and incontinence than did nonimpotent men. They also found different patterns of sweating in impotent, partially impotent, and normally potent men with MS. They suggested that this could be due to a loss of central control of the SNS, possibly in the ventral reticulospinal tracks between the hypothalamus and thoracolumbar cord.

In a series of 217 patients, Valleroy and Kraft found that men with MS most commonly complained of erectile dysfunction followed by decreased genital sensation, fatigue, and decreased libido.[77] They found that bladder dysfunction was associated with sexual dysfunction. Patients complained of weakness and spasticity, which interfered with their ability to have intercourse. Kirkeby et al. found penile inflow and outflow to be normal in 29 men with MS.[78] Pudendal evoked potentials were abnormal in 26, and 8 had abnormal BCRs. Pudendal evoked potentials and BCR were normal in 6 men without erectile problems. NPT testing was normal in 11 men, and 9 of these had abnormal pudendal evoked potentials or BCR. They concluded that NPT could be normal in spite of probable evidence of neurogenic impotence and disagreed with Kaneko and Bradley[69] that NPT could discriminate between psychogenic and organic ED.

TABLE 7–6
Idiopathic Neuropathies

1. Guillain-Barré syndrome
2. Chronic polyradiculoneuropathy
3. Steroid-responsive polyneuropathy
4. Fisher's syndrome
5. Shoulder girdle neuropathy

From Kraft GH. Peripheral neuropathies. In: Johnson EW, ed. *Practical Electromyography*, 2nd ed. Baltimore: Williams & Wilkins, 1988:246–318. © 1988.

Parkinson's Disease

Parkinson's disease is commonly associated with sexual dysfunction. Parkinson's may be con-

TABLE 7–7
Diseases Associated with Autonomic Neuropathy

I. The acute autonomic neuropathies
  A. Acute panautonomic neuropathy (pandysau-tonomia)
  B. Acute paraneoplastic autonomic neuropathy
  C. Acute cholinergic neuropathy
  D. Guillain-Barré syndrome
  E. Botulism
  F. Porphyria
  G. Drug-induced acute autonomic neuropathies
    1. Cisplatin
    2. Vincristine
    3. Vacor
    4. Amiodarone
    5. Perhexilene maleate
  H. Toxic acute autonomic neuropathies
    1. Heavy metals
    2. Organic solvents
    3. Acrylamide
II. The chronic autonomic neuropathies
  A. Distal sympathetic neuropathies
    1. Distal small-fiber neuropathy
    2. Peripheral neuropathies
  B. Pure cholinergic neuropathies
    1. Lambert-Eaton myasthenic syndrome
    2. Chronic idiopathic anhidrosis
    3. Adie's syndrome
    4. Chagas' syndrome
  C. Pure adrenergic neuropathy
  D. Combined sympathetic and parasympathetic failure: autonomic dysfunction clinically important
    1. Amyloid neuropathy
      a. Sporadic systemic amyloid neuropathy
      b. Multiple myeloma-associated amyloid neuropathy
      c. Familial amyloidotic polyneuropathy
    2. Diabetic autonomic neuropathy
    3. Chronic panautonomic neuropathy
    4. Chronic paraneoplastic autonomic, including pandysautonomic neuropathy
    5. Sensory neuropathy with autonomic failure
    6. Pure autonomic failure
    7. Familial dysautonomia

  E. Combined sympathetic and parasympathetic failure: autonomic dysfunction usually clinically unimportant
    1. Hereditary neuropathies
      a. Hereditary motor and sensory neuropathy (Charcot-Marie-Tooth disease)
      b. Friedreich's ataxia
      c. Hereditary sensory neuropathy
      d. Adrenomyeloneuropathy
      e. Fabry's disease
    2. Connective tissue disease
      a. Rheumatoid arthritis
      b. Systemic lupus erythematosus and mixed connective tissue diseases
    3. Infections
      a. Leprosy
      b. AIDS
    4. Immune-mediated disorders: chronic inflammatory demyelinating polyradiculoneuropathy
    5. Metabolic: uremia
    6. Nutritional deficiencies
      a. Subacute combined degeneration
      b. Alcoholic neuropathy
    7. Dysautonomia of old age
    8. Amyotrophic lateral sclerosis
  F. Paroxysmal or intermittent acral dysautonomia
    1. Paroxysmal hyperhidrosis
    2. Raynaud's syndrome
    3. Erythromelagia
  G. Disorders of reduced orthostatic tolerance
    1. Vasovagal syncope
    2. Prolonged bedrest
    3. Dysautonomia sometimes associated with mitral valve prolapse
    4. Postural orthostatic tachycardia syndrome
    5. Prolonged weightlessness
    6. Postexercise syncope

Reprinted with permission from Low PA, McLeod JG. The autonomic neuropathies. Evaluation and Management. In: Low PA, ed. Clinical Autonomic Disorders. Little, Brown and Company, Boston, copyright 1992:395–421.

fused with idiopathic orthostatic hypotension and progressive autonomic failure (PAF), a degenerative disorder of peripheral and autonomic nervous systems that may be associated with parkinsonian features. These patients lose cells in the intermedial lateral columns, with loss of small myelinated fibers in ventral horn and loss of neurons in the dorsal vagal nuclei. Blake et al. found impotence in 60.4% of patients with Parkinson's disease compared to 35.7% in age-matched controls.[79]

Temporal Lobe Pathology

Temporal lobe pathology often is associated with sexual disorders. Seizures were manifest by syncope, fugue states, vertigo, hallucination, and abdominal pain. Spark et al. diagnosed previously unrecognized temporal lobe epilepsy in 11 of 16 hyposexual men.[80] Six of these had hypogonadism, and 4 had increased prolactin. Some had improved sexual performance with anticonvulsives alone. The temporal lobe modulates sexual, reproductive, and endocrine function in animals. It was thought that sexual behavior could be modified by such seizures. Ellison found sexual aberrant behavior to be frequent and varied in patients with temporal lobe epilepsy.[81] Behaviors he found included sexual arousal, orgasm, and exhibitionism. Herzog et al. found 20 men with temporal lobe seizures with sexual and reproductive dysfunction.[82] Fifty-five percent had diminished sexual interest and reduced potency. Hierons and Sanders reported that sexual function was poor in two thirds of 36 temporal lobe epileptics but in no patients with other types of epilepsy.[83]

Stroke (Cerebrovascular Accident)

Some physicians have found that men with cerebrovascular accidents experience sexual dysfunction. This seems to be particularly common in right hemispheric stroke. Agarwal and Jain studied 14 patients with stroke.[83a] Half of the patients had decreased libido. Reduced potency was found in 86%. Right hemispheric stroke patients had significantly higher reduction in libido than did left hemispheric stroke patients. The authors suggested that the libido may have more specific cortical and limbic representation in the right cerebral hemisphere and that right hemispheric stroke affected sexual arousal by affecting perception of complex visual stimuli, emotions, and emotionally related visual stimuli. None of their patients had hemiplegic neglect. Weinstine found decreased libido in 75% of men with right hemispheric lesions.[83b]

Alcoholism

Impotence is commonly associated with chronic alcoholism. Causes of alcoholic impotence have been attributed to endocrine dysfunction, liver dysfunction, psychologic causes, and alcoholic neuropathy. Villalta et al. found that 5 of 70 men with chronic alcoholism had symptoms of autonomic neuropathy.[83c] Fourteen of 70 had abnormal R-R interval testing. They found a strong correlation between abnormal deep breathing indices and total alcohol intake and motor conduction of velocity in the lower limbs. It appeared that alcohol exercised a dose-related toxic effect on both autonomic and peripheral nervous systems. After abstinence, 12 of 14 men with abnormal breathing tests were evaluated at 1 year. Eleven who reported complete abstinence had an improvement in R-R intervals and

conduction times, and 9 reached the normal range. They concluded that autonomic neuropathy may reverse in patients who manage to abstain from alcohol.

Chronic Pain Syndromes

Chronic pain is a problem for 20 to 50 million Americans. Men and women with chronic pain often experience sexual dysfunction.[84–86] Sjogren and Fugl-Meyer found that 54% of men and 52% of women with back pain had decreased sexual satisfaction.[87] Thirty-seven percent of men had ED, and 23% had difficulty reaching orgasms. Reasons were pain, fear of pain, and fatigue. Ferguson and Figley found that 54% of a group of 70 arthritic women and 56% of a group of 38 men with arthritis had sexual problems.[88] Commonly associated reasons were pain, weakness, fatigue, and limited range of motion. Blake et al. investigated 169 patients with arthritis and 130 age-matched controls.[79] Marital unhappiness was not associated with arthritis but was associated with sexual dysfunction. Impotence was found in 62% of patients and 42% of controls. Little systematic work has been done in patients with chronic back pain to determine the extent, if any, of neurologic impairment in this group.

Sleep Apnea

The syndrome of sleep apnea has been found to be associated with impotence. Hirshkowitz et al. reported that impotence was associated with sleep apnea in 48% of patients.[89] Among those with erectile dysfunction, a high percentage also had sleep apnea. Hypertension was associated with sleep apnea, and treated hypertensives had less sleep apnea than those whose blood pressure remained high.

AGING

The association between the decreased function of most organ systems and aging is obvious to even the casual observer of the human condition. Whether or not aging is a cause of impotence has to be determined. We are certain of these two facts: sexual function (including erectile function) decreases with age in all individuals, and there is a great degree of association between aging and impotence.

Kenney[90] states that aging changes within organ systems can be categorized as follows: total loss of function, as with reproductive function in women, decreased function caused by loss of anatomic units, with surviving units unchanged (i.e., kidney nephrons), decreased anatomic unit efficiency (i.e., nerve fibres), and secondary aging changes, exemplified by the loss of feedback control, leading to increased serum gonadotropin levels.

Erectile function is a multifactorial process made up of vascular, neurologic, endocrine, and structural components. The types of changes that occur in these component parts, as well as the rates of change, vary among body systems and individuals. Interindividual heterogeneity in organ function (and in overall function) begins to increase in late middle age, then decreases in late old age. Characterizing how aging affects organ system function is further complicated by the accumulation of one or more chronic illnesses by most individuals as they age.

For these and other reasons, researchers in the area of geriatrics have stopped trying to describe normal aging and instead have shifted their attention to describing successful aging. Impotence is not (we hope) part of anyone's definition of successful aging. Is impotence a culmination of aging changes or of pathologic ones or of both?

We begin our discussion of these possibilities by summarizing what is known about aging changes in the four areas described. The cardiovascular system undergoes many well-recognized changes with age. Cardiac output decreases by about 1% per year between 20 and 80 years of age. Total peripheral resistance increases about 1% per year after age 40, although this increase is variable among organ systems.[90] Aging also brings with it greater levels of overt or occult cardiovascular disease, which may modify these general trends positively or negatively.[91]

Nervous system changes include decreased pressure, touch, tactile discrimination, and vibratory sense, the last of these being the most greatly altered with age. Reductions in reaction time seen with older age are most affected by decreases in muscle and joint function. Nerve conduction time only slows minimally. Centrally, increased conduction velocity and synaptic delay result in slower processing times in the older adult. Increased monoamine oxidase inhibitor concentrations result in decreased norepinephrine levels, which may affect gonadotropin-releasing factors. Dopamine and beta-adrenergic binding sites decrease with age as well. Sleep disturbances increase in the elderly, and although total sleep time decreases with age, the percent of time spent in rapid eye movement (REM) sleep does not change.[90]

Testosterone levels begin to decrease in men after early adulthood, and its circadian rhythm of release is decreased by older age. Older men have increased levels of LH and FSH. Fibrous tissue in the intertubular spaces of the testicles increase with little change in actual testicular weight. Sperm counts in 80- to 90-year-olds are generally 50% of those in young adult males, and the percentage of abnormal forms increases.[90]

Elastin and other connective body fibers are steadily replaced by less elastic collagen with age. Absolute and relative refractory periods of muscle increase. Muscle fibers are reduced in number, and the size of motor units is reduced.[90]

Studies examining the effects of aging on sexual function take two basic forms. The first type is organ based, using either animal or human models of sexual functioning to measure biologic parameters. The second type is population-based studies, which are of two general types. Cross-sectional studies evaluate selected subjects on one occasion. These studies represent aging at one particular age and date. Longitudinal (or cohort) studies follow individuals over a period of time and note changes that occur at given intervals. The obvious advantages of longitudinal studies to detect changes with time (and, by inference, with age) are frequently outweighed by the expense and time needed to conduct them.

There is only limited laboratory research relating impotence to aging. This may be because of the difficulty in designing and conducting studies that have any generalizability to the general population of older men. Christ et al.[92] examined tissue from the corpora cavernosum of 17 men undergoing penile prosthesis implantation and 1 man undergoing a sex change operation. They found that older subjects had greater responsiveness to alpha-adrenergic receptors that led to greater baseline tone in the corpora. They suggested that this may be an aging change that could help bring about impotence in some men.

Lal et al.[93] found that 17 of 28 impotent men studied attained full erection in response to subcutaneously administered apomorphine, a dopaminergic agonist. None of the men responded to placebo. Neither of the 2 patients with Parkinson's disease and only 2 of the 6 with diabetes responded. Of 9 men placed on oral bromocriptine, 3 reportedly returned to normal function and 3 reported improved function. The authors suggested that impotence in some older men could be secondary to a decline in dopaminergic function.

Conti and Virag[94] histologically evaluated the penises of 7 human embryos, 12 stillborns, and 12 male autopsy subjects ranging in age from 2 to 86 years. They also evaluated various penile pathologic specimens from 80 surgical subjects. They described a gradual vasculosclerosis of the penile veins and arteries over time, becoming complete after age 65. The intracavernal trabeculae were seen as becoming more and more fibrotic over time after age 50, eventually becoming entirely nonvascular. They also noted that impotent subjects underwent these processes prematurely. The authors did not control for underlying illnesses or do any statistical analysis of their data. Nonetheless, the large amount of material evaluated and the difficulty of performing such a study make it an important one. Their findings suggest that these are changes secondary to aging and that they may contribute to the onset of impotence. Possible hypercoagulability due to elevated thromboxane A_2 levels in older men (especially diabetics) has been suggested as a possible cause for arterial changes such as these.[95]

Androgens play an important role in sexual function through their effects on libido and seminal emissions. They are not, however, essential for penile erection.[96] It is quite possible that men with low libido are less likely to come in for an evaluation of their erectile dysfunction.[97] Lower levels of bioavailable testosterone, often found in older men,[97] have been reported to be associated with less frequent and less rigid nocturnal erections. They have not been found to be associated with impotence.

The prevalence of impotence in selected elderly populations of men has been estimated at various levels by various investigators: 28% by Cogen and Steinman,[98] 34% by Slag et al.,[99] 36% by Weitzman and Hart,[100] and 40% by Diokno et al.[101] While they are a seemingly diverse group of estimates, they have a lot in common. The study by Slag et al.[99] was done on a representative sample of men attending a Veteran's Administration hospital and could be generalized to this population. However, none of these studies can be thought of as being representative of the population of older men as a whole. They all found the prevalence of impotence increased by a large percentage after age 70, and to some extent, their divergent estimates represent the differing proportions of such men in their sample. Finally, all these authors would agree that impotence in their populations was either caused by or associated with comorbid conditions that affected vascular and neurologic function as it relates to erection.

These authors' results more or less confirm the results Kinsey et al. arrived at in their groundbreaking work in 1948.[102] They collected information about erectile impotence on only 4108 males under 60 years of age and interviewed only 126 males over the age of 60. They found a geometric increase in the prevalence of self-reported age of onset of impotence in their study sample, from 2% at age 40 to 75% at age 80.

Kinsey's group found that the median frequency of intercourse for married men decreased steadily with age, from about three times per week at 40 years of age to less than once a week at age 60. Multiple orgasm was reported by 15% to 20% of men in their teens and 20s. This number steadily

declined until about age 45, where it leveled off at about 3%. Angles of erection increased until age 26 to 30 and then steadily declined. Precoital seminal emissions increased to age 21 to 25, then declined as well.

Kinsey's data were indirectly confirmed by the prospective Duke Longitudinal Study of Normal Aging.[103] They found that sexual activity and sexual interest declined with increased age. Sexual activity was reported by 67% to 71% of male subjects at age 60 to 65 and by only 21% to 39% at age 78+. Sexual interest was present in 77% to 88% of men aged 60 to 65 but in only 50% to 72% of those aged 78+. In their discussion, the authors attribute this decline in large part to physical infirmity or illness.

Busse and Maddox,[104] commenting on the Duke Longitudinal Study, noted an increasing homogeneity in the sexual activity of men in their 70s and 80s. This is consistent with what we know about other body systems, such as circulation and respiration. They also commented that sexual interest began to decline in the fifth decade of life.

Evidence of the association of comorbid conditions with impotence is well demonstrated by the study of Mulligan et al.[105] of three age-stratified groups of VA hospital outpatient attenders. Subjects were mailed questionnaires, and consenting subjects were sent a medical records review. They found that self-reported poor health status was their most significant predictor of sexual dysfunction. They also found that the prevalence of erectile dysfunction was about the same in a subgroup of men 65 to 75 years (27%) as in a group of younger men with comparable rates of comorbid illnesses (26%).

The idea that impotence is most frequently the effect of an underlying pathologic condition was supported by two other studies. Mulligan and Katz[106] reported on a series of 121 male veterans between the ages of 60 and 85 who chose to have their impotence evaluated diagnostically. They found the causes of impotence in this subject population to be the following: neurologic and vascular disorders combined 30.3%, vascular 21.1%, diabetic neuropathy 17.1%, nondiabetic neuropathy 10.5%, psychogenic 9.2%, drug effects 3.9%, hypogonadism 2.6%, Peyronie's disease 1.3%, and idiopathic 3.9%.

Slag et al.[99] conducted a hallmark study of 1180 men attending an outpatient VA hospital medical clinic. The age range of their subjects was not reported, but the average subject's age for two of the three subgroups reported on were 56 and 59 years (SD 1.3 years for each). Forty-seven percent of the 401 men who were impotent chose to be fully evaluated for this problem. They found the causes of impotence in this select group to be the following: medication effect 25%, psychogenic

14%, neurologic 7%, urologic 6%, primary and secondary hypogonadism 19%, diabetes mellitus 9%, hypothyroidism 5%, hyperprolactinemia 4%, miscellaneous 5%, and unknown 7%.

The differences in diagnostic findings between these two studies may be accounted for by the following reasons. First, the population in Mulligan and Katz's study[106] was older and thus more likely to be manifesting the adverse effects of chronic illness, such as diabetes. Second, both studies depended on expert diagnoses from more than one clinician to determine the causes of impotence in their subjects. This is unavoidably susceptible to the type of bias caused when different investigators (both within and among studies) use different diagnostic criteria when defining the causes of impotence in their subject populations.

What these studies have in common is that they both found idiopathic impotence to account for no more than 4% to 7% of their cases. This implies that even if aging is a direct cause of impotence, it is a minor cause overall. These results await the conduct of a large-scale population-based study for confirmation.

REFERENCES

1. Williams PL, Warwick R. Gray's Anatomy, 36th ed. Philadelphia: WB Saunders Co, 1980.
2. Krane RJ, Siroky MB. Neurophysiology of erection. Urol Clin North Am 8:91, 1981.
3. Kaneko S, Bradley W. Penile electrodiagnosis: penile peripheral innervation. J Urol 30:210, 1987.
4. Eckhard C. Untersuchungen uber die Erection des Penis beim Hunde. Beitr Anat Physiol 3:123, 1869.
5. Walsh PC, Donker PJ. Impotence following radical prostatectomy: insight into etiology and prevention. J Urol 128:492, 1982.
6. Lue T, Zeineh SJ, Schmidt RA, et al. Neuroanatomy of penile erection: its relevance to iatrogenic impotence. J Urol 131:273, 1984.
7. Bennett C, Seager SW, Vasher EA, et al. Sexual dysfunction and electroejaculation in men with spinal cord injury: review. J Urol 139:453, 1988.
8. Roos WS, Bard P. The mediation of feline erection through sympathetic pathways with some remarks on sexual behavior after differentiation of the genitalia. Am J Physiol 150:80, 1947.
9. Andy OJ. Hypersexuality and limbic system seizures. Pavlov J Biol Sci 12:187, 1977.
10. Klüver H, Bucy PC. Preliminary analysis of functions of the temporal lobes in monkeys. Arch Neurol Psychiatry 42:979, 1939.
11. MacLean PD, Ploog DW. Cerebral representation of penile erection. J Neurophysiol 25:29, 1962.
12. Dua S, MacLean PD. Localization for penile erection in medial frontal lobe. Am J Physiol 207:1425, 1964.
13. Haerer AF, DeJong RN. The Neurologic Examination, 5th ed. Philadelphia: JB Lippincott, 1992.
14. Rowland DL, Greenleaf W, Mas M, et al. Penile and finger sensory thresholds in young, aging, and diabetic males. Arch Sex Behav 18:1, 1989.
15. DeTejada ID, Goldstein I. Diabetic penile neuropathy. Urol Clin North Am 15:17, 1988.
16. Beckett SD, Hudson RS, Walker DF, et al. Effect of local anesthetic of the penis and dorsal penile neurectomy on the mating ability of bulls. J Mam Bet Med Assoc 1973:838, 1978.
17. Zuckerman M, Neeb M, Ficher M, et al. Nocturnal penile tumescence and penile responses in the waking state in diabetic and nondiabetic sexual dysfunctionals. Arch Sex Behav 14:109, 1985.
18. Opsomer RJ, Guerit JM, Wese FX, et al. Pudendal cortical somatosensory evoked potentials. J Urol 135:1216, 1986.
19. Vodusek DB. Pudendal SEP and bulbocavernosus reflex in women. Electroencephalogr Clin Neurophysiol 77:134, 1990.
20. Haldeman S, Bradley WE, Bhatia N. Evoked responses from the pudendal nerve. J Urol 128:974, 1982.
21. Gerstenberg TC, Nordling J, Metz P. Bulbocavernosus reflex latency in the investigation of diabetic impotence [Letter]. Br J Urol 62:95, 1988.
22. Guerit JM, Opsomer RJ. Bit-mapped imaging of somatosensory evoked potentials after stimulation of the posterior tibial nerves and dorsal nerve of the penis/clitoris. Electroencephalogr Clin Neurophysiol 80:228, 1991.
23. Vas CJ. Sexual impotence and some autonomic disturbances in men with multiple sclerosis. Acta Neurol Scand 45:166, 1969.
24. Ertekin C, Akürekli O, Gürses AN, et al. The value of somatosensory-evoked potentials and bulbocavernosus reflex in patients with impotence. Acta Neurol Scand 71:48, 1985.
25. Herman CW, Weinberg HJ, Brown J. Testing for neurogenic impotence: a challenge. Urology 27:318, 1986.
26. Tackmann W, Porst H, vanAhlen H. Bulbocavernosus reflex latencies and somatosensory evoked potentials after pudendal nerve stimulation in the diagnosis of impotence. J Neurol 235:219, 1988.
27. Parys BT, Evans CM, Parsons KF. Bulbocavernosus reflex latency in the investigation of diabetic impotence [see comments]. Br J Urol 61:59, 1988.
28. Rushworth G. Diagnostic value of the electromyographic study of reflex activity in man. Electroencephalogr Clin Neurophysiol S25:65, 1967.
29. Kaneko S, Park YC, Yachiku S, et al. Evoked central somatosensory potentials after penile stimulation in man. J Urol 21:58, 1983.
30. Krane RJ, Siroky MB. Studies on sacral-evoked potentials. J Urol 124:872, 1980.
31. Vodusek DB, Janko M. The bulbocavernosus reflex. Brain 113:813, 1990.
32. Ertekin C, Reel F. Bulbocavernosus reflex in normal men and in patients with neurogenic bladder and/or impotence. J Neurol Sci 28:1, 1976.
33. Bilkey WJ, Awad EA, Smith AD. Clinical application of sacral reflex latency. J Urol 129:1187, 1983.

34. Vodusek DB, Janko M, Lokar J. Direct and reflex responses in perineal muscles on electrical stimulation. J Neurol Neurosurg Psychiatry 46:67, 1983.

35. Lavoisier P, Proulx J, Courtois F, et al. Bulbocavernosus reflex: its validity as a diagnostic test of neurogenic impotence. J Urol 141:311, 1989.

36. Blaivas JG, Zayed AAH, Labib KB. The bulbocavernosus reflex in urology: a prospective study of 299 patients. J Urol 126:197, 1981.

37. Vodusek DB, Janko M, Lokar J. EMG, single fibre EMG and sacral reflexes in assessment of sacral nervous system lesions. J Neurol Neurosurg Psychiatry 45:1064, 1982.

38. Dick HC, Scott SB, Bradley WE, et al. Pudendal sexual reflexes: electrophysiological investigations. Urology 3:376, 1974.

39. Vodusek DB, Zidar J. Pudendal nerve involvement in patients with hereditary motor and sensory neuropathy. Acta Neurol Scand 76:457, 1987.

40. Lue TF, Tanagho EA. Hemodynamics of erection. In: Tanagho EA, Lue TF, McClure RD, eds. Contemporary Management of Impotence and Infertility. Baltimore: Williams & Wilkins, 1988.

41. De Groat WC, Steers WD. Neuroanatomy and neurophysiology of penile erection. In: Tanagho EA, Lue TF, McClure RD, eds. Contemporary Management of Impotence and Infertility. Baltimore: Williams & Wilkins, 1988.

42. Eardley I, Quinn NP, Fowler CJ, et al. The value of urethral sphincter electromyography in the differential diagnosis of parkinsonism. Br J Urol 64:360, 1989.

43. Onufrowicz B. Notes on the arrangement and function of the cell groups in the sacral region of the spinal cord. J Nerv Ment Dis 26:498, 1899.

44. Kirby R, Fowler C, Gosling J, et al. Urethrovesical dysfunction in progressive autonomic failure with multiple system atrophy. J Neurol Neurosurg Psychiatry 49:554, 1986.

45. McCulloch DK, Campbell IW, Wu FC, et al. The prevalence of diabetic impotence. Diabetologia 18:279, 1980.

46. Genovely H, Pfeifer M. R-R variation: the autonomic test of choice in diabetes. Diabetes/Metab Rev 4:255, 1988.

47. Fagius J. Syndromes of autonomic overactivity: clinical presentation, assessment, and management. In: Low PA, ed. Clinical Autonomic Disorders: Evaluation and Management. Boston: Little, Brown, and Co, 1992:197–208.

48. Low PA. Laboratory evaluation of autonomic failure. In: Low PA, ed. Clinical Autonomic Disorders: Evaluation and Management. Boston: Little, Brown, and Co, 1992:169–192.

49. Wagner G, Gerstenberg T, Levin RJ. Electrical activity of corpus cavernosum during flaccidity and erection of the human penis: a new diagnostic method? J Urol 142:723–725, 1989.

50. Steif CG, Djamilian M, Anton P, et al. Single potential analysis of cavernous electrical activity in impotent patients: a possible diagnostic method for autonomic cavernous dysfunction and cavernous smooth muscle degeneration. J Urol 146:771, 1991.

51. Stief CG, Thon WF, Djamilian M, et al. Single potential analysis of cavernous electrical activity. Urol Res 19:277, 1991.

52. Ellenberg M. Sexual function in diabetic patients. Ann Intern Med 92:331, 1980.

53. McCulloch DK, Young RJ, Prescott RJ, et al. The natural history of impotence in diabetic men. Diabetologia 26:437, 1984.

54. Braunstein GD. Impotence in diabetic men. Mt Sinai J Med 54:236, 1987.

55. Jensen SB. Sexual customs and dysfunction in alcoholics: Part I. Br J Sex Med 53:29, 1979.

56. Jensen SB, Olsen PS, Ronne HR. Seksuel dysfunktion i almen praksis. Ugeskrift Laeger 142:401, 1980.

57. Newman HF, Marcus H. Erectile dysfunction in diabetes and hypertension. Urology 26:135, 1985.

58. Robinson LQ, Woodcock JP, Stephenson TP. Results of investigation of impotence in patients with overt or probable neuropathy. Br J Urol 60:583, 1987.

59. Hirshkowitz M, Karacan I, Rando KC, et al. Diabetes, erectile dysfunction, and sleep-related erections. Sleep 13:53, 1990.

60. Lipson LG. Treatment of hypertension in diabetic men: problems with sexual dysfunction. Am J Cardiol 53:47a, 1984.

61. Bancroft J, Bell C, Ewing DJ, et al. Assessment of erectile function in diabetic and non-diabetic impotence by simultaneous recording of penile diameter and penile arterial pulse. J Psychosom Res 29:315, 1985.

62. Faerman I, Vilar O, Rivardama MA, et al. Impotence and diabetes. Studies of androgenic function in diabetic impotent males. Diabetes 21:23, 1972.

63. Daniels JS. Abnormal nerve conduction in impotent patients with diabetes mellitus. Diabetes Care 12:449, 1989.

64. Devathasan G, Cheah JS, Puvanendran K. The bulbocavernosus reflex in diabetic impotence. Singapore Med J 25:181, 1984.

65. Sarica Y, Karacan I. Bulbocavernosus reflex to somatic and visceral nerve stimulation in normal subjects and in diabetics with erectile impotence. J Urol 138:55, 1987.

66. Fowler CJ, Ali Z, Kirby RS, et al. The value of testing for unmyelinated fibre, sensory neuropathy in diabetic impotence. Br J Urol 61:63, 1988.

67. Barron SA, Mazliah J, Hoch Z, et al. A non-invasive electrophysiological indicator of organic impotence in diabetic men. Electromyogr Clin Neurophysiol 28:39, 1988.

68. Desai KM, Dembny K, Morgan H, et al. Neurophysiological investigation of diabetic impotence. Are sacral response studies of value? Br J Urol 61:68, 1988.

69. Kaneko S, Bradley WE. Penile electrodiagnosis. Value of bulbocavernosus reflex latency versus nerve conduction velocity of the dorsal nerve of

the penis in diagnosis of diabetic impotence. J Urol 137:933, 1987.

70. Frimodt-Moller C. Diabetic cystopathy: epidemiology and related disorders. Ann Intern Med 92:318, 1980.

71. Buvat J, Lemaire A, Buvat-Herbaut M, et al. Comparative investigations in 26 impotent and 26 nonimpotent diabetic patients. J Urol 133:34, 1985.

72. Ertekin C, Ertekin N, Mutlu S, et al. Skin potentials (SP) recorded from the extremities and genital regions in normal and impotent subjects. Acta Neurol Scand 76:28, 1987.

73. Rothschild AH, Weinberg CR, Hatter JB, et al. Sensitivity of R-R variation and Valsalva ratio in assessment of cardiovascular diabetic autonomic neuropathy. Diabetes Care 10:735, 1987.

74. Quadri R, Veglio M, Flecchia D, et al. Autonomic neuropathy and sexual impotence in diabetic patients: analysis of cardiovascular reflexes. Andrologia 21:346, 1989.

75. Ewing DJ, Campbell IW, Clarke BF, et al. Vascular reflexes in diabetic autonomic neuropathy. Lancet 2:601, 1976.

76. Goldstein I, Seròky MB, Sax DS, et al. Neurourologic abnormalities in multiple sclerosis. J Urol 128:541, 1982.

77. Valleroy ML, Kraft GH. Sexual dysfunction in multiple sclerosis. Arch Phys Med Rehabil 65:125, 1984.

78. Kirkeby HJ, Poulsen EU, Paterson T, et al. Erectile dysfunction in multiple sclerosis. Neurology 38:1366, 1988.

79. Blake DJ, Maisiak R, Kaplan A, et al. Sexual dysfunction among patients with arthritis. Clin Rheumatol 7:50, 1988.

80. Spark RF, Wills CA, Royal H. Hypogonadism, hyperprolactinaemia, and temporal lobe epilepsy in hyposexual men. Lancet 1:413, 1984.

81. Ellison JM. Alterations of sexual behavior in temporal lobe epilepsy. Psychosomatics 23:499, 1982.

82. Herzog AG, Seibel MM, Schomer DL, et al. Reproductive endocrine disorders in men with partial seizures of temporal lobe origin. Arch Neurol 43:347, 1986.

83. Hierons R, Sanders M. Impotence in patients with temporal lobe lesions. Lancet 467:761–763, 1966.

83a. Agarwal A, Jain DC. Male sexual dysfunction with stroke. J Asso Physcians India 37:505–507, 1989.

83b. Weinstine I. Effects of brain damage on sexual behavior. Med Aspects Hum Sex 15:158–164, 1981.

83c. Villalta J, Estruch R, Atunez E, et al. Vagal neuropathy in chronic alcoholics: relation to ethanol consumption. Alcohol Alcohol 24:421, 1989.

84. Infante MC. Sexual dysfunction in the patient with chronic back pain. Sex Disabil 4:173, 1981.

85. Roy R. Chronic pain and marital difficulties. Health Social Work 10:199, 1985.

86. Turk D, Meichenbaum D, Genest M. Pain and Behavioral Medicine: A Cognitive-Behavioral Perspective. New York: Guilford Press, 1983.

87. Sjogren K, Fugl-Meyer A. Chronic back pain and sexuality. Int Rehab Med 3:19,1981.

88. Ferguson K, Figley B. Sexuality and rheumatic disease: a prospective study. Sex Disabil 2:130, 1979.

89. Hirshkowitz M, et al. Hypertension, erectile dysfunction, and occult sleep apnea. Sleep 12:223, 1989.

90. Kenney RA. Physiology of Aging, 2nd ed. Chicago: Year Book Medical Publishers, 1989.

91. Lakatta EG. Heart and circulation. In: Finch CE, Schneider EL, eds. The Biology of Aging. New York: Van Nostrand Reinhold, 1985:377–413.

92. Christ GJ, Maayani S, Valcic M, Melman A. Pharmacological studies of human erectile tissue: characteristics of spontaneous contractions and alterations in alpha-adrenoceptor responsiveness with age and disease in isolated tissues. Br J Pharmacol 101:375, 1990.

93. Lal S, Tesfaye Y, Thavundayil JX, et al. Apomorphine: clinical studies on erectile impotence and yawning. Prog Neuropsychopharmacol Biol Psychiatry 13:329, 1989.

94. Conti G, Virag R. Human penile erection and organic impotence: normal histology and histopathology. Urol Int 44:303, 1989.

95. Kim SC, Choi IG, Oh CH, Cha YJ. Prostacyclin-to-thromboxane A_2 ratio in arteriogenic impotence. J Urol 144:1373, 1990.

96. Lue TF. Physiology of penile erection. In: Jonas U, Thon WF, Stief CG, eds. Erectile Dysfunction. Berlin: Springer-Verlag, 1991:44–56.

97. Kaiser FE, Viosca SP, Morley JE, et al. Impotence and aging: clinical and hormonal factors. J Am Geriatr Soc 36:511, 1988.

98. Cogen R, Steinman W. Sexual function and practice in elderly men of lower socioeconomic status. J Fam Pract 31:162, 1990.

99. Slag MF, Morley JE, Elson MK, et al. Impotence in medical clinic outpatients. JAMA 249:1736, 1983.

100. Weitzman R, Hart J. Sexual behavior in healthy married elderly men. Arch Sex Behav 16:39, 1987.

101. Diokno AC, Brown MB, Herzog AR. Sexual function in the elderly. Arch Intern Med 150:197, 1990.

102. Kinsey AC, Pomeroy WB, Martin CE. Sexual Behavior in the Human Male. Philadelphia: WB Saunders Co, 1948.

103. Verwoerdt A, Pfeiffer E, Wang H. Sexual behavior in senescence: changes in sexual activity and interest of aging men and women. J Geriatr Psychiatry 2:163, 1969.

104. Busse EW, Maddox GL. The Duke Longitudinal Studies of Normal Aging 1955–80: Overview of History, Design, and Findings. New York: Springer Publishing Co, 1985.

105. Mulligan T, Retchin SM, Chinchilli VM, Bettinger CB. The role of aging and chronic disease in sexual dysfunction. J Am Geriatr Soc 36:520, 1988.

106. Mulligan T, Katz PG. Why aged men become impotent. Arch Intern Med 149:1365, 1989.

CHAPTER 8

Impotence and Chronic Renal Failure

Culley C. Carson

Chronic renal failure (CRF) and subsequent uremia are commonly associated with erectile dysfunction, diminished libido, and infertility.[1-3] A variety of problems contribute to this overall sexual dysfunction, including uremia, changes associated with dialysis, medication used to control underlying disease processes, and renal failure-associated conditions, as well as the sequelae of renal transplantation.

PREVALENCE

Abnormalities in male sexual and reproductive function have been widely reported in patients with CRF. Studies in which patients and spouses were interviewed or evaluated by questionnaire have demonstrated decreased sexual activity and potency in 38% to 80% of uremic men and complete erectile dysfunction and impotence in 20% to 60% of patients surveyed.[4-9] Although both Kinsey et al.[10] and Masters and Johnson[11] reported the incidence of impotence in normal men in their 40s as less than 5%, Sherman[7] identified more than 50% of patients with uremeia on hemodialysis in the same age group as having significant sexual dysfunction and impotence.

Procci et al. combined questionnaires and nocturnal penile tumescence monitoring (NPT) to further evaluate the incidence of erectile dysfunction in uremic males (Fig. 8–1).[12] The NPT monitoring technique has been demonstrated by Karacan and others to differentiate organic from psychogenic causes of erectile dysfunction by observing erection during rapid eye movement (REM) sleep.[13] If neurovascular, hormonal, or pharmacologic factors are responsible for impotence, patients should have altered NPT results. If, however, psychologic factors are primarily responsible for erectile dysfunction in uremia, NPT would be expected to be normal. Procci's results demonstrated a significant abnormality in NPT recordings in 50% of uremic patients on hemodialysis.[12] Questionnaires quantitating frequency of intercourse correlated with NPT findings in this group of patients. Interestingly, the incidence of depression common in uremic patients did not correlate with NPT findings or frequency of intercourse. Thus, this study strongly suggests an organic or physiologic cause for erectile dysfunction identified in uremic patients on hemodialysis.

ETIOLOGIC FACTORS IN IMPOTENCE IN UREMIC MEN

As a result of the multisystem disease processes present in many uremic men, it is apparent that the pathogenesis of impotence is most likely multifaceted. Uremic men variously complain of loss of libido, loss of potency, inadequate or lost ejaculation, and decreased penile sensation. Each of these functional changes may be caused by different and separate, although linked, physiologic mechanisms.[14,15] Factors to be considered include decreased arterial blood flow, venous occlusive incompetence, altered smooth muscle function, neurogenic abnormalities, and hormonal disturbances. These physiologic functions may be supplemented by significant psychologic stresses and abnormalities resulting from chronic illness and generalized changes in body function (Fig. 8–2).

ARTERIAL ABNORMALITIES

In 1923, Leriche described the association of obstructive vascular disease and erectile impotence.[16] The pelvic steal syndrome has long been associated with erectile dysfunction, as have abnormalities in distal, arterial, and vascular obstructive processes.[17] Dalal et al. have reported a hemodialysis patient with penile vascular calcification.[18]

It is well known that patients with uremia on chronic hemodialysis have accelerated atherosclerosis associated with both large vessel and small vessel occlusive disease. Vasculogenic impotence can be suspected in these patients regardless of age.[19] The multifactorial nature of vascular insufficiency in uremic patients makes specific treatment of these patients difficult. Diabetes mellitus, smoking, hypertension, hyperlipidemia, and multiple

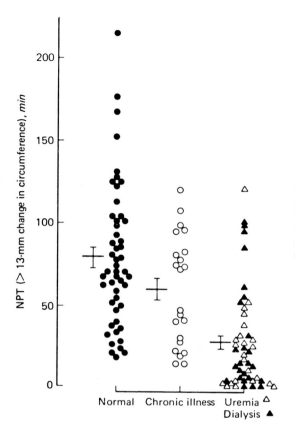

Figure 8–1. Nocturnal penile tumescence (NPT) in normal subjects, patients with chronic illness and normal renal function, those with advanced renal failure (uremia), and dialysis patients. The brackets represent the mean ± SEM. (From Procci WR, Goldstein DA, Adelstein J, Massry SG. Sexual dysfunction in the male patient with uremia: a reappraisal. Kidney Int 19:317–323, 1981.)

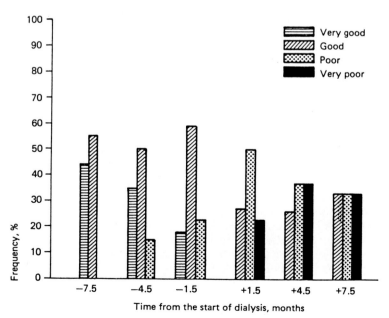

Figure 8–2. Sexual performances relative to the start of dialysis in 26 uremic patients during an 18-month follow-up. (From Di Paolo N. Capotondo L, Gaggiotti E, Rossi P. Sexual function in uremic patients: 18 months follow-up in 26 subjects. Contrib Nephrol 77:34–44, 1990.)

medications are all factors producing arterial insufficiency in these patients. Virag et al. have demonstrated these factors as causes for erectile dysfunction in uremic as well as nonuremic individuals.[20] Since many dialysis patients have long-term hypertension and as many as 50% require continuous antihypertensive therapy, one can strongly suspect hypertension and its treatment medications as contributing to arterial erectile dysfunction. Since as many as 15% of uremic patients are diabetic, diabetic vascular changes also can be suspected to contribute to erectile dysfunction.

Additionally, those patients who have undergone renal transplantation may have vascular compromise to their lower extremities and genitalia. These vascular changes can be documented using Doppler sonography and are well reported.[21]

As a result of recent developments in the understanding of the physiology of erectile dysfunction, one must consider not only arterial inflow but also venous outflow abnormalities in the vascular assessment of erectile dysfunction.[22-24] Although these considerations have not been specifically isolated to patients with uremia and hemodialysis, these vascular abnormalities are well known causes of erectile dysfunction. Venoocclusive dysfunction as a cause of erectile problems probably results from a combination of venous vascular abnormalities associated with peripheral smooth muscle function of the corpora cavernosa. Standard investigation techniques for this abnormality include dynamic infusion, pharmacocavernosometry, and pharmacocavernosography. These studies, combined with color Doppler evaluation of arterial inflow, are necessary to identify specific vascular abnormalities producing erectile dysfunction.[22] Because most uremic patients have predominantly arterial inflow abnormalities, venoocclusive studies have not been performed widely.[22,23]

NEUROGENIC IMPOTENCE

Autonomic control of erectile smooth muscle tissue is critical in the maintenance of erectile function. Penile smooth muscle tone is controlled primarily by adrenergic and cholinergic neurotransmitters and regulates blood flow within the corpora cavernosa.[24] Since autonomic nerve dysfunction is a common problem with uremic patients on hemodialysis, a significant role for autonomic neuropathy in the impotent hemodialysis patient can be suspected.[25,26] Campese et al. studied the autonomic nervous system in uremic patients by monitoring heart rate response to Valsalva.[27] This technique can, to some extent, measure the integrity of the afferent parasympathetic and efferent sympathetic pathways. They correlated this response

with NPT results and intercourse frequency by questionnaire. In the 12 uremic men studied, there was a significantly abnormal Valsalva ratio that corresponded to significant abnormalities in NPT and a significant decrease in frequency of intercourse. These data suggest that autonomic nervous system dysfunction is an etiologic factor in impotence associated with uremia. Kersh et al. reported significant vascular instability and hypotension in patients with uremia, further suggesting autonomic insufficiency in their patients.[28]

Peripheral neuropathy frequently is associated with erectile dysfunction. Peripheral neuropathy that occurs most commonly in patients with diabetes mellitus also can be seen in patients with nondiabetic uremia. Measured abnormalities in bulbocavernosus reflux have been demonstrated in this group of patients.[29] Although there are few satisfactory neurophysiologic tests to identify patients with neurogenic impotence, clinical neurophysiology can be useful in assessing patients with defects in somatic nervous system pathways to the sacral segments affected by uremia, diabetes, or other metabolic disease processes. There are, however, no satisfactory direct methods for assessing autonomic nervous system function, and only secondary evidence for autonomic neuropathy is available.[30]

PSYCHOLOGIC FACTORS

The psychologic impact of uremia and its treatment and management have a significant role in sexual dysfunction in patients with CRF. Patients with uremia, especially those on hemodialysis, have a significant incidence of psychiatric and depressive illness compared with the normal population.[8] These psychologic abnormalities will certainly add to the already significant physiologic abnormalities in these patients. The psychologic conditions identified include low self-esteem, lack of a sense of well-being, a significant increase in stress from chronic illness, job loss, and financial concerns, and a documented increase in depression and marital discord. Procci et al. have identified a higher incidence of depressive episodes in patients on hemodialysis in comparison with a normal population.[12] Glass et al. studied the psychologic impact of CRF, dialysis, and renal transplantation and found that dialysis patients were more likely to be depressed than transplant patients, whereas transplant patients showed a greater level of anxiety.[9] Marital discord rates were higher in all patients with CRF, and they were especially marked in those patients on hemodialysis. The findings of Glass et al., which demonstrated impotence in many patients in whom physiologic erectile function could be measured, suggested that psychologic stresses and abnormalities were a significant part of uremic sexual dysfunction.

PHARMACOLOGIC FACTORS

Because of the underlying conditions that have produced erectile dysfunction in patients with CRF, close attention must be paid to erectile abnormalities associated with medications. Pharmacologic treatment of conditions associated with CRF may produce side effects causing or increasing impotence and diminished libido (Table 8-1). Such agents may produce abnormalities in central, neuroendocrine regulation or in the neurovascular control of erectile function either in the corpora cavernosa or at a central level.[31] Agents that increase prolactin or are associated with other central neurologic abnormalities are likely to reduce libido. Antihypertensive agents, which are commonly used in patients with CRF, are well-known causes for erectile dysfunction. Impotence has been associated with virtually all available antihypertensive medications.[32-34] These antihypertensive medications added to the associated physiologic arterial changes noted to occur with atherosclerosis magnify the problem of erectile dysfunction in these individuals. Although calcium channel blocking agents, alpha-adrenergic blocking agents, and ACE inhibitors are least likely to impair physiologic erectile response, the sympatholytics, beta-adrenergic blocking agents, and vasodilators are strongly associated with local effects that overcome the normal physiologic response of the smooth muscles of the corpora cavernosa and locally as well as centrally inhibit erectile function.[32,33] Patients with hypertension and erectile dysfunction who can be appropriately controlled are best treated with selective alpha$_1$-blocking agents, such as prazosin, doxazosin, and terazosin. Cases of priapism have been reported with alpha$_1$-adrenergic blocking agents, such as prazosin.[3,4] Many dialysis patients are treated with sympatholytic medications such as methyldopa and clonidine, beta-blockers such as propranolol, and vasodilators such as hydralazine and can be expected to exhibit physiologic erectile dysfunction as a result of the local cavernosal effects of these agents.[33] Alpha$_2$-adrenergic antagonists, such as clonidine, may produce central cavernosal artery constriction or limit its dilation potential, decreasing cavernosal perfusion and diminishing erectile function.[35]

ENDOCRINE FACTORS

The kidney plays an integral role in endocrine function. Hormonal effects on the kidney are well known, and the kidney provides significant hormonal metabolism. CRF, therefore, can be ex-

TABLE 8-1

Agents Frequently Used in CRF-Associated with Male Sexual Dysfunction

Antihypertensives
  Sympatholytics
    Methyldopa (Aldomet)
    Clonidine (Catopres)
    Reserpine (Serpasil, Sandril)
    Guanethidine (Ismelin)
  Beta-adrenergic antagonists
    Propranolol (Inderol)
    Pindolol (Vislein)
    Atenolol (Tenormin)
    Metoprolol (Lopressor)
    Labetalol (Trandate, Normadyne)
  Vasodilators
    Hydralazine (Apresoline)
  Diuretics
    Thiazides (Diuril)
    Spironolactone (Aldactone)
Cimetidine (Tagomet)
Digoxin
Clofibrate (Atromid-S)
Metodopramide (Reglan)
Antidepressants (depress libido)

pected to produce profound changes in endocrine function and hormone balance that affect many bodily functions, including male sexual activity. Impairment of the hypothalamic-pituitary testicular axis in men with CRF has been well documented (Fig. 8-3).[36-39] Semen analyses in these patients demonstrate low or absent sperm count with abnormalities in both morphology and motility.[25] These abnormalities are supported by testicular histologic abnormalities on biopsy, including abnormalities in both spermatogenesis and interstitial cell morphology.[40] Interstitial cell abnormalities can be correlated with reduced testosterone secretion.[41-43] Most male patients with CRF on dialysis have low serum testosterone levels, although many may be in the low normal range.[40] Low testosterone levels are most likely caused by decreased testosterone production, but there is evidence for elevated metabolic clearance of testosterone in addition to decreased production.[36,38,40] As a result of normal testicular binding capacity, free testosterone and salivary testosterone levels also are low.[36,39,41,44] These abnormalities have been identified in patients despite differing methods of dialysis, including hemodialysis and peritoneal dialysis (CAPD).[42,43] Some dialysis patients have elevated levels of testosterone-binding globulin, and some patients have normal testosterone and free testosterone levels.[45-47] These low free and total testosterone

Sexual Function in Uremic Patients

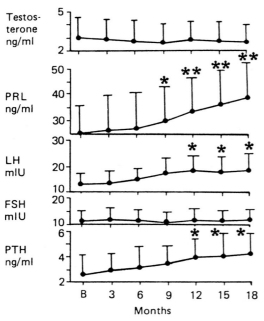

Figure 8–3. Behavior of serum hormones in males during 18-month follow-up. *p < 0.05, **p < 0.001 vs basal (B). (From Di Paolo N, Capotondo L, Gaggiotti E, Rossi P. Sexual function in uremic patients: 18 months follow-up in 26 subjects. Contrib Nephrol 77:34–44, 1990.)

levels remain low despite attempted stimulation with the administration of exogenous human chorionic gonadotropin (HCG).[48] These data strongly suggest that testosterone deficiency is a result of decreased hormone production and secretion. Investigation of patients immediately after initiation of dialysis in early uremia demonstrates an initial elevation in testosterone levels, suggesting that circulating toxins may be important in uremic testicular failure.[38] Unfortunately, however, testicular function is only temporarily restored, and men with CRF on hemodialysis or CAPD fail to experience restoration of hormone production satisfactory to restore fertility or potency. Although the exact level of testosterone synthesis deficiency remains controversial, recent evidence points to abnormalities in the production of dehydroisoandrosterone (DHA) from 17-hydroxypregnenolone via the enzyme catalyzed reaction with desmolase C17-20. Restoration of testosterone levels with exogenous testosterone administration in patients with deficient circulating testosterone frequently, however, fails to restore adequate sexual functioning and fertility.[36,48]

Most uremic males demonstrate abnormalities

of pituitary hormone secretion. These abnormalities include LH, FSH, and prolactin changes. LH levels are characteristically increased in males with uremia on maintenance dialysis. This increase is caused by both an increase in secretion and reduced metabolic clearance of the hormone.[49,50] It has been estimated that LH levels exceed 20% of normal in many of these patients probably as a result of decreased testosterone levels caused by hypogonadism. Evaluation of FSH levels likewise demonstrates abnormalities. However, FSH is usually only increased in patients with significantly diminished spermatogenesis.[50] Holdsworth et al. have suggested that the FSH levels in patients with uremia can be used as prognostic indicators for return of fertility following renal transplantation.[50] If FSH levels are significantly elevated and spermatogenesis is grossly abnormal, patients are unlikely to have a return of semen analyses consistent with expected fertility.[50] Occasionally, pituitary abnormalities can be suggested by low LH levels despite low testosterone concentrations.[51,52] More commonly, however, pituitary response to gonadotrophin-releasing hormone (GNRH) with increased FSH and LH production is quite normal.[47,50,52,53] Rodger et al. have suggested that testosterone secretion is further effected by the loss of pulsatile rhythm of luteinizing hormone-releasing hormone (LHRH), resulting in diminished LH peak levels.[47]

A probable proposed cause of sexual dysfunction in patients with chronic renal failure is hyperprolactinemia. Sexual dysfunction is commonly experienced by patients with hyperprolactinemia caused by pituitary neoplasms or pharmacologic abnormalities with normal renal function. Although the mechanism of sexual dysfunction caused by hyperprolactinemia remains controversial, loss of libido, decreased erectile function, and infertility have been widely associated with elevations in prolactin.[54] The cause of sexual dysfunction in those patients with elevated prolactin may be a result of disordered hypothalamic pituitary axis or a direct peripheral gonadal effect of prolactin. Hyperprolactinemia without renal failure usually results in increased levels of LH and hypogonadism. This response differs from the usual low testosterone and the low LH associated with the hyperprolactinemia of CRF. There is evidence to suggest that the elevation in prolactin in uremic men is a result of not only increased secretion but also reduced degradation of secreted prolactin.[55]

Hyperprolactinemia is identified in more than 50% of CRF patients on dialysis.[56,57] Increased prolactin levels also can be a result of medications used in patients with CRF. These medications include methyldopa, digoxin, cimetidine, and metoclopramide. There are numerous reports of improvement of erectile dysfunction and fertility when hyperprolactinemia alone is treated.[56]

Other endocrinologic abnormalities can strongly contribute to erectile dysfunction in patients with CRF on dialysis treatment. Most common among these is diabetes mellitus, which is one of the most common causes of erectile dysfunction with or without renal failure. Vascular changes in long-term insulin-dependent diabetics are well known and cause corporal arterial insufficiency and veno-occlusive dysfunction. In younger patients with normal vascular function, diabetic renal complications frequently are associated with autonomic peripheral neuropathy and neuropathic dysfunction, resulting in inadequate erectile response. These abnormalities significantly increase the neurologic abnormalities associated with erectile dysfunction previously described.[58,59]

Other hormonal abnormalities that contribute to erectile dysfunction in uremic men include abnormalities in parathyroid hormone. Massry et al. have suggested that elevated parathyroid hormone levels are an integral part of uremic male erectile dysfunction.[60] They report 2 impotent dialysis patients in whom sexual function was restored following parathyroidectomy without other changes in CRF management.[60] These investigators have suggested that elevated PTH may result in both peripheral and central nervous system defects that decrease erectile function. Akmal et al., in a laboratory study using a canine uremic model, demonstrated significantly decreased serum testosterone levels, which could be prevented by parathyroidectomy before producing experimental uremia.[61]

OTHER FACTORS ASSOCIATED WITH ERECTILE DYSFUNCTION

Zinc deficiency and abnormal zinc metabolism in uremic patients associated with gonadal dysfunction have been reported but remain controversial.[62–64] Because of the difficulty in assessing true tissue zinc levels and the effect of these levels on erectile function, it cannot be satisfactorily concluded that serum or tissue zinc levels are directly responsible for erectile dysfunction, and it cannot be concluded that zinc administration could be expected to produce improvement in sexual function, fertility, or libido.[65–67]

DIAGNOSIS OF UREMIC IMPOTENCE

It is clear from the foregoing discussion that the causes of erectile dysfunction and infertility in uremic men can be multifactorial. As a result, a careful history, physical examination, and appropriate laboratory studies are necessary to provide specific, tailored, and adequate treatment for these individuals. A careful history to identify psychologic factors, such as significant depression, must be carried out by a qualified mental health care professional. A careful physical examination, including studies for the identification of peripheral neuropathy and vascular abnormalities, is also helpful. The use of NPT monitoring in patients with marginal erectile dysfunction may be helpful in differentiating those patients with clear organic causes for their erectile dysfunction from patients with a significant psychogenic diagnosis. In patients in whom venoocclusive incompetence or arterial abnormalities are suspected by Doppler screening studies, dynamic infusion, pharmacocavernosometry and cavernosography along with colored Doppler arterial response studies may be helpful, especially if surgical intervention is planned.

A hormone profile to include testosterone, LH, prolactin, and FSH should be performed. Although provocative studies using LHRH or thyroid-releasing hormone (TRH) may be academically interesting, their importance in treatment programs remains controversial. Communication with nephrologist and transplant surgeon is essential, as transplantation may reverse many of the previously mentioned abnormalities of uremia, and initiation of specific impotence treatment modalities may be delayed until after transplantation is carried out in some patients.

TREATMENT ALTERNATIVES
Medical Treatment

Patients with deficient testosterone levels may be treated with testosterone replacement therapy with benefit to some patients. Most commonly, testosterone replacement therapy improves libido without significant impact on potency or fertility. Although testosterone can be replaced using oral medication, it is usually most effectively administered with sustained-release injectable testosterone preparations.[68,69] Many studies, however, have demonstrated that even the use of 100 to 200 mg of testosterone injected weekly produces only variable improvement in sexual function.[70,71] Other methods of raising serum testosterone have been more effective. These methods include clomiphene (100 mg/day) and HCG (500 IU/week).[72,73]

Pharmacologic methods for decreasing hyperprolactinemia also appear to be effective in some males with uremic-associated sexual dysfunction. Dopaminergic agonists, such as bromocryptine or lisuride hydrogen maleate, have been effective in some patients.[57,74,75] Bromocryptine can be administered in doses of 1.25 to 5 mg daily, and lisuride can be given at doses from 0.05 to 0.2 mg daily, with expected decrease in prolactin levels to the low normal range. Subsequent rises in plasma testosterone with expected improvement in sexual function result from these medications. Side effects from bromocriptine, including hypotension, nausea, and dizziness, are intolerable to some patients but seem to be less frequent with lisuride.[74]

Zinc therapy with administration of zinc through the dialysate or oral administration remains controversial. Further studies with dialysis and zinc administration are necessary before firm conclusions can be drawn about the effectiveness of zinc replacement and restoration of sexual function.[76,77]

CRF and uremia frequently are associated with profound anemia, which may result in psychologic erectile dysfunction caused by weakness, fatigue, and anxiety. The association of anemia and hormonal abnormalities is also the subject of some controversy.[78] Treatment of anemia with recombinant human erythropoietin in male uremic patients has been reported to improve sexual performance and fertility and to increase serum testosterone and FSH levels. Although the studies on recombinant human erythropoietin are preliminary, there appears to be some salutary effect of this method of treatment in some uremic patients.[79,80]

Intracavernosal Injection of Vasoactive Agents

Since the majority of uremic patients on hemodialysis in the younger age group have adequate vascular supply to their corpora cavernosa, injection of vasoactive agents into the corpora cavernosa can be expected to result in return of erectile function. Some patients with vascular problems, such as diabetic microangiopathy, mild to moderate arteriosclerosis, and partial arterial dysplasia, may respond to higher doses of intracavernosal injection. Patients with concomitant venoocclusive incompetence, however, may not respond to these agents and may require surgical intervention or other therapeutic techniques. As noted in other discussions in this text, treatment with papaverine, papaverine and phentolamine, prostaglandin E_1, or combinations of these agents may be effective for long-term treatment of erectile dysfunction, with few complications. Successful injection of older patients has been reported, with expected higher dosage requirements but comparative success rates without increased complications.[81] Long-term use of these intracavernosal vasoactive agents has been demonstrated to be effective with few long-term complications in patients following renal transplantation.[82] No other abnormalities or effect on the transplanted kidney have been identified with this treatment technique, and it can be expected to be safe and effective.

Vacuum Constriction Devices

Vacuum constriction devices have been widely reported as effective in patients who are impotent with a variety of etiologies. These devices, which appear to be effective in diabetic males as well as in patients with other causes for erectile dysfunction, are rarely associated with morbidity but are difficult for some patients to use and to tolerate. Vacuum constriction devices, however, can be an alternative for motivated patients who find this method of treatment satisfactory.[83]

SURGICAL TREATMENT OF ERECTILE IMPOTENCE

A variety of surgical procedures have been proposed for arterial insufficiency causing erectile dysfunction. Although the success rates of these procedures are variable, their use in patients with CRF before transplantation may be associated with significant morbidity. Because most patients with CRF and uremia associated with erectile dysfunction have significant large and small vessel disease, adequate response from arterial bypass procedures cannot be expected. In selected patients, however, balloon dilatation of pelvic arteries may be helpful, with expected low morbidity.[17]

Implantation of Penile Prostheses

Implantation of penile prostheses in these patients may be expected to be successful, with low morbidity. Although there are few reports of penile prosthesis implantation in hemodialysis patients, penile implants are used commonly in patients with CRF following renal transplantation.[86] These surgical procedures are best left to patients who have undergone transplantation, since many patients will find return of sexual function, potency, and fertility after reversal of the toxic effects of uremia by renal transplantation. If, however, underlying disease processes preclude the return of normal erectile function, penile prosthesis implantation can be expected to be successful in many of these men. There is little question, however, that the immunocompromised patient is at increased risk for complications of prosthesis implantation, with a likely higher risk of prosthesis infection. Despite this increased risk, however, successful implantation and function can be expected in the vast majority of patients, with little morbidity.[87,88]

SEXUAL FUNCTION IMPROVEMENT AFTER RENAL TRANSPLANTATION

As a result of normalization of metabolic and hormonal function in patients after successful renal transplantation, many patients report improved

MANAGEMENT OPTIONS FOR PATIENTS
WITH CRF AND IMPOTENCE

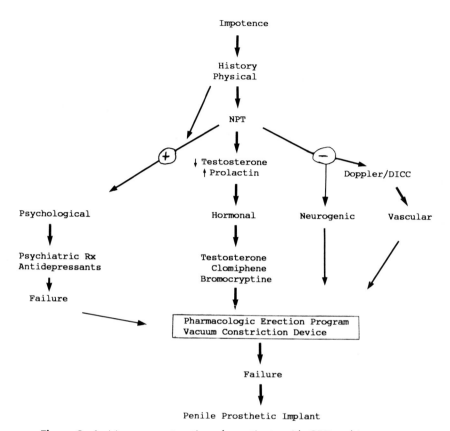

Figure 8–4. Management options for patients with CRF and impotence.

sexual function. Within 2 to 3 months of transplantation, testosterone levels frequently return to a normal range, with a concomitant normalization of LH, FSH, and prolactin levels. Lim and Fang reported a return of normal sperm count and motility 9 to 16 months after transplantation in 4 of 5 patients.[51] Gonadal resistance to gonadotropin stimulation also improves when hemodialysis and renal transplantation are successful. A more normal HCG stimulation with a higher testosterone response is observed in transplanted patients compared with those on hemodialysis. Salvatierra et al. studied a group of patients with CRF.[89] Their results demonstrate a 66% potency rate before the onset of CRF, declining to only 22% during dialysis. Following successful renal transplantation, however, 84% of patients with functioning renal allografts resumed preuremia potency within 3 years. Psychologic problems of hemodialyzed patients improved after transplantation, although there continued to be some increased anxiety despite decreased depression.[90]

Many patients, however, remain impotent after transplantation. Causes of posttransplant impotence include failure to resolve hormonal abnormalities, underlying disease processes that have resulted in continued erectile dysfunction, and the effects of the renal transplant itself.[91] As many as 87% of patients will continue to be impotent following transplantation.[92,93] The causes for this erectile dysfunction vary. The majority of patients will have restoration of hormone values, and no specific posttransplant diagnosis is consistent with erectile dysfunction. Reports of marked increase in erectile dysfunction following bilateral renal transplantation may be a result of changes in pelvic hemodynamics resulting from decreased penile blood flow, although reports of patients potent following interruption of bilateral hypogastric arteries are common. Impotence following sequential bilateral renal transplantation, however, appears to be increased as a result of decreased blood flow associated with ligation of both internal iliac arteries. Because of the difficulties with underlying vascular disease, multiple surgical interventions, and patient risk factors, revascularization may result in higher potential morbidity than the use of a penile implant in these complex surgical patients.[21,94,95] Billet et al., however, reported a successful saphenous vein bypass graft between the external iliac and internal iliac arteries in a patient impotent following bilateral renal transplantation.[94] Their patient demonstrated substantial improvement in penile blood flow and reported subjective return of erections and sexual function.

CONCLUSION

Patients with CRF, uremia, hemodialysis, and transplantation frequently suffer from loss of libido, erectile dysfunction, and infertility (Fig. 8–4). This multifactorial condition results in psychologic, hormonal, neurologic, vascular, and pharmacologic effects, all of which combine to limit sexual activity. Although pharmacologic manipulation of hormonal abnormalities may improve libido, erectile dysfunction is more difficult to resolve. Renal transplantation appears to be the most effective method for improving sexual function in the majority of patients. Despite renal transplantation and the resolution of hormonal abnormalities, however, underlying medical problems frequently continue the chronic erectile dysfunction. Treatment alternatives must, therefore, be directed not only at the CRF but also at the specific causes of erectile dysfunction. Treatment alternatives, in addition to pharmacologic manipulation, include intracorporal injection of pharmacoactive agents, vacuum constriction devices, and penile prosthesis implantation. Although revascularization posttransplant is an option, it should be considered only in highly selected patients.

REFERENCES

1. DiPaola N, Capotondo L, Gaggiotti E, Rossi P. Sexual function in uremic patients. Contrib Nephrol 77:34–44, 1990.
2. Abram HS, Hester LR, Sheridan WF, Epstein GM. Sexual functioning in patients with chronic renal failure. J Nerv Ment Dis 160:220, 1975.
3. Waltzer WC. Sexual and reproductive function in men treated with hemodialysis and renal transplantation. J Urol 126:713, 1981.
4. Rodger RSC, Fletcher K, Dewar JH, et al. Prevalence and pathogenesis of impotence in 100 uremic men. Uremia Invest 8:89, 1984.
5. Massry SG, Goldstein DA, Procci WR, Kletzky OA. On the pathogenesis of sexual dysfunction of the uremic male. Proc Eur Dial Transplant Assoc 17:139, 1980.
6. Levy NB. Sexual adjustment and maintenance, hemodialysis and renal transplantation. National survey by questionnaire: preliminary report. Trans Am Soc Artif Intern Organs 9:138, 1973.
7. Sherman FP. Impotence in patients with chronic renal failure on dialysis: its frequency and etiology. Fertil Steril 26:221, 1975.
8. Procci WR. The study of sexual dysfunction in uremic males: problems for patients and investigators. Clin Exp Dial Apheresis 7:289, 1983.
9. Glass CA, Fielding DM, Evans C, Ashcroft JB. Factors related to sexual functioning in male patients undergoing hemodialysis and with kidney transplants. Arch Sex Behav 16:189, 1987.
10. Kinsey AC, Pomeroy WB, Martin CE, eds. Sexual Behavior in the Human Male. Philadelphia: WB Saunders Co, 1948:86.
11. Masters WH, Johnson VE, eds. Human Sexual Inadequacy. Boston: Little, Brown, and Co, 1970.
12. Procci WR, Goldstein DA, Adelstein J, Massry SG. Sexual dysfunction in the male patient with uremia: a reappraisal. Kidney Int 19:317, 1981.
13. Karacan I. NPT/rigidometry. In: Kirby RS, Carson CC, Webster GD, eds. Impotence: Diagnosis and Management of Erectile Dysfunction. Boston: Butterworth, Heinemann, 1991:62–71.
14. Krumlovsky FA, Madsen JD. Mechanism and therapy of impotence associated with chronic renal failure and chronic dialysis. J Dial 3:395, 1979.
15. Pacitti A, Segoloni GP, Gallon EG, et al. An outpatient approach to sexual problems in uremic patients. Contrib Nephrol 77:45, 1990.
16. Leriche R. Des obliterations arterialles haules (obliteration de la termination de l'aorte) comme cause d'insuffisance circulatore des mambre inferieures. Bull Mem Soc Chir Paris 49:1404, 1923.
17. Goldwasser B, Carson CC, Braun SD, McCann RL. Impotence due to the pelvic steal syndrome: treatment by iliac transluminal angioplasty. J Urol 133:860, 1985.
18. Dalal S, Gandhi VC, Yu AW, et al. Penile calcification in maintenance hemodialysis patients. Urology 40:422, 1992.
19. Lindner A, Charra B, Sherrar D, Scribner BH. Accelerated atherosclerosis and prolonged maintenance hemodialysis. N Engl J Med 290:697, 1974.
20. Virag R, Bouilly P, Frydman D. Is impotence an arterial disorder? Lancet 1:181, 1985.
21. Ngheim DD, Corry RJ, Mendez GP, Lee HM. Pelvic hemodynamics and male sexual impotence after renal transplantation. Am Surg 48:532, 1982.
22. Carson CC. Impotence: new diagnostic modalities. Urol Annu 6:229, 1992.
23. Rudnick J, Becker HC. Present state of diagnostic management in venoocclusive dysfunction. Urol Int 49:9, 1992.
24. Saenz de Tejada I. Etiology of impotence. Contemporary Urology. Oradell, NJ: Medical Economics Co.
25. Fraser CL, Arief AI. Nervous system complications in uremia. Ann Intern Med 109:143, 1988.
26. Nogues MA, Starkstein S, Davolas M, et al. Cardiovascular reflexes and pudendal evoked responses in chronic hemodialysis patients. Funct Neurol 6:359, 1991.

27. Campese VM, Procci WR, Levitan D, et al. Autonomic nervous system dysfunction and impotence in uremia. Am J Nephrol 2:140, 1982.
28. Kersh ES, Kronfield SJ, Unger A, et al. Autonomic insufficiency in uremia as a cause of hemodialysis-induced hypotension. N Engl J Med 290:650, 1974.
29. Waltzer WW. Sexual and reproductive function in men treated with hemodialysis and renal transplantation. J Urol 126:713, 1981.
30. Eardley I, Kirby RS, Fowler CJ. Neurophysiological testing. In: Kirby RS, Carson CC, Webster GD, eds. Impotence: Diagnosis and Management of Male Erectile Dysfunction. Boston: Butterworth, Heinemann, 1991:109.
31. Wein AJ, van Arsdalen KN. Drug-induced male sexual dysfunction. Urol Clin North Am 15:23, 1988.
32. Stevenson JG, Umstead GS. Sexual dysfunction due to antihypertensive agents. Drug Intel Clin Pharm 18:113, 1984.
33. Kim JY, Park HY, Kerfoot WW, et al. Local effects of antihypertensive agents on isolated corpus cavernosum. J Urol (in press).
34. Jandhyala BS, Clarke DE, Buckley JP. Effects of prolonged administration of certain antihypertensive agents. J Pharm Sci 63:1497, 1974.
35. Hedlund H, Andersson KE. Comparison of the responses to drugs acting on adrenoreceptors and muscarinic receptors in human isolated corpus cavernosum and cavernous artery. J Autonomic Pharm 5:81, 1985.
36. Copolla A, Cuomo G. Pituitary testicular evaluation in patients with chronic renal insufficiency in hemodialysis treatment. Min Med 81:461, 1990.
37. Menchini-Fabris GF, Turchip-Giorgi PM, Canale D. Diagnosis and treatment of sexual dysfunction in patients affected by chronic renal failure on hemodialysis. Contrib Nephrol 77:24, 1990.
38. Stewart-Bently M, Gans D, Horton R. Regulation of gonadal function in uremia. Metabolism 23:1065, 1974.
39. Ramirez G, Butcher D, Bruggenmyer CD, Gungangly A. Testicular defect: the primary abnormality in gonadal dysfunction of uremia. South Med J 80:698, 1987.
40. Corvol B, Beretagna X, Bedrossian J. Increased steroid metabolic clearance rate in anephric patients. Acta Endocrinol 75:756, 1974.
41. DeVries CP, Gooren LJG, Oe PL. Hemodialysis and testicular function. Int J Androl 7:97, 1984.
42. Gokal R, Utley L. A collection of problems in CAPD. Adv Perit Dial 5:76, 1989.
43. Altman JA. Sex hormones and chronic renal failure of the diabetic. Ann Endocrinol 49:412, 1988.
44. Muir JW. Bromocryptine improves reduced libido and potency in men receiving maintenance hemodialysis. Clin Nephrol 20:308, 1983.
45. Bommer J, Kugel M, Schwobel B, et al. Improved sexual function during recombinant human erythropoitin therapy. Nephrol Dial Transplant 5:204, 1990.
46. Rodger RSC, Morrison L, Dewar JH, et al. Loss of pulsatile luteinizing hormone secretion in men with chronic renal failure. Br Med J 291:1598, 1985.
47. Rodger RSC, Dewar JH, Turner SJ, et al. Anterior pituitary dysfunction in patients with chronic renal failure treated by hemodialysis or continuous peritoneal ambulatory dialysis. Nephron 43:169, 1986.
48. Rager K, Bundschu H, Gupta D. The effect of HCG on testicular androgen production in adult men with chronic renal failure. J Reprod Fertil 42:113, 1975.
49. Zumoff B, Walter L, Rosenfeld RS. Subnormal plasma adrenal androgen levels in men with uremia. J Clin Endocrinol Metab 51:801, 1980.
50. Holdsworth S, Atkins RC, deKretsker DM. The pituitary testicular axis in men with chronic renal failure. N Engl J Med 296:1245, 1977.
51. Lim VS, Fang VS. Gonadal dysfunction in uremic men: a study of hypothalamo-pituitary-testicular axis before and after renal transplantation. Am J Med 58:655, 1975.
52. LeRoith D, Danovitz G, Trestian S, Spitz JM. Dissociation of pituitary glycoprotein response to releasing hormones in chronic renal failure. Acta Endocrinol 93:277, 1980.
53. Distiller LA. Pituitary gonadal function in chronic renal failure: the effect of luteinizing hormone-releasing hormone and the influence of dialysis. Metabolism 24:711, 1975.
54. Spark RE. Hyperprolactinemia in males with and without pituitary microadenomas. Lancet 2:129, 1982.
55. Sieverstein GD, Lim VS, Nakawates EC. Metabolic clearance and secretion rates of human prolactin in normal subjects and in patients with chronic renal failure. J Clin Endocrinol Metab 50:846, 1980.
56. Vircburger MI, Prelevick GM. Testosterone levels after bromocryptine treatment in patients undergoing long-term hemodialysis. J Andro 6:113, 1985.
57. Bommer J, del Pozo E, Ritz E, Bommer G. Improved sexual function in male hemodialysis patients on bromocryptine. Lancet 2:496, 1979.
58. Saenz de Tejada I, Goldstein I. Diabetic penile neuropathy. Urol Clin North Am 15:17, 1988.
59. Brindley GS. Neurophysiology. In: Kirby RS, Carson CC, Webster GD, eds. Impotence: Diagnosis and Management of Erectile Dysfunction. Boston: Butterworth, Heinemann, 1991:27.
60. Massry SG, Goldstein DA, Procci WR, Kletzky OA. Impotence and patients with uremia. A possible role for parathyroid hormone. Nephron 19:305, 1977.
61. Akmal M, Goldstein DA, Kletzky OA, Massry SG. Hyperparathyroidism and hypotestosteronemia of acute renal failure. Am J Nephrol 8:166, 1988.
62. Rodger RS, Sheldon WL, Watson MJ, et al. Zinc deficiency and hyperprolactinemia are not reversible causes of sexual dysfunction in uremia. Nephrol Dial Transplant 4:888, 1989.
63. Condon CJ, Freeman RM. Zinc metabolism in renal failure. Ann Intern Med 73:531, 1970.
64. Mahajan SK, Abbasi DA, Prasad AA, et al. Effect of oral zinc therapy on gonadal function in hemodialysis patients. Ann Intern Med 97:357, 1982.
65. Ritz E, Bommer J. Discussion. Zinc metabolisms. Contrib Nephrol 38:126, 1984.

66. Sprenger KB, Schmitz J, Hetzel D, et al. Zinc and sexual dysfunction. Contrib Nephrol 38:119, 1984.

67. Rodger SC, Brook AC, Muirhead N, Kerr DNS. Zinc metabolism does not influence sexual function in chronic renal insufficiency. Contrib Nephrol 38:112, 1984.

68. van Coeverden A, Stolear JC, dHaen EM, et al. Effect of chronic oral testosterone on the pituitary testicular axis on hemodialyzed male patients. J Clin Nephrol 26:48, 1988.

69. Barton CH, Mirahamadi MK, Vairi ND. Effects of long-term testosterone administration on pituitary testicular axis and end-stage renal failure. Nephron 31:61, 1982.

70. Lim VS. Reproductive function in patients with renal insufficiency. Am J Kidney Dis 4:363, 1987.

71. Foulks CJ, Cushner HM. Sexual function in the male dialysis patient. Pathogenesis, evaluation and therapy. Am J Kidney Dis 4:211, 1986.

72. Lim VS, Fang VS. Restoration of plasma testosterone levels in uremic men with clomiphene citrate. J Clin Endocrinol Metab 43:1370, 1976.

73. Canale D. Human chorionic gonadotropin treatment of male sexual inadequacy in patients affected by chronic renal failure. J Androl 5:120, 1984.

74. Ruilope L, Garcia-Robles R, Paya C, et al. Influence of lisuride and dopaminerigic agonists on the sexual function of male patients with chronic renal failure. Am J Kidney Dis 3:182, 1985.

75. Muir JW, Besser GM, Edwards CRW, et al. Bromocryptine improves reduced libido and potency in men receiving maintenance hemodialysis. Clin Nephrol 20:308, 1983.

76. Brook AC, Johnston DG, Ward MK, et al. Absence of therapeutic effect of zinc in sexual dysfunction of hemodialysis patients. Lancet 2:618, 1980.

77. Mahajan SK, Handburger RJ, Flamenbaum W, et al. Effect of zinc supplementation and hyperprolactinemia in uremic men. Lancet 2:750, 1985.

78. Campese VM, Liu CL. Sexual dysfunction in uremia. Contrib Nephrol 77:1, 1990.

79. Imagawa A, Kawanish Y, Numata A. Is erythropoietin effective for impotence in dialysis patients? Nephron 54:95, 1990.

80. Schaefer RM, Kokot F, Wernze H, et al. Improved sexual function in hemodialysis patients on recombinent erythropoietin: a possible role for prolactin. Clin Nephrol 31:1, 1989.

81. Kerfoot WJ, Carson CC. Pharmacologically induced erections among geriatric men. J Urol 146:1022, 1991.

82. Rodriguez Antolin A, Morales JM, Andres A, et al. Treatment of erectile impotence in renal transplant patients with intracavernosal vasoactive drugs. Transplant Proc 24:105, 1992.

83. Wiles PG. Successful noninvasive management of erectile impotence in diabetic men. Br Med J 296:161, 1988.

84. Whitherington R. External penile appliances for management of impotence. Semin Urol 8:124, 1990.

85. Kim JH, Carson CC. Peyronie's disease as a complication of the use of vacuum constriction device. J Urol (in press).

86. Kabalin JN, Kessler R. Successful implantation of penile prostheses in organ transplant patients. Urology 33:282, 1989.

87. Walther PJ, Andriani RT, Maggio MI, Carson CC. Fornier's gangrene: a complication of penile prosthetic implantation in a renal transplant patient. J Urol 137:299, 1987.

88. Carson CC. Infectious complications of genitourinary prostheses. Prob Urol (In press).

89. Salvatierra O, Fortmann JL, Belzer FO. Sexual function in males before and after renal transplantation. Sobhma Abd el Hamidia At tamg Refaief: Effect of erythropoietin on sexual potency in chronic hemodialysis patients. Scand J Urol Nephrol 26:181, 1992.

90. Charmet GP. Sexual function in dialysis patients: psychological aspects. Contrib Nephrol 77:15, 1990.

91. Reinberj Y, Bumgardner GL, Aliabadi H. Urological aspects of renal transplantation. J Urol 143:1087, 1990.

92. Dillard FT, Miller BS, Sommer BG, et al. Erectile dysfunction posttransplant. Transplant Proc 21:3961, 1989.

93. Brannen GE, Peters TG, Hambridge KM, et al. Impotence after kidney transplantation. Urology 15:138, 1980.

94. Billet A, Dagher FJ, Querell A. Surgical correction of vasculogenic impotence in a patient after bilateral renal transplantation. Surgery 91:108, 1982.

95. Gittes RF, Waters WB. Sexual impotence: the overlooked complication of a second renal transplant. J Urol 121:719, 1979.

CHAPTER 9

Iatrogenic Causes of Impotence

Eric L. Martin
Alan H. Bennett

Penile tumescence is an intricate process that relies on an intact neurologic system, arterial and venous vascular tree, and local endothelium-derived transmitters. As medical knowledge has progressed, procedures that in the past would render the patient impotent with high frequency can be performed in a potency-preserving fashion. Although potency cannot be spared in all cases, advances in intracavernosal injection therapy have made iatrogenic impotence easily treatable.

NORMAL ANATOMY

The complexity of the vascular and nervous supply to the penis leaves many points of vulnerability to injury during surgical procedures. The penis receives its somatic supply from the dorsal nerve of the penis, which arises from the pudendal nerve. Interruption of the dorsal nerve will result in diminished afferent sensation and affect both reflexogenic and tactile erection.

CHOLINERGIC INNERVATION

Preganglionic cholinergic fibers arise from S2–S4 to join the pelvic plexus posterior to the rectum. From the pelvic plexus, they join the cavernous nerve fibers, which, as described by Walsh and Donker, are located outside of Denovilliers' fascia dorsolaterally between the rectum and the prostate.[1] The peripheral cholinergic neurotransmitter, acetylcholine, has only limited direct effects on human erection and likely acts through an endothelium-derived factor now thought to be nitric oxide. Nitric oxide stimulates production of guanosine monophosphate, leading to relaxation of smooth muscle and increased arterial inflow, as well as increased sinusoidal compliance.

SYMPATHETIC INNERVATION

Sympathetic tonus results in detumescence. Preganglionic fibers arise from spinal levels T11–T12 as well as S2–S4. Sympathetic fibers enter the inferior mesenteric plexus and superior hypogastric plexus, then join the hypogastric nerve to the pelvic plexus. From the pelvic plexus, they join the cavernous nerve, which courses as described.

ARTERIAL SUPPLY

The pudendal artery arises from the hypogastric artery and contributes the dorsal artery and the corporal and spongiosal arteries. As end-arteries, these vessels are especially sensitive to the effects of nicotine, diabetes, lipid disorders, and trauma.

VENOUS DRAINAGE

Venous drainage begins with the emissary veins, which drain the sinusoids and penetrate the tunica albuginea of the corpora cavernosa. Abnormalities of the tunica that prevent occlusion of the emissary veins or sinusoids may result in venogenic impotence. Additionally, abnormal communications between the corpora cavernosa and corpora spongiousam may result in venogenic impotence.

SURGICAL CAUSES OF IMPOTENCE
Prostatectomy for Benign Disease

Impotence after prostatectomy is a recognized, although relatively poorly studied, complication of one of urology's most common procedures. Although some authors have attributed postprostatectomy impotence to psychogenic factors,[2] most studies have found that patients with postoperative impotence had underlying erectile dysfunction before their procedure, and it is this group who are at highest risk of postprostatectomy impotence.[3–5]

Age appears to play a major role in the patient's potency after prostatectomy for benign disease. Men who become impotent after prostatectomy are slightly older than those who retain erectile function.[6] Men under 60 who were potent before operation had an 89% postprostatectomy potency rate in a study by Finkle and Moyers, and men over 60 who underwent prostatectomy had an overall 58% postoperative potency rate.[7] Supporting this finding are additional data from Gold and Hotchkiss, who found an overall potency rate of 80% for men under 60 in their study group, whereas only 32% and 34% of men over age 60 and 70, respectively, were potent.[8] Of note in their study, only 10% of men under age 60 reported worse potency postoperatively, whereas 62% and 66% of men over 60 and 70, respectively, reported worse potency, as measured by desire, quality of erection, frequency of intercourse, and ejaculation.[8] The actual overall incidence of impotence remains controversial, with widely disparate reports in the literature from 0% to 40%.[9,10]

In addition to age and preoperative sexual function, the type of operative intervention required to alleviate the patient's obstruction appears to have a direct effect on postoperative onset of impotence.[7,10] In two reports, Finkle et al. confirmed that simple perineal prostatectomy is associated with a 29% to 34% impotence rate, and suprapubic prostatectomy led to impotence in 14% to 25%. In the two studies, TURP had the lowest impotence rate at 4%.[9,11] Whereas simple perineal prostatectomy is associated with high impotence rates, other authors have failed to find significant differences in the frequency of postoperative impotence after TURP, suprapubic prostatectomy, or simple retropubic prostatectomy.[5]

It is clear that impotence can result from prostatectomy, and as noted previously, some authors believe that there is a psychologic component to postprostatectomy impotence. Zohar et al. assessed 15 potent men with a structured interview, and mini-Minnesota Multiphasic Personality Inventory (mini-MMPI) preoperatively and 6 months postoperatively and found three main differences between the potent and impotent men. Anxiety regarding the operation and its outcome correlated highly with postoperative impotence. In addition, the explanation the patient receives regarding the surgery and the expected outcome, with reassurance that he can expect normal erectile function with a low risk of impotence, appears to be an important factor in determining postoperative sexual function. Finally, the patient's general satisfaction with life, his relationships, sense of well-being, security, and optimism all appear to have some impact on postoperative sexual function.[2]

Several authors have noted worsening erectile dysfunction in patients with preexisting partial erectile dysfunction or risk factors (e.g., diabetes).[4,12,13] Lue hypothesized that these patients have "borderline neural and vascular function pre-operatively, and a minor change in neural conduction or arterial or venous flow was sufficient to jeopardize the erectile neuro vascular event."[14]

Numerous mechanisms can be postulated to account for erectile failure postprostatectomy. During perineal prostatectomy, the neurovascular bundles may be injured easily as they course within millimeters of the prostatic apex. During transurethral resection of prostate, thermal injury may occur to the cavernous nerves, which are intimately apposed to the prostatic capsule at the 5 and 7 o'clock positions near the apex. Spot cauterization of bleeding points, avoidance of perforation of the capsule, and limiting extravasation of irrigant may all help to lessen impotence.

Additionally, Lue has suggested that during simple retropubic prostatectomy, the capsular incision should be made near the bladder neck to avoid tearing into the region of the neurovascular bundles.[14] During simple retropubic prostatectomy, dissection should be limited to the midline as much as possible to avoid damage to the neurovascular bundles laterally.

Prostatectomy for Malignancy

Before description of the nerve-sparing radical prostatectomy, few patients maintained potency postoperatively. Walsh and Donker described the anatomy of the pelvic plexus and cavernous nerves in 1982, and since that time, the technique of radical prostatectomy has been modified to allow preservation of the neurovascular bundles either bilaterally or unilaterally and thus maintain potency in selected individuals.[1]

As previously outlined, the autonomic innervation of the erectile bodies of the penis arises from the pelvic plexus, including fibers from the anterior branches of S2–S4 as well as sympathetic fibers from T11–T12. In an elegant study, Lepor et al. described the precise location of the autonomic nerves to the corpora cavernosum. In this study the autonomic nerves were identified in the lateral pelvic fascia outside the prostatic fascia. Fortunately, the nerves are associated with capsular vessels of the prostate and, in general, lie lateral to these vessels within the lateral pelvic fascia some 1.5 mm to 3.0 mm from the prostatic capsule posterolateral to the prostate, allowing their identification and sparing intraoperatively.[15]

The technique of nerve-sparing radical prostatectomy and, by extension, radical cystoprostatectomy begins with incision of the endopelvic fascia at its reflection on to the pelvic sidewall. The puboprostatic ligaments are then carefully divided at their insertion on the pubis, avoiding medial dissection, which could result in bleeding from the deep dorsal bundle. At this point, either the deep dorsal bundle is controlled with suture ligatures passed anterior to the urethra, or alternatively, a right angle clamp may be passed around the dorsal vein complex anterior to the urethra and the dorsal vein complex may be ligated with a heavy absorbable suture. A suture ligature passed through the prostate proximal to the apex may decrease back bleeding and improve visualization as the anterior urethra is divided just distal to the prostatic apex. A right angle clamp can be placed behind the urethra after the intact bands of the lateral pelvic fascia have been separated from the urethra. After division of the urethra, the rectourethralis is divided in the midline, avoiding lateral dissection, which may injure the neurovascular bundles. The plane between prostate and rectum is opened bluntly, and the lateral pelvic fascia is released anteriorly from the prostatic capsule. The lateral pedicles are taken near the prostate, allowing the neurovascular bundles to fall away from the prostate posteriorly.

Indications for wide excision of the neurovascular bundle include surgery on an impotent male, lateral induration on examination, induration of the lateral pelvic fascia found intraoperatively, and fixation of the neurovascular bundle to the prostatic apex[16] (Tables 9–1, 9–2).

After the seminal vesicles have been reached, a plane of dissection can be developed between the seminal vesicles and bladder, facilitating excision of the prostate from the bladder neck. Finally, the seminal vesicles are dissected free and their vascular pedicles are ligated and divided. Similarly, the ampulary vas are ligated and divided.[16–18]

If both neurovascular bundles are preserved, a potency rate of 76% can be expected at 1 year postoperatively, and if one neurovascular bundle is preserved, 56% potency has been reported. In men less than age 50, potency was similar with unilateral or bilateral preservation of the neurovascular bundles.[19]

Recently, Leach conducted a prospective study of men aged 45 to 70 who underwent nerve-sparing radical prostatectomy. Patients were evaluated by interview with the patient and partner in 30 of 43, as well as by Doppler blood flow after injection of PGE_1, and NPT monitoring. In this study, at 6 months, 35% of men were potent, although most reported moderate to weak erections. At 12

TABLE 9–1
Indications for Nerve Sparing Radical Prostatectomy or Radical Cystoprostatectomy

Patient potent
Clinically localized disease
Stage B prostate cancer (may require unilateral excision of neurovascular bundle)

TABLE 9–2
Contraindications to Nerve-Sparing Radical Prostatectomy or Radical Cystoprostatectomy

Impotent patient
Patient with impaired preoperative potency
Tumor involvement of neurovascular bundle
Induration of lateral pelvic fascia
Carcinoma involving urethra
Extensive tumor involvement of seminal vesicles
Uncontrollable bleeding
Extraprostatic or extravesical tumor extension

months, 42% of men were potent, with no improvement at 18 months.[20] As noted previously by Walsh, postoperative potency was higher in men who had both neurovascular bundles spared.[1]

Quinlan et al. have shown that postoperative potency is related to several factors. Patient age over 70 is a poor prognostic sign for return of potency. Even with bilateral nerve sparing, only 22% of the patients over 70 years of age will remain potent, whereas in men less than 50 years of age, there is no influence on potency with unilateral excision. Clinical stage B2 or C disease results in a twofold increase in impotence.[19] Additionally, injury to accessory vessels from the obturator and vesicle arteries during radical prostatectomy may contribute toward arterial insufficiency.[19]

In a detailed report, Breza et al. described the variability of the arterial supply to the corporal bodies.[17] They found that an accessory internal pudendal artery was present in 7 of 10 cadaver dissections that coursed inferiorly on the bladder and then on the anterolateral surface of the prostate. In 1 cadaver, this vessel was present bilaterally, and in 6 it was present unilaterally, providing supplemental corporal blood supply in 5 of 6 specimens. In 1 cadaver, this accessory artery provided the only arterial supply to the left side of the penis. In this study, the origin of the accessory pudendal artery was variable but included the ipsilateral obturator vessel in the majority, the inferior vesicle artery in 3, and the superior vesicle artery in 1. Since this vessel ends as the cavernous artery in 3 of 4 cases, it is apparent that inadvertent injury to this accessory vessel or ligation of its vessel of origin (e.g., the obturator artery) may contribute to postoperative arteriogenic impotence.[17]

Cystoprostatectomy and Urinary Diversion

The technique used to preserve the neurovascular bundles during radical prostatectomy has been successfully applied to cystoprostatectomy.

Marshall et al. described their experience with an ileocolic neobladder after a potency-preserving cystoprostatectomy.[21] In this series, potency was maintained in 71% of patients. This high potency rate was likely affected by the large number of young patients in the study group (average age 52 years).

A technique for potency-preserving urethrectomy has been described by Brendler based on Walsh and Donker's original description of the anatomy of the pelvic plexus and cavernous nerves to the penis. In anatomic dissections, Brendler showed that the cavernous nerves travel posterolateral to the membranous urethra as they course through the urogenital diaphragm. From the urogenital diaphragm, the cavernous nerves appear to course to the crura of the corpora cavernosa. The observation was made that injury to the cavernous nerves during urethrectomy likely occurred during mobilization of the membranous urethra.[22]

Potency-preserving urethrectomy begins with a nerve-sparing approach to the prostate. After ligation of the dorsal bundle, the urethra is encircled and bluntly dissected from the urogenital diaphragm, with displacement of the neurovascular bundles posterolaterally. After the membranous urethra has been freed, the urethra is transected and the remaining prostatic and bladder pedicles are ligated and divided. Brendler recommends delaying the perineal dissection 2 weeks to decrease mobilization of the cavernous nerves. However, if frozen sections of the urethra are positive, urethrectomy should be completed at the time of cystoprostatectomy. Completion urethrectomy continues in the standard fashion with the patient in an exaggerated lithotomy position.[22]

Urethral Disruption

The management of urethral disruption remains controversial, with many advocating immediate realignment and others advocating initial suprapubic cystotomy followed by delayed urethral realignment. Part of this controversy has centered around potency after surgical intervention. In a review of 15 series of patients suffering urethral disruptions, Webster reported that 56% of patients treated by primary urethroplasty were impotent, whereas in 236 patients treated with delayed urethroplasty, only 11.6% were impotent.[23] More recent studies, however, have shown little difference in potency rates, 47% and 53%, between patients treated by immediate realignment or delayed urethroplasty.[24] Immediate urethroplasty, rather than simple realignment, is likely associated with an increased risk of postoperative impotence.[25] This may be secondary to extensive dissection undertaken at the time of acute injury or damage to vascular structures at the time of urethroplasty. Impotence following urethral disruption may be a result of the initial injury rather than intervention. At the time of pelvic fracture, many men are rendered impotent by damage to sacral nerve roots. Damage appears to be especially associated with sacroiliac fractures, extensive pelvic dissection to control bleeding, and prostatic dissection.[26] In a study of patients who became impotent after blunt perineal or pelvic trauma, Levine et al. reviewed 20 impotent patients who underwent selective internal pudendal arteriography. In patients with immediate impotence after pelvic trauma, arteriography revealed lesions in arteries within the hypogastric and cavernous arterial beds, with occlusive disease in the cavernous and dorsal arteries.[27] In patients who had suffered perineal trauma, significant lesions were identified in only 35% of the hypogastric cavernous beds. These patients more commonly had occlusive disease of the common penile artery, cavernous artery, or dorsal arteries.[27] Additionally, in reviewing a larger group of patients with a history of blunt pelvic or perineal trauma, these same authors found that either form of trauma was a risk factor for future impotence.

Optical Internal Urethrotomy

Rarely a cause of impotence, optical internal urethrotomy (OIU) has nonetheless been reported as a cause of iatrogenic impotence in small numbers of patients. McDermott et al. reported on 179 patients who had undergone OIU, of which 4 developed permanent or temporary impotence. Two of these patients had preexisting erectile impairment. Urethrotomy was performed at the 12-o'clock position and extended into the underlying spongiosum to allow passage of a 30F sound. Each patient had significant penile edema at the end of the procedure secondary to extravasation, and 1 patient developed a high-flow priapism.[28] After reviewing their experience, these authors suggested limiting urethrotomy to create a channel of approximately 22F. In addition to extravasation of irrigant, OIU may create abnormal venous communications between the corpus spongiosum and corpus cavernosum, allowing venous shunting and impaired turgidity, and large amounts of scar tissue generated by multiple urethrotomies may impair erectile ability. By limiting extravasation, scarring may be minimized.

Peyronie's Disease

Peyronie's disease covers a broad spectrum of lesions from small, insignificant plaques to severe bilateral involvement with impaired or absent erectile ability. Treatment centers around three interventions. The Nesbitt procedure has been shown to be safe and effective therapy for Peyronie's disease in men who maintain erectile ability. Alternatively, autologous dermal or tunica vaginalis grafts may be used to repair the area of plaque. It has been shown that plaque excision can be associated with the onset of postoperative venogenic impotence in 12% to 100% of patients undergoing the procedure.[29-33] Dalkin and Carter reported on 3 patients who had undergone plaque excision and dermal grafting and subsequently became impotent.[33] In evaluating these patients, they found venous leakage to be the primary factor responsible for the onset of postoperative impotence. No clear etiology for postplaque excision/grafting has been developed, but possible etiologies include scarring at the site of the graft, allowing emissary veins in that region to remain fixed and open. In men undergoing plaque excision, numbness may occur if the dorsal bundle is injured during dissection. For impotent patients with Peyronie's disease, a penile prosthesis can be considered to both correct curvature and provide rigidity. Chapter 11 gives a complete discussion of Peyronie's disease.

Penile Carcinoma

Large, bulky, or invasive tumors of the penis will require partial or complete penile amputation. Penis-sparing surgery has been shown to be effective for T1 and small T2 tumors.[34] Treatment modalities for T1 and small T2 tumors include surgery, laser fulgaration, and external beam radiation, all having near equivalent efficacy. The neodymium:YAG (Nd:YAG) laser has been recommended because of minimal tissue changes associated with its use. Conservation of the penis should result in continued potency. However, penis-conserving therapy should only be instituted when long-term follow-up can be assured, as recurrences have been reported as late as 8 years.[34]

Priapism

Priapism may be associated with impotence in up to 50% of men regardless of treatment. Priapism may result from sickle cell anemia, acute leukemia, trauma, alcohol or drug ingestion, hyperalimentation, or infection or be idiopathic (Table 9–3). As intracavernosal injection of vasoactive drugs has become more common, priapism resulting from injection therapy has occurred. Several strategies are available for treatment of postinjection priapism, including early use of oral terbutaline if erection persists for greater than 4 h.[35] Should this fail, cavernosal aspiration and irrigation with saline, dilute epinephrine, or phenylephrine solution is indicated. To perform corporal irrigation for treatment of priapism, a closed aspiration-irrigation system is used, consisting of a length of IV tubing connected to a three-way stopcock connected to a 19-gauge butterfly needle. Many patients will require oral or IM analgesics before aspiration-irrigation. After sterile preparation and draping, the corpora is cannulated midshaft with a 19-gauge butterfly needle. The corporal body is aspirated until partial detumescence occurs. The aspirate should be observed. Dark venous-appearing blood indicates low-flow priapism, whereas high-flow priapism is characterized by bright red returning on aspiration. One ampule of 1 ml of 1: 1000 epinephrine is mixed with 1 L of saline. Aspiration-irrigation is performed via the three-way stopcock, placing 20 ml of solution in the corporal body and waiting several minutes. The sequence can be repeated until detumescence occurs. If detumescence is not attained after 15 cycles or systemic toxicity occurs, a formal shunting procedure may be necessary.[36]

Patients with high-flow priapism may constitute a special subset of patients who have injury to the arterial system, allowing increased inflow while sinusoidal relaxation does not occur and pathologic corporal distention is absent. These patients may present after perineal trauma, and Das and Leidinger identified eight clinical characterisics of high-flow priapism.[37] (1) The patient will give a history of trauma, (2) the onset of priapism was prolonged, (3) the erection is not painful, (4) the penis is nontender and is not woody, (5) the aspirated blood is bright red with a PO2 consistent with arterial blood, (6) on aspiration-irrigation there is prompt detumescence followed by recurrent priapism, (7) the cavernosal artery signals are readily apparent on Doppler examination, and (8) on cavernosography there is no restriction to flow through the penile veins. In these patients, Das and others recommend selective pudendal arteriography, followed by embolization of abnormal arterial sinusoidal communications.[37,38] Other authors have recommended

TABLE 9–3
Causes of Priapism

Idiopathic
Drug induced
  Phenothiazines
  Trazadone
  Prazosin
  Guanethidine
Sickle cell disease/trait
Acute leukemia
Posttraumatic
Hyperalimentation
Prolonged pharmacologic erection

direct ligation of vessels providing the abnormal arterial blood flow to the sinusoidal space.[39]

Most cases of priapism are of idiopathic origin. Again, initial treatment consists of aspiration and irrigation. If this fails, creation of a glans/cavernosal fistula should be performed preferably within the first 24 h.[40] Patients with sickle cell disease are treated with hydration, oxygenation, alkalinization, and exchange transfusion. Patients with sickle cell disease may respond to aspiration-irrigation therapy if medical therapy fails. If priapism persists, a shunt procedure can be considered.

Renal Transplantation

Patients on dialysis are commonly impotent, with rates of 45% to 80% reported.[41,42] After transplantation, improvement in sexual function occurs in 50% of patients.[43,44] Several etiologies for post-transplantation impotence have been identified, including hypogonadism, hyperprolactinemia, autonomic neuropathies, and atherosclerotic cardiovascular disease.[45–47] Of special note is end-to-end anastomosis of the internal iliac artery to renal artery, which may result in impotence in men with preexisting arteriosclerosis. Gittes and Waters suggested avoiding the use of end-to-end internal iliac to renal artery anastomosis and instead employing an end-to-side renal artery to hypogastric artery anastomosis during transplantation if it is necessary to use the hypogastric artery as an inflow source.[48] Evaluation and treatment are similar to that of the nontransplant patient, although avoidance of implants should be strongly considered, since immunosuppressed patients will be at increased risk of prosthetic-associated infection.[49]

Colorectal Surgery

Both erectile and ejaculatory failure may occur after low anterior resection and abdominoperineal resection for colorectal carcinoma. Santangelo et al. reviewed a group of 25 potent men who underwent either abdominoperineal resection, low anterior resection, or high anterior resection. In the abdominoperineal group, 44% of patients became impotent postoperatively. For the high anterior group, no patients became impotent, and for low anterior resection patients, a 33% impotence rate was identified.[50] Other authors have reported similar findings.[51] Bernstein and Bernstein reported on the incidence of impotence in 122 patients under 65 years old who underwent abdominoperineal excision of rectal cancers at various clinics. The incidence of impotence varied from 53% to 100%, with an average rate of 76%.[52] Injury causing impotence may occur during the perineal phase of the abdominoperineal resection if the nervi erigentes

are torn from the sacral nerve roots. More likely, the injury occurs at the level of the periprostatic plexus as the neurovascular bundle courses posterolateral to the prostate along the rectum. Santangelo et al. suggested that in low-stage rectal carcinomas, potency may be preserved by limiting dissection near the periprostatic plexus. For more advanced tumors, wide resection remains necessary, with an increased risk of postoperative impotence.[50] As more lesions are deemed resectable via an anterior approach, thus avoiding a perineal dissection, higher preservation of postoperative potency may be possible.

Vascular Surgery

Aortofemoral reconstruction with synthetic grafts may influence postoperative erectile function. In a prospective study, Nevelsteen et al. examined the effects of aortofemoral reconstruction in 62 men with aortoiliac occlusive disease. Seventy-seven percent of their patients experienced no change from preoperative sexual function, 11.3% of patients had improved erectile function, and 20.5% of patients reported deterioration. Only 1 patient with normal preoperative erections became impotent in the postoperative period. However, in men with impaired preoperative erectile ability, 31% developed postoperative impotence. These authors proposed that postoperative impotence could be limited by nerve-sparing aortic dissection as well as attempting to restore pelvic bloodflow.[53]

Gorssetti et al. reported on 148 patients with preoperative impotence and aortoiliac disease. All patients had abnormal penile–brachial indices. On angiography, 80% of these patients had unilateral or bilateral hypogastric occlusive disease as well as more proximal lesions. Three operative interventions were undertaken. In 106 patients, standard aortofemoral bypass was performed without attempts at revascularization of the hypogastric arteries. Twenty-two (20.7%) of these patients regained erectile function. An additional 24 patients underwent aortofemoral bypass with distal anastomosis to the common iliac artery. Of this group, 18 (75%) regained erectile function. Finally, 18 patients had an additional graft on one side to the hypogastric artery, and 14 (77.7%) of these patients became potent. Only 13% of diabetic patients responded to revascularization. These authors concluded that in patients with severe vascular disease, impotence is often of vascular origin, and when feasible, revascularization of the hypogastric arteries should be undertaken.[54] Preservation of the inferior mesenteric artery also may play a role in preservation of collateral pelvic blood flow and, thus, improve postoperative potency.[55] Others have advocated direct arterial anastomosis between the vascular graft and a penile dorsal vessel in patients with Leriche's syndrome.[56]

Segraves and Rutherford suggested that in patients with recurrent impotence or buttock claudication after aortoiliac reconstruction, the bypassed iliac segment may be occluded. Selected patients may benefit by thromboendarterectomy of the proximal hypogastric artery or by direct hypogastric artery revascularization.[57]

Occlusion of the hypogastric arteries may result in arteriogenic impotence. During reconstruction of the aortofemoral segment, impotence can occur. However, preserving or restoring flow to the hypogastric arteries may restore erectile function.

Radiation Therapy

Patients treated with radiation therapy for prostatic or pituatary tumors are at risk of developing impotence. After radiation therapy for pituitary adenomas, hypogonadatrophic hypogonadism may occur and may respond to hormonal replacement.[58] Patients undergoing radiation therapy for prostate cancer who are potent before radiotherapy are reported to have an initial potency rate of 73% to 86%.[59,60] With time, the impotence rate approaches 50%.[60] Goldstein et al. reported that 79% of men noted decreased sexual function after radiation treatment for prostate cancer and thought the etiology may be vascular in origin.[61] Mittal has evaluated a small group of men pre- and postradiation therapy for prostate cancer and did not detect a change in penile blood flow.[62] In men with reduced sexual function before radiation therapy (intercourse less than three times per month), the postradiation potency preservation rate has been reported to be 43%.[60] Patients with postradiation impotence have responded well to intracavernosal injection therapy, with all patients in a recent report attaining erections sufficient for intercourse after injection therapy was instituted.[58]

Lumbar Spine Surgery

Impotence and failure of emission have been reported sporadically after anterior approaches to the spine.[63-66] During anterior approaches to the spine, only the sympathetic nerve fibers contained within the superior hypogastric plexus appear to be at risk. To injure the parasympathetic fibers responsible for erection, one would have to carry the anterior dissection below the pelvic brim and injure the nerve fibers as they exit S2–S4.[67] In young men who undergo sympathectomy, prolonged penile erection or priapism may occur whereas in older men, impotence has been reported after lumbar sympathectomy.[67,68] Impotence is rare after lumbar surgery and implies extended dissection be-

low the pelvic rim. Ejaculatory disturbances are more common and reflect disturbance of the sympathetic fibers in the hypogastric plexus.

Penile Amputation

Most cases of penile amputation are the result of psychotic episodes, where in response to hallucinations, the patient may amputate his genitalia. Others may suffer from severe personality disorders and perform autoemasculization while intoxicated. The rest of such individuals likely suffered from an assault and subsequent amputation.[69,70] Self-mutilation is not a contraindication for replantation. Greilsheimer and Groves reviewed 40 patients recovering after autoemasculanization. Of the 40 patients, 1 repeat attempt at emasculation and 1 suicide were reported.[69]

Current techniques of penile reimplantation are based on microvascular reapproximation of the dorsal neurovascular structures. Hypothermic ischemic times of up to 16 h have been reported with successful reimplantation.[71] Jordan and Gilbert suggest that hypothermic ischemic times of 24 h or more do not preclude successful reimplantation.[72] The technique of microreimplantation begins with debridement as necessary followed by spatulated, two-layer, end-to-end urethral anastomosis. If the amputation is proximal, the cavernosal arteries can be approximated. Next, the tunica of the corporal bodies are carefully reapproximated, and the dorsal neurovascular structures are sequentially reanastomosed. The fascia and skin are closed, with splinting of the urethral anastomosis and placement of a suprapubic tube.[72] If microreimplantation is not available and the patient cannot be transported to a suitable center, an alternative is corporal reapproximation and penile reattachment. Some authors recommend degloving of the penis and burying the corporal bodies in the scrotum when microvascular techniques are unavailable.[73,74]

Pediatric Urologic Procedures

Approximately 85% of male infants born between 1977 and 1979 underwent neonatal circumcision.[75] Complications of circumcision range from 1.5% to 5% and include concealed penis, penile torsion, chordee, and slough of the penis, all of which may impair a male's future erectile function.[76,77] Prevention of complications is most important in this population. The repair of concealed penis and penile torsion is similar. The penis is degloved, and in the case of concealed penis, sutures are passed into the tunic of the corporal bodies and then to distal Buck's fascia in several quadrants, thus releasing the penis and fixing the penile skin in place to prevent retraction. In a similar fashion, penile torsion requires degloving of the penis and again suture fixation of the corporal bodies to Buck's fascia once the true rotational orientation of the penis is attained. When chordee tissue is present, repair depends on resection of all chordee tissue to attain a normal erection. In some cases, intraoperative artificial erection may be useful during resection of the chordee tissue.

Complications of surgery for hypospadias are relatively common, with residual chordee most likely to affect future potency.[78] As with correction of chordee secondary to circumcision injury, the goal is to remove all residual chordee tissue. Again, the use of intraoperative artificial erection may be helpful. If residual bend is present, either Nesbit tucks may be used or dorsal plication sutures may be helpful to fully straighten the erection.[79] Many authors recommend completion of surgical intervention before 2 years of age to help reduce the psychologic trauma to the child.[80]

REFERENCES

1. Walsh PC, Donker PJ. Impotence following radical prostatectomy: insight into etiology and prevention. J Urol 128:492, 1982.
2. Ozhar J, Meiraz D, Moaz B. Factors influencing sexual activity after prostatectomy: a prospective study. J Urol 116:332, 1976.
3. Wasserman MD, Pollack CP, Spielman AJ. Impaired nocturnal erections and impotence following transurethral prostatectomy. Urology 15:552, 1980.
4. Bolt JW, Evans C, Marshal VR. Sexual dysfunction after prostatectomy. Br J Urol 58:319, 1986.
5. Hargreave TB, Stephenson TP. Potency and prostatectomy. Br J Urol 49:683, 1977.
6. Windle R, Roberts JBM. Ejaculatory function after prostatectomy. Proc R Soc Med 67:1160, 1974.
7. Finkle AL, Moyers TG. Sexual potency in aging males: status of private patients before and after prostatectomy. J Urol 84:1952, 1960.
8. Gold FM, Hotchkiss RS. Sexual potency following simple prostatectomy. NY State J Med 69:2987, 1969.
9. Hauri D. Life after prostatectomy. Urol Int 37:271, 1982.
10. Debacker E, Lauwerijns A, Willem C. Sexual behavior after prostatectomy. Eur Urol 3:295, 1977.
11. Finkle AL, Prian DV. Sexual potency in elderly men before and after prostatectomy. JAMA 196:139, 1966.
12. Cytron S, Simon D, Segenreich E. Changes in the sexual of couples after prostatectomy: a prospective study. Eur Urol 13:35, 1987.
13. Malone PR, Cook A, Edmonson R. Prostatectomy: patient's perceptions and long-term follow-up. Br J Urol 61:234, 1988.
14. Lue TF. Impotence after prostatectomy. Urol Clin North Am 17:613, 1990.
15. Lepor H, Gregerman M, Crosby R, et al. Precise localization of the autonomic nerves from the pelvic plexus to the corpora cavernosa: a detailed anatomical study of the adult male pelvis. J Urol 133:207, 1985.
16. Walsh PC. Radical retropubic prostatectomy with preservation of sexual function. Norwich Eaton Audio-Visual Library, 1988.
17. Breza J, Aboseif SR, Orvis BR, et al. Detailed anatomy of penile neurovascular structures: surgical significance. J Urol 141:437, 1989.
18. Walsh PC. Radical prostatectomy, preservation of sexual function, cancer control: the controversy. Urol Clin North Am 14:663, 1987.
19. Quinlan DM, Epstein JI, Carter BS, et al. Sexual function following radical prostatectomy, influence of preservation of neurovascular bundles. J Urol 145:998, 1991.
20. Leach GE. Potency evaluated after radical retropubic prostatectomy. AUA 92 Clin Persp 5:1, 1992.
21. Marshall FF, Mostwin JL, Radebaugh LC, et al. Ileocolic neobladder post-cystectomy: continence potency. J Urol 145:502, 1991.
22. Brendler CB, Schlegel PN, Walsh PC. Urethrectomy with preservation of potency. J Urol 144:270, 1990.
23. Webster GD. Perineal repair of membranous urethral stricture. Urol Clin North Am 16:303, 1989.
24. Husmann DA, Wilson WT, Boone TB, et al. Prostatomembranous urethral disruptions: management by suprapubic cystostomy and delayed urethroplasty. J Urol 144:76, 1990.
25. Turner-Warwick R. Prevention of complications resulting from pelvic fracture urethral injuries and from their surgical management. Urol Clin North Am 16:335, 1989.
26. Devine CJ, Jordan GH, Devine PC. Primary realignment of the disrupted prostatomembranous urethra. Urol Clin North Am 16:291, 1989.
27. Levine FJ, Greenfield AJ, Goldstein I. Arteriographically determined occlusive disease within the hypogastric-cavernous bed in impotent patients following blunt perineal and pelvic trauma. J Urol 144:1147, 1990.
28. McDermott DW, Bates RJ, Heney NM, et al. Erectile impotence as complication of direct vision cold knife urethrotomy. Urology 13:467, 1981.
29. Hicks CC, O'Brien DP, Bostwick J, et al. Experience with the Horton-Devine dermal graft in the treatment of Peyronie's disease. J Urol 119:504, 1978.
30. Palomar JM, Halikiopoulos H, Thomas R. Evaluation of surgical management of Peyronie's disease. J Urol 123:680, 1980.
31. Melman A, Holland TF. Evaluation of the dermal graft inlay technique for the surgical treatment of Peyronie's disease. J Urol 120:421, 1978.
32. Wild RM, Devine CJ, Horton CE. Dermal graft repair of Peyronie's disease: survey of 50 patients. J Urol 121:47, 1979.
33. Dalkin DL, Carter MF. Venogenic impotence following dermal graft repair for Peyronie's disease. 146:849, 1991.

34. Horenblas S, Tinteren H, Delemarre JFM, et al. Squamous cell carcinoma of the penis II: treatment of the primary tumor. J Urol 147:1533, 1992.

35. Fouda A, Hassouna M, Beddoe E, et al. Priapism: an avoidable complication of pharmacologically induced erection. J Urol 142:995, 1989.

36. Barada JH, Bennett AH. Therapeutic penile detumescence by corporal irrigation. Contemp Urol 3:40, 1991.

37. Das S, Leidinger RJ. Percutaneous embolization therapy of high-flow priapism. J Endourol 6:459, 1992.

38. Walker TG, Grant PW, Goldstein I, et al. "High-flow" priapism: treatment with superselective transcatheter embolization. Radiology 174:1053, 1990.

39. Ricciardi R, Bhatt GM, Cynamon J, et al. Delayed high-flow priapism: pathophysiology and management. J Urol 149:119, 1993.

40. Winter CC, McDowell G. Experience with 105 patients with priapism: update review of all aspects. J Urol 140:980, 1988.

41. Abram HS, Hester LR, Sheridan WF, et al. Sexual function in patients with chronic renal failure. J Nerv Ment Dis 160:220, 1975.

42. Nghiem DD, Corry RJ, Picon-Mendez G, et al. Factors influencing male sexual impotence after renal transplantation. Urology 21:49, 1983.

43. Procci WR, Hoffman KI, Chatterjee SN. Sexual functioning of renal transplant recipients. J Nerv Ment Dis 166:402, 1978.

44. Salvatierra O Jr, Fortmann JL, Belzer FO. Sexual function in males before and after renal transplantation. Urology 5:64, 1975.

45. Foulks CJ, Cushner HM. Sexual dysfunction in the male dialysis patient: pathogenesis, evaluation, and therapy. Am J Kidney Dis 8:211, 1986.

46. Sidi AA, Peng W, Sanseau C, et al. Penile prosthesis surgery in the treatment of impotence in the immunosuppressed man. J Urol 137:681, 1987.

47. Waltzer WC. Sexual and reproductive function in men treated with hemodialysis and renal transplantation. J Urol 126:713, 1981.

48. Gittes RF, Waters WB. Sexual impotence: the overlooked complication of a second renal transplant. J Urol 121:719, 1979.

49. Reinberg YR, Bumgardner GL, Aliabadi H. Urologic aspects of renal transplantation. J Urol 143:187, 1990.

50. Santangelo ML, Romano G, Sassaroli C. Sexual function after resection for rectal cancer. Am J Surg 154:502, 1987.

51. Weinstein M, Roberts M. Sexual potency following surgery for rectal carcinoma. Ann Surg 185:295, 1977.

52. Bernstein WC, Bernstein EF. Sexual dysfunction following radical surgery for cancer of the rectum. Dis Colon Rectum 9:328, 1966.

53. Nevelsteen A, Beyens G, Duchateau J, et al. Aorto-femoral reconstruction and sexual function: a prospective study. Eur J Vasc Surg 4:247, 1990.

54. Gossetti B, Gattuso R, Irace L, et al. Aorto-iliac/femoral reconstructions in patients with vasculogenic impotence. Eur J Vasc Surg 5:425, 1991.

55. Kawai M. Pelvic hemodynamics before and after aortoiliac vascular reconstruction: the significance of penile blood pressure. Jpn J Surg 18:514, 1988.

56. Krotovsky GS, Turpitko SO, Gerasimov VB, et al. Surgical treatment and prevention of vasculopathic impotence in conjunction with revascularization of the lower extremities in Leriche's syndrome. J Cardiovasc Surg 32:340, 1991.

57. Segraves A, Rutherford RB. Isolated hypogastric artery revascularization after previous bypass for aortoiliac occlusive disease. J Vasc Surg 5:472, 1987.

58. Pierce DJ, Whittington R, Hanno PM. Pharmocologic erection with intracavernosal injection for men with sexual dysfunction following irradiation: a preliminary report. Int J Radiat Oncol Biol Phys 21:1311, 1991.

59. Banker FL. The preservation of potency after external beam irradiation for prostate cancer. Int J Radiat Oncol Biol Phys 15:219, 1988.

60. Bagshaw M, Cox R, Ray G. Status of radiation treatment of prostate cancer at Stanford University. NCI Monogr 7:47, 1988.

61. Goldstein I, Feldman M, Deckers P, et al. Radiation-associated impotence, a clinical study of its mechanism. JAMA 251:903, 1984.

62. Mittal B. A study of penile circulation before and after radiation in prostate cancer and its effects on impotence. Int J Radiat Oncol Biol Phys 11:1121, 1985.

63. Duncan HJM, Jonck LM. The presacral plexus in anterior fusion of the lumbar spine. S Afr J Surg 3:93, 1965.

64. Goldner JL, McCollum DE, Urbaniak JR. Anterior disc excision and interbody spine fusion for chronic low back pain. In: AAOS Symposium on the Spine. St. Louis: CV Mosby Co, 1969:111.

65. Sacks S. Anterior interbody fusion of the lumbar spine. Clin Orthop 44:163, 1966.

66. Stauffer RN, Coventry MB. Anterior interbody lumbar spine fusion, analysis of Mayo Clinic series. J Bone Joint Surg 54A:756, 1972.

67. Johnson RM, McGuire EJ. Urogenital complications of anterior approaches to the lumbar spine. Clin Orthop 154:114, 1981.

68. Whitelaw GP, Smithwick RH. Some secondary effects of sympathectomy with particular reference to disturbance of sexual function. N Engl J Med 245:121, 1951.

69. Greilheimer H, Groves JE. Male genital self-mutilation. Arch Gen Psychiatry 36:441, 1979.

70. Hall DC, Lawson BZ, Wilson LG. Command hallucinations and self-amputation of the penis and hand during the first psychotic break. J Clin Psychiatry 42:322, 1981.

71. Wei FC, Mckee NH, Huerta FJ, et al. Microsurgical replantation of a completely amputated penis. Ann Plast Surg 20:317, 1983.

72. Jordan GH, Gilbert DA. Management of amputation injuries. Urol Clin North Am 16:359, 1989.

73. Bhanganada K, Chayavatana T, Pongnumkul C, et al. Surgical management of an epidemic of penile amputations in Siam. Am J Surg 146:376, 1983.

74. McRoberts JW, Chapman WH, Ansell JS. Primary anastomosis of the traumatically amputed penis: case report and summary of literature. J Urol 100:751, 1968.

75. Metcalf TJ, Osborn LM, Mariani EM. Circumcision: a study of current practices. Clin Pediatr 22:575, 1983.

76. Kaplan GW. Complications of circumcision. Urol Clin North Am 10:543, 1983.

77. AAP Task Force on Circumcision. Report of the task force on circumcision. Pediatrics 84:338, 1989.

78. Duckett JW. Hypospadias. In: Walsh PC, ed. Campbell's Urology, 5th ed. Philadelphia: WB Saunders Co, 1986:1969–1999.

79. Livne PM, Gibbons MD, Gonzales ET. Meatal advancement and glanuloplasty: an operation for distal hypospadias. J Urol 131:95, 1984.

80. Cromie WJ. Genital anomalies and their implications on potency. In: Bennett AH, ed. Management of Male Impotence. Baltimore: Williams and Wilkins, 1982:143–161.

CHAPTER 10

The Pharmacology of Impotence

Alvaro Morales

Jeremy W.P. Heaton

Michael Condra

The understanding of the pharmacology of impotence has shown a steady improvement over the last 15 years. This improvement has resulted in a better appreciation of the neurovascular mechanisms of the erectile process and the introduction of increasingly more effective medication to correct deficiencies in sexual performance. Intracavernosal therapy is dealt with in Chapter 17. Although our knowledge of the mechanisms of erection and libido is still deficient, a great deal has been clarified recently, and worldwide research in this area is continuing. It is anticipated that further definition of the interactions of central and peripheral mechanisms in sexual desire and performance will, in turn, result in more effective and simpler treatment approaches.

The current state of knowledge on the effect of drugs on libido and erectile function is built on a complex foundation. Coupled with methodologically sound research in some areas, most notably in treatment outcomes, there is also a patchwork of poorly designed studies, uncontrolled trials, clinical impressions, and single case reports. Because of the ease with which wide public interest is generated, the field is also replete with misinformation.

ERECTOLYTIC AGENTS

Although a large portion of the literature dealing with agents that negatively affect the erectile mechanisms of the penis is anecdotal, there is reliable evidence that a number of drugs consistently exhibit erectolytic activity (Table 10–1). The mechanisms of action of many of the drugs are not clearly understood. Furthermore, they are consistently or reliably accepted as etiologic agents in the development of male sexual dysfunction. A systematic approach to classification of these drugs can be started under the general subheading of recreational and therapeutic agents.

Recreational Agents

Most of these drugs are not only addictive but are frequently abused and exhibit a variety of physiologic and psychologic effects that may be devastating to sexual performance, particularly in individuals already victims of well-recognized predisposing factors. A series of problems exists in reaching conclusions about the impact of recreational drugs on erectile functioning. Among these problems are the tendency for polydrug use (e.g., alcohol and tobacco), delineation of chronic vs acute effects, and extreme variability in the quality of illicit substances. The compounds most commonly abused and recognized for their erectolytic effects are tobacco, alcohol, and cannabis.

Tobacco

The observation that smoking negatively affects erectile function is not new. As early as 1919, abstinence from tobacco smoking was considered part of an effective treatment for impotence.[1] However, a causal relationship has become more firmly accepted in the last decade. Several investigators[2,3] have provided evidence that smoking is a significant risk factor in erectile dysfunction, and its effects are evident in the small vasculature. Acute clinical experiments have shown clearly that smoking two cigarettes immediately before testing prevents the induction of an erection and markedly diminishes intracorporeal pressures following intracavernosal administration of papaverine.[4] As could be anticipated, the use of tobacco appears to work synergistically in aggravating the detrimental effect of intercurrent medical conditions (e.g., hypertension, diabetes) on potency.[5–7]

Alcohol

The consumption of alcoholic beverages has long been associated with the induction of erectile

TABLE 10–1
Erectolytic Drugs

Legal
Tobacco
Alcohol

Illegal
Cannabis
LSD
Cocaine

Iatrogenic
Endocrine
    Estrogens
    Antiandrogens
    LHRH analogues
    5-alpha-reductase inhibitors
Antihypertensives
    Diuretics
    Methyldopa
    Beta-blockers
    Calcium antagonists (?)
Psychotropics
    Major tranquilizers
    MAO inhibitors
    Tricyclic antidepressants
Other
    Histamine receptor antagonists
    Antihyperlipidemics

difficulties. Both central and peripheral mechanisms are involved in their development. Among the central mechanisms, there is convincing evidence that alcoholic liver disease is accompanied by profound alterations in the function of the pituitary-gonadal axis. The primary mechanism appears to be an increase in hepatic aromatization of androgens, as well as an enhanced activity of hepatic microsomal 5-alpha-reductase.[8] The fundamental influence of chronic alcoholic liver disease was documented elegantly and conclusively by the studies of Van Thiel et al.,[9] showing that liver-transplanted men with nonalcoholic hepatocellular disease had normal FSH, LH, and testosterone levels pre- and posttransplantation. By contrast, alcoholic men had abnormal endocrine function, which improved after successful transplantation. Further central mechanisms are independent of the hormonal milieu. There is extensive anecdotal evidence that potent men develop temporary inability to achieve an erection following the acute ingestion of large amounts of alcohol. A likely mechanism for this phenomenon is the physiologic activity of ethanol on the dopaminergic system.[10] Experimental evidence to support this hypothesis has been

provided by one of us (JPWH) in an animal model in which rats subjected to the acute administration of 0.5 mg/kg of ethyl alcohol exhibited an almost complete abolition of erectile activity.[11]

Among the peripheral mechanisms implicated in the causal relationship between alcohol and impotence, the most commonly accepted is the development of peripheral autonomic neuropathy.[12,13] The concept of peripheral neuropathy is widely but not universally accepted and has been challenged by at least one study. Using the electrophysiologic method of sympathetic skin potentials recorded from the genital skin and also by electrically inducing the bulbocavernous reflex, Ertekin et al.[14] found no difference in results between normal controls and impotent chronic alcoholics.

Alcohol abuse produces behavioral and interpersonal effects that are observed early in the domain of sexual performance. Chronic alcoholism is undoubtedly a major factor in the etiology of marital and psychologic alterations frequently found in couples in which one or both partners abuse alcohol.[15]

Cannabis

Convincing evidence is available indicating that both large acute doses and chronic use of marijuana seriously interfere with normal erectile function. The detrimental effects of the drug were found initially to be secondary to a depression in plasma testosterone.[16] This view is further supported by the significant reduction in fertility documented in users of cannabis. Tetrahydrocannabinol has been found to act as a dopamine agonist, with a number of central effects that may affect sexual functioning.[17] As with alcohol and other recreational substances, a number of psychologic and marital alterations are identified with cannabis use.

Other legal (Demerol) and illegal drugs have been implicated in the genesis of erectile failure. There is little reliable information on the widely believed but purely anecdotal association of cocaine and increased sexual enjoyment and sensitivity.

Therapeutic Agents

A large number of drugs used for therapeutic purposes exhibit, as a significant side effect, the induction of difficulties in sexual performance. For the purpose of this chapter, only those associated with recognized erectolytic activity or that are known to decrease sexual desire are included. As mentioned previously, a large body of literature exists that implicates a variety of therapeutic agents in hindering erectile function. Unfortunately, consistent and convincing evidence in support of those claims is the exception rather than the rule. For the purpose of convenience, they are listed by groups, highlighting the most representative of each class.

Hormones

The fundamental importance of androgens in the maintenance of normal sexual activity in men can be altered readily by many agents that are endocrinologically active. These substances are most often employed in the treatment of men with carcinoma of the prostate. Estrogenic compounds (diethylstilbestrol, ethinylestradiol) rapidly and effectively diminish both libido and erections. However, these hormones enjoy much less popularity nowadays due to their effects on the cardiovascular system. Antiandrogens have a major adverse effect on potency and libido. Flutamide, although inducing an increase in levels of total serum testosterone, has been associated with impotence and decreased libido, since it blocks the access of testosterone to all relevant target cells.[18] Recently, however, it was reported that a new, nonsteroidal, pure antiandrogen does not interfere with the frequency or quality of nocturnal erections.[19] Cyproterone acetate, on the other hand, is clearly detrimental to sexual function, and this characteristic has been exploited to treat sex offenders.[20] LHRH analogs (goserelin and leuprolide acetate) also are effective depressors of sexual function in males.[21]

A great deal of interest exists in the treatment of benign prostatic hyperplasia with compounds exhibiting endocrinologic activity. Progestins (medroxyprogesterone and hydroxyprogesterone), the early representatives of this group of drugs, are known to decrease libido and erectile function.[22] Finasteride (Proscar), a specific competitive inhibitor of the enzyme 5-alpha-reductase inhibitor, has been approved by the Food and Drug Administration for the treatment of benign prostatic hyperplasia. Although initial reports indicate that its effect on potency is minimal (0.2%),[23] a much larger and detailed experience is needed to confirm this early finding.

Antihypertensives

This class of drugs has long been implicated in the induction of erectile failure. A significant component of erectile dysfunction in hypertensive males is their inability to develop a rapid arterial vasodilatation commonly secondary to arterial wall hypertrophy, fixed vasomotor tone, or atherosclerotic plaques. Treatment of hypertension with diuretics or beta-blockers does not cause vasodilatation and may further impair penile tumescence and rigidity.[24] In fact, the development of erectile problems is one of the most common causes for noncompliance in the treatment of hypertension. There is an obvious difficulty in identifying the causal effect of an antihypertensive agent on a specific patient. The occurrence of hypertension commonly coincides with many factors related to age (diabetes, atherosclerosis) and prolonged history of substance abuse (tobacco, alcohol). There is a paucity of studies using rigid controls. Nevertheless, almost every antihypertensive medication has been implicated more or less frequently in the production of impotence. The information presented here, however, is hardly conclusive and should be interpreted with caution.

DIURETICS

These are commonly used as the first-line treatment for hypertension. It is believed by some[25] that with the exception of spironolactone, most diuretics alone are rarely the cause of serious erectile disturbances. Spironolactone appears to have a marked effect on libido at high doses (400 mg/day), whereas its effect as an erectolytic drug is much less marked.[26] Thiazides (hydrochlorothiazide, chlorthalidone, bendroflumethiazide) are the class of compounds most commonly associated with sexual disturbances, with a reported incidence ranging between 3% and 36%.[27,28]

METHYLDOPA (ALDOMET)

This synthetic derivative related to natural dopa has been implicated repeatedly in the induction of a variety of disturbances in sexual function, including impotence.[29] The variety of central and peripheral effects of this drug suggests that it is a major culprit and should be replaced by other agents if its administration coincides with the onset of erectile problems.

BETA-ADRENOCEPTOR BLOCKERS

These drugs are used for a variety of cardiovascular abnormalities, including hypertension. They have been included among the compounds affecting erectile function adversely. The Medical Research Council study[26] on antihypertensives and erectile dysfunction reported the incidence of impotence to be significantly higher on propranolol (13.8%) than on placebo. Again, in the presence of a temporal relationship between the administration of a beta-blocker and the development of impotence, the drug should be replaced with one of a different class.

ARTERIAL VASODILATORS

Hydralazine is the most commonly used of this class of compounds. Its primary mechanism of action is diminution of peripheral vascular resistance. It is seldom used as a single agent, and its role in erectile difficulties, therefore, is difficult to establish. Minoxidil, on the contrary, has been used to generate tumescence (see section on Erectogenic Drugs).

CALCIUM ANTAGONISTS

Treatment with arterial vasodilators is a sensible approach to the treatment of hypertension but generally requires concomitant diuretic or beta-blocker therapy, which carries adverse effects on penile tumescence. In a review of the effects of drugs on sexual function,[30] calcium antagonists were named as drugs not being reported to cause sexual dysfunction. There are, however, a few publications indicating that such a view may require reassessment. A single case focused on the development of impotence in a patient receiving verapamil.[31] Another cites the development of impotence in 3 of 14 subjects undergoing treatment of angina with verapamil.[32] These drugs are gaining increasing attention, since they are effective when used as single agents and induce vasodilatation as well as prevent further development of arterial wall abnormalities. Their effects on sexual function require additional study.

OTHER ANTIHYPERTENSIVES

It appears that almost every available antihypertensive agent has been, at one time or another, given putative erectolytic capacity. The only ones that have not been implicated as detrimental to sexual functioning are angiotensin-converting enzyme (ACE) inhibitors (Captopril) and minoxidil (mentioned among the vasodilators). ACE inhibitors do not impair quality of life by metabolic alterations, as has been reported with some beta-blockers and diuretics. In fact, ACE inhibitors may, over the long term, reverse vascular wall hypertrophy,[33] thus improving blood supply to the vasculature of the corpora and, probably, enhancing erectile capacity.

Psychotropic Agents

"As with antihypertensive agents, cases of male sexual dysfunction have been reported in at least some patients using virtually every psychiatric drug."[29] Identifying the direct cause (i.e., the patient's emotional state or the medication) is problematic.

ANTIPSYCHOTIC AGENTS

Most classes of major tranquilizers have been found to exhibit undesirable side effects in the area of sexual performance. Fluphenazine, thioridazine, and thiothixene were reported to inhibit erections in association with a decrease in libido. Chlorpromazine[34] and trazodone[35] are recognized

for their capacity to induce priapism. In the case of trazodone, this probably occurs through its adrenoceptor-blocking and dopaminergic agonistic properties.

Monoamine oxidase inhibitors (isocarboxazid, phenelzine, tranylcypromine) and tricyclic antidepressants (amitriptyline, clomipramine, imipramine) have been reported frequently as agents capable of inhibiting both erection and ejaculation. Lithium used as monotherapy has little effect on erections, but when used in combination with benzodiazepines, it was associated with sexual dysfunction in a large proportion of patients.[36] Fluoxetine (Prozac) is a frequently used antidepressant whose action is linked to its ability to inhibit the neuronal reuptake of serotonin. A recent prospective study found the development of sexual dysfunction in over one third of patients after successful antidepressant treatment with this drug. Interestingly, in the same report, 90% of the patients developing sexual dysfunction following the administration of fluoxetine and concomitantly treated with yohimbine reported an improvement in their sexual performance.[37] Recent indirect evidence indicates that lithium, fluoxetine, and imipramine exert a powerful downregulating effect in sexual behavior. It was reported that sexual addictions in paraphilic and nonparaphilic men respond promptly to the administration of these drugs.[38]

ANXIOLYTIC AGENTS

There is little evidence that minor tranquilizers interfere with sexual function. Early studies have shown that chlorazepate and diazepam exhibit no more activity against sexual function than placebo.[39] More recently, however, a meager report associated diazepam with sexual dysfunction.[40] Once more, these two reports illustrate the enormous difficulties in establishing a causal relationship between drugs and sexual functioning. The physician is forced to make a difficult decision and to be prepared to search for alternative therapies if a temporal relationship is found. Even in such situations, the suspect drug may not be the culprit, since the placebo effect has been so frequently found to be significant.

Other Drugs

A large variety of pharmacologic agents continue to be implicated in the induction of erectile difficulties. Included here are only those reported to affect erectile function and that are commonly used in medical practice. For some, a possible or definitive pharmacologic mechanism of action has been documented. The rest are included only because sufficient reports exist in the literature to make them suspect in the production of sexual difficulties.

DIGOXIN

Digoxin is still widely employed as first-line treatment for congestive heart failure. It has long been suspected of being an erectolytic agent.[41] As the most likely causal mechanism, it has been noted that chronic administration of the drug is associated with endocrine disturbances, including a decrease in serum testosterone with simultaneous increases in circulating estrogens.

CIMETIDINE

Cimetidine is another extremely popular drug with remarkable effectiveness in the treatment of duodenal ulcer. Cimetidine and ranitidine have been strongly associated with erectile difficulties.[42] It appears that this undesirable side effect disappears promptly after discontinuation of the drug.[43] The observations on the detrimental effects of cimetidine and related compounds are given additional support by the hypothesis that histamine H_2 receptor antagonists inhibit libido and interfere with erections by increasing prolactin levels and acting as antiandrogens.

ANTIHYPERLIPIDEMICS

A variety of this class of agents with specific indications is available in the market. All of them have been recognized for their tendency to depress libido. Clofibrate (Atromid) and gemfibrozil (Lopid) have been reported to induce impotence.[44] The mechanism(s) of interference on sexual behavior is not clear, but it is suspected that there is a relationship with steroidogenesis of hormonal precursors and also with the liver metabolism of sex steroids.

As new drugs become available, many will be labeled as erectolytic. The perspicacious physician must evaluate the evidence carefully. If an alternative treatment for the primary condition is not available, it is necessary to discuss with the patient the possible cause of his problems and the consequences of discontinuing the medication. The emphasis, of course, is on the reliability of the data implicating a drug in the etiology of impotence. The myriad of single case reports or inconclusive studies must be viewed with skepticism, the same type as one exhibits when confronted with the many drugs, potions, and incantations that are reported to cure or improve impotence.

ERECTOGENIC DRUGS

Other chapters of this book refer to the significant amount of progress achieved over the last decade in the diagnosis and treatment of erectile failure. Surgical techniques have proven effective in dealing with some vascular problems, and the intracavernosal administration of vasoactive drugs has been shown to be capable of producing erections of sufficient quality for intercourse in many situations. However, there is still a large group of patients who may not be, or choose not to be, candidates for these invasive forms of treatment. In the case of vasoactive medication, some men reject long-term use because of pain, fibrosis, or more frequently, dissatisfaction with the results. The number of patients in this last category is not small.

Unquestionably, an oral medication effective in restoring or improving the quality of erections in impotence would be a most welcome addition to the urologic armamentarium. Although many attempts have been made at finding systemic agents with activity in men with erectile failure, conclusive positive results have been elusive. Nevertheless, our improved understanding of the physiology of penile tumescence (and detumescence) augers well for the possible discovery of effective compounds. This optimism is somewhat tempered by recognition of the complexity of clearly identified, as well as putative, neurohormonal pathways involved in erectile function.[45] It appears entirely reasonable, therefore, to anticipate that a combination of agents could provide the best results. At this early stage in the search for an effective, easily administered pharmacologic cure, however, it is mandatory to investigate the individual merits of various drugs and later to determine their synergistic activity.

Hormones

A serum testosterone determination or a complete hormone screening is part of the assessment of an impotent man.[46] From the therapeutic standpoint, endocrine abnormalities are amenable to effective treatment. Unfortunately, they are also a relatively rare finding in impotence. Current methods allow the clinician to pinpoint defects in the hypothalamic-pituitary-gonadal axis with a high degree of accuracy and to institute specific therapy for the abnormality present.

Hormonal abnormalities most commonly associated with erectile disturbances are hyperprolactinemia and hypogonadism.

Hyperprolactinemia

This is an exceedingly uncommon cause of impotence, with an estimated incidence of less than 5%. In most cases, the elevation in serum prolactin levels is the result of medication known to induce an excessive production of prolactin, most commonly estrogens or alpha-methyldopa. The initial treatment, of course, includes the appropriate changes in medication. A small number of individuals with hyperprolactinemia are found to harbor pituitary tumors (prolactinomas). Most of these patients have microadenomas, which respond to the judicious use of bromocriptine. It is commonly agreed that only those with large tumors that do not respond adequately to administration of the drug require hypophysectomy. Bromocriptine is normally started at small doses because it frequently induces gastric intolerance. The dose is progressively increased until a total daily dose of 5 to 7.5 mg is reached. These patients require periodic determinations of serum prolactin, radiologic evaluation of the sella turcica, and visual-field examinations. Normalization of serum prolactin may not be sufficient to bring back normal erections. Some of these patients require supplemental androgens, and as in most cases of organic impotence, varying degrees of counseling are necessary before satisfactory restoration of function is achieved. Despite isolated views in the literature, we and others remain firmly convinced that modest elevations in serum prolactin do not require the hasty administration of bromocriptine but require first a thorough investigation to rule out other subtle causes of the dysfunction.[47]

Hypogonadism

Both hypergonadotropic and hypogonadotropic hypogonadism require administration of exogenous androgens. For androgen replacement, preference should be given to the injectable preparations: testosterone enanthate 300 mg IM every 3 to 4 weeks (or 200 mg IM every 2 weeks). The amount and frequency of administration vary and may require adjustments with chronic use. The sublingual and oral administration of testosterone is simpler and more readily acceptable to the patient. Unfortunately, drug absorption by these routes is somewhat unpredictable. Newer preparations may provide a more stable absorption of the hormone by the gut. Investigations suggest that transcutaneous administration of testosterone may be a simpler viable alternative.[48] The transscrotal route has been used with promising results. In our experience, oral administration of androgens is associated with a large increase in the serum levels of total testosterone but not with a proportional enhancement of the bioavailable fraction. This startling phenomenon is under further scrutiny.

Nonhormonal Therapy

Patients with organic impotence rarely are candidates for hormonal manipulation, and as a general rule, such an approach should be limited to those in whom hormonal deficiencies are thoroughly documented. There is, therefore, a large population of men with erectile dysfunction in whom other organic factors (vascular, neurologic) are the underlying cause of their problem and who could benefit from nonhormonal pharmacologic treatment. Furthermore, a significant group of impotent men with a predominantly psychogenic etiology could derive significant benefit from pharmacologic therapy. A number of studies have been carried out in an effort to elucidate the value of drugs thought to be effective, and research is being conducted to find new compounds that may be useful in the treatment of one or more causes of erectile failure. A few drugs have been investigated in small phase I or II clinical trials, in some cases with encouraging results. Among the preparations tested were glyceryl trinitrate,[49] zinc,[50] oxytocin,[51] and luteinizing hormone-releasing hormone (LHRH).[52] None of these, however, has found a place in the armamentarium. On the other hand, the introduction of intracavernosal therapy has fundamentally changed our approach to the treatment of impotence. The injection of single or multiple agents is the first therapeutic choice for many patients. Slower and much less dramatic progress is being made in developing noninvasive, preferably oral, alternatives. However, basic research is providing an increasing understanding of the physiology of libido and erection, which is evolving into significant therapeutic developments.

For instance, detailed studies have resulted in identification of zones in the medial preoptic area (MPOA) of the diencephalon that are strongly associated with erectile function and sexual behavior. Other studies have resulted in identification of a peripheral neural network controlling sexual reflex responses. Equally important has been the determination of the fundamental role of adrenergic, dopaminergic, and serotonergic activities in the regulation of erections in men. These developments are beginning to provide a basis for the development of effective pharmacologic therapy in erectile failure. There is, for instance, convincing evidence that alterations in catecholamine metabolism result in alteration of sexual behavior, thus suggesting an important participation of both adrenergic and dopaminergic receptors in sex drive.

CENTRAL MECHANISMS
Adrenergic Receptor Antagonists

A large number of compounds are included in this group. The most commonly used have been phentolamine and yohimbine. Phentolamine is employed either alone or in combination with papaverine by intracorporeal administration (Chapter

17). Very preliminary evidence indicating that oral phentolamine exhibits erectogenic activity was presented by Gwinup.[53] This finding has received support by a large study recently reported by Zorgniotti.[54] Further investigations of this compound should provide a better understanding of its effectiveness.

Yohimbine, on the other hand, has received much attention as an oral treatment for impotence. It is an indole alkaloid with well-defined properties as an alpha$_2$-adrenoceptor antagonist, with profound central and peripheral effects in animals and humans.[55] It has been widely touted as an aphrodisiac for over a century, but it was not properly investigated until relatively recently. The early reports on the effectiveness of yohimbine, which were quite remarkable,[56] were later supported by Wolpowitz and Barnard.[57] Despite its early promise in these and other trials, the drug produced no significant clinical impact. Several reasons account for the waning of interest in the role of yohimbine in the treatment of impotence. Most important, early uses of the drug were entirely empirical, and its pharmacology was poorly understood. Further damage to its reputation was caused by combining it with other drugs (testosterone, caffeine, strychnine, vitamin E), thus making it impossible to determine its individual effectiveness. Finally, the procedures used to establish the etiologic diagnosis of impotence were inappropriate even for those days and certainly unacceptable for today. There was, however, sufficient evidence in the literature to justify a careful and objective look at the effects of yohimbine in sexual function.

A pilot investigation on the treatment of impotence with yohimbine was published in 1982.[58] The study found a positive response in 43% of the sample of impotent men with a predominantly organic etiology. Of these, 26% became able to achieve full, sustained erections. Although the findings were significantly lower than those reported in earlier studies, there was enough activity attributable to the drug to justify further trials. A controlled randomized study in patients with organic impotence receiving 6 mg of yohimbine orally three times a day for 10 weeks vs placebo demonstrated a response similar to the one noted in the pilot study: 42% of the patients experienced a positive response, which, in half of them, was complete recovery of erectile function. Thirteen percent of the patients receiving placebo also experienced a positive response. Although the trend was in favor of the active compound, the differences between yohimbine and placebo did not reach statistical significance. A more reliable differentiation of response to yohimbine was found in a controlled study of patients with a diagnosis of psychogenic

impotence. The positive response in the yohimbine cohort was 62%, whereas in the control group it was only 16%. This difference was statistically highly significant.[59] Further controlled studies have indicated that yohimbine favorably affects erectile function in impotent patients and have rekindled interest in the development of new alpha$_2$-adrenoceptor antagonists with improved selectivity.[60] These agents are still at the investigational level, and it may be several years before their activity is known.

It is evident from available studies that, under the best circumstances, yohimbine is of limited effectiveness. The drug, however, is well tolerated, and it can be recommended as the first line of treatment. It is possible that larger amounts (i.e., 30 mg daily in divided doses) may be more effective. Recently, an empirical combination of yohimbine and the serotonergic agonist, trazodone, has been reported to be more effective than yohimbine alone. At our center, very early experience with this approach tends to support this concept, but a larger study is needed to determine the synergistic value of the two drugs. Additional support of this concept was provided by the report of Hollander and McCarley,[61] demonstrating in a small, uncontrolled study that administration of yohimbine on demand counteracts the detrimental effects of serotonin blockers on sexual activity.

Although the mechanism of action of yohimbine on sexual functioning has not been established, some evidence indicates that its effects are primarily central. Clark[62] conducted a series of revealing experiments on rats in which complete inhibition of sexual performance (mounting, intromission, and ejaculation) was achieved by administration of clonidine into the MPOA. Total restoration of sexual functioning was accomplished by administration of yohimbine either systemically or directly into the MPOA. Clark concluded from these studies that alpha$_2$-adrenoceptors are important in the control of male sexual behavior and that alterations of adrenergic mechanisms in the MPOA may underlie sexual dysfunctions from multiple etiologies. It is conceivable that in this portion of the diencephalon, there is integration of a number of neurotransmitter interactions that are important in the regulation of penile erections.

Dopamine Receptor Agonists

As mentioned previously, numerous studies have documented some of the details of the central neurotransmitter systems contributing to the control of sexual behavior. In addition to norepinephrine, interest has focused on the role of dopamine, which is also widely distributed in brain tissues.[63]

Dopamine has long been recognized to be a facilitator of male copulatory performance in animals, and administration of dopamine-blocking agents inhibits their copulatory behavior. Administration of the dopamine agonist apomorphine has been shown to induce bouts of yawning and penile erections both in animals and in humans. This effect has permitted the development of important animal models for the investigation of potency.[64] Clinical studies have indicated that apomorphine may play a role in the treatment of erectile dysfunction in men. Lal et al. have shown that apomorphine induces erections in both impotent and nonimpotent men[65] when administered subcutaneously. Trials are in progress to determine the effectiveness of apomorphine and other dopaminergic agonists (i.e., bromocriptine) in the treatment of impotence from various causes. Table 10–2 provides additional examples of the many dopaminergic agonists that have been investigated as possible erectogenic compounds.

TABLE 10–2
Systemic Therapy for Impotence

Neuropharmacotherapy
Dopaminergic agonists
 L-dopa
 Amphetamine
 Deprenyl
 Apomorphine
 Pergolide
 Quinelorane
 Methylenedioxy-propyl-noraporphine
 Fenfluramine
Adrenergic antagonists
 Yohimbine
 Phentolamine
Serotonergic agonists
 Trazodone
 Methysergide
Opiate antagonists
 Naltrexone
 Naloxone

Hormonal
Hypogonadism
 Testosterone
Hyperprolactenemia
 Bromocriptine

Vascular
Nitric oxide derivatives
Pentoxifylline
Minoxidil

Serotonergic Receptors

An additional system with a recognized major involvement in the erectile process includes serotonin-related compounds. Serotonergic compounds appear more complex to study than either the adrenergic or dopaminergic ones, since they seem to have an inhibitory effect on sex drive centrally but an erectogenic effect peripherally. The enhancement of serotonergic activity has been implicated as the mechanism of action of trazodone in normal and impotent patients. More recently, however, Saenz de Tejada et al.[66] suggested that an alternative possible mechanism would be related to the alpha-adrenergic blocking properties of trazodone by interference with the sympathetic control of penile detumescence. It is evident that much more needs to be understood about serotonergic receptors and the drugs affecting them. They appear to play an important role in the erectile process, and their pharmacologic manipulation may translate into a significant avenue of treatment in disturbances of sexual function.

Other receptors are believed to be involved in the human penile response. For example, opiate antagonists, such as naloxone, can enhance sexual performance and induce erections. It has been suggested[67] that the additive effect of a psychopharmacologic agent, such as yohimbine, and a neuropharmacologic agent, such as naloxone, may be a fruitful approach to treatment. Although this hypothesis is attractive, categorization of drugs as neuropharmacologic or psychopharmacologic agents is artificial, probably inappropriate, and certainly confusing. Regardless of nomenclature, reliable information about the synergistic effect of class compounds is, unfortunately, lacking, but it is a crucial consideration to be discussed later. In any case, the simultaneous use of two or more agents may be necessary, since there is evidence indicating that an adequate hormonal environment is mandatory for the occurrence of an appropriate response to a neuropharmacologic agent.[68]

PERIPHERAL MECHANISMS

Oral and transcutaneous drugs may have profound effects on the penis. There is undisputable and not surprising evidence that nitric oxide (NO) mediates the relaxation of cavernosal smooth muscle, as it does in other vascular beds. Organic nitrates and nitrites are well-recognized vasodilators, which have a relaxant effect on vascular smooth muscle.[69] Among the best known of these compounds is nitroglycerin, which is readily absorbed after topical administration.

Several years ago, we thought that nitroglycerin deserved to be investigated in patients with impotence. Initially, a pilot study was conducted under laboratory conditions,[70] and this was followed by a further assessment also performed in the laboratory.[71] In the latter, the effect of 2% nitroglycerin paste applied to the penile shaft of impotent subjects was evaluated in a placebo-controlled double-blind study. After application of nitroglycerin paste or a placebo ointment, base penile tumescence was recorded while subjects viewed an erotic video presentation. Relative to the placebo paste, the number of patients demonstrating an increase in penile circumference after nitroglycerin administration was significantly larger than all other outcome possibilities. In an additional study, it was shown that topical administration of nitroglycerin to the penile shaft is rapidly followed by a significant dilatation of the cavernosal arteries, with a concomitant increase in blood flow.[72] Although other investigators have confirmed these observations,[73] nitroglycerin and related compounds have not been fully and systematically investigated outside laboratory conditions, and their effect in the treatment of impotence remains speculative. It is anticipated, however, that their main role would be in the treatment of those patients with an underlying vascular etiology. Nevertheless, the discovery of the role of NO or endothelium-derived relaxing factor (EDRF) as a powerful vasodilator with a putative role in cavernosal physiology[74] has opened new avenues for therapeutic research. Overwhelming evidence suggests that EDRF and NO[75] are identical. Thus, the trickle down from mainstream vascular physiology and pharmacology may open new possibilities in manipulating the penile vascular bed with NO-derived or other simple nitrogen-based compounds.[76]

Cavallini[77] presented the intriguing results of a study in which the topical application of minoxidil (best known for its capacity to reverse alopecia androgenetica) was found to be more effective than nitroglycerin in enhancing penile tumescence in impotent men. These results have not yet been reproduced by other investigators. Confirmation of such findings would further support the value of local vasodilatation. Needless to say, an erection requires more than simple vasodilatation. However, if a deficiency in blood supply is the main or a significant contributor to the problem, this could be treated with a relatively simple, local measure thus circumventing the potential side effects of systemic therapy.

CONCLUSION

It is evident that any effective pharmacologic agent requires at least some preservation of the erectile mechanisms in the penis. It would be absurd to anticipate, for instance, any response from a penis with severely occluded cavernosal arteries. On the other hand, we suspect that until recently undue emphasis has been given to the pharmacologic events at the level of the target organ (penis), leading to considerable neglect of mechanisms at higher centers. This imbalance is understandable given the relative accessibility of the former for a variety of animal and clinical investigations. It is our contention, however, that a more comprehensive and integrated approach is mandatory in the search for successful strategies in treating male sexual dysfunction.

We seem to have come in a complete circle to the therapies advocated in the 1960s, when multiple ingredients were combined in a single tablet for the generic treatment of impotence, reportedly with good results. The level of understanding of the mechanisms of sexual functioning has increased considerably in three decades, and the sophistication of the diagnostic process has changed dramatically. The multipronged approach to treatment of impotence should be considered carefully again. A list of drugs with recognized erectogenic properties is shown in Table 10-2.

Discovery of a noninvasive pharmacologic cure for erectile failure has proven to be difficult. Part of the problem may be the enormous complexity of mechanisms involved in the development of an erection. As examples, one can think of the finding of regularization of substantia nigra dopamine cell firing by adrenergic neurotransmitters[78] or the effect of adrenergic antagonists on hydroxytryptamine receptor-mediated inhibition in the same area of the brain of experimental animals.[79] Findings such as these suggest a scenario in which all neurotransmitters influencing sexual behavior work in a very close and interdependent fashion. Certainly, there is a multiplicity of central and peripheral neurotransmitter systems involved in the sexual human response. Therefore, it is likely that a combination of agents or a highly specific diagnostic process with a specifically defined therapeutic objective will be needed for successful treatment.[1] A combined treatment approach may be most appropriate until the individual contributions of each of the various central and peripheral systems are better understood.

REFERENCES

1. Herman JR. Impotence through the ages. J Am Soc Psychosom Dent Med 16:3, 1969.
2. Wabreck AJ, Shelley MM, Horowitz L, et al. Noninvasive penile arterial evaluation in 120 males with erectile dysfunction. Urology 22:230, 1983.
3. Forsberg L, Hederstrom E, Olsson AM. Severe ar-

terial insufficiency in impotence confirmed with an improved angiographic technique: the impact of smoking and some other etiologic factors. Eur Urol 16:357, 1989.

4. Glina S, Reichelt AS, Puech-Leao P, DosReis JMSM. Impact of cigarette smoking on papaverine-induced erection. J Urol 140:523, 1988.
5. Muller SC, el-Damanhoury H, Ruth J, Lue TF. Hypertension and impotence. Eur Urol 19:29, 1991.
6. Rosen MP, Greenfield AJ, Walker TG, Grant P. Cigarette smoking: an independent risk factor for atherosclerosis in the hypogastric-cavernous arterial bed of men with arteriogenic impotence. J Urol 145:759, 1991.
7. Forsberg L, Hederstrom E, Olsson AM. Severe arterial insufficiency in impotence confirmed with an improved angiographic technique: the impact of smoking and some other etiologic factors. Eur Urol 16:357, 1989.
8. Rubin E. Prolonged ethanol consumption increases testosterone metabolism in the liver. Science 191:563, 1976.
9. Van Thiel DH, Kumar S, Gavaler JS, Tarter RE. Effect of liver transplantation on the hypothalamic-pituitary-gonadal axis of chronic alcoholic men with advanced liver disease. Alcohol Clin Exp Res 14:478, 1990.
10. Nutt D, Glue P. Monoamines and alcohol. Br J Addiction 81:327, 1986.
11. Heaton JPW, Varrin S. The impact of alcohol ingestion on erections in rats as measured by a novel bioassay. J Urol 145:192, 1991.
12. Novak DJ, Victor M. The vagus and sympathetic nerves in alcoholic neuropathy. Arch Neurol 30:273, 1974.
13. Villalta J, Estruch R, Antunez E, Urbano-Marquez A. Vagal neuropathy in chronic alcoholics: relation to ethanol consumption. Alcohol 24:421, 1989.
14. Ertekin C, Almis S, Ertekin N. Sympathetic skin potentials and bulbocavernosus reflex in patients with chronic alcoholism and impotence. Eur Neurol 30:334, 1990.
15. Nirenberg TD, Liepman MR, Begin AM, et al. The sexual relationship of male alcoholics and their female partners during periods of drinking and abstinence. J Stud Alcohol 51:565, 1990.
16. Kolodny RC, Masters WH, Kolodny RM. Depression of plasma testosterone levels after chronic intensive marijuana use. N Engl J Med 290:872, 1974.
17. Gardner EL, Lowinson JH. Marijuana's interaction with brain reward systems: update 1991. Pharmacol Biochem Behav 40:571, 1991.
18. Pavone-Macaluso M, Serreta V, Daricello G, Pavone C. Is there a role for pure antiandrogens in the treatment of advanced prostatic cancer? Prog Clin Biol Res 350:149, 1990.
19. Migliari R, Muscas G, Usai E. Effect of casodex on sleep-related erections in patients with advanced carcinoma of the prostate. J Urol 148:338, 1992.
20. Berlin F, Meinecke F. Treatment of sex offenders with antiandrogen medication. Am J Psychiatry 138:601, 1981.
21. Oesterling JE. LHRH agonists. A non-surgical treat-

ment for benign prostatic hyperplasia. J Androl 12:381, 1991.
22. Meiraz D, Margolin Y, Lev-Ran A, Lazebnik J. Treatment of benign prostatic hyperplasia with hydroxy-progesterone-caprovate. Urology 9:144, 1977.
23. Roehrborn CG, McConell JD, Eddy DM. Outcome analysis after treatment for benign prostatic hyperplasia by various modalities: a confidence profile analysis. Presented at AUA Meeting, Toronto, 1991.
24. Bansal S. Sexual dysfunction in hypertensive men: a critical review of the literature. Hypertension 12:22, 1988.
25. Munjack DJ. Sex and drugs. Clin Toxicol 15:75, 1979.
26. Zarren HS, Black PM. Unilateral gynecomastia and impotence during low-dose spironolactone administration in men. Mil Med 140:417, 1975.
27. Yendt ER, Gray GF, Garcia DA. The use of thiazides in the prevention of renal calculi. Can Med Assoc J 102:614, 1970.
28. Medical Research Council Working Party on mild to moderate hypertension. Lancet 2:539, 1981.
29. Hogan MJ, Wallin JD, Baer RM. Antihypertensive therapy and male sexual dysfunction. Psychosomatics 12:234, 1980.
30. Wein AJ, Van Arsdalen KN. Drug-induced male sexual dysfunction. Urol Clin North Am 15:23, 1988.
31. Fogelman J. Verapamil caused depression, confusion and impotence [Letter]. Am J Psychiatry 145:380, 1988.
32. King BD, Pitcho R, Stern RH. Impotence during therapy with verapamil. Arch Intern Med 143:1248, 1983.
33. Cruickshank JM. What does the future hold for ACE inhibitors? J Hum Hypertension 5:(Suppl 2):41, 1991.
34. Dawson-Butterworth K. Priapism and phenothiazines. Br Med J 4:118, 1970.
35. Lal S, Rios O, Thavundayil JX. Treatment of impotence with trazodone: a case report. J Urol 143:819, 1990.
36. Ghadirian AM, Annable L, Belanger MC. Lithium, benzodiazepines and sexual function in bipolar patients. Am J Psychiatry 149:801, 1992.
37. Jacobsen FM. Fluoxetine-induced sexual dysfunction and an open trial of yohimbine. J Clin Psychiatry 53:119, 1992.
38. Kafka MP. Successful anti-depressant treatment of nonparaphilic sexual addictions and paraphilias in men. J Clin Psychiatry 52:60, 1991.
39. Magnus RV, Dean BC, Curry SH. Chlorazepate: double-blind crossover comparison of a single nightly dose with diazepam thrice daily in anxiety. Dis Nerv Syst 38:317, 1977.
40. Balon R, Ramesh C, Pohl R. Sexual dysfunction associated with diazepam but not with clonazepam. Can J Psychiatry 34:947, 1989.
41. Neri A, Aygen M, Zuckerman Z. Subjective assessment of sexual dysfunction of patients in long-term administration of digoxin. Arch Sex Behav 9:343, 1980.

42. Barth JA. Can ulcer treatment with cimetidine and other H_2 receptor antagonists induce sexual dysfunctions and other endocrine disorders? Zentralbl Gynakol 113:667, 1991.

43. Gifford LM, Aeugle ME, Myerson RM, Tannenbaum PJ. Cimetidine postmarket outpatient surveillance program. JAMA 243:1532, 1980.

44. Bain SC, Lemon M, Jones AF. Gemfibrozil-induced impotence [Letter]. Lancet 336:1389, 1990.

45. Morales A, Condra MS, Owen JE, et al. Oral and transcutaneous pharmacological agents in the treatment of impotence. Urol Clin North Am 15:87, 1988.

46. Leonard M, Nickel JC, Morales A. Hyperprolactinemia and impotence: why, when and how to investigate. J Urol 142:992, 1989.

47. Leonard M, Nickel JC, Morales A. Re: hyperprolactenemia and impotence: why, when and how to investigate [Letter]. J Urol 146:1380, 1991.

48. Carey PO, Howards SS, Vance ML. Transdermal testosterone treatment of hypogonadal men. J Urol 140:76, 1988.

49. Muddi JW. Impotence response to glyceryl trinitrate. Am J Psychiatry 134:922, 1977.

50. Antonio L, Shalhoub R, Sudhkar T. Reversal of uremic impotence by zinc. Lancet 2:895, 1977.

51. Lidberg L, Sternthal V. A new approach to the hormonal treatment of impotentia erections. Pharmacopsychiatry 10:21, 1977.

52. Levit N, Vinik A, Sive A. Synthetic LHRH in impotent male diabetics: a double-blind crossover trial. S Afr Med J 59:10, 1981.

53. Gwinup G. Oral phentolamine in nonspecific erectile insufficiency. Ann Intern Med 109:162, 1988.

54. Zorgniotti AW. "On demand" oral drugs for erection on impotent men. J Urol 147:308A, 1992.

55. Grunhaus L, Tiongco D, Zelnik T. Intravenous yohimbine. Selective enhancer of norepinephrine and cortisol secretion and systolic blood pressure in humans. Clin Neuropharmacol 12:106, 1989.

56. Margolis A, Prieto P, Stein L. Statistical summary of 10,000 male cases using Afrodex in the treatment of impotence. Curr Ther Res 13:616, 1971.

57. Wolpowitz A, Barnard CN. Impotence in heart transplantation. S Afr Med J 53:693, 1978.

58. Morales A, Surridge DH, Marshall PG, Fenemore J. Nonhormonal pharmacological treatment of organic impotence. J Urol 128:45, 1982.

59. Reid K, Surridge DH, Morales A, et al. Double-blind trial of yohimbine in treatment of psychogenic impotence. Lancet 2:421, 1987.

60. Susset JG, Tesier CD, Wincze J, et al. Effect of yohimbine hydrochloride on erectile impotence: a double-blind study. J Urol 141:1360, 1989.

61. Hollander E, McCarley A. Yohimbine treatment of sexual side effects induced by serotonin reuptake blockers. J Clin Psychiatry 53:207, 1992.

62. Clark JT. Suppression of copulatory behavior in male rats following central administration of clonidine. Neuropharmacology 30:373, 1991.

63. Crowley WR, Zelman FP. The neurochemical control of mating behavior. In: Adler NT, ed. Neuroendocrinology of Reproduction, Physiology and Behavior. New York: Plenum, 1981:451.

64. Heaton JPW, Varrin S, Morales A. The characterization of a bio-assay of erectile function in a rat model. J Urol 145:1099, 1991.

65. Lal S, Larya E, Thavunadyil JX, et al. Apomorphine-induced penile tumescence in impotent patients—preliminary findings. Progr Neuropsychopharmacol Biol Psychiatry 11:235, 1987.

66. Saenz de Tejada I, Ware JC, Blanco R, et al. Pathophysiology of prolonged penile erection associated with trazodone use. J Urol 145:60–64, 1991.

67. Foreman MN, Wenicke JF. Approaches for the development of oral drug therapies for erectile dysfunction. Semin Urol 8:107, 1990.

68. Heaton JPW, Varrin SJ, Gee SP, Morales A. Manipulation of the hormonal milieu and penile tumescence: effects of castration, diethylstilbestrol, flutamide and cyproterone acetate. J Urol (in press)

69. Needleman P, Corr PB, Johnson EM Jr. Drugs used for the treatment of angina: organic nitrates, calcium channel blockers and β-adrenergic antagonists. In: Gilman AG, Goodman LS, Rall TW, Murad F, eds. The Pharmacological Basis of Therapeutics. New York: Macmillan, 1985:806.

70. Morales A. Clinical use of systemic erectile agents. J Urol 135:31A, 1986.

71. Owen JA, Saunders F, Harris C, et al. Topical nitroglycerin: a potential treatment for impotence. J Urol 141:546, 1989.

72. Heaton JPW, Morales A, Owen J, et al. Topical glyceryltrinitrate causes measurable penile arterial dilatation in impotent men. J Urol 143:729, 1990.

73. Claes H, Baert L. Transcutaneous nitroglycerin therapy in the treatment of impotence. Urol Int 44:309, 1989.

74. Vanhoutte PM. Vascular physiology: the end of the quest? Nature 327:459, 1987.

75. Palmer RM, Ferrige AG, Moncada S. Nitric oxide release accounts for the biological activity of endothelium-derived relaxing factor. Nature 327:524, 1987.

76. Aronson WJ, Trigo-Rocha F, Ignarro LJ, Rajfer J. The role of nitric oxide and cyclic GMP in mediating pelvic nerve stimulation induced erections in dogs. J Urol 147:454A, 1992.

77. Cavallini G. Minoxidil versus nitroglycerin: a prospective double-blind controlled trial in transcutaneous erection facilitation for organic impotence. J Urol 146:50, 1991.

78. Grenhoff J, Svensson TH. Clonidine regularizes substantia nigra dopamine cell firing. Life Sci 42:2003, 1988.

79. Schoeffter P, Hoyer D. 5-Hydroxytriptamine 5-HT1B and 5-HT1D receptors mediating inhibition of adenylate cyclase activity. Pharmacological comparison with special reference to the effects of yohimbine, rauwolscine, and some beta adrenoceptor antagonists. Nauyn Schmiedebergs Arch Pharmacol 340:285, 1989.

Bends of the Penis, Peyronie's Disease, and Other Problems

Charles J. Devine, Jr.
Gerald H. Jordan

ANATOMY OF THE PENIS

The shaft of the penis is composed of three erectile bodies and their enveloping fascial layers, nerves, and vessels, covered by skin[1] (Fig. 11–1). All of these structures continue into the perineum. The penis is fixed at its base by the attachment of the crura of the corpora cavernosa to the underside of the pubis. Distally, the crura fuse to form a single blood space containing erectile tissue within a compliant sheath of connective tissue, called the tunica albuginea. The tunica albuginea consists of two layers of elastic fibers, the outer being longitudinal and the inner circular. A midline septum formed by multiple strands of similar elastic fibers separates the two corpora cavernosa. At their attachment dorsally and ventrally, these fibers fan out and are interwoven with the strands of the inner, circular layer of the tunica albuginea. These strands are critical for proper rigidity of the erect penis.

The erectile tissue consists of arteries and venous sinuses encompassed by smooth muscle. There are also nerves and an intracavernosal fibrous framework, which also contributes to the rigidity of the erect penis.[2] This tissue is separated from the tunica albuginea by a thin layer of areolar connective tissue[3] containing the veins that drain the venous sinuses of the erectile tissue, another relationship important in the physiology of erection.

The corpora cavernosa make up the bulk of the penis. The corpus spongiosum, containing the urethra, lying in a groove in its ventral midline, expands at the distal end of the penis to form the glans covering the tips of the corpora cavernosa. The edge of the glans forms the corona, with the loose skin of the frenulum filling a distally pointed V in the ventral midline. The vertically oriented slit of the urethral meatus is just distal to this. The tunica of the corpus spongiosum is thinner, and there is less elastic tissue.

The deep dorsal vein of the penis is located in a less shallow groove in the dorsal midline of the corpora cavernosa. Lateral to the dorsal vein on either side, the coiled dorsal arteries and multiple branches of the dorsal nerves run the length of the penile shaft loosely attached to the underside of Buck's fascia. Distally, Buck's fascia is attached to the undersurface of the glans penis. It surrounds the penile shaft, splitting ventrally to contain the corpus spongiosum. On each side of the corpus spongiosum, thickenings of the fascia fix that structure to the corpora cavernosa. Superficial to Buck's fascia, the loose layer of the dartos fascia separates the two layers of the prepuce and allows the proximal skin to slide on the shaft of the penis.

As the penis engorges with blood during erection, it expands its girth and extends its length until the tissues of the tunica and the strands of the septum have been stretched to the limit of their elasticity. In the normal penis, the tissues are symmetrically elastic, and the erection will be straight. Chordee, a bend of the penis, may be congenital or acquired. In most cases, it is caused by a decrease in the elasticity of one or more of the fascial layers of the penile shaft shortening the involved aspect of the penis during erection. Such a bend may be dorsal, ventral, lateral, or complex. Disproportion in the size of the corpora cavernosa may result in a lateral bend of the penis, almost always to the left. We have seen only three to the right.

CONGENITAL ANOMALIES

Development of the male external genitalia depends on testosterone produced by the developing testes. Testosterone is converted into dihydrotestosterone by the enzyme 5-alpha-reductase within

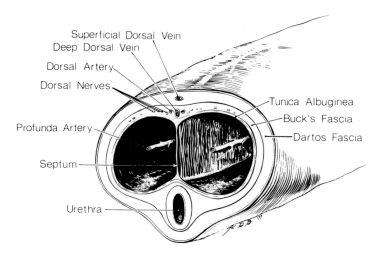

Figure 11–1. Transverse section of the penis in midshaft. The septum is not a solid structure but is made up of multiple strands of compliant tissue attached to the inner surface of the tunica albuginea of the corpora cavernosa in the dorsal and ventral midlines. (From Devine CJ Jr. Surgery of the penis and urethra. In: Campbell's Urology, 6th ed. Philadelphia: WB Saunders Co, 1992.)

the cells of the genital structures. This hormone produces the growth of the penis with the urethra on its ventral surface. Chordee caused by dysgenetic development is usually associated with hypospadias or epispadias, but chordee can occur without these abnormalities of the urethra.[4] Mesenchyme, which would have formed the normal structures surrounding the urethra, becomes an inelastic fascial layer deep to, or lateral to, the urethra, and this tissue must be removed to correct the deformity. In most cases, these anomalies will have been taken care of during childhood and will not influence an adult patient's sexual function.

However, persistent or recurrent chordee has been present in 71 of 190 patients we treated for the complications of hypospadias repairs from 1979 to 1991. Most of these patients had other anomalies in addition to the chordee.[5] Figure 11–2 is an algorithm outlining the treatment of chordee in those patients.

We have seen a number of young men with a ventral bend of the penis that has been present as long as they can remember. Often, however, their parents remember only straight erections during childhood. Most of these young men have a penis with a stretched length above the median (13.3 ±

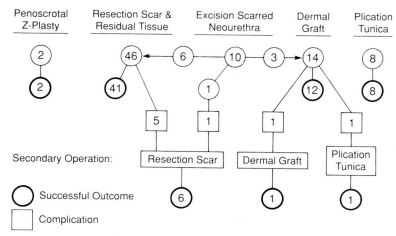

Figure 11–2. Algorithm illustrating our choice of surgical treatment of recurrent or residual chordee. By itself, excision of the scarred neourethra was ineffective. Plication of the tunica was used when we did not want to disturb a satisfactory neourethra. At times, scarring did not involve the tunica albuginea and could be resected without opening the erectile space, but if the tunica was involved, opening the space was necessary, and the defect was closed with a dermal graft.

1.6 cm).[6] We ask each patient to bring Polaroid photographs of his erection, and these show a gradual downward curvature of 30 degrees to 60 degrees throughout the length of the shaft. The ventral side of the penis may be flattened, and there may be some lateral curvature as well. Some patients have been able to have intercourse, though with some difficulty and embarrassment. When the flaccid penis is stretched, a dense band of tissue can be felt on the ventral side deep to the corpus spongiosum. The restrictive effect of this tissue can be noted in that the dorsal aspect of the shaft will still be loose while the ventral side has been stretched taut. At surgery, this fibrous band involves Buck's fascia on the ventral aspect of the corpora cavernosa and often the tunica itself. At the time of surgery, we have biopsied this tissue as well as tunica from the dorsal side of the penis, and there seems to be a deficiency of 5-alpha-reductase in the ventral fibrotic tissue. To date, the values are inconclusive (C. J. Devine, Jr., and G. Pepe, unpublished observations). However, the bend may be the result of dysgenetic growth in this area of the penis during the changes brought about by puberty.

Corrective surgery has been successful. In only 2 of 26 patients in a 2-year period was a second operation necessary to achieve a straight penis.[7] In some cases, we have straightened the penis by sharply excising the dysgenetic tissue from the ventral side of the penis, mobilizing the very elastic corpus spongiosum (Fig. 11–3). In most patients, however, an artificial erection at the conclusion of this dissection will still demonstrate curvature due to lack of elasticity in the ventral aspect of the corpora cavernosa. To equalize the lengths of the ventral and dorsal aspects of the corporal bodies, it has been necessary to excise one or more ellipses of dorsal tunica albuginea (Fig. 11–4).

Most of the patients have been circumcised, and because the pattern of venous and lymphatic drainage of the skin will have been established by that procedure, we make the incision through the circumcision scar, even if it is halfway down the shaft of the penis. The skin is reflected by dissecting in the dartos fascia layer. An artificial erection will then demonstrate the extent of the curvature. We excise the fibrous tissue and mobilize the corpus spongiosum and urethra. If at that time an artificial

Figure 11–3. Release of tissue causing ventral chordee. **A,** Artificial erection demonstrating curvature. **B,** Dysgenetic dartos fascia elevated. This will be excised. **C,** Dysgenetic Buck's fascia undermined. **D,** Corpus spongiosum is mobilized by excising the inelastic fascia. **E,** Correctin of chordee demonstrated by repeat artificial erection. (From Devine CJ Jr. Surgery of the penis and urethra. In: Campbell's Urology, 6th ed. Philadelphia: WB Saunders Co, 1992.)

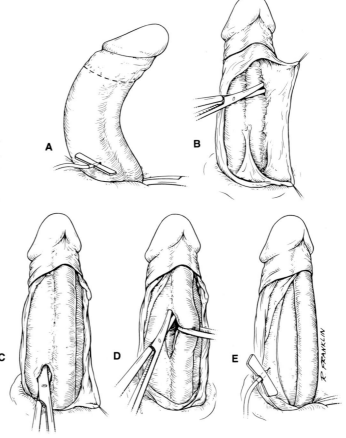

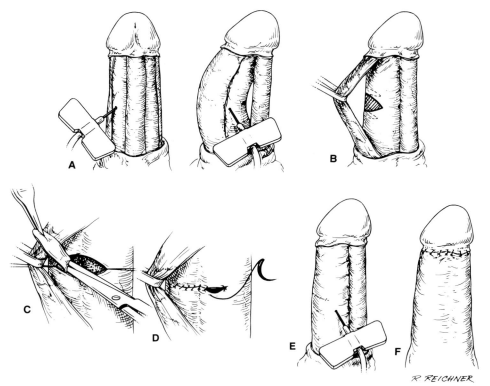

Figure 11–4. Release of chordee caused by dysgenetic ventral aspect of corpora cavernosa. **A,** Ventral and lateral views of artificial erection at conclusion of surgery depicted in Figure 11–3. Chordee persists; the elastic urethra is not the cause of this bend. The point of maximum concavity has been marked. **B,** An ellipse of tunica has been marked opposite the point of maximum concavity. Two alternative smaller ellipses are shown. **C,** Excision of ellipse of tunica. **D,** Closure of edges of tunica. **E,** Artificial erection demonstrates straight penis. **F,** Skin closure. (From Devine CJ. Bent penis. Semin Urol 5:4, 1987.)

erection shows the penis to be straight, this is the end of the operation. However, in most patients, although expansion of the circumference of the penile shaft will be improved, the ventral aspect of the tunica will be fibrotic and the curvature will persist. There are now two options for surgical correction: (1) to lengthen the ventral aspect of the penis by making one or more transverse incisions in the tunica with placement of a dermal graft(s) or (2) to shorten the dorsal aspect of the penis by mobilizing Buck's fascia and the neurovascular bundle, excising an ellipse or several ellipses of the dorsal tunica albuginea and closing the defect(s) in a watertight fashion (the Nesbit procedure[8]). Because the penis is longer than average in most of these cases and the recovery period is much shorter than after the placement of a graft, we usually have chosen the Nesbit procedure. However, we employ a dermal graft if the patient has a short penis.[9]

Lateral penile curvature due to a disparity in the size of the corpora cavernosa is rare in postadolescent males. It is usually uncomplicated, but

there may be an upward or downward component. Repair of lateral curvature (Fig. 11–5) is similar to that of ventral curvature. After induction of anesthesia, an artificial erection is accomplished to delineate the deformity. As this is carried out before the skin incision, placing the needle through the glans is associated with fewer problems. After marking the point of maximum concavity on the short side of the penis, we make a longitudinal incision in the skin of the longer side opposite that mark. The dartos fascia and Buck's fascia with the dorsal neurovascular bundle are mobilized to expose the tunica albuginea, and we place two prolene sutures, one near the corpus spongiosum and the other directly above on the dorsal surface of the tunica. Then, while maintaining an artificial erection and placing opposing tension on the two prolene sutures, we push on the glans to straighten the shaft of the penis. This generates a fold in the tunica between the two prolene sutures. The edges of this fold are marked and when the erection is released, these marks define the ellipse of tunica

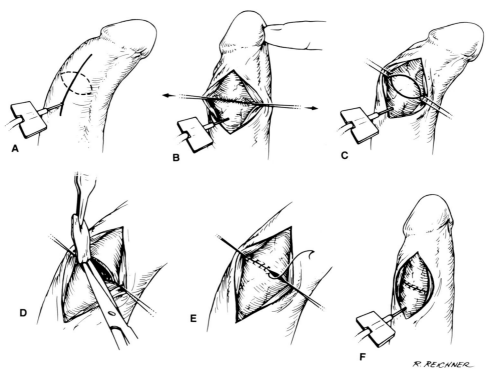

R. REICHNER

Figure 11–5. Correction of lateral curvature. **A,** Artificial erection demonstrates the curvature. The incision and the potential ellipse of tunica are illustrated. **B,** Prolene sutures have been placed in the exposed tunica at the ventral and dorsal tips of the potential ellipse. The edges of the fold produced by straightening the erected penis while maintaining traction on the sutures will be marked. **C,** With the erection relaxed, the marks are connected to outline the ellipse to be incised. **D,** The tunica is removed. **E,** The edges are approximated. **F,** The penis is straight. The fascia and skin will be closed. (From Devine CJ Jr. Surgery of the penis and urethra. In: Campbell's Urology, 6th ed. Philadelphia: WB Saunders Co, 1992.)

to be excised. If the ellipse is wider than 1 cm, it would be better to outline two ellipses.

If the curvature is more gradual or is complex, more of the shaft of the penis must be exposed. Therefore, a circumcising incision is made, and the skin is reflected to the base of the penis by dissection in the plane between the dartos fascia and Buck's fascia. While maintaining the artificial erection, we identify the location of multiple ellipses that will be necessary to straighten the penis. To be sure that the correct amount of tissue will be excised, we plicate the edges of these ellipses with prolene sutures and establish another artificial erection. Some surgeons would imbricate the tissue with these sutures as the definitive procedure. We have not chosen to leave the nonabsorbable suture material in the penile shaft. We remove the ellipses and approximate the edges with interrupted and running sutures of 5-0 PDS (Ethicon-Inc., Somerville, NJ). This suture is monofilament and retains its strength as it is absorbed by hydrolysis over a period of 6 months. By the time the suture

has been absorbed, the suture line is strong enough to withstand the tension of erection and the added stress of intercourse.

ACQUIRED CHORDEE

Acquired chordee may follow trauma, such as injury or inflammation resulting in a scar in the tunica albuginea. Correction of this deformity involves surgery of the corpus cavernosum similar to that described for Peyronie's disease.

Peyronie's disease is not rare. We have seen it in about 1% of the men in two groups of physicians. Most patients have been middle-aged, but the youngest was 19. As many as 25% of our patients also had Dupuytren's contracture, a similar lesion in the palmar fascia, or Ledderhose disease, in which the plantar fascia is involved. There has been a familial relationship, with relatives having Peyronie's disease or these other conditions in which an inelastic lesion has formed in tissues that require elasticity to function.[10,11]

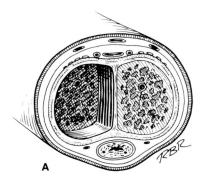

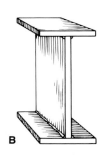

Figure 11–6. A, Diagram of cross-section of penis illustrating the function of the septum. Plaques of Peyronie's disease occur in the tunica at the sites of attachment of the septal strands. **B,** Diagram of an I-beam, illustrating the configuration of the septum responsible for the ultimate rigidity of the penile erection. (From Devine CJ, Jordan GH, Somers KD. Peyronie's disease: cause and surgical treatment. AUA Today 2(5), Sept/Oct 1989.)

Peyronie's disease is named for Francois de la Peyronie.[12] In this condition, a plaque, an area of inelastic scar in the compliant tunica albuginea of the corpora cavernosa, restricts expansion of the involved aspect of the penis, causing the erection to be bent. The etiology of this condition has not been well understood. In 1966, Smith[3] described its pathology and attributed it to the perivascular inflammation that he found in the space between the tunica and the erectile tissue. However, he was never able to define the cause of this inflammation.[13] Inflammation is present in this space beneath the plaque, but it is also present in and beneath Buck's fascia overlying the lesion. We believe that the inflammation is a result, not the cause, of the lesion in the tunica. The plaque is a scar, not the result of an inflammatory or autoimmune process. Trauma in a susceptible individual, possibly during sexual intercourse, has been proposed as its cause.[14–17] We agree with that view.[18]

The cross-section of the penis demonstrates the anatomic factors that contribute to the occurrence of Peyronie's disease (Fig. 11–6A). When the penis fills with blood, the tissues of the penis are stretched to the limit of their elasticity. The septal strands and their attachments to the inner circular layer of the tunica albuginea in the dorsal and ventral midline assume the configuration of an inflated I-beam (Fig. 11–6B), resisting upward or downward bending and imparting the ultimate rigidity to the penile shaft. As in an I-beam, when during intercourse the penis is bent dorsally or ventrally, the attachments of the septal fibers to the tunica (Fig. 11–7A) are stressed, generating tension on the convex side. In young men, despite the turgor of the erection and the vigor of the intercourse, the elasticity of the tissues will permit the structures to deform and rebound without damage. However, as a man ages, his tissues become less elastic, and the tension associated with this same degree of distortion can delaminate the circular, inner fibers of the tunica where they are interlaced with the fibers of the septal strands (Fig. 11–7B). This tear causes microvascular injury, bleeding, and clot for-

mation. Many patients will have a vivid memory of this having happened a month or so before their discovery of the lump and the bend. Other patients do not have an acute episode. Though continuing to have what they and their partner consider to be satisfactory intercourse, they will have lost some of the turgor of their erection, and the less rigid shaft of the penis flexes. This action generates tissue fatigue, further reducing, over time, the elasticity of the connections of the septal strands to the tunica. Eventually, this produces multiple tears, with multiple smaller collections of blood clot (Fig. 11–7C). Clots in the tissue spaces lead to the deposition of fibrin. Fibrin is associated with fibroblast activation and proliferation, enhanced blood vessel permeability, and generation of chemotactic factors for inflammatory cells (histiocytes). The lesion fails to resolve due to retention of fibrin in the not well vascularized tunica albuginea or to further deposition after further trauma. Inflammation persists, collagen is trapped, and pathologic fibrosis ensues.* Diminution of the elasticity of the aging tissues of the penis plays a major part in the pathogenesis of Peyronie's disease. The rapidity of this change may be genetically determined, accounting for the familial association that has been noted.

The course of the active process lasts for 1 year to 18 months. During this time, the body is attempting to remodel the scar. In some cases, the plaque has disappeared completely. In many patients the disease appears suddenly; one erection will be straight and the next one will be bent with little or no further progression. Other men may first have pain, then a lump, with minimal curvature that is slowly progressive, eventually reaching an end point. Pain, which often has been considered pathognomonic of Peyronie's disease, is associated with the inflammation present in the active phase

---

*The investigation that led to these conclusions was carried out under grant 1546055378A2 from the National Institutes of Health, Bethesda, MD, to K.D.S.

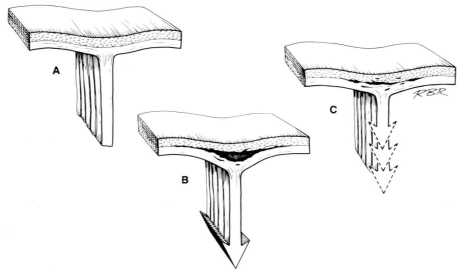

Figure 11–7. A, Diagram of normal situation. Fibers of the septum fan out and are interwoven with the inner, circular layer of fibers of the tunica albuginea. **B,** Diagram illustrating the acute occurrence of Peyronie's disease. Tension generated by bending the erect penis out of column has delaminated the fibers of the tunica albuginea. Bleeding into this tissue space has produced a clot. Fibrin forms, and the scar resulting from the response of the tissue to this trauma becomes the plaque of Peyronie's disease. **C,** Diagram demonstrating the chronic occurrence of Peyronie's disease. Flexion of the less turgid penis results in tissue fatigue at the junctions of the septal strands with the tunica, further reducing the compliance of the tissue. There are multiple tears in the circular fibers of the tunica, where collections of blood produce multiple scars. (From Devine CJ, Jordan GH, Somers KD: Peyronie's disease: cause and surgical treatment. AUA Today 2(5), Sept/Oct 1989.)

of the condition. It has been present in only one third of the patients we have seen, and with resolution of the inflammation, it disappears (R. Snow and C.J. Devine, Jr., unpublished observations). Because of this, medical therapy directed at the inflammation may help early in the course of the disease.

Peyronie's plaques are located in either the dorsal or ventral midline, where they are associated with the insertion of the septal fibers. On the dorsal aspect of the penis, a plaque will cause the shaft to bend upward, whereas a ventral plaque will produce a downward bend. Asymmetry of the plaque in either location will cause a deviation to the most involved side. If both aspects of the shaft are involved, the effect of the plaques will be balanced, with the penis being straight or having a lateral curve but shortened, with its circumference reduced in the involved area. Often this causes the shaft to be flail, and there is loss of turgor distal to the constriction.

Patients with an upward bend of 45 degrees or less can usually continue sexual function satisfactory to both partners. With a lateral or ventral bend, this critical angle is 30 degrees. Patients with greater distortion can continue sexual activity, but

despite attaining a firm erection, with the penis this far out of column, attempts at intromission will be met with further bending and failure. Patients with Peyronie's disease may complain of impotence. Often a man may be able to attain an erection but may lose it quickly, especially if pain is present. Peyronie's disease does not cause impotence. However, loss of elasticity in the structures of the penis is also associated with venous occlusive incompetence (venous leak), which may be concurrent with Peyronie's disease. Indeed, a minimal degree of this may be a factor in the genesis of the chronic onset of Peyronie's disease.

When the patient notices that the penis proximal to the plaque is firm whereas the shaft distal to the plaque is soft, he may presume, and often may have been told by a physician, that the plaque has blocked blood flow into the penis. However, the plaque of Peyronie's disease involves only the tunica albuginea. It does not extend into the erectile tissue, although the inflammation does, and Doppler flow studies usually are normal distal to the plaque. The tunica and the attached extensions of the intracavernosal fibrous framework must be stretched to the limit of their elasticity to maintain the turgor of the erection. The plaque resists this stretch, and though the involved portion of the penis cannot be made turgid by physiologic arterial inflow, this can be accomplished by an artificial erection.

When the active remodeling process of the scar in the tunica has run its course, the effects of the lesion may remain static or recede. Occasionally, usually in young men, the process will resolve completely. During the 1 year to 18 months that it takes for the situation to resolve and for the scar to become fixed, most patients have been able to maintain sexual activity, but they will never be the same as they were before the onset of Peyronie's disease. When the scar has matured, there is no further change in the configuration of the penis,[19] and no medical therapy will help the situation. If the patient and his partner are satisfied with their sexual function, they should be advised that no surgery should be done. However, if the distortion does not allow intercourse that is satisfactory for both, surgery is indicated. Maturation of the scar can arrive without calcification, but calcification is a sure sign of the end-stage of the disease, and this may be present in 6 months.

EVALUATION

We insist that a man's wife or sex partner accompany him at an early visit so that we may give an explanation of the condition to both of them. However, the trauma that originated in the process may have involved another sex partner, so the initial interview is with him alone. We ask each patient to bring Polaroid photographs of his erect penis that define the angle of bend and the character of the erection. The bend will increase as the turgor of the erection increases. The history and character of the lesion usually will provide the diagnosis.

Physical examination of the penis must be precise. The plaque is located in the dorsal or ventral midline and confined to the tunica albuginea. A dorsoventral squeeze of the penis may reveal the lesion, but it will not define its extent. The glans penis must be grasped with one hand and the penis stretched to the limit. The edges of the lesion can then be palpated between the index finger and the thumb of the other hand placed laterally on the shaft. Dorsal plaques can be differentiated easily from ventral plaques, and the presence of concomitant dorsal and ventral plaques will be evident.

Extensive studies are not necessary for diagnosis of Peyronie's disease, but an x-ray to discern calcification will aid in the prognosis. The lesion has been calcified in a quarter of the patients we have seen, and in a quarter of these there has been bone formation. Xeroradiography, which is more complex and costly, cannot demonstrate the extent of an uncalcified lesion. Ultrasound can show the plaque, but this study adds little to digital examination.[20] It can identify calcification, but the sonic shadow of the lesion obscures the spongy tissue beneath it. This has been interpreted as evidence of involvement of the erectile tissue, but the erectile tissue has not been involved in any of the many patients we have operated on. Simple corpus cavernosography can delineate the extent of the plaque but will not furnish information useful in therapy. Magnetic resonance imaging (MRI) is expensive and has contributed nothing to our understanding of the disease or of the situation in individual patients. In young patients, there is a possibility of sarcoma, but it is necessary to biopsy the lesion only if it is uncharacteristic.

After the examination, we explain the disease and discuss the situation with the couple, drawing diagrams and explaining the process by which this has come about. Jordan has produced a television tape for this purpose. We assure them that this is not the end of their sex life. We discuss therapy, noting that there is no quick cure for the lesion—just slow healing of a scar in the tunica albuginea. If they are still functioning sexually, we prescribe vitamin E and arrange for follow-up evaluation. Most patients and their partners can understand this explanation, and they ask discerning questions. Formerly, this may have been the first time that the couple will have discussed the problem, but this is not so much so at the present. Some wives indicate that sex is not the big thing in their lives and that the decision as to therapy is the man's to make. Others are greatly distressed. Most of the couples also have the benefit of consultation with a sex therapist who understands Peyronie's disease.[21]

In 1978 and 1979 we saw 200 patients, 75 of whom required surgery. The others, some of whom had sufficient distortion to be nonfunctional but who had had the condition for less than 6 months, were sent home with vitamin E and encouragement. In 1981, Snow, who was our fellow at the time, was able to contact 105 of these patients (R. Snow and C.J. Devine, Jr., unpublished observations) (Fig. 11–8). Overall, 66% of them were happy with their situation, 3% considered themselves normal, 10% were improved, and the rest were able to function well without disability or pain and intercourse was satisfactory for both partners. Some of these patients noted that partner cooperation was necessary for penetration, but they did not feel that this degree of disability warranted further treatment. Thirty-four percent of the 105 patients needed further treatment: 11% were having good erections but the bend precluded sex and 6 of these went on to satisfactory dermal graft surgery, 8% were impotent—initially 4% had been impotent—3 of these had a penile prosthesis implanted, but the other 5 patients declined. The other

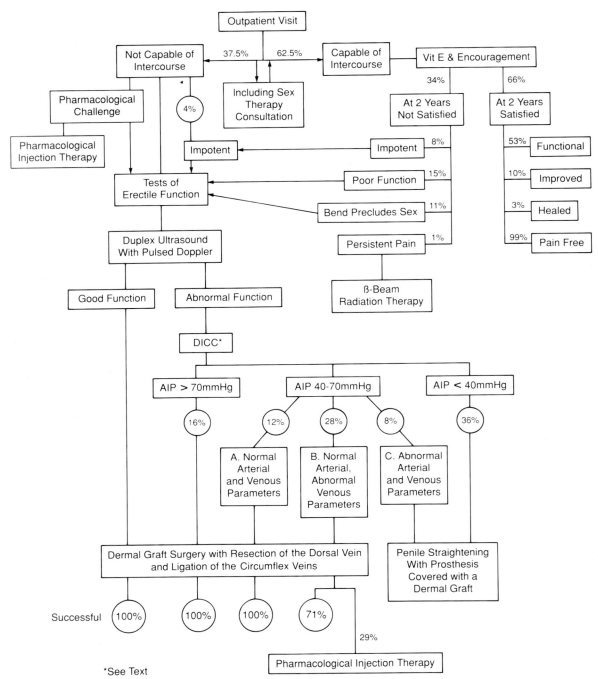

Figure 11–8. Algorithm illustrating the course of Peyronie's disease therapy. About one third of patients have been candidates for surgical treatment. At the end of 2 years, the same proportion holds. The prognosis for success of the surgery depends on measurements of erectile function, and the treatment proposed is based on the results of these tests.

15% had poor function—some had flaccidity distal to the bend, others had a generally soft erection with a bend, and others complained of shortening of the penis. All of these patients would have benefited from an evaluation using the tests of function

that are available now. Of interest in this group of nonfunctional patients is the fact that their performance ability had been toward the lower end of the spectrum at their initial presentation. It was unusual for a person who had been functioning well to have deteriorated to this degree over the 2-year period.

Treatment is aimed at maintenance of recovery of sexual function. Having established the diagnosis, most medical therapy during the acute phase (e.g., DMSO, ultrasound, injection and iontophoresis of steroids, or radiation) is designed to control inflammation. These treatments may help to relieve the discomfort associated with Peyronie's disease, but it is unlikely that they will influence the outcome. Some of our patients have reported that terfenadine (Seldane), an antihistamine without sedative side effects, helped to relieve painful erections in this phase of the disease. No controlled studies have been done. Collagenase injections sound reasonable,[22] but a double-blind evaluation did not encourage continuation of this therapy.[23] Potaba (P-aminobenzoate) has been described as specific therapy for "the bent spike." However, it is expensive and requires extensive dosage, and there is no evidence that it is effective. We do not inject plaques with steroids, having seen little benefit from this. In some patients, the injections have led to tissue atrophy, worsening the lesion. We have seen tissue atrophy after radiation therapy delivered with the high-energy sources sometimes reported in the literature. Radiation is not likely to affect the outcome of the healing process in the scar, but if pain persists or is particularly troublesome, a small dose of radiation delivered by a soft modality (450 rad by the beta beam of a linear accelerator), much as is used to treat a keloid (A. M. El-Mahdi, personal communication, 1990) can relieve residual pain.

Though we do not know the mechanism, we have found that Peyronie's disease resolved, improved, or became static with continuing functioning in two thirds of our patients taking vitamin E, 200 mg (iu) with each meal or 400 mg (iu) twice a day, and we continue to prescribe this treatment.[23a]

In some patients the inability to have intercourse is due to the loss of turgor of the erection rather than to the distortion of the penis. These patients are given a challenge dose of the medication necessary to establish a pharmacologic erection. If the patient achieves a firm enough erection and he and his partner conclude that the bend will not interfere with intromission, we discourage surgery and recommend that he be maintained on a pharmacologic erection program. If not, we proceed with our evaluation (Fig. 11–8).

If the plaque has been present for at least a year or is calcified and the distortion precludes intercourse, we offer the patient surgical treatment consisting of excision of the plaque and patching of the defect with a graft of the dermal layer of the skin.[24,25] The operation, first described in 1973, has been modified over the years.[26] Other materials have been used for this patch by other surgeons. Full-thickness skin is unacceptable because buried epithelium will form a cyst. Tunica vaginalis has been used as a graft[27] or as a flap (J. L. Lockhart, personal communication, 1992). Though we found in dogs that arterial and venous segments and pieces of fascia tended to contract and form scars,[24] temporalis fascia[28] and the dorsal vein of the penis (T. F. Lue, personal communication, 1992) have been used successfully to patch transverse incisions placed so that they lengthen the involved surface of the tunica albuginea. Gore-Tex and other synthetic materials have been used to patch incisions in the tunica after insertion of prosthetic devices, but they are not elastic, though they are flexible, and inflammatory collections of collagen form beneath them when they are used as a substitute for a dermal graft. The Nesbit procedure[8] has been employed for correction of the bend in Peyronie's disease.[29] We would not like to further shorten the penis of a man already distressed by its size, but if the problem that incapacitates a man without a regular sex partner is merely the presence of a bend rather than its severity, minimal distortion can be corrected by a Nesbit tuck or two on the long side of the penis opposite the bend. We have used plication to complete the repair when the penis still has a minimal bend after a dermal graft operation.

Having decided that surgery is necessary, we plan the approach. The Polaroid photographs demonstrate the distortion. Palpation of the stretched penis locates the plaque, and x-ray identifies calcification. Because impotence has been a postoperative problem in some patients, all patients receive a detailed evaluation of their erectile potential, and to a certain extent, the results of this study can predict the functional outcome of the surgery (Fig. 11–8). A duplex ultrasound scan with pulsed Doppler[30] is used to evaluate an erection induced by injection of 0.5 to 1.0 ml of a mixture of papaverine 18 mg, phentolamine 1.0 mg, and prostaglandin E_1 12.5 mg/ml. If this study is normal,[31] with good pulsatile arterial inflow achieving a turgid erection at which time venous flow ceases, we do no further testing. If any aspect of the Doppler flow study is abnormal, we proceed to dynamic infusion corpus cavernosometry and corpus cavernosography (DICC).[32,33]

Though normal values have been developed for various phases of DICC, a man does not have to measure up to these to have satisfactory sexual relations. We record the time it takes after the pharmacologic injection to attain maximum accumulated intracorporal pressure (AIP) and the level of this pressure. As the saline infusion is begun, the flow necessary to maintain intracorporal pressures of 90, 120, and 150 mm Hg are noted, and the pressure is recorded 30 sec after the flow is stopped. Also, the pressure necessary to occlude the pulse in the cavernosal arteries is recorded, and cavernosography x-rays are made to record the presence and location of venous leaks. In patients with Peyronie's disease, we consider as normal an equilibrium AIP of at least 90 mm Hg, a maintenance flow rate of less than or equal to 5 ml/min, and a 30 sec pressure fall of 45 mm Hg (1.5 mm Hg/sec) or less. Cavernosal artery systolic occlusion pressure of at least 90 mm Hg or a penile/systemic gradient of 35 mm Hg or less is considered adequate. Based on the initial equilibrium AIP after pharmacologic injection at the time of DICC, patients can be divided into three groups: (1) AIP 70 mm Hg or more, (2) AIP 40 to 69 mm Hg, and (3) AIP less than 40 mm Hg (Fig. 11–8). In 25 consecutive patients seen and evaluated by Jordan and Angermeier,[34] there were 4 patients in group 1, 12 in group 2, and 9 in group 3. In 19 of these, there was evidence of corporal venoocclusive dysfunction, and there was abnormal arterial inflow in 11.

A dermal graft operation with resection of the dorsal vein was successful in all 4 of group 1. Group 2 was divided into three subgroups: (a) 3 patients who had normal venous and arterial parameters, (b) 7 patients with abnormal venous parameters yet adequate arterial studies, and (c) 2 patients who had abnormal venous and arterial evaluation. The 3 patients in group 2a had dermal graft surgery, 2 of them with dorsal vein resection. All of these were successful. The patients in 2b and 2c also had dermal graft surgery with dorsal vein resection. Five of the 7 patients in 2b had successful results, with 1 of the failures having had his penile rigidity restored with pharmacologic injection therapy. One patient in group 2c was straight and functional, and 1 has responded to the pharmacologic erection program.

In group 3, 1 patient had dermal grafting without vein surgery. Three had dermal grafting with extensive penile vein ligation,[35] and in 5, the plaque was excised, a prosthesis installed, and the defect in the tunica covered with a dermal graft. The 5 patients with prostheses have done well. One of the patients who had extensive vein ligation did well but has been lost to follow-up. The others are straight but impotent. These patients illustrate our recommendations for therapy (Fig. 11–8). If the Doppler flow study is normal and if during DICC the patient can maintain a pressure of at least 70 mm Hg, or if he can maintain at least 40 mm Hg and evidences good arterial and venous function, he is likely to have a good result from dermal graft surgery with resection of the dorsal vein. If he has a good arterial flow and can maintain at least 40 mm of intracavernosal pressure despite some evidence of a venous leak, after dermal graft surgery and resection of the dorsal vein, he is likely to do well, though there is a chance that he will need to begin a pharmacologic injection program or perhaps have a prosthesis placed as a later procedure. Our dermal graft operation does not preclude this. If, however, he has poor arterial flow, he will probably do poorly despite being able to attain 40 mm Hg intracavernosal pressure. These patients and those who cannot maintain at least that much pressure should have a prosthesis implanted at the time the penis is straightened.

We began to resect the dorsal vein and to approach dorsal plaques through its bed because we were concerned that because of the acquisition of new vessels by each face of the graft, venous connections that were not controlled by the normal venous occlusive mechanism could occur. Resection of the dorsal vein has improved postoperative function, but to obviate all venous short circuits, it has been necessary to ligate the circumflex veins at their junction with the deep veins that run parallel to the corpus spongiosum. When the plaque is on the ventrum, we do not excise the deep dorsal vein but do ligate the circumflex and periurethral veins in mobilizing the corpus spongiosum.

SURGERY

The incision depends on the location of the lesion. Most patients will have been circumcised, and for a dorsal plaque involving the midshaft or distal shaft, we make an incision through that scar (Fig. 11–9A) and mobilize the skin to the base of the penis. When the plaque is more proximal or when we plan extensive venous ligation, we deliver the penile shaft through an incision in the scrotum lateral to the base of the penis (Fig. 11–10). To protect the penile skin from trauma, it is laid to the side, covered with a warm saline sponge. At the end of the operation, the shaft is replaced within the sleeve of skin. This technique also helps to reduce edema in uncircumcised patients who do not wish to have their foreskin removed and can be used to expose a ventral plaque, though usually we make a ventral midline incision and mobilize the corpus spongiosum, carefully ligating the circumflex veins as we encounter them (Fig. 11–11).

In the past, after reflecting the skin, we exposed dorsal plaques by making incisions in the lateral aspects of Buck's fascia, and dissecting beneath it with blunt-tipped scissors, we protected the dorsal neurovascular bundle while elevating it along with the fascia. Where the underlying tunica is normal, the fascia can be lifted easily by spreading the tips of the scissors, but the inflammation in this tissue plane where it overlies the Peyronie's disease

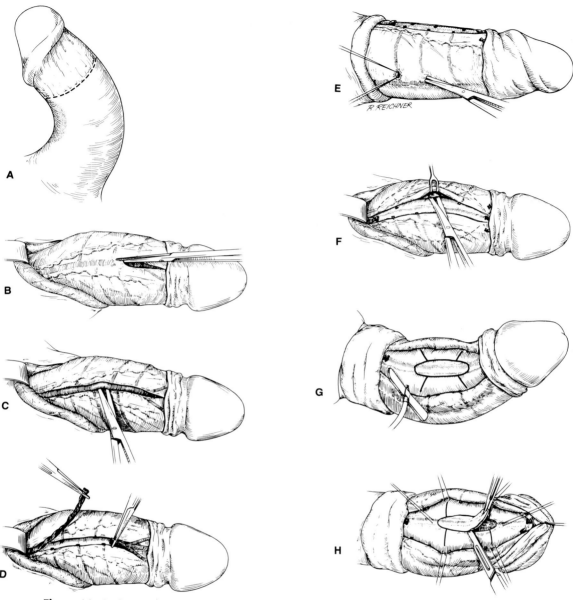

Figure 11–9. Surgical treatment of a dorsal Peyronie's disease plaque. **A,** An erection demonstrates the curve. The circumcision scar is marked. **B,** The skin is reflected, and Buck's fascia is opened to expose the deep dorsal vein. The coiled dorsal arteries and the circumflex veins are illustrated. **C,** The deep dorsal vein is mobilized. **D,** The transected vein is dissected proximally, ligating and dividing the communicating veins. Distally, the veins draining the glans will also be ligated and divided. Dissection of the plaque will be in the plane beneath these vessels. **E,** The circumflex veins are ligated on each side where they join the deep ventral veins running lateral to the corpus spongiosum. **F,** Buck's fascia is elevated from the plaque. The area of dissection outlined by the dashed line continues proximal, lateral, and distal to the plaque at a distance sufficient to avoid distraction injury to the arteries and nerves, which are clearly seen and can be avoided during this dissection. **G,** An artificial erection demonstrates the effect of the plaque outlined on the tunica, along with the planned stellate releasing incisions. **H,** Prolene sutures placed proximal and distal to the plaque and lateral to the ends of the stellate incisions afford control of the tunica as the plaque is removed. An incision has been made around the plaque, the tip of which has been elevated as the erectile tissue is dissected away sharply.

Continued on following page

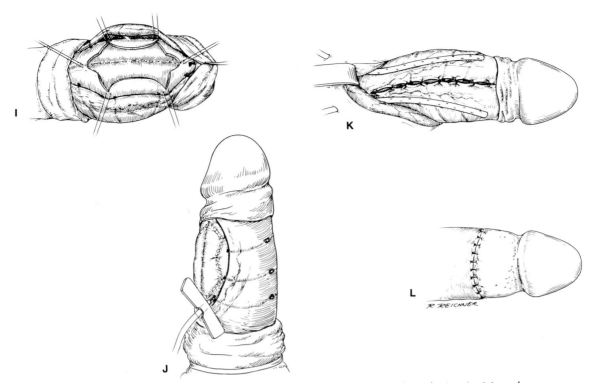

Figure 11-9 *Continued* **I,** The plaque has been removed and the relaxing incisions have allowed expansion of the defect. The ends of the septal strands can be seen in the midline. The defect is now measured to determine the size of the dermal graft that will be needed as a patch. **J,** The graft has been obtained (Fig. 11–12) and applied (Fig. 11–13). The penis is straight. **K,** Buck's fascia is loosely reapproximated in the midline, and two small suction drains are in place. **L,** The skin closure is completed. A Bioclusive dressing will be applied, and a light pressure Kling wrap is left on for 3 to 4 h. A 14 Foley catheter remains until the following morning. (From Devine CJ Jr. Surgery of the penis and urethra. In: Campbell's Urology, 6th ed. Philadelphia: WB Saunders Co, 1992.)

Figure 11–10. Atraumatic mobilization of the full length of the penile shaft. **A,** Two incisions are marked, one to circumcise the penis and the other lateral to the base of the penis and carried down into the scrotum. **B,** The shaft of the penis has been freed by dissecting close to Buck's fascia and leaving most of the dartos fascia with the skin. The penis is delivered into the scrotal incision.

Continued on following page

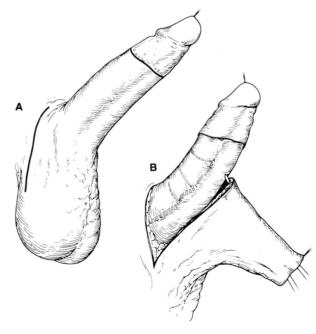

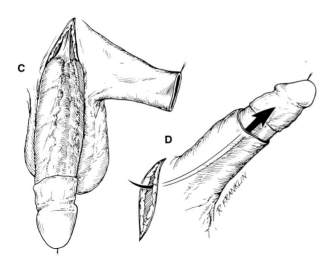

Figure 11-10 *Continued* **C,** After minimal dissection, traction on the penis affords visualization of the suspensory ligaments. With further dissection, complete resection of the dorsal vein can be accomplished. **D,** After the procedure, the shaft of the penis is replaced within the relatively untraumatized sleeve of skin. (From Devine CJ Jr. Surgery of the penis and urethra. In: Campbell's Urology, 6th ed. Philadelphia: WB Saunders Co, 1992.)

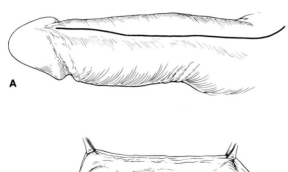

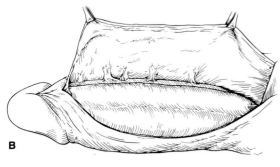

Figure 11–11. Exposure of a ventral plaque. **A,** The ventral midline incision is marked. This may be continued into the scrotum to approach a more proximal plaque. **B,** The skin is elevated to expose Buck's fascia covering the corpus spongiosum. **C,** The corpus spongiosum is elevated after incising Buck's fascia on each side. The plaque is easily seen in the midline, and because of the inflammation, sharp dissection was necessary to complete this step. The connections between the circumflex veins and the deep ventral veins lateral to the corpus spongiosum were ligated during this process.

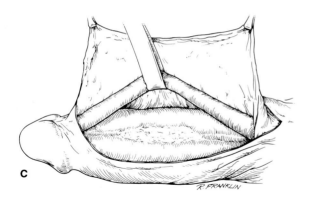

Continued on following page

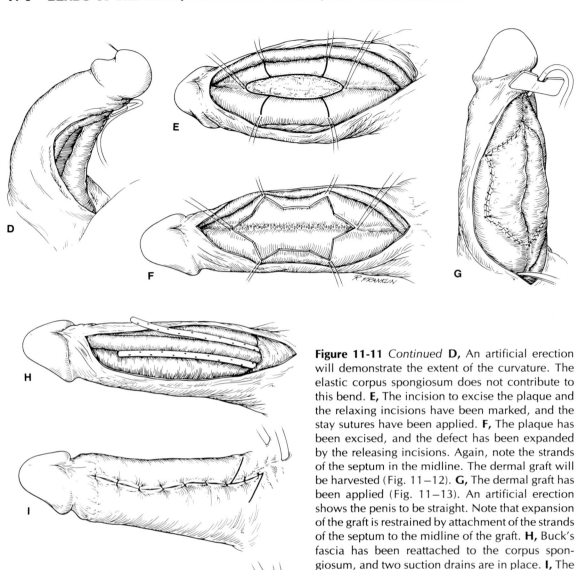

Figure 11-11 *Continued* **D,** An artificial erection will demonstrate the extent of the curvature. The elastic corpus spongiosum does not contribute to this bend. **E,** The incision to excise the plaque and the relaxing incisions have been marked, and the stay sutures have been applied. **F,** The plaque has been excised, and the defect has been expanded by the releasing incisions. Again, note the strands of the septum in the midline. The dermal graft will be harvested (Fig. 11–12). **G,** The dermal graft has been applied (Fig. 11–13). An artificial erection shows the penis to be straight. Note that expansion of the graft is restrained by attachment of the strands of the septum to the midline of the graft. **H,** Buck's fascia has been reattached to the corpus spongiosum, and two suction drains are in place. **I,** The skin is approximated, and a Z-plasty has been marked where the incision crosses the penoscrotal junction. The suction drains can be seen as they exit the scrotum. **J,** Closure is complete. A Bioclusive dressing will be applied with a Kling wrap for 3 to 4 h. A 14F Foley catheter will be removed the next morning.

plaque makes it necessary to use sharp dissection, keeping the tips of the scissors against the plaque. Today, to approach a dorsal plaque, we remove the deep dorsal vein and dissect through its bed, but the same techniques apply. Retracting the tunica with hooks while lifting Buck's fascia with atraumatic Beasley forceps defines a sharp angle between the tissue layers, facilitating the dissection.

We excise the deep dorsal vein from its origin at the retrocoronal plexus, where the veins draining the glans come together, to the level of the suspensory ligament proximally (Fig. 11–9D). Often, there is not a single vein but several veins running together and anastomosing with each other. It is not unusual to find a connection between a deep dorsal vein and a superficial vein. We ligate the circumflex veins and the emissary veins where they enter the deep dorsal vein. We also expose the circumflex veins where they join the deep ventral veins that run lateral to the corpus spongiosum. We make small openings in Buck's fascia with the tips of the dissecting scissors and coagulate the small veins or ligate the larger veins with 4-0 silk sutures (Fig. 11–9E).

By dissecting laterally from the bed of the deep dorsal vein, we are able to expose the entire plaque and uninvolved tunica lateral to it (Fig. 11–9F). Mobilization is continued proximal and distal to the plaque so that the dorsal nerves will not be stretched as the fascia is retracted during resection of the plaque. The extent of the fibrosis can be determined easily because of the consistency of the tunica and the roughness of its surface. An artificial erection will define the curvature (Fig. 11–9G). Incisions are planned to excise the plaque and release the tunica at the margins of the defect. We place midline prolene stay sutures proximal and distal to the plaque and at the tips of the lateral incisions. The incision is made through the full thickness of the tunica around the plaque.

The tip of the plaque is lifted, and with a knife or scissors, erectile tissue is mobilized (Fig. 11–9H). The lesion does not extend into it, but because of the inflammation, the erectile tissue will be adherent to the undersurface of the plaque. The erectile tissue should not be injured during this dissection. The septal strands, however, will be attached to the undersurface of the plaque and must be cut across. The ends will lie prominently in the midline of the defect after the plaque has been removed (Fig. 11–9I). We make matching lateral incisions by undermining the tunica and cutting with a knife, expanding the area of the defect to 1.5 to 2 times the size of the plaque that has been removed.

A tourniquet is not necessary for this dissection. When the penis is flaccid, blood flow in the erectile space is limited and can be controlled by pressure on the underside of the shaft, but the level of anesthesia must be as deep as for an abdominal operation or the stimulus associated with surgery will initiate the erection reflex and bleeding will be excessive. Should this happen, stop and deepen the anesthesia before proceeding.

We measure the defect while stretching it first longitudinally and then laterally, allowing a little extra for the roundness of the penis. We prefer the skin of the abdomen just above the iliac crest and lateral to the hairline as a donor site for the dermis (Fig. 11–12). We usually remove the epidermis freehand and discard it. Trying to close the defect by applying the epidermis as a split-thickness graft will generate an ugly scar. The dermal graft will

be about 1 mm thick. To harvest this, an incision is made around the dermal patch, leaving a few millimeters of dermal cuff on the skin to aid in closure. One end of the dermis is elevated, and the patch is removed by excising the fat from its underside, exposing the subdermal vascular plexus. The defect is closed full thickness, placing 5-0 Vicryl sutures in the dermal cuff and using a pullout subcuticular suture of 3-0 prolene. This suture is removed in 3 weeks, leaving a narrow scar that will widen a little with time.

The graft is placed in the defect in the tunica with the subdermal plexus deep. Tacking sutures of 4-0 PDS are placed, securing the graft at the proximal and distal midline and at the tips of the releasing incisions on one side (Fig. 11–13). Using a cutting needle, a running suture of 5-0 PDS is placed, producing an edge-to-edge closure of the graft to the tunica with no overlap. When the first side has been secured, the graft is folded, and its midline is marked so that we will not lose the relationship as we place another line of 5-0 PDS to attach the deep surface of the graft to the cut ends of the septal strands. The graft is unfolded, and the other edge is secured as was the first. When the sutures have been placed, another artificial erection demonstrates that the penis is straight and that the suture line is watertight (Fig. 11–9J). Any leaks are oversewn. If the penis is straight, we close the superficial layers. However, if curvature persists, the incisions have to be extended and further grafts applied.

On the dorsal side, closure begins by approximating Buck's fascia in the midline with interrupted 5-0 PDS sutures, carefully avoiding the dorsal arteries and nerves (Fig. 11–9K). Small suction drains are placed superficial to Buck's fascia but deep to the dartos layer. The skin incisions are closed, or if the penis has been removed from the sheath of skin, it is replaced and the skin incisions closed with 5-0 chromic gut (Fig. 11–10D). On the ventral side, Buck's fascia is reattached to the corpus spongiosum (Fig. 11–11H). Suction drains are placed lateral to that structure, and the skin is closed in two layers, approximating the dartos with interrupted Vicryl sutures and the skin with 5-0 chromic sutures.

We dress the penis with Bioclusive semipermeable dressing (Johnson & Johnson, New Brunswick, NJ), applying it loosely, extending from the base of the penis to the level of the midglans. This serves as a pressure dressing, and because it is transparent, we are able to visualize the condition of the skin during the healing process. It stays for about 5 days. We leave a 14F Foley catheter until the patient ambulates the next morning. The suction drains are removed at 24 and 48 h. Erections are suppressed with diazepam and amylnitrate

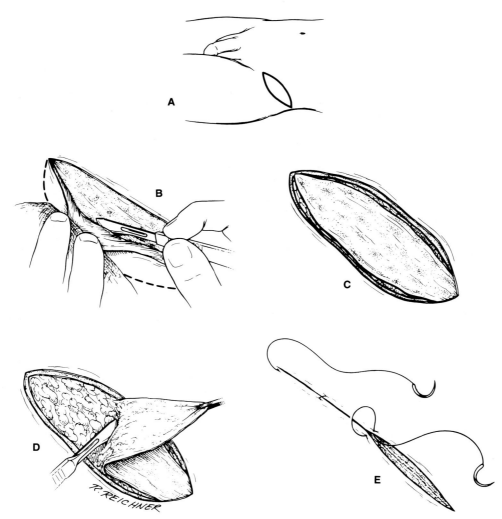

Figure 11–12. Harvesting a dermal graft. **A,** The donor site is marked above the iliac crest, lateral to the hairline. **B,** The epidermis is removed freehand with a No. 10 blade. **C,** An incision is made around the dermal patch, leaving a narrow cuff of dermis to aid in skin closure. **D,** The graft is elevated while fat is trimmed off its undersurface. **E,** The skin is closed. Vicryl sutures in the dermis approximate the edges. Using a running, double-ended suture of nylon or prolene, the subcuticular closure is begun at the midpoint. Each needle is passed from the outside in, leaving a loop of suture on the outside to aid in its removal in about 3 weeks. Sewing is continued to the two ends, bringing another loop to the surface halfway along. The ends of the suture are tied together loosely, and a Bioclusive dressing is applied. (From Devine CJ Jr. Surgery of the penis and urethra. In: Campbell's Urology, 6th ed. Philadelphia: WB Saunders Co, 1992.)

pearls. Patients are discharged on the third to the fifth day.

Dermal grafts go through maturation as do other grafts. They are first nourished by imbibition of tissue fluids from the graft bed while blood vessels in the bed, in response to growth factors produced by the graft, bud to form vessels that penetrate the graft and hook up with the blood vessels in the graft. This process, called inosculation, is complete by the fifth day. The dermis continues to undergo remodeling for 6 months to 1 year. At first, it contracts, and during this period, some rebending may occur, but after 3 months, it softens, and as remodeling progresses, the shape of the penis improves.

After the first 2 weeks, we encourage erections

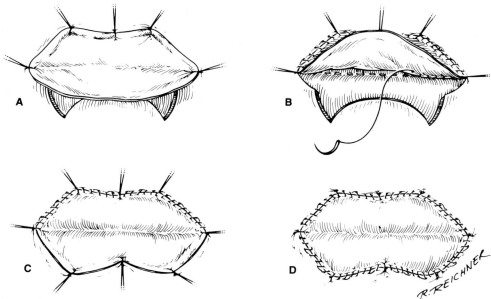

Figure 11–13. The dermal graft is placed into the incision with its fat side down. **A,** Sutures of 4-0 PDS are placed to secure the graft at the proximal and distal midlines of the defect and at the tips of the releasing incisions on one side of the defect. **B,** The edge of the graft has been sewn to the edge of the defect with a running 5-0 PDS suture, locking every third throw. The graft has been folded, and its midline, marked with brilliant green, is being sewn to the strands of the septum with a running 5-0 PDS suture. **C,** Stay sutures are applied to secure the other edge of the graft. **D,** Placement of the graft is completed by sewing this side in the same manner as was the first side, making a watertight closure. (From Devine CJ Jr. Peyronie's disease. In: Glen JF, ed. Urologic Surgery, 4th ed. Philadelphia: JB Lippincott Co, 1991: 873.)

that will stretch the graft but discourage intercourse for another month. During that time, the erect penis should be manipulated so that the skin will not become adherent to the deeper tissue layers. We ask the patient's sex partner to carry out this physical therapy—which is also sex therapy, involving both of them in the patient's rehabilitation. When the suture line can stand the stress, this activity can lead directly to intercourse. We have the patient continue taking vitamin E 400 mg bid with vitamin B_1 150 mg daily and vitamin C 500 mg bid. At least 75% of our patients have been happy after the surgery.[36,37] This experience compares well with the results of other penile surgery.

REFERENCES

1. Devine CJ Jr, Angermeier KW. Anatomy of the penis and male perineum: Part I. A.U.A. Update Series (in press).
2. Goldstein AM, Padma-Nathan H. The microarchitecture of the intracavernosal smooth muscle and the cavernosal fibrous skeleton. J Urol 144:1144, 1990.
3. Smith BH. Peyronie's disease. Am J Clin Pathol 45:670, 1966.
4. Devine CJ Jr, Horton CE. Chordee without hypospadias. J Urol 110:264–271, 1973.
5. Secrest CL, Jordan GH, Winslow BH, et al. The repair of complications of hypospadias surgery (in press).
6. Schonfeld WA, Beebe GW. Normal growth and variation in the male genitalia from birth to maturity. Am J Dis Child 64:759, 1942.
7. Devine CJ Jr, Blackley SK, Horton CE, Gilbert DA. The surgical treatment of chordee without hypospadias in postadolescent men. J Urol 146:325–329, 1991.
8. Nesbit RM. Congenital curvature of the phallus: a report of three cases with description of corrective operation. J Urol 93:230, 1965.
9. Devine CJ Jr, Horton CE. Use of dermal graft to correct chordee. J Urol 113:56, 1975.
10. Nyberg LM, Bias WB, Hochberg MC, Walsh PC. Identification of an inherited form of Peyronie's disease with autosomal dominant inheritance and association with Dupuytren's contracture and histo-

compatibility B7 crossreacting antigens. J Urol 128:48, 1982.

11. Leffell MS, Devine CJ Jr, Horton CE, et al. Non-association of Peyronie's disease with HLA B7 crossreactive antigens. J Urol 127:122, 1982.

12. Peyronie F de la. Sur quelques obstacles qui s'opposent a l'ejaculation naturelle de la semence. Mem Acad Chir 1:318, 1743.

13. Smith BH. Subclinical Peyronie's disease. Am J Clin Pathol 52:385, 1969.

14. DeSanctis PN, Furey GA. Steroid injection therapy for Peyronie's disease: a 10-year summary and review of 38 cases. J Urol 97:114, 1967.

15. McRoberts JW. Peyronie's disease. Surg Gynecol Obstet 12:1291, 1969.

16. Godec CJ, Van Beek AL. Peyronie's disease is curable—is it also preventable? Urology 21:257, 1983.

17. Hinman F Jr. Peyronie's disease: etiological considerations. Prog Reprod Biol Med 9:5–12, 1983.

18. Devine CJ Jr, Somers KD, Wright GL Jr, et al. A working model for the genesis of Peyronie's disease derived from its pathobiology (Abstract 495). J Urol 139:286A, 1988.

19. Gelbard MK, James K, Dorey F. The natural history of Peyronie's disease. J Urol 114:1376–1379, 1990.

20. Altaffer LF III, Jordan G. Sonographic demonstration of Peyronie's plaques. Urology 17:292, 1981.

21. Jones WJ Jr, Horton CE, Stecker JF Jr, et al. The treatment of psychogenic impotence after dermal graft repair for Peyronie's disease. J Urol 131:286, 1984.

22. Gelbard MK, Linder A, Kaufman JJ. The use of collagenase in the treatment of Peyronie's disease. J Urol 134:280, 1985.

23. Gelbard MK, James K, Riach P, Dorey F. Collagenase versus placebo in the treatment of Peyronie's disease: a double-blind study. J Urol 149:56, 1993.

23a. Devine CJ Jr. Peyronie's disease. In: Hurst JW, ed. Medicine for the Practicing Physician, 3rd ed. Boston: Butterworth, 1992:1249–1351.

24. Horton CE, Devine CJ Jr. Plication of the tunica albuginea to straighten the curved penis. Plast Reconstr Surg 52:32, 1973.

25. Devine CJ Jr, Horton CE. The surgical treatment of Peyronie's disease with a dermal graft. J Urol 110:264–271, 1973.

26. Devine CJ, Jordan GH, Schlossberg SM. Surgery of the penis and urethra. In: Walsh PC, Retik AB, Stamey TA, Vaughan ED, eds. Campbell's Urology. Philadelphia: WB Saunders Co, 1991:2957–3032.

27. Das S, Maggio AJ. Tunica vaginalis autografting for Peyronie's disease. An experimental study. Invest Urol 17:186, 1979.

28. Gelbard MK, Hayden B. Expanding contractures of the tunica albuginea due to Peyronie's disease with temporalis fascia free grafts. J Urol 145:722–776, 1991.

29. Pryor JP, Fitzpatrick JM. A new approach to the correction of the penile deformity in Peyronie's disease. J Urol 122:622, 1979.

30. Lue TF, Hricak H, Marich KW, Tanagho EA. Vasculogenic impotence evaluated by high-resolution ultrasonography and pulsed Doppler spectrum analysis. Radiology 155:777, 1985.

31. Jordan GH, Kodama RT, Rowe DF, Devine CJ Jr. Interpretation of penile duplex ultrasound wave forms and measurements in pharmacologically induced erections (Abstract 33). J Urol 143:197A, 1990.

32. Padma-Nathan H. Evaluation of the corporal veno-occlusive mechanism: dynamic infusion cavernosometry and cavernosography. Semin Intervent Radiol 6:205–211, 1989.

33. Goldstein I. Penile reconstruction. Urol Clin North Am 14:805, 1987.

34. Jordan GH, Angermeier KW. Preoperative evaluation of erectile function with dynamic infusion cavernosometry/cavernosography (DICC) in patients undergoing surgery for Peyronie's disease: correlation with postoperative results. J Urol (in press).

35. Lue TF. Penile venous surgery. Urol Clin North Am 16:607–611, 1989.

36. Wild RM, Devine CJ Jr, Horton CE. Dermal graft repair of Peyronie's disease. Survey of 50 patients. J Urol 121:47–50, 1979.

37. Horton CE, Sadove RC, Devine CJ Jr. Peyronie's disease. Ann Plast Surg 18:121–127, 1987.

CHAPTER 12

Sexual Dysfunction and Spinal Cord Injury

Subbarao V. Yalla
Martyn A. Vickers, Jr.
Maryrose P. Sullivan
Mehdi Sarkarati

Spinal cord injuries (SCI) dramatically and adversely affect sexual function. Each year, there are approximately 10,000 new cases of SCI in the United States. The social impact of this injury is particularly disturbing when one considers that the majority of these patients are less than 30 years of age. Since sexual interest and activity are often well preserved in these patients, restoration of sexual function is critical to their successful overall rehabilitation. The severity of the sexual dysfunction depends on the level and completeness of the cord lesion and on the duration of the injury.[1]

SEXUAL DYSFUNCTION OF SPINAL CORD INJURY PATIENTS

Before Talbot's classic report on sexual function in paraplegics, there was a general belief that all of these unfortunate patients were permanently and completely impotent and sterile. His 1949 work, based on questioning and observing 200 paraplegic males, revealed that 36.5% were unable to have erections, 42.5% had reflex erections evoked by local stimulation, and 21% had erections resulting from both local and psychic stimulation. Forty-six of these patients had vaginal intercourse. Of these, 32 reached orgasm, and 20 were able to ejaculate.[2] Subsequent studies confirmed the presence of erectile and ejaculatory capacity in patients with SCI (Table 12–1). Bors and Comarr highlighted the impact of the level and completeness of cord transection on ultimate erectile and ejaculatory function[3] (Fig. 12–1). A subsequent study by Comarr reported that patients with incomplete lesions were more likely to achieve vaginal penetration (87% of those who attempted), ejaculate (33%), and experience orgasm (33%) than those with complete lesions—50%, 1%, and less than 1%, respectively[4] (Table 12–2). Further, patients with upper motor neuron lesions (normal external

sphincter tone and intact bulbocavernosus reflex) were more likely to have reflex erections (induced by penile manipulation, 77%) than psychic erections (induced by nontactile erotic sensory stimuli, 24%). Conversely, patients with lower motor neuron lesions frequently had psychogenic erections but did not experience reflex erections.

The relationship between the type of erection and the causative cord lesion was clarified by the study by Chapelle et al. of 149 men with complete SCI.[5] Reflex erection involved the corpus cavernosum and spongiosum if the lower level of the injury was above T10–T12 and involved only the corpus cavernosum if the lesion was caudal to T10–L2. Psychogenic erection may occur when the upper level of the cord injury is caudal to T12. From this work and that of others, it became apparent that the efferent factors capable of organizing a psychogenic erection leave the spinal cord at myelomeres T11 and T12.

NEUROANATOMY

Knowledge of the gross neuroanatomy of the spinal cord allows the diagnostician to accurately predict neurogenic defects based on review of lumbosacral films, CT scan, or MRI. The adult spinal cord is a 41 to 45 cm cylindrical organ that terminates at the level of the intervertebral disc between the first and second lumbar vertebra. The dural sac and the subarachnoid space extend to the second sacral vertebral level. In the lumbar area, the dural sac contains only the spinal rootlets (cauda equina).

Each vertebral segment consists of a portion of the spinal cord and its anterior and posterior roots, which join to form the associated pair of spinal nerves. There are 31 spinal segments: 8 cervical, 12 thoracic, 5 lumbar, 5 sacral, and 1 coccygeal. Because of the difference in the length of the spinal

TABLE 12–1
Sexual Function in Spinal Cord Injury Patients

Author (year)	No. of Patients	Erection (%)	Ejaculation (%)	Coitus (%)
Talbot (1955)	40	60	11.5	23
Zeitlin et al. (1957)	100	94	3.0	33
Tsuji et al. (1961)	638	54	9.0	15
Comarr (1970)	150	82	11.0	38

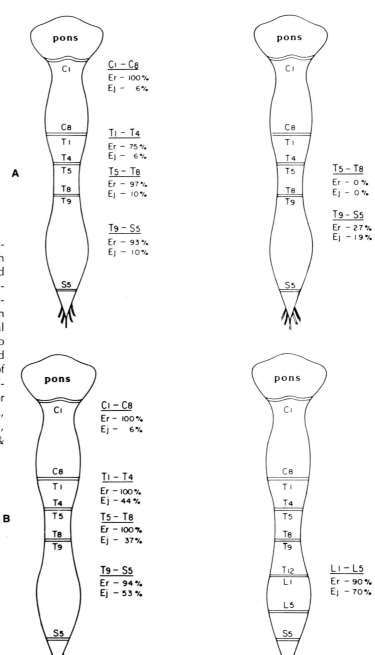

Figure 12–1. The incidence of erections and ejaculations in patients with complete **(A)** and incomplete **(B)** cord lesions. Upper neuron lesions are illustrated on the left and right, respectively. Complete lower motor neuron lesions with involvement of proximal cord segments T5–T8 usually lead to complete absence of erections and ejaculations. A higher incidence of erections and ejaculations are associated with incomplete lesions (upper or lower motor neuron). (From Bennett A, ed. Management of Male Impotence, pp 183–184. ©1982, the Williams & Wilkins Co., Baltimore.)

176

TABLE 12–2
Correlation of Erection, Ejaculation, and Intercourse with Level and Severity of Cord Lesion

	Cord Lesion	Reflexogenic Erections (%)	Psychogenic Erections (%)	Successful Coitus (%)	Ejaculation (%)
Upper motor neuron lesions (115)	Complete (75)	92	9	66	1
	Incomplete (40)	93	48	86	22
Lower motor neuron lesions (119)	Complete (109)	0	24	33	15
	Incomplete (10)	0	1	100	100

cord and the spinal column, the rootlets may emerge perpendicular or oblique to the cord, depending on their origin (Fig. 12–2).

The penis has both somatic and autonomic innervation. Afferent somatic fibers, originating in the free nerve endings in the penis, scrotum, and pubis, course within the pudendal nerve and enter the spinal cord through the dorsal roots of S2–S4. These fibers ascend in the posterior columns to the contralateral thalamus, terminating in the contralateral primary sensory strip deep within the interhemispheric fissure. The somatic efferent pathways originate in the motor strip of the interhemispheric fissure. On entering the cord, they descend in the most medial corticospinal pathway and emerge from the ventral roots of S2–S4 to innervate the bulbocavernosus, ischiocavernosus, striated urethral sphincter, and perineal muscles via the pudendal nerve.

Injury of the afferent somatosensory fibers (dorsal nerve impotence) is characterized by an inability to sustain an erection during coitus. Injury of the efferent somatic pathway may prevent achievement of suprasystolic penile rigidity just before ejaculation.[6]

The autonomic penile innervation has been thought to originate in various areas of the brain: the hypothalamus, paraventricular nucleus, median forebrain bundle, gyrus rectus, septum pellucidum, mamillothalamic tracts, cingulate gyrus, and hippocampus. Efferent fibers traverse in the intermediate gray matter (intermediolateral column). The spinal nuclei, located in segments T10–L2 and S2–S4,[7] constitute the respective origins of sympathetic innervation to the smooth muscles of the vas deferens, seminal vesicles, bladder neck, prostate and penile blood vessels, and the parasympathetic supply to the prostate, corpora cavernosa,

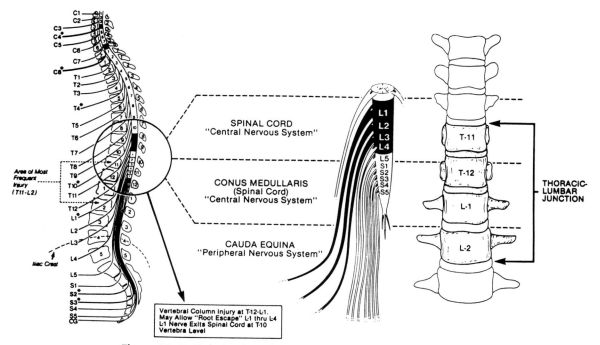

Figure 12–2. Relationship of thoracolumbar spine to spinal nerves.

and detrusor. The peripheral component of this system—the pelvic–cavernosal pathway—exits the cord through their respective ventral rootlets. The neurophysiology of the cavernosal system is described in detail in Chapter 2.

Injury to the autonomic system is characterized by the inability to achieve or sustain penile rigidity during sexual stimulation.

PATHOPHYSIOLOGY OF SPINAL CORD TRAUMA

Open or closed trauma to the spinal cord can cause damage or destruction of nerve fibers and neuronal cell bodies. Immediately after injury, the spinal cord swells and becomes rounded and tense within the leptomeninges and dura. Adjacent hemorrhage and displaced bony fragments can increased pressure on the cord. The result is a fusiform region of softening that affects one or more segments and tapers above and below the injury, producing a small rounded area of necrosis usually situated in the posterior columns.[8]

After 2 to 3 weeks, a reparative phase begins and can continue for at least 2 years. The edema and hemorrhage gradually subside as phagocytes clear the product debris. In severely damaged areas, the glia, neuron, cell bodies, and their processes are destroyed. Within 5 years, this region is replaced by connective tissue.

In rare instances, an upward progression of the spinal lesion can occur long after the initial injury despite an extended period of neurologic stability. In this case, the cavitation (syrinx) at the site of the original trauma extends upward, occasionally to the level of the medulla.

Depending on the site of spinal injury, partial or complete lesions of the cord occur. Cord injuries proximal to the conus medullaris usually produce an upper motor neuron lesion after recovery from spinal shock.[9-11] Injuries that involve the conus medullaris and cauda equina may lead to lower motor neuron lesions, with loss of the sacral cord segment (S2,S3,S4) and their reflexes. Injuries at T12 and L1 vertebrae do not conform to any one of these two classic patterns, namely, upper and lower motor neuron lesions. Mixed lesions, a combination of upper and lower motor neuron lesions, may follow the injuries at this level. All neurologic lesions proximal to the sacral cord segments (S2–S4) produce an upper motor neuron type of bladder and striated sphincter. Ischemic cord changes can occur distal to the proximal cord lesions and may later lead to a lower motor neuron type of bladder and sphincter. Lesions involving S2–S4 cord segments or the sacral nerve roots of the pelvic and pudendal nerves or both may lead to complete and incomplete patterns of injuries.

CLINICAL DIAGNOSIS OF SPINAL CORD INJURY

There are five neurologic abnormalities present in patients with spinal cord disease.[12] The most prominent is pain. Shortly after injury, pain is experienced over the vertebral column at the level of the involved spinal segment. A less common type of pain may occur months after cord injury and is experienced in the buttocks, feet, and legs regardless of the site of the SCI. The second abnormality is motor deficit. This will occur if more than 50% of the ascending motor pathways or more than 50% of the anterior horn cells have been destroyed. The third neurologic finding is abnormal sensory phenomena, i.e., paresthesia, lack of sensation, the perception of pain during gentle testing for sensory integrity. Abnormalities of reflexes in muscle tone are the fourth finding. Immediately after injury, the patient will encounter a period of spinal shock, characterized by areflexia, atonia, and nonresponsiveness to plantar stimulation. Commonly, in patients with upper motor lesions, the tendon reflexes return within several weeks and then become spastic. The bulbocavernosus reflex returns almost immediately. Finally, the ultimate type of urinary bladder dysfunction (spastic or flaccid) depends on the site of the cord lesion.

SPINAL SHOCK

Immediately after spinal injury, all skeletal and visceral reflexes are suppressed below the level of the cord injury. During this period, which can last from a few hours to several weeks, it is impossible to predict the extent of sexual impairment. Reflex penile erection, ejaculation, and bulbocavernosus and scrotal reflexes are absent or severely depressed. Passive engorgement of the corpora cavernosa, secondary to interruption of vasoconstrictor pathways, may cause penile enlargement in patients with complete lesions.[13] The return of normal erectile function (NEF) coincides with the return of other tendon and visceral reflexes. Eighty percent of patients who eventually regain erectile function do so within 1 year of injury, and another 5% recover after 2 years. The probability of recovery of normal erectile function is greater in patients with cervical and thoracic lesions than in those with lumbar injury.

EFFECT OF SPHINCTEROTOMY ON ERECTIONS

External sphincterotomy is the procedure of choice in patients with striated sphincter dyssynergia[14,15] to relieve bladder outlet obstruction, minimize the incidence of urinary infections, eliminate vesicoureteral reflux, and prevent upper tract deterioration. One of the major complications of this procedure is alterations in erection. Bilateral sphincterotomy (3 and 9 o'clock positions) has been associated with a high incidence (2% to 56%) of erectile dysfunction, perhaps caused by vascular insult to the dorsal arteries of the corpora cavernosa during electrocoagulation[16] or division of autonomic nerves traversing the urethra. With the adoption of the anteromedian sphincterotomy, reported rates of erectile incompetence have dramatically improved (0 to 5%).[17]

DIAGNOSTIC EVALUATION OF ERECTILE DYSFUNCTION IN PATIENTS WITH SPINAL CORD INJURY

Assuming that spinal cord recovery is unlikely and the patient is unable to maintain penile rigidity sufficient for at least 5 min of vaginal intercourse, what diagnostic tests are necessary to clarify the cause of erectile dysfunction and aid in its treatment?

Motor Deficits and Abnormalities of Reflexes and Motor Tone

The evaluation begins with a thorough history of the patient's premorbid sexual capacity and behavior. A general neurologic examination will confirm the level of cord injury. A majority of these patients will have reflex or psychogenic erections, yet both the patients and their partners usually are unsatisfied with the quality of these erections. Pharmacologic testing with low doses of vasoactive substances will allow the patient to assess the pharmacologic treatment option and permit the physician to confirm the neurogenic cause of the erectile dysfunction. Doubts concerning the primary origin of the dysfunction can be resolved by sleep testing with the penile tumescence and rigidity monitor.[18]

Approximately 80% of spastic supraconal SCI patients at our center experience rigid reflexogenic erections. However, 10% to 20% of these patients fail to maintain an erection that is adequate for vaginal penetration. Patients with cauda equina and conus lesions do not experience reflexogenic erection, but some patients with conus lesions below S2 have claimed to have functional psychogenic erections.

Sensory Deficits and Isolated Bladder Dysfunction

Again, the evaluation begins with a thorough history. Serum testosterone, blood glucose, cholesterol, creatinine, and liver function studies are performed. Afferent somatic pathways are evaluated with a biothesiometer.[19] The somatic loop is assessed by testing the bulbocavernosus reflex. Bulbocavernosus reflex latency times or dorsal nerve somatic sensory evoked potentials or both can be performed if the origin of the problem remains in question.[20,21] The integrity of the efferent autonomic component has remained difficult to determine. Work by Wagner et al. and Stief et al., assessing electromyelographic activity of cavernosal muscle, offers hope that a simple reliable test soon will be developed.[22,23] Both penile monitoring with visual sexual stimulation and sleep studies with penile tumescence and rigidity monitor are methods of evaluating the integrity of both the somatic and autonomic components. The amount of vasoactive substance administered to provoke a rigid erection and the time delay between injection and penile rigidity can be used to confirm neurogenic injury.[24]

If the primary organic cause of the erectile dysfunction remains uncertain after this evaluation, penile ultrasonography and dynamic pharmacocavernosometry can be used to rule out a possible vascular cause.[25,26]

THERAPEUTIC OPTIONS FOR NEUROGENIC ERECTILE DYSFUNCTION

There are four practical options for treatment of neurogenic erectile dysfunction and one option that has proved successful in laboratory animals.

Pharmacologic Erection Program (PEP)

This therapy has been used widely in SCI patients. The patient or his sexual partner is taught a sterile technique (Fig. 12–3) for injection of papaverine (a smooth muscle relaxant producing vasodilatation and relaxation of the sinusoidal spaces), a combination of papaverine and phentolamine (an alpha-adrenergic blocking agent producing vasodilation), or PGE_1 into the corpus cavernosum.[27–29]

The vasoactive pharmacologic agents are injected on the lateral aspect of the base of the penile shaft (Fig. 12–4). External compression is applied to the injection site for 3 to 5 min to prevent hematoma formation. Initial test dosages are papaverine 10 mg, papaverine/phentolamine 9 mg/0.15 mg, or PGE_1 3 to 5 µg. These doses are increased gradually until a rigid erection is induced that lasts 30 to 60 min. The denervated tissue in this group of patients seems to be supersensitive to these vasoactive substances, so that erections are more rigid and sustained than those in patients with vascular impotence. Drug-induced priapism can be treated successfully with sympathomimetic agents (phenylephrine and epinephrine), which should be initiated within 4 h of onset of penile rigidity. If initial

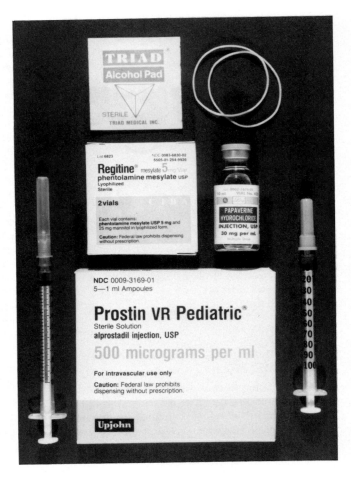

Figure 12–3. Supplies for the pharmacologic erection program.

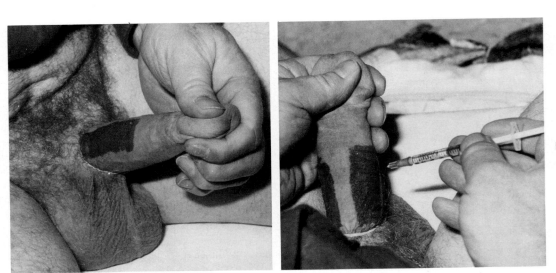

Figure 12–4. Injection technique. **A,** The area of injection has been darkened on the penis. **B,** The syringe is held like a dart, and the needle enters the corpus cavernosum at a right angle.

testing with low doses induces priapism, repeat testing with half the dose usually will induce functional nonpriapismic erections.

At our institution, over 50 SCI patients use intracavernous pharmacotherapy for the restoration of erectile function. We have not observed any incidences of autonomic dysreflexia, cavernosal fibrosis, or hepatic dysfunction, even in patients followed for over 5 years. Other investigators have reported a general acceptance (71%) of this approach in motivated SCI patients with genital sensation and cooperative partners.[30]

Vacuum Erectile Device (VED)

This therapy has gained general acceptance in the SCI patient.[31,32] By pumping air away from the enclosed penis, a negative pressure is created within the cylinder that increases the inflow of arterial blood and the backflow of venous blood (see Chapter 18). Once the cavernosal sinusoids have been filled and penile ridity is obtained, constriction bands are placed at the base of the penis to maintain penile rigidity for up to 30 min. The constricting band has the additional advantage of preventing urinary leakage but has the disadvantage of blocking antegrade ejaculation. Although most SCI patients can produce adequate erections with vacuum devices, complications may include penile edema and ecchymosis. The partner frequently complains that the penis is cold. Unsuitable candidates for this device include SCI patients taking anticoagulant medication and those with bleeding disorders.

Oral and Transcutaneous Agents

Retrospective studies have demonstrated that transcutaneous nitroglycerin applied to the penile shaft induced erections sufficient for vaginal penetration in 25% of SCI patients in whom papaverine had induced rigid erections.[33] Levodopa has been used in SCI patients. Fifty-five to sixty percent of these patients achieved rigid erections.[34] Although the use of these agents appears to be an appealing, noninvasive alternative treatment with minimal side effects (headache, allergic dermatitis), their therapeutic efficacy has to be proven through prospective double-blinded studies.

Penile Prosthesis

The penile prosthesis has been the cornerstone of treatment for the SCI patient. Its use has decreased gradually due to two factors: (1) recognition of the frequency of complications—infection of the prosthesis requiring its removal, erosion through the tunica albuginea and urethra, and me-

chanical failure,[35] and (2) the simplicity, safety, efficacy, and relative cost saving of the PEP and the VED. There remains a subset of SCI patients in whom the penile implant is the best option. These include patients with dysfunctional penile curvature and patients with psychologic problems (needle phobia or extreme dislike of the mechanical pump) that preclude election of these less invasive options. Sensory deficiency and lack of pain perception may complicate the use of prosthetic devices in patients with SCI, who are particularly at risk for chronic bacteriuria and decubitus ulcers. Inflatable, self-contained, and semirigid prostheses are available commercially. However, the inflatable penile prosthesis (see Chapter 19) is preferred over the semirigid device in these patients, since it is less likely to cause pressure necrosis and eventual erosion.

An erection pacemaker has been tested successfully in monkeys and used on a very restricted basis in humans.[36,37] The limiting factor may be the half-life of the electrodes and the risk of cavernosal neural pressure or devascularization injury induced by the electrodes.

SEXUAL FUNCTION AND AUTONOMIC DYSREFLEXIA

Although there is a possibility that autonomic dysreflexia (flushed face, throbbing headache, muscle spasms, bradycardia, and severe hypertension) could occur during sexual activity in patients with spinal injuries at or above T4–T6, only one of our patients has had such an episode (M. A. Vickers and M. Sarkarati, unpublished observations). As a precaution, patients are reminded to evacuate their bladder and bowel before sexual activity and are taught to become quiet and elevate the head in the event of severe headaches during sexual activity. If the headache does not promptly subside, the physician should be notified. Sublingual nifedipine is our first-line drug but is given only with blood pressure monitoring and the availability of agents to treat drug-induced hypotension.

Profound episodes of autonomic dysreflexia in patients with high spinal cord lesions have been reported with ejaculations provoked by intrathecal injection of neostigmine[38] and electroejaculation. Intravenous infusion of prostaglandin E_2[39] or sublingual nifedipine[40] prophylaxis has been used to prevent severe elevation of blood pressure.

EJACULATORY DYSFUNCTION

The ability to ejaculate is profoundly impaired by SCI. In those patients who are capable of successful ejaculation, the sensation of orgasm may be absent, and retrograde ejaculation often occurs.

Less than 5% of patients with complete upper motor neuron lesions retain ejaculatory function. Ejaculation rates are higher (18%) in patients with both lower motor neuron lesions and an intact sympathetic outflow. The incidence of ejaculation has been reported as 32% in patients with incomplete upper motor neuron lesions and 70% in those with incomplete lower motor neuron lesions.

Various techniques of obtaining semen from SCI men with ejaculatory dysfunction have been promoted. Intrathecal neostigmine and subcutaneous physostigmine have been used to induce ejaculation. However, the dangerous side effects and the unacceptable risk of autonomic dysreflexia associated with these agents have led to their widespread rejection.

Electroejaculation provides a safe method of obtaining semen through electrical stimulation of myelinated efferent sympathetic fibers of the hypogastric plexus, resulting in seminal emission into the posterior urethra. The electrode mount is inserted into the rectum and connected to a stimulator that typically delivers 30 stimulations of 15 V and 314 mA. Seminal fluid subsequently is recovered from the posterior urethra by milking the bulbous urethra and catheterizing the posterior urethra. The success rate of electroejaculation in a recent survey of 48 men with SCI was reported as 71%, with many documented pregnancies.[41] Recovery of motile semen was slightly more successful in patients with thoracic or complete lesions, whereas sperm count and motility were higher in those with incomplete lesions.[42]

Vibratory stimulation has been used successfully to obtain semen from 52% to 59% of male SCI patients. This technique induces a reflexogenic event involving the sacral roots as well as the ejaculatory coordination center in the upper thoracolumbar cord. Brindley[41,43] has reported that the most effective and tolerable parameters to provoke ejaculation are at vibratory frequencies of 60 and 80 Hz with an amplitude of 2.5 mm. Vibratory stimulation is preferable to electroejaculation in patients for whom either technique can be used successfully, since retrograde emission is less likely and semen quality is often superior. However, electroejaculation may be safer for patients at risk of autonomic dysreflexia, and it provides a feasible method for patients who lack intact lower thoracic and sacral segments.

Hypogastric plexus stimulation and cannulation of the vas deferens have been proposed for patients in whom vibratory stimulation fails and electroejaculation is impractical. In 7 SCI patients, platinum electrodes were implanted around the hypogastric plexus and connected to a subcutaneous radio receiver.[43] Using an appropriate radio transmitter, semen containing motile spermatozoa was obtained, and 3 successful pregnancies have resulted.

In a small number of SCI patients, a cannula implanted into the vas deferens and connected to a subcutaneous capsule has been used to obtain semen for insemination. Although no pregnancies were reported, semen containing motile spermatozoa has been withdrawn from the implanted capsule of at least 1 patient for over a year.[41,43]

SEMEN QUALITY

Impaired fertility following SCI can be caused not only by ejaculatory dysfunction but also by low sperm count and diminished sperm motility. Probable explanations for poor semen quality include chronic urinary tract infection, sperm contact with urine, chronic use of various medications, raised scrotal temperature (due to prolonged sitting), and stasis of prostatic fluid. Histologic examination of testicular biopsies has revealed a wide range of testicular dysfunction, including hypospermatogenesis, maturation arrest, atrophy of the seminiferous tubules, germinal cell hypoplasia, interstitial fibrosis, and Leydig cell hyperplasia. In addition, prostatitis (secondary to prolonged catheterization), epididymitis, and epididymoorchitis can precipitate obstructive ductal lesions and testicular damage.

SEXUAL DYSFUNCTION IN FEMALE SPINAL CORD INJURY

The pathophysiologic effect of SCI on female sexuality has received considerably less attention than the effect on the male. The paucity of reliable information on this subject may be a consequence of several factors, including the assertion that only a minority of SCI patients are women (18%), the expectation that the disabled patient becomes asexual, and the misconception that erectile and ejaculatory dysfunction and infertility, which are more easily quantifiable with measurable parameters, warrant more attention. Unfortunately, these misleading attitudes have stymied interest and research regarding the female equivalent of male erection—vaginal lubrication, swelling of the labia, and clitoral erection—all of which can be dramatically impaired following SCI.

Permanent hormonal changes following SCI have not been described. Thus, these patients may continue to have libido and arousal responses. In fact, several recent studies suggest that sexual activity certainly persists and can be enjoyed by many female SCI patients. However, the extent of these sexual responses depends on the severity of the damage to the low thoracic, lumbar, and sacral cord segments.

Loss of sensation of the external genitalia occurs with injury to the spinal cord above S2. Voluntary control of the pelvic floor is maintained in some female patients with incomplete lesions in the S2–S5 region of the spinal cord. Incomplete lesions in this area and complete lesions above the conus medullaris and the cauda equina result in spasticity of the pelvic floor, levator ani, and constrictor vulvae muscles during anal or clitoral stimulation. Reflex and psychogenic lubrication may occur in patients with incomplete cord lesions at all levels except those between T10 and T12. Patients with complete lesions above T10 can experience reflex lubrication, whereas those with lesions below T12 exhibit psychogenic lubrication. Reflex congestion of the external genitalia may occur in patients with incomplete injuries or complete injuries above T10. Although sensation during sexual stimulation can be perceived by female patients with lesions above T10 and below T12, it may emulate a sense of bladder fullness or feel markedly attenuated. Sensation is absent in patients with spinal cord lesions between T10 and T12. Patients with complete lesions above T6 and those with cervical SCI may experience headaches and bradycardia analogous to symptoms of autonomic hyperreflexia. Orgasm in patients with high complete lesions is associated with hyperreflexia followed by complete relaxation. In patients with lesions below T12, diminished sensation can be intensified by concomitant stimulation of erogenous zones above the level of the injury.

For the female patient with SCI, many obstacles—some of which can be psychologically devastating—can impede pleasurable sexual intercourse. These may include loss of lubrication, bladder and bowel incontinence, and increased urinary tract infections. Spasticity of the pelvic floor and adductor muscles that restricts penetration can be reduced with benzodiazepines.

Although SCI women may experience little sensation during intercourse, their fertility, despite denervation of the ovaries, and their ability to have children usually are unaffected. Successful pregnancies have been reported in many of these patients with increasing frequency as postinjury rehabilitation improves. Appropriate preparation and an understanding of the potential complications can facilitate an uneventful pregnancy and delivery.

Most female patients experience a period of amenorrhoea usually lasting 3 to 9 months after SCI. The level and completeness of the injury do not correlate with the duration of menstrual interruption, thus suggesting that the temporary interruption in some women is probably caused by the physical and psychologic stress imposed by the SCI. During this anovulatory phase, ovulation can be highly unpredictable before the first menstruation. Since pregnancy is still possible during this phase, anticonceptional precautions may be advisable.

Pregnancy in SCI patients can be complicated by urinary tract infection, constipation, thrombophlebitis, edema of the legs, decubitus ulcers, premature labor, and immobilization-induced osteoporosis. The risk of toxemia of pregnancy increases with repeated urinary tract infections and residual albuminuria. Hypertension, which can be dangerous for the fetus, should be prevented with alpha-blockers or calcium antagonists. Since uterine innervation arises from T10–T12 levels of the spinal cord, patients with complete lesions above T10 lack perception of uterine contractions or movement of the fetus.

For female patients with SCI above the level of T10, labor normally progresses without incident. However, patients with lesions above T6 should be effectively premedicated to prevent episodes of autonomic hyperreflexia during childbirth. Although uterine contractions develop in patients with lesions above T10, paralysis of the abdominal muscles may impede expulsion of the fetus, thus requiring the use of forceps and an episiotomy.[44] In patients with lesions below T12 who retain perception of the uterus during labor, perineal insensitivity promotes tears during the expulsion phase and damage to the perineal musculature. Indications for cesarean section are essentially the same as for non-SCI woman, since hormonally controlled reflex contractions occur even with complete motor and sensory loss.[45]

A recent survey of 231 women with SCI aged 18 to 45 revealed a two-thirds reduction in pregnancy rate following SCI compared with preinjury rates. More pregnancies were reported in patients with incomplete lesions than in those with complete lesions, probably due to the decreased rate of sexual activity in women with complete lesions. Almost three fourths of the pregnant women in this study had vaginal deliveries, and nearly half required no anesthesia.[46]

ULTIMATE OUTCOMES: SEXUAL RELATIONSHIPS

Major impediments still remain for both male and female SCI patients to attain a stable sexual relationship.[47] These include low self-esteem as a result of their motor deficits, hesitancy to seek such a relationship due to embarrassment or concern about reflex urination, defecation, or sympathetic crisis during sexual activity, or, finally, difficulty in finding a suitable partner. Adequate sexual rehabilitation must address these very important issues.

REFERENCES

1. Yalla SV. Sexual dysfunction in the paraplegic and quadriplegic. In: Bennett AH, ed. Management of Male Impotence. Baltimore: Williams & Wilkins, 1982:181–191.
2. Talbot HS. A report on sexual function in paraplegics. J Urol 61:265, 1949.
3. Bors E, Comarr AE. Neurological disturbances of sexual function with special reference to 529 patients with spinal cord injury. Urol Surv 10:191, 1960.
4. Comarr AE. Sexual function among patients with spinal cord injury. Urol Int 25:134, 1970.
5. Chapelle PA, Durand J, Lacert P. Penile erection following complete spinal cord injury in man. Br J Urol 52:216, 1980.
6. Goldstein I. Evaluation of penile nerves. In: Tanagho E, Lue TF, McClure RD, eds. Contemporary Management of Impotence and Infertility. Baltimore: Williams & Wilkins, 1988.
7. Lue TF, Zeinch SJ, Schmidt RA, Tanagho EA. Neuroanatomy of penile erection. Its relevance to iatrogenic impotence. J Urol 131:273, 1984.
8. Hughes JT. Neuropathology of the spinal cord. Neurol Clin 9:562, 1991.
9. Bors E, Comarr AE. Neurological Urology. Baltimore: University Park Press, 1971:181–184.
10. Hardy AG, Rossier AB. Spinal Cord Injuries: Orthopedic and Neurological Aspects. Stuttgart: George Theime Publishers, 1975.
11. Fam BA, Sarkarati M, Yalla SV. Spinal cord injury. In: Yalla SV, McGuire EJ, Elbadawi A, Blaivas JG, eds. Neurourology and Urodynamics: Principles and Practice. New York: Macmillan, 1988:291–302.
12. Woolsey RM, Young RR. The clinical diagnosis of disorders of the spinal cord. Neurol Clin 9:573–578, 1991.
13. Biering-Sørensen F, Sønksen J. Penile erection in men with spinal cord or cauda equina lesions. Semin Neurol 12:98, 1992.
14. Yalla SV, Fam BA, Gabilondo FB, et al. Anteromedian external sphincterotomy: technique, rationale and complications, J Urol 117:489, 1977.
15. Yalla SV, Blunt KJ, Fam BA, et al. Detrusor urethral sphincter dyssynergia. J Urol 118:1025, 1977.
16. Carrion HM, Brown BT, Politano VA. External sphincterotomy at the 12 o'clock position. J Urol 121:462, 1979.
17. Whitmore WF, Fam BA, Yalla SV. Experience with anteromedian (12 o'clock) external urethral sphincterotomy in 100 male subjects with neuropathic bladder. Br J Urol 50:99, 1978.
18. Vickers M, DeNobrega A, Dluhy R. Diagnosis and treatment of psychogenic erectile dysfunction in a urological setting: outcome of eighteen consecutive patients. J Urol 149:1258, 1993.
19. Padma-Nathan H, Levine F. Vibratory testing of the penis. J Urol 137:210A, 1987.
20. Scherb W, Bähren W, Gall H, Thai W. Neurophysiologic parameters in evaluation of erectile dysfunction. Acta Urol Belg 56:154–161, 1988.
21. Opsomer R, Queril J, Wese F. Pudendal cortical somatosensory evoked potentials. J Urol 135:1216, 1986.
22. Wagner G, Gerstenberg T, Levin R. Electrical activity of corpus cavernosum during flaccidity and erection of the human penis: a new diagnostic method? J Urol 142:723, 1989.
23. Stief G, Djamiban M, Schaebsdau F, et al. Single potential analysis of cavernous electric activity—a possible diagnosis of autonomic impotence? World J Urol 8:75, 1990.
24. Wagner G, Uhrenholdt A. Blood flow measurement by the clearance methods in the human corpus cavernosum in the flaccid and erect states. In: Zorgniotti A, Rossi G, eds. Vasculogenic Impotence. Proceedings of the First International Conference on the Corpus Cavernosum Revascularization. Springfield, Ill: Charles C Thomas, 1980:41–46.
25. Benson CB, Arumy JE, Vickers MA. Correlation of duplex sonography with arteriography in patients with erectile dysfunction. Am J Radiol 160:71, 1993.
26. Vickers MA, Benson CB, Dluhy R, Ball RA. The current cavernosometric criteria for corporo-venous dysfunction are too strict. J Urol 147:614, 1991.
27. Virag R. Intracavernous injection of papaverine for erectile failure. Lancet 2:938, 1982.
28. Zorgniotti A, Lefleur R. Autoinjection of the corpus cavernosum with a vasoactive drug combination for vasculogenic impotence. J Urol 133:39, 1985.
29. Waldhauser N, Schramek P. Efficiency and side effects of prostaglandin E_1 in the treatment of erectile dysfunction. J Urol 140:525, 1988.
30. Sidi AA, Cameron JS, Dykstra DD, et al. Vasoactive intracavernous pharmacotherapy for the treatment of erectile impotence in men with spinal cord injury. J Urol 138:539, 1987.
31. Nadig P, Ware J, Blumoff R. Noninvasive device to produce and maintain an erection-like state. Urology 27:126, 1986.
32. Heller L, Keren O, Aloni R, Davidoff G. An open trial of vacuum penile tumescence: constriction therapy for neurological impotence. Paraplegia 30:550, 1992.
33. Sonksen J, Biering-Sorensen F. Transcutaneous nitroglycerin in the treatment of erectile dysfunction in spinal cord injured. Paraplegia 30:554, 1992.
34. Leyson JFJ. Controversies and research in male sexuality. In: Leyson JFJ, ed. Sexual Rehabilitation of the Spinal Cord Injured Patient. Clifton, NJ: Humana Press, 1991:504–505.
35. Rossier A, Fam BA. Indications and results of semirigid penile prosthesis in spinal cord injury patients: long-term follow-up. J Urol 131:59, 1984.
36. Lue TF, Tanagho E. Erection pacemaker. In: Tanagho E, Lue TF, MClure RD, eds. Contemporary Management of Impotence and Infertility. Baltimore: Williams & Wilkins, 1988:157–159.
37. Brindley G, Polkey C, Ruskton D, Cardozo L. Sacral anterior root stimulators for bladder control in paraplegia: the first 50 cases. J Neurol Neurosurg Psychiatry 49:1104, 1986.
38. Rossier AB, Ziegler WH, Duchosal PW, Meylan J.

Sexual function and dysreflexia. Paraplegia 9:51, 1971.

39. Frankel HL, Mathias CJ. Severe hypertension in patients with high spinal cord lesions undergoing electro-ejaculation management with prostaglandin E$_2$. Paraplegia 18:293, 1980.

40. Steinberger RE, Ohl DA, Bennett CJ, et al. Nifedipine pretreatment for autonomic dysreflexia during electroejaculation. Urology 36:228, 1990.

41. Brindley GS. Sexual and reproductive problems of paraplegic men. Oxford Rev Reprod Biol 8:214, 1986.

42. Ohl DA, Bennett CJ, McCabe M, et al. Predictors of success in electroejaculation of spinal cord injured men. J Urol 142:1483, 1989.

43. Brindley GS. The actions of parasympathetic and sympathetic nerves in human micturition, erection and seminal emission, and their restoration in paraplegic patients by implanted electrical stimulators. Proc R Soc Lond 235:111, 1988.

44. Berard EJJ. The sexuality of spinal cord injured women: physiology and pathophysiology. A review. Paraplegia 27:99, 1989.

45. McCluer S. Reproductive aspects of spinal cord injury in females. In: Leyson JFJ, ed. Sexual Rehabilitation of the Spinal Cord Injured Patient. Clifton, NJ: Humana Press, 1991:181–206.

46. Charlifue SW, Gerhart KA, Menter RR, et al. Sexual issues of women with spinal cord injuries. Paraplegia 30:192, 1992.

47. Leyson JFJ. Sociosexual and marital relationships. In: Leyson JFJ, ed. Sexual Rehabilitation of the Spinal Cord Injured Patient. Clifton, NJ: Humana Press, 1991:319–339.

CHAPTER 13

Disorders of Ejaculation

Jeffrey P. Buch

The male sexual response includes the physiologic events of erection, emission, ejaculation, and orgasm. Although the physiology and occurrence of each of these events are intimately related, each one may occur independent of the other, especially in pathologic states. The physiology of erection has been presented in detail. Currently, a clear understanding of orgasmic physiology is lacking, although these subjective feelings are largely linked to the process of seminal emission and urethral bulb distention.[1] The purpose of this chapter is to present the anatomy and physiology of ejaculation and to define how the causes of abnormal ejaculation are diagnosed and treated.

Further discussion regarding ejaculation requires a few working definitions. Although ejaculation has been viewed traditionally as a single event comprised of emission, ejaculation, and orgasm, these are truly three distinct events. Emission is the deposition of semen from the ejaculatory ducts into the posterior urethra. Ejaculation is the propulsion of semen from the posterior urethra distally and outward through the urethral meatus. Orgasm is a cerebral event, with significant subjective variations, that typically occurs simultaneously with emission or ejaculation. This chapter evaluates and presents what is currently known about emission and ejaculation in normal and pathologic states, including some mention of how a man's psyche, libido, and lifestyle may affect these functions.

To accomplish these goals, the material progresses from gross anatomy and physiology to neuroanatomy and neurophysiology. The impact of endocrinology is discussed. Techniques employed in the diagnosis of specific causes of ejaculatory dysfunction and background discussions of these pathologic states follow. The range of treatments applied to ejaculatory dysfunction and their comparative success rates are presented.

ANATOMY AND PHYSIOLOGY

The anatomy and physiology of emission and ejaculation have been well described in prior reviews.[2-5] Herein, the highlights of anatomy and physiology are presented while incorporating the most current additions to the understanding of emission and ejaculation. Much of the data have resulted from the study of mechanisms in animal models and observations from human pathologic states.

The gross anatomic components of the ejaculatory apparatus include the testis, epididymis, vas deferens, seminal vesicles, prostate, and urethra (Fig. 13–1). The flow of seminal fluid in emission is described commonly as beginning with contractions in the tail of the epididymis and convoluted portion of the vas deferens. However, contractions may begin as proximal as the efferent ducts[6] or even at the level of the tunica albuginea of the testis.[7] This contractile wave propels the mature sperm from the epididymis and vas deferens through the ejaculatory ducts into the posterior (prostatic) urethra. The bladder neck must be closed during emission to prevent retrograde ejaculation.[8] During emission, concomitant closure of the external urethral sphincter creates a pressure chamber effect in the prostatic urethra that is associated with a feeling of the inevitability of ejaculation.[2,6]

Ejaculation follows emission as a series of events beginning with relaxation of the external sphincter while the internal sphincter (bladder neck) remains closed. Rhythmic contractions of the prostate combine with straightening of the pendulous urethra and strong rhythmic periurethral and pelvic floor contractions of the bulbocavernosus and ischiocavernosus muscles, respectively.[3,6,9,10] The bolus of semen is propelled forward through the urethra and out of the urethral meatus. The force of human ejaculation can result in forward projection of semen a distance of 1 to 2 feet from the urethral meatus.[2,6] It is believed that part of the pleasurable sensation in orgasm is derived from the proportionate size of the semen bolus and its ability to distend the urethral bulb.[2,6]

Brief mention of the embryology involved with the ejaculatory apparatus will benefit subsequent discussion of the anatomic causes of abnormal ejaculation. There is evidence that the testicle and the head of the epididymis have a common origin from the cells of the genital ridge.[11,12] The seminal vesicles, vas deferens, body, and tail of the epididymis alternatively arise from the wolffian (mesenteric) duct.[11,13] The vas deferens extends a distance of 35

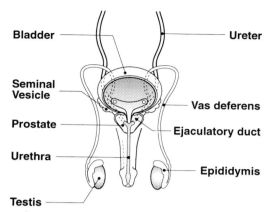

Figure 13–1. Gross anatomy of the male reproductive tract.

to 40 cm from the tail of the epididymis in the scrotum to the ampullary portion, where it connects with the duct of the seminal vesicle to form its respective ejaculatory duct, bilaterally. The ejaculatory ducts traverse the prostate from posterior to anterior and from lateral to medial directions before they exit from either side of the midline of the verumontanum (Fig. 13–2). The verumontanum is a mullerian duct remnant that occasionally is prone to forming blind ending cysts, with resultant congenital ejaculatory duct obstruction.[14] The male urethra is the end result of the combination of androgens and mullerian inhibiting substance (MIS) exerting their effects on the genital tubercle.[15,16] The bulbocavernosus and ischiocavernosus are striated muscles of the perineum, which support and surround the urethra developing in conjunction with the genitalia. The bulbocavernosus

arises from the central tendon, surrounds the corpus spongiosum, and extends to the corpus cavernosum.[3] The ischiocavernosus extends from the inner surface of the ischial tuberosity to surround and insert into the crura of the corpora.[3]

NEUROANATOMY

Seminal emission and ejaculation are controlled primarily by adrenergic mechanisms acting through the sympathetic nervous system.[2–6] The afferent stimuli for these ejaculatory pathways are processed at either the cerebral or spinal cord levels or both. Visual and other nontactile erotic stimuli are processed at the cerebral level. Tactile genital stimulation, on the other hand, may result in emission and ejaculation mediated directly through the emission (T10–L2) and ejaculatory (S2–S4) centers of the spinal cord without any cerebral modification, as in cases of complete spinal cord transection above these cord levels.[3–5,17] Tactile sensation of the genitalia is transmitted by the dorsal penile nerves, onward to the sensory division of the pudendal nerves, and then back to the sacral cord. Afferent signals from the male accessory sex organs reach the sacral cord via the pelvic splanchnic nerves.[18] Distension of the posterior urethra with seminal emission yields an afferent signal along these pathways that results in a spinal-mediated reflex ejaculation.[19]

Cerebral efferent signals for ejaculation apparently are mediated through anterior thalamic nuclei, preoptic hypothalamic nuclei, and median forebrain bundles before transmission down the spinal cord in the lateral gray matter.[20,21] Observations in the human by Learmonth[22] and in the cat by Semans and Langworthy[23] support the

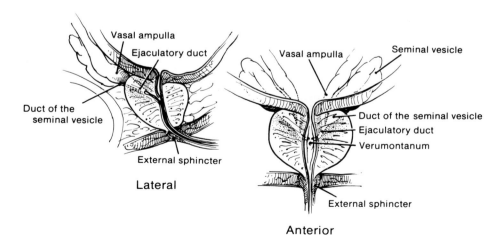

Lateral

Anterior

Figure 13–2. Anatomy of the male accessory sex organs. (From Shaban SF. Treatment of abnormalities of ejaculation. In: Lipshultz LI, Howards SS, eds. Infertility in the Male, 2nd ed. St. Louis: Mosby-Year Book, 1991.)

presence of an emission center in the cord at the T10–L2 level. The ejaculatory center of the spinal cord mediates efferent signals at the S2–S4 level.[3,4,22]

Peripheral transmission of efferent sacral ejaculatory signals occurs via somatic pathways in the motor division of the pudendal nerve.[3,4,22] The network of peripheral nerves carrying efferent signals from the emission center of the cord (T10–L2) is more complex (Figs. 13–3 and 13–4).

Based on human data from lumbar sympathectomy (ablation of L2–L4 paraspinal sympathetic ganglia) with subsequent preservation of emission, Learmonth concluded that the L1 ganglion was critical for efferent transmission to the superior hypogastric plexus (presacral nerve), which then gives rise to the hypogastric nerves.[22] Similar conclusions have been drawn from animal data.[23] Direct stimulation of either hypogastric nerve results in seminal emission.[22,23] Inferior to the superior hypogastric plexus, the hypogastric nerves coalesce with sacral parasympathetic branches.[24] From this point, the hypogastric nerve branches synapse with a series of short adrenergic neurons in ganglia located in the adventitia of the end-organs they innervate.[2,4,25,26] Recent evidence presented by Sato

et al.[27] suggests three possible efferent signal transmission routes for seminal emission from the L1 paravertebral sympathetic ganglion: (1) hypogastric nerves, (2) sympathetic nerve fibers through the lumbosacral sympathetic trunk, and (3) spermatic nerves. Furthermore, these investigators were able to achieve seminal emission through direct stimulation of nerves in the tail of the epididymis.[27] These observations help to explain the resilience of the seminal emission mechanism to neural injury. Apparently, human seminal emission is prevented only when the L1 ganglion is completely ablated bilaterally.

NEUROPHYSIOLOGY

The cerebral centers for emission and ejaculation are controlled in a positive manner by dopaminergic stimulation[28] and in a negative manner by serotonergic stimulation.[29] Peripherally, the efferent signals for seminal emission are carried from the sympathetic chain onward to their end-organs, which are controlled largely by adrenergic stimuli.[25,30] Although some cholinergic innervation of the vas deferens has been noted,[31] experimental parasympathetic stimulation has resulted in only

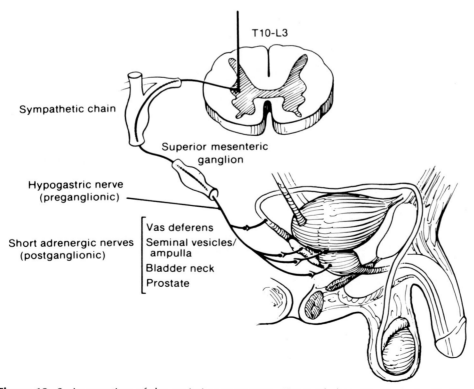

T10–L3

Sympathetic chain

Superior mesenteric ganglion

Hypogastric nerve (preganglionic)

Short adrenergic nerves (postganglionic)

Vas deferens
Seminal vesicles/ ampulla
Bladder neck
Prostate

Figure 13–3. Innervation of the emission apparatus. (From Shaban SF, Lipshultz LI. Electroejaculation. In: Rajfer J, ed. *Common Problems in Infertility and Impotence.* Chicago: Year Book, 1989.)

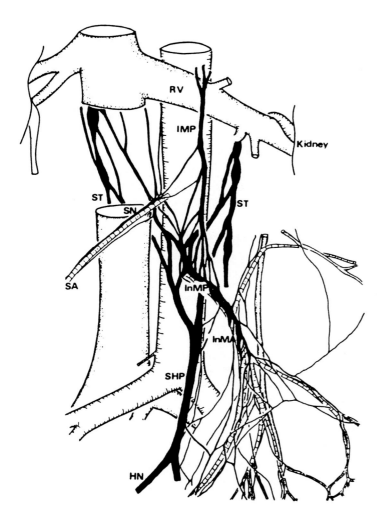

Figure 13–4. Schematic diagram of the gross neuroanatomy of human emission. Spermatic nerve (SN) originates from the right lumbar sympathetic trunk (ST) and intermesenteric plexus (IMP). Autonomic fibers are indicated by solid black lines. RV, renal vein; InMP, inferior mesenteric plexus; InMA, inferior mesenteric artery; SA, spermatic artery; SHP, superior hypogastric plexus; HN, hypogastric nerve. (From Sato K, Kihara K, Ando M, et al. Seminal emission by electrical stimulation of the spermatic nerve and epididymis. Int J Androl 14:461, 1991.)

minimal contraction of the vasa and seminal vesicles.[32] The main neurotransmitter for vas deferens contraction apparently is norepinephrine.[33] Likewise, the bladder neck contains both cholinergic and adrenergic receptors, with a predominantly adrenergic mechanism of closure.[34] Alternatively, the ejaculatory mechanism (perineal and periurethral muscles) is innervated by somatic branches from the pudendal nerve, which originate in the sacral cord (S2–S4).[2–6] Thus, emission and ejaculation are largely the result of complementary sympathetic and somatic innervation. Evidence suggests that these functions are affected also by serum androgen level and age-related factors.[4,6]

EVALUATION AND CAUSES

An exact estimate of the incidence of ejaculatory dysfunction in the general population is not available. However, when patients go to the urologist for evaluation of ejaculatory abnormalities, their clinical pictures can vary significantly. The complaints may be of total ejaculatory failure, premature ejaculation, or diminishing ejaculatory volumes, just to name a few. Fertility status may or may not be an issue. The causes of the dysfunction are variable, ranging from traumatic neural disruption to medication side effects to manifestations of a systemic disorder, such as diabetes. Because of the variable nature of the dysfunction and its causes, a detailed history is critical to the evaluation.

Evaluation

As with the history for erectile function, a series of questions is asked that correlate sexual function with risk factors for dysfunction. A careful description of the problem in the patient's own words is elicited. Comorbid medical history is documented to assess for conditions that affect emission and ejaculation, such as prior pelvic or retroperitoneal surgery, neuropathy, spinal cord injury, diabetes, congenital anomalies of the genitalia, prior urinary infections, metabolic disorders, and medications. The patient is questioned about his emotional and psychologic stability as well as relationship issues and libido. In this manner, functional (psychogenic) causes of ejaculatory dysfunction may also be defined.

The physical examination may be guided by the history. Primarily, evidence of neurologic impairment of the genitalia or anatomic variations from the norm are noted and recorded. Assessment of penile sensation and evaluation of the bulbocavernosus reflex are important. The phallus and testes are inspected and palpated for detection of any abnormalities. A rectal examination that documents chronic inflammation of the prostate, for instance, can help to diagnose a specific cause for the dysfunction.

Additional testing is of limited value except in specific cases. Simple neurologic testing of the penis with the Biothesiometer has been proposed as a method for documenting neurogenic impotence.[35] This technique may also help document neurogenic ejaculatory dysfunction, which is not apparent by history or physical examination. A serum testosterone level is routinely determined to rule out hypogonadism.

When fertility is an issue, it is especially important to record antegrade semen volumes and to rule out complete or partial retrograde ejaculation with evaluation of the postejaculatory urine. In addition, overall fertility parameters of semen are recorded, including sperm density, motility, and morphology. Transrectal ultrasonography may be important when ejaculatory duct obstruction is suspected.

Causes

On the basis of evaluation, Shaban[4] has suggested three broad categories of causes of ejaculatory dysfunction: neuropathic, anatomic, and functional. Neuropathic etiologies include surgical nerve ablation, spinal cord injury (SCI), diabetes, generalized neurologic disorders (i.e., Parkinson's disease and multiple sclerosis), medication, and idiopathic. Anatomic etiologies are both congenital and acquired, including atresia or absence of the vas deferens or seminal vesicles or both, ejaculatory duct obstruction, epispadias/hypospadias, congenital anomalies of the prostatic urethra, and prior bladder neck or prostate surgery. Functional problems include premature and retarded ejaculation.

Neuropathic Causes
SURGICAL NERVE ABLATION

The most common postsurgical cause of either ejaculatory failure or retrograde ejaculation is extended retroperitoneal lymph node dissection (RLND) for testicular cancer. However, excision of the rectum for benign or malignant disease also may have this result by affecting the hypogastric nerves below the aortic bifurcation.[36] In the era of extended RLND for testis tumor patients, bilateral sympathectomy at the L2 level, combined with iliac dissections, resulted in a 40% incidence of ejaculatory dysfunction.[37–38] However, more recent efforts to modify the lymph node dissection through nerve-sparing techniques, which stay above the level of the inferior mesenteric artery, have resulted in preservation of ejaculation in 80% or more of patients.[4,39,40]

SPINAL CORD INJURY

It is estimated that 10,000 new cases of SCI occur in the United States each year, with the majority of patients being men in their reproductive years.[41] Natural fertility is present in only 5% to 10% of SCI men, and ejaculatory failure is present in up to 90% of SCI men.[42] The ejaculatory failure is compounded by a relatively high incidence of erectile dysfunction.[43] Various techniques have been successful in procuring semen from SCI men with ejaculatory dysfunction, including intrathecal neostigmine,[44,45] vibratory stimulation,[17,46,47] and electroejaculation.[42,47–50]

DIABETES AND OTHER NEUROPATHIES

In diabetes, the neuropathy is predominantly somatic and peripheral, but autonomic manifestations do occur. Erectile dysfunction has been reported in up to 50% of diabetic men.[51] Emission or ejaculatory abnormalities have been reported in up to 32% of diabetic men.[4,51–53] The most common dysfunction is retrograde ejaculation rather than complete failure of emission. Other systemic neuropathic conditions, such as Parkinson's disease and multiple sclerosis, may predispose an individual to ejaculatory dysfunction. In such cases, erectile function may persist in the presence of ejaculatory dysfunction, or vice versa, or both functions may be lost simultaneously.

MEDICATION

Since the physiology of emission and ejaculation is largely under sympathetic (adrenergic) control, medications that affect the autonomic nervous system (ganglionic blockers) or those that function by alpha-adrenergic receptor blockade can cause ejaculatory dysfunction. These actions are noted in many antidepressants (both tricyclics and monoamine oxidase inhibitors) and in many antihypertensives (ganglionic blockers and alpha-adrenergic blockers).[4,54] Antipsychotic (psychotropic) medications and benzodiazepines have been associated with ejaculatory dysfunction as well.[55] Presumably, this is on the basis of sedative effects and modification of cerebral sensory input processing. For a more extensive list of such medications, see Shaban.[4]

IDIOPATHIC

Total failure of ejaculation can be idiopathic or functional in nature. More commonly, however, retrograde ejaculation is idiopathic.[56] This form of retrograde ejaculation responds to therapy just as well as retrograde ejaculation secondary to diabetes or surgical nerve ablation.

Anatomic Causes
CONGENITAL ABSENCE OF VAS DEFERENS

Absence of one vas deferens or both may be noted in up to 1% of men requesting fertility evaluation.[57] This condition is often associated with congenital abnormalities of the seminal vesicles and occasionally with unilateral renal agenesis. Due to the potential association of this anomaly with unrecognized cystic fibrosis (CF) or with the CF carrier state, genetic counseling is important before attempts at conception with sperm harvested from the epididymis.[58]

EJACULATORY DUCT OBSTRUCTION

Typically, the man with ejaculatory duct obstruction comes for fertility evaluation with low volume (< 1.0 ml) azoospermia. His testicular examination is normal, he has no endocrine abnormalities, and his postejaculatory urine is negative for sperm. However, partial (high-grade) ejaculatory duct obstruction can occur as low-volume oligoasthenospermia. These obstructions may be either congenital anomalies of the prostatic utricle (mullerian duct cyst) or acquired secondary to prostatitis or urethral instrumentation.[59–61] Transrectal ultrasonography may be very helpful in the preoperative evaluation.

Treatment involves resection of the ejaculatory ducts, including the verumontanum, either with or without simultaneous vasography. If sperm fail to return to the ejaculate in spite of increased semen volume posttreatment, there may be an associated epididymis obstruction.[61] To avoid such a missed diagnosis, some authors advise routinely performing vasography with vasotomy and vas fluid examination for sperm at the time of resection, so that microscopic vasoepididymostomy also may be performed when indicated.[61]

URETHRAL ABNORMALITIES

Both congenital and acquired urethral abnormalities can be associated with abnormal ejaculation. Severe cases of hypospadias and the epispadias/exstrophy complex may be associated with

anomalies of the ejaculatory ducts or retrograde ejaculation or both.[62] Most certainly, surgery that alters the bladder neck closure mechanism (such as Y-V urethroplasty or transurethral prostatectomy) often results in retrograde ejaculation.[63] Additionally, urethral strictures can result in restricted or painful ejaculation.

Psychogenic (Functional) Dysfunction
RETARDED EJACULATION

Psychogenic failure to ejaculate in spite of adequate erection and stimulation has acquired the interesting name, "retarded ejaculation." Although this is a relatively uncommon problem, it can be quite frustrating to the man and his partner. It is reported to occur in up to 4% of all men with sexual dysfunction.[64] Psychologic reasons for this disorder may include fear of pregnancy, religious concerns, and other types of anxiety reaction to the thought of ejaculation.[64,65]

PREMATURE EJACULATION

Arguably, the most common type of ejaculatory dysfunction is premature ejaculation. Exact definitions vary, but classically this term represents ejaculation that either precedes vaginal entry or occurs immediately after vaginal entry. Proposed causes include performance anxiety, subconscious unresolved conflicts, marital difficulties, and infrequent intercourse.[64,66] Treatment primarily has involved sex therapy and counseling, although the penile-squeeze technique often is helpful.[64] Psychotropic medications (phenothiazines and anxiolytics), local anesthetic jelly or condoms, and oral phenoxybenzamine all have been of reported benefit.[4,67,68]

TREATMENT OF EJACULATORY DYSFUNCTION

It is generally unnecessary to treat abnormalities of ejaculation unless the individual's fertility is of concern. However, in those men whose ejaculatory dysfunction is due to medication, especially when associated with anorgasmia, treatment by altering medical regimens is beneficial. The only other abnormality of ejaculation that is not usually related to fertility concerns is premature ejaculation. The treatment of premature ejaculation has already been discussed.

Ejaculatory duct obstruction can be treated only by surgical resection with or without concomitant vasography.[59,60] Similarly, congenital absence of the vas deferens can be treated only through surgical means. In this case, the options are either microscopic epididymal sperm aspiration[58] or creation of an alloplastic spermatocele for delayed transscrotal sperm retrieval.[69] Either of these two treatment options requires appropriate sperm processing and assisted reproductive techniques (i.e., intrauterine insemination or in vitro fertilization, IVF) to achieve pregnancy.

All other forms of ejaculatory dysfunction generally are of a nature that will respond to an overall treatment algorithm progressing from simpler to more complex therapies. These therapies include oral sympathomimetics, harvesting and processing of retrograde ejaculates, intrathecal neostigmine, vibratory stimulation, and rectal probe electroejaculation (RPE).

Oral Sympathomimetics

Oral alpha-adrenergic agonists, such as pseudoephedrine and imipramine, can be effective in converting failure of emission to retrograde ejaculation and in converting retrograde ejaculation to antegrade ejaculation.[70–73] Pseudoephedrine (60 mg PO qid for 2 weeks) is the typical initial therapy. Should this fail, imipramine (25 mg PO qid for 2 weeks) has been shown to be 40% successful in converting retrograde ejaculation to antegrade ejaculation.[70] If antegrade ejaculation cannot be achieved, harvesting and processing of the retrograde ejaculate should be considered in conjunction with intrauterine insemination (IUI).

Harvesting and Processing of Retrograde Ejaculate

Retrograde ejaculates can be harvested with noninvasive or invasive methods.[74–77] Both methods involve urinary alkalinization with oral sodium bicarbonate (325–975 mg PO qid) beginning 24 to 48 h before planned sperm retrieval. The noninvasive method relies on the man to void to near completion before masturbation and subsequent collection of the postejaculatory voided urine. The invasive method assures an optimum bladder environment for sperm survival, but this requires preejaculatory catheterization for bladder washing with an appropriate sperm-processing buffer, such as modified HTF (Irvine Scientific, Irvine, CA). After bladder washing, approximately 30 ml of buffer is left behind before proceeding to masturbation and collection of the postejaculatory voided specimen. Regardless of the method, all retrograde ejaculates must be processed to remove cellular contaminants and to isolate a concentrated highly motile sperm sample for insemination. Density gradient centrifugation with Percoll (Pharmacia, Uppsala, Sweden) is a favored technique.[78] Accurate determination of ovulation is critical to successful timing of the insemination.[76] Since success rates

with these techniques have improved considerably over the past decade, there is little justification for attempts at surgical correction of retrograde ejaculation due to anatomic bladder neck incompetence.

Intrathecal Neostigmine

Intrathecal injection of neostigmine has been used successfully to induce ejaculation in otherwise anejaculatory SCI men.[44,45] However, these patients can have significant autonomic dysreflexia and resultant hypertensive crises associated with this treatment. This treatment has been abandoned in favor of safer and more reproducible techniques.

Vas Deferens Sperm Retrieval

Retrieval of sperm from the vas deferens of SCI men was first reported by Berger et al. in 1985.[79] Conception using this technique was reported by Bustillo and Rajfer shortly thereafter.[80] Although this procedure is minimally invasive and can be repeated on multiple occasions, its proper role is limited to those anejaculatory men who fail either vibratory ejaculation or RPE.

External Vibratory Massage

Electric vibrators have been employed in the ejaculation of SCI men with success rates of up to 50% in selected populations.[46,47] Potential predictors of successful vibratory massage include hip flexion response to stimulation of the sole of the foot.[46] Limiting features of this technique include the unpredictability of response in many individuals, as well as frequent problems with autonomic dysreflexia and associated hypertension.

Rectal Probe Electroejaculation (RPE)

The use of electric current to induce ejaculation in humans was first reported in SCI men by Horne et al. in 1948.[49] Since that time, many of the improvements in instrumentation arose from the use of electroejaculation in veterinary medicine. The first human live birth resulting from electroejaculation was not reported until 1978.[81] In the subsequent 15 years, several studies have reported successful semen retrieval and pregnancies with RPE.[7,46,47–50,82–84] Semen has been obtained through RPE from up to 90% of all SCI men evaluated, and the procedure is nearly 100% reliable on multiple occasions with a given man once ejaculation has been achieved.[83] Although several different devices have been designed and used successfully in humans,[46,50,82,84] they all function by direct regional stimulation of the ejaculatory nerves in proximity

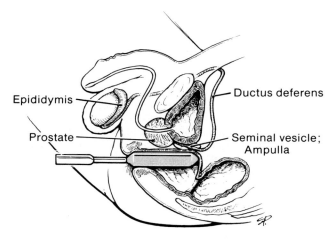

Epididymis

Ductus deferens

Prostate

Seminal vesicle; Ampulla

Figure 13–5. Sagittal view showing rectal probe placement for electroejaculation. (From Shaban SF, Seager SWJ, Lipshultz LI. Clinical electroejaculation. Med Instrum 22:78, 1988.)

to the posterolateral surface of the prostate (Fig. 13–5). The most common device in use is the apparatus designed by Seager (G&S Instruments, Washington, DC).[7,82,83] A significant addition to the safety and efficacy of this procedure was the introduction of pretreatment with sublingual nifedipine to control the hypertension associated with autonomic dysreflexia during RPE.[85] Sublingual nifedipine is used in many external vibratory protocols as well.

A simplified protocol is as follows. Patients are pretreated with broad-spectrum antibiotics for at least 48 h before the procedure to sterilize the bladder environment. Alkalinization and bladder washing are performed as previously described for retrograde ejaculation. The patient is turned in the lateral decubitus position, and preprocedure proctoscopy is carried out. Rectal probe electrostimulation is carried out until either antegrade ejaculation is observed or a maximum of 30 V is achieved or elevation of the systolic blood pressure above 200 mm Hg forces termination of the procedure. Caution must be exercised in advancing the voltage too quickly and in monitoring probe temperature as voltage increases, since rectal burns may occur. Average voltage required to achieve ejaculation with the G&S Instruments probe is between 15 and 20 V. Postprocedure proctoscopy is performed to assure rectal mucosa integrity. After collection of the antegrade ejaculate, the patient is returned to the supine position for catheterization of the bladder for any retrograde ejaculate. It is imperative to monitor systolic blood pressure frequently during the stimulation phase so that the procedure may be terminated when the systolic pressure reaches 200 mm Hg.

Although RPE has effectively obtained semen from SCI men and men with ejaculatory failure secondary to RLND,[86] a persistent problem is the frequently observed low motility of the sperm ob-

tained.[42,50,83] In detailed fertility testing of ejaculates from RPE in 16 SCI men, we have noted normal fertility potential in 25%, subfertility in 50%, and near-sterility in 25%.[83] These figures correlate well with reported pregnancy rates of 25% to 40% in some series.[42,83] It is hoped on the basis of these data that with improvements in assisted reproductive techniques, we can achieve pregnancy rates in excess of 50% from semen obtained by RPE. Certainly, this is a significant improvement when compared with the 5% to 10% fertility rate for SCI men without medical assistance.

Assisted Reproductive Techniques

Since the semen obtained by RPE often has high numbers of sperm with low motility contaminated by cellular debris, the methods of sperm processing are important. Equally important to achieving pregnancy in these couples is appropriate management of the female partner, both to correct any fertility problems and to monitor ovulation accurately. Many pregnancies may be achieved through IUI in natural cycles. However, most pregnancies reported with semen from RPE have involved fertility drug administration combined with ovulation monitoring for the female partner. The problem in achieving pregnancy is no longer a lack of semen but rather how best to extend the limited fertility potential of these ejaculates. It is likely that pregnancy rates from RPE beyond 25% will require a sophisticated team approach involving the urologist/andrologist, gynecologist/reproductive endocrinologist, and a quality-controlled andrology laboratory for sperm processing. It is quite possible that by combining appropriate use of IVF with or without sperm-egg microinjection,[87,88] we can approach pregnancy rates of 60% to 75% with semen from RPE.

SUMMARY

Normal sexual function often is taken for granted. Only when conditions arise that result in ejaculatory dysfunction is there incentive to define the physiologic mechanisms involved and how to compensate for the dysfunction. We are fortunate to have made great strides in our understanding of the neural-chemical mechanisms involved with ejaculatory function and, therefore, in how to treat ejaculatory dysfunction. Much is still lacking in our understanding of the cerebral mechanisms responsible for emission, ejaculation, and orgasm. In addition to the potential for future development of implantable pelvic nerve pacemakers for ejaculatory dysfunction, future efforts will likely progress toward delineation of the cerebral mechanisms responsible for orgasm.

REFERENCES

1. Masters WH, Johnson VE. The sexual response of the human male: gross anatomic considerations. West J Surg 71:85, 1963.
2. Rivard DJ. Anatomy, physiology, and neurophysiology of male sexual function. In: Bennett AH, ed. Management of Male Impotence. Baltimore: Williams & Wilkins, 1982:1–25.
3. Benson GS, McConnell J. Erection, emission, and ejaculation: physiologic mechanisms. In: Lipshultz LI, Howards SS, eds. Infertility in the Male, 2nd ed. St. Louis: Mosby–Year Book, 1991:155–176.
4. Shaban SF. Treatment of abnormalities of ejaculation. In: Lipshultz LI, Howards SS, eds. Infertility in the Male, 2nd ed. St. Louis: Mosby–Year Book, 1991:409–426.
5. Thomas AJ. Ejaculatory dysfunction. Fertil Steril 39:445, 1983.
6. Masters WH, Johnson VE. Human Sexual Response. Boston: Little, Brown & Co, 1970.
7. Johnson AL, Howards SS. Intratubular hydrostatic pressure in testis and epididymis before and after long-term vasectomy in the guinea pig. Biol Reprod 14:371, 1976.
8. Koraitim M, Schafer W, Melchior H, et al. Dynamic activity of bladder neck and external sphincter in ejaculation. Urology 10:130, 1977.
9. Kollberg S, Peterson I, Stener I. Preliminary results of an electromyographic study of ejaculation. Acta Chir Scand 123:478, 1962.
10. Peterson I, Stener I. An electromyographical study of the striated urethral sphincter, the striated anal sphincter, and the levator ani muscle during ejaculation. Electromyography 1:23, 1970.
11. Buch JP, Cromie WJ. Advances in the diagnosis and management of the undescended testis. In: Whitaker RH, Woodard JR, eds. Pediatric Urology. London: Butterworth & Co, 1985:1–13.
12. Marshall FF, Shermeta DW. Epididymal abnormalities associated with undescended testis. J Urol 121:341, 1979.
13. Wilson JD, George FW, Griffin JE. The hormonal control of sexual development. Science 211:1278, 1981.
14. Elder JS, Mostwin JL. Cyst of the ejaculatory duct/urogenital sinus. J Urol 132:768, 1984.
15. Duckett JW. Hypospadias. In: Gillenwater JY, et al, eds. Adult and Pediatric Urology, 2nd ed. St. Louis: Mosby-Year Book, 1991:2103–2140.
16. Donahoe PK, Budzik GP, Trelstad R, et al. Mullerian inhibiting substance: an update. Recent Prog Horm Res 38:279, 1982.
17. Brindley GS. Reflex ejaculation under vibratory stimulation in paraplegic men. Paraplegia 19:299, 1981.
18. Newman HF, Reiss H, Northrup JD. Physical basis of emission, ejaculation and orgasm in the male. Urology 19:341, 1982.
19. McConnell JA, Benson GS, Wood J. Distribution of autonomic fibers to pelvic/perineal viscera of the human male. Anat Rec 190:475, 1978.
20. MacLean PD, Dua S, Denniston RH. Cerebral localization for scratching and seminal discharge. Arch Neurol 9:485, 1963.
21. Herberg LJ. A hypothalamic mechanism causing seminal ejaculation. Nature 1:218, 1963.
22. Learmonth JR. A contribution to the neurophysiology of the urinary bladder in man. Brain 54:147, 1931.
23. Semans JH, Langworthy OR. Observations on the neurophysiology of sexual function in the male cat. J Urol 40:836, 1938.
24. Fletcher TF, Bradley WE. Neuroanatomy of the bladder–urethra. J Urol 119:153, 1978.
25. Sjostrand NO. The adrengeric innervation of the vas deferens and the accessory male genital glands. Acta Physiol Scand 65:257, 1965.
26. Owman CH, Sjoberg NO. The importance of short adrenergic neurons in the seminal emission mechanism of rat, guinea pig and man. J Reprod Fertil 28:379, 1972.
27. Sato K, Kihara K, Ando M, et al. Seminal emission by electrical stimulation of the spermatic nerve and epididymis. Int J Androl 14:461, 1991.
28. Kimura Y, Kisaki N, Sakurada S, et al. On the brain monoaminergic systems relating to ejaculation. I. Brain dopamine and ejaculation. Andrologia 8:313, 1976.
29. Kimura Y, Kisaki N, Sakurada S, et al. On the brain monoaminergic systems relating to ejaculation. II. Brain serotonin and ejaculation. Andrologia 9:50, 1977.
30. Birmingham AT. The human isolated vas deferens: its response to electrical stimulation and to drugs. Br J Pharmacol 34:692, 1968.
31. Baumgarten HG, Holstein AF, Rosengren E. Arrangement, ultrastructure, and adrenergic innervation of smooth musculature of the ductuli efferentes, ductus epididymis, and ductus of man. Z Zellforsch 120:37, 1971.
32. Sweden G. Studies on neurotransmission mechanisms in the rat and guinea pig vas deferens. Acta J Physiol Scand (Suppl) 83:369, 1971.
33. McConnell JA, Benson GS, Wood J. Distribution

of autonomic fibers to pelvic/perineal viscera of the human male. Anat Rec 190:475, 1978.

34. Raezer DM, Wein AJ, Jacobowitz D, et al. Autonomic innervation of canine urinary bladder: cholinergic and adrenergic contributions and interaction of sympathetic and parasympathetic nervous systems in bladder function. Urology 2:211, 1973.

35. Padma-Nathan H, Levine F. Vibration testing of the penis. J Urol 4:201A, 1987.

36. Goligher JC. Sexual function after excision of the rectum. Proc R Soc Med 44:824, 1951.

37. Whitelaw GP, Smithwick RH. Some secondary effects of sympathectomy with particular reference to disturbances of sexual function. N Engl J Med 245:121, 1951.

38. Kedia KR, Markland C, Fraley EE. Sexual function following high retroperitoneal lymphadenectomy. J Urol 114:237, 1975.

39. Colleselli K, Poisel S, Schachtner W, Bartsh G. Nerve-preserving bilateral retroperitoneal lymphadenectomy: anatomical study and operative approach. J Urol 144:293, 1990.

40. Donohue JP, Foster RS, Rowland RG, et al. Nerve-sparing retroperitoneal lymphadenectomy with preservation of ejaculation. J Urol 144:287, 1990.

41. Collins WF, Pipemeier J, Ogle E. The spinal cord injury problem—a review. J Neurotrauma 3:317, 1986.

42. Bennett CJ, Seager SW, Vasher EA, et al. Sexual dysfunction and electroejaculation in men with spinal cord injury: review. J Urol 139:453, 1988.

43. Comarr AE. Sexual function among patients with spinal cord injury. Urol Int 25:134, 1970.

44. Chapelle PA, Jondet M, Durand J, et al. Pregnancy of the wife of a complete paraplegic by homologous insemination after an intrathecal injection of neostigmine. Paraplegia 14:173, 1976.

45. Guttman L, Walsh JJ. Prostigmin assessment test of fertility in spinal man. Paraplegia 9:39, 1970.

46. Brindley GS. The fertility of men with spinal injuries. Paraplegia 22:337, 1984.

47. Sarkarati M, Rossier A, Fam BA. Experience in vibratory and electroejaculation techniques in spinal cord injury patients: a preliminary report. J Urol 138:59, 1987.

48. Brindley GS. Electroejaculation: its technique, neurological implications and uses. J Neurol Neurosurg Psychiatry 44:9, 1981.

49. Horne HW, Paull DP, Munro D. Fertility studies in the human male with traumatic injuries of the spinal cord and cauda equina. N Engl J Med 239:959, 1948.

50. Perkash I, Martin DE, Warner H, et al. Reproductive biology of paraplegics: results of semen collection, testicular biopsy and serum hormone evaluation. J Urol 134:284, 1985.

51. Templeton A, Mortimer D. Successful circumvention of retrograde ejaculation in an infertile diabetic man: case report. Br J Obstet Gynaecol 89:1064, 1982.

52. Greene LF, Kelalis PP. Retrograde ejaculation of semen due to diabetic neuropathy. J Urol 98:693, 1968.

53. Klebanow D, MacLeod J. Semen quality and certain disturbances of reproduction in diabetic men. Fertil Steril 11:255, 1960.

54. Kedia K, Markland C. The effect of pharmacologic agents on ejaculation. J Urol 114:569, 1975.

55. Munjack DJ, Crocker B. Alprazolam-induced ejaculatory inhibition. J Clin Psychopharmacol 6:57, 1986.

56. Sandler B. Idiopathic retrograde ejaculation. Fertil Steril 32:474, 1979.

57. Wagenknecht LV, Lotzin CF, Sommer JH, et al. Vas deferens aplasia: clinical and anatomical features of 90 cases. Prog Reprod Biol Med 12:162, 1985.

58. Silber SJ, Ord T, Balmaceda J, et al. Congenital absence of the vas deferens: the fertilizing capacity of human epididymal sperm. N Engl J Med 323:1788, 1990.

59. Goldwasser BZ, Weinerth JL, Carson CC. Ejaculatory duct obstruction: the case for aggressive diagnosis and treatment. J Urol 134:964, 1985.

60. Pryor JP, Hendry WF. Ejaculatory duct obstruction in subfertile males: analysis of 87 patients. Fertil Steril 56:725, 1991.

61. Silber SJ. Ejaculatory duct obstruction. J Urol 124:294, 1980.

62. Hanna NK, Williams DI. Genital function in males with vesical exstrophy and epispadias. Br J Urol 44:169, 1972.

63. Ochsner MG, Burns E, Henry HH. Incidence of retrograde ejaculation following bladder neck revision as a child. J Urol 104:596, 1970.

64. Masters WH, Johnson VE. Human Sexual Inadequacy. Boston: Little, Brown & Co, 1970.

65. Munjack DJ, Kanno PH. Retarded ejaculation: a review. Arch Sex Behav 8:139, 1979.

66. Spiess WFJ, Geer JH, O'Donohue WT. Premature ejaculation: investigation of factors in ejaculatory latency. J Abnorm Psychol 93:242, 1984.

67. Boneff AN. Topical treatment of chronic prostatitis and premature ejaculation. Int Urol Nephrol 4:1183, 1971.

68. Shilon M, Paz GF, Hommonai ZT. The use of phenoxybenzamine treatment in premature ejaculation. Fertil Steril 42:659, 1984.

69. Belker AM. Alloplastic spermatocele: an update. In: Lipshultz LI, Howards SS, eds. Infertility in the Male, 2nd ed. St. Louis: Mosby-Year Book, 1991:370–375.

70. Brooks ME, Berezin M, Braf Z. Treatment of retrograde ejaculation using imipramine. Urology 18:633, 1981.

71. Lynch JH, Maxted WC. Use of ephedrine in post-lymphadenectomy ejaculatory failure: a case report. J Urol 129:379, 1983.

72. Proctor KJ, Howards SS. The effect of sympathomimetic drugs on post-lymphadenectomy aspermia. J Urol 129:837, 1983.

73. Stockamp K, Schreiter F, Altwein JE. Adrenergic drugs in retrograde ejaculation. Fertil Steril 25:817, 1984.

74. Rieser C. The etiology of retrograde ejaculation and

a method for insemination. Fertil Steril 12:488, 1961.

75. Mahadevan M, Leeton JF, Trounsen AO. Noninvasive method of semen collection for successful artificial insemination in a case of retrograde ejaculation. Fertil Steril 36:243, 1981.

76. Urry RL, Middleton RG, McGavin S. A simple and effective technique for increasing pregnancy rates in couples with retrograde ejaculation. Fertil Steril 46:1124, 1986.

77. Zavos PM, Wilson EA. Retrograde ejaculation: etiology and treatment via the use of a new noninvasive method. Fertil Steril 42:627, 1984.

78. Gellert ST, Clarke GN, Baker HWG, et al. Evaluation of Nycodenz and Percoll density gradients for the selection of human motile spermatozoa. Fertil Steril 49:335, 1988.

79. Berger RE, Muller C, Smith D, et al. Operative recovery of vasal sperm from anejaculatory men: preliminary report. J Urol 135:948, 1986.

80. Bustillo M, Rajfer J. Pregnancy following insemination with sperm aspirated directly from vas deferens. Fertil Steril 46:144, 1986.

81. Francois N, Maury M, Jouannet D, et al. Electroejaculation of a complete paraplegic followed by pregnancy. Paraplegia 216:248, 1978.

82. Halstead LS, VerVoort SM, Seager SWJ. Rectal probe electrostimulation in the treatment of anejaculatory spinal cord injured men. Paraplegia 25:120, 1987.

83. Buch JP, Zorn BH. Evaluation and treatment of infertility in spinal cord injured men through rectal probe electroejaculation. J Urol 149:1350, 1993.

84. Blank W, Batzofin J, Tran CT, et al. The use of electroejaculation and zygote intrafallopian transfer to achieve a pregnancy after a major gunshot wound to the abdomen: a unique application. Fertil Steril 54:950, 1990.

85. VerVoort SM, Donovan WH, Dykstra DD, et al. Increased current delivery and sperm collection using nifedipine during electroejaculation in men with high spinal cord injury. Arch Phys Med Rehabil 69:595, 1988.

86. Bennett CJ, Seager SWJ, McGuire EJ. Electroejaculation for recovery of semen after retroperitoneal lymph node dissection: case report. J Urol 137:513, 1987.

87. Brody S, Gibbons WE, Lamb DJ. Assisted reproductive techniques in the treatment of male infertility. In: Lipshultz LI, Howards SS, eds. Infertility in the Male, 2nd ed. St. Louis: Mosby-Year Book, 1991:427–447.

88. Cohen J, Schlegel P, Goldstein M. Gamete micromanipulation and epididymal micropuncture for male factor infertility. Adv Urol 5:237–254, 1992.

CHAPTER 14

Dysfunction of the Venoocclusive Mechanism

Tom F. Lue
Craig F. Donatucci

Normal male sexual function is dependent on the integrity of penile erection. A careful balance between blood flow into and out of the erectile bodies is essential in providing penile rigidity of sufficient strength to allow for vaginal intromission. Maintenance of inflow is a function of arterial health. Outflow regulation is dependent on the integrity of corporal venoocclusive mechanism. Abnormal penile venous drainage has long been recognized as a cause of impotence. Operative attempts at correcting abnormal venous leakage were reported as early as 1908.[1] With the exception of patients with pure arterial insufficiency, varying degrees of venoocclusive dysfunction are present in the majority of patients with vasculogenic impotence. Our understanding of venoocclusive dysfunction is incomplete, and this deficit in our knowledge is reflected in the inconsistent results of penile venous surgery. Although operative penile vein ligation was promising initially, follow-up of patients over time shows that restoration of normal potency has been limited.[2]

DEFINITION AND CAUSES

The introduction of intracavernous vasoactive agents revolutionized the diagnosis and treatment of erectile dysfunction. Therapeutic self-injection regimens have had significant success. However, some patients do not respond to intracavernous injection due to the presence of moderate to severe venous leakage. In fact, the clinical definition of venous dysfunction rests on the inability to respond to intracavernous agents. If a patient does not respond to injection with a complete and rigid erection and vascular evaluation reveals excellent arteries, the patient is defined as suffering from venoocclusive dysfunction. The dysfunction may be primary or secondary and the result of several pathophysiologic processes. Occlusive dysfunction may result from (1) degeneration of sinusoidal smooth muscle, preventing sufficient expansion and compression of the subtunical venules, probably the most common but least recognized cause of venoocclusive dysfunction, (2) the presence or development of large venous channels through the corpora cavernosa, which may result in excessive blood drainage with loss of erection, (3) degeneration or trauma to the tunica albuginea, resulting in inadequate compression of the subtunical and emissary veins, (4) insufficient or inadequate parasympathetic neurotransmitter release, which can result in poor sinusoidal relaxation and failure of the venoocclusive mechanism, as will excessive sympathetic tone, and (5) acquired venous shunts, which are the result of operative correction of priapism or Peyronie's disease, causing failure of the venoocclusive mechanism.

PATHOPHYSIOLOGY

The veins of the penis drain into three systems.[3] In the superficial system, the superficial dorsal veins are small venous channels in the subcutaneous layer draining the skin and subcutaneous tissue of the penis, which usually empty into the saphenous vein. In the intermediate system (deep dorsal vein and circumflex veins), venous blood from the corporal sinusoids drains initially into tiny venules under the tunica albuginea. This subtunical venular plexuses then penetrates the tunica albuginea as the emissary veins. The emissary veins course obliquely through the tunica albuginea to join the deep dorsal vein, which in turn drains into periprostatic veins. In the deep system (cavernous and crural veins), the proximal third of the penis is drained by the cavernous and crural veins. These paired veins arise from the penile hilum and crura on the dorsomedial surface of each corpus cavernosum and drain into the internal pudendal vein.

The anatomic changes of the corporal tissue that result in activation of the corporal venoocclusive mechanism have been described.[4] During erection, the smooth muscles of the sinusoids and the arterioles relax, resulting in a large increase in arterial flow and rapid filling of the sinusoidal spaces. The arteries and arterioles become straight and larger, leading to markedly distended, smooth-appearing sinusoids. As the sinusoids distend, the subtunical venules between the sinusoidal walls and the tunica albuginea are compressed. In addition, stretching of the layers of the tunica also compresses the emissary veins, thus reducing venous flow to a minimum, resulting in a rigid erection.

The smooth muscles of the cavernous trabeculae and the arterioles control tumescence and detumescence of the penis. The state of contraction of the cavernous smooth muscle is regulated by impulses from both the sympathetic and parasympathetic nervous systems. Cholinergic transmission supports penile tumescence, but the noncholinergic, nonadrenergic neurotransmitter nitric oxide appears to play the central role in erection.[5,6] Nitric oxide release involves both endothelium-dependent and endothelium-independent mechanisms and may be disturbed by certain disease states. Tejada et al. demonstrated an impairment in neurogenic and endothelium-dependent corporal smooth muscle relaxation in diabetics.[7] Failure of the venoocclusive mechanism on this basis may be common.

Adrenergic impulses are important in detumescence. Norepinephrine released from postganglionic sympathetic nerve endings causes contraction of the sinusoidal smooth muscle, opening the subtunical venular plexus, which results in prompt drainage of intracavernous blood and detumescence. Excessive norepinephrine release due to anxiety may lead to failure of venous occlusion and is the probable cause of psychogenic impotence.[8] Kim and Oh recently demonstrated that the intracavernous levels of norepinehrine were much higher in psychogenic patients compared to controls and patients with vasculogenic impotence.[9] Further, norepinephrine levels were significantly higher in psychogenic patients who failed to respond to papaverine injection than in psychogenic patients with full response to papaverine.

DIAGNOSIS

Initial patient evaluation should start with a detailed history. A patient with pure venous leak may report normal onset of erection but an inability to maintain the erection. The medical history may reveal chronic conditions, such as diabetes, hypertension, and hyperlipidemia, that may predispose to vascular impotence. Physical examination with appropriate laboratory investigation is performed as necessary. Hypogonadism, an uncommon cause of erectile dysfunction, is excluded through determination of serum testosterone, free testosterone, and prolactin levels.[10,11] Nocturnal penile tumescence studies may be performed when indicated to confirm or exclude the diagnosis of psychogenic impotence.

Cavernosometry and Cavernosography

Direct measurement of venous function is by cavernosometry and cavernosography. Dynamic infusion cavernosometry was introduced by Virag et al.[12] and Wespes et al.,[13] who proposed the maintenance flow rate after inducing artificial erection by saline perfusion as a measure of penile venous function. Because the physiologic venoocclusive mechanism is not activated, larger fluid volumes are required to achieve and maintain penile erection than the amount needed in a natural erection. This fluid load may be harmful in patients with compromised cardiovascular function. To obviate this problem, Lue et al.[14] and Wespes et al.[15] suggested that venous studies be performed after activation of the venoocclusive mechanism by intracavernous injection of vasodilators. The major advantages of the cavernosometry after intracavernous vasodilator injection are (1) the saline required to induce and maintain penile erection is much reduced, and (2) there is diminution or elimination of psychologic norepinephrine-mediated inhibition by vasodilators. Pharmacologic cavernosometry bypasses the neurotransmitters and their receptors. The test can easily overshadow minor arterial or venous insufficiency by paralyzing the intracavernous smooth muscles. Because of concern over the inaccuracy of maintenance flow rates in determining venous leak, Goldstein introduced the concept of the initial decompression rate.[16] Heparinized saline is infused after activation of the venoocclusive mechanism with intracavernous vasoactive agents to raise intracorporal pressure to suprasystolic levels. A value of 150 mm Hg is used for standardization. Infusion is then halted, and the resultant pressure drop over a defined observation period, usually 30 sec, is recorded. The degree of pressure drop is directly related to the severity of venous outflow. A number of additional parameters of corporal venoocclusive function have been used by investigators (Table 14–1).

The diagnosis of venoocclusive dysfunction is problematic. Normal results on cavernosometry cannot rule out an occult neural (or receptor) disorder or minor smooth muscle dysfunction. Abnormal results do not necessarily assure venous leakage because the study can be affected by psychologic inhibition. False positive results due to extreme apprehension of the patient occur even af-

TABLE 14–1
Parameters of Cavernosometry

Author	Parameter
Bookstein et al.[17,18]	Pressure/volume response Pharmacologic maintenance erection flow
Bennett and Garofalo[19]	Maintenance flow
Goldstein et al.[16]	Rate of fall of corporal body pressure from a control pressure over a defined observation period
Lewis[20,21]	Maintenance flow
Stief et al.[22]	Maintenance flow
Wespes et al.[13,15]	Flow to create maintenance flow

ter maximal amounts of papaverine and phentolamine are injected. Therefore, the urologist must always use caution in interpreting the test result.

Although the performance of cavernosometry with intracavernous vasodilators has been widely accepted, there is no consensus on the best intracavernous regimen to activate the venoocclusive mechanism (Table 14–2). At our institutions, cavernosometry is performed as follows. A rubber band is placed around the penile shaft at the penoscrotal junction. A 23-gauge scalp vein needle is inserted into the corpus without anesthesia, through which 0.5 ml of a combination of papaverine 12 mg/ml, phentolamine 1 mg/ml, and prostaglandin E_1 9 mg/ml is injected. The rubber bands are removed after 2 min, and a second 23-gauge butterfly is inserted into the same corpus 10 min after injection. Initial intracorporal pressure is measured. Using a Cavropump (LifeTech, Houston, Tx), infusion of nonheparinized sterile saline is begun at 10 ml/min. Intracorporal pressure is recorded after it has stabilized for 15 sec. The infusion is increased at 10 to 20 ml/min rates until an intracorporal pressure of 150 mm Hg is reached or an infusion rate of 100 ml/min is exceeded. Fall in intracavernous pressure is measured at 30 sec intervals for 5 min, after which flow to maintain an intracorporal pressure of 90 mm Hg is measured. Patients are considered to have moderate venous leakage for a maintenance rate of >25 ml/min and a drop to below 40 mm Hg from an intracorporal pressure of 150 mm Hg over 5 min. Patients unable to achieve an intracorporal pressure of at least 80 mm Hg with 100 ml/min saline infusion are considered to have severe venous leak. Cavernosography is performed using 50% diluted contrast. Nondilute contrast may cause osmotic injury to the

cavernous tissue and result in priapism. Right oblique, left oblique, and anteroposterior pelvic views are taken, and points of venous leakage are documented.

Vickers et al. have criticized current criteria used in cavernosometry as being too strict and leading to overdiagnosis of clinical venoocclusive disease.[23] They investigated a group of six patients and found individuals who met the criteria for corporal occlusive dysfunction yet had normal erections while being monitored in the sleep laboratory. No individual parameter of cavernosometry was better than another in its specificity.

Gravity Cavernosometry

Puech-Leo et al. have proposed an alternative method of performing cavernosometry by gravity infusion.[24] The corpora cavernosa are infused by saline infusion placed at a predetermined height. When the intracorporal pressure equals the infusion pressure, a steady state is reached. The degree of venous leakage is determined by the value of the intracorporal pressure. The larger the venous leak, the lower will be the intracorporal pressure measured at constant infusion. This technique requires less complicated technology and is less expensive. Meulemann et al. have documented equivalent use of the measurements obtained by gravity cavernosometry when directly compared to those obtained by infusion cavernosometry.[25] They found good correlation between the parameters of cavernosometry as measured by pump infusion and those measured by gravity.

CIS Test

We used the combined intracavernous injection and stimulation (CIS) test as our initial diagnostic

TABLE 14–2
Regimens for Pharmacologic Cavernosometry and Cavernosography

Author	Regimen
Bookstein[17]	Papaverine 60 mg/phentol- amine 1 mg
Bennett and Garofalo[19]	Papaverine 30 mg/phentol- amine 1 mg
Goldstein et al.[16]	Papaverine 45 mg/phentol- amine 2.5 mg
Lewis[20,21]	Papaverine 45 mg/phentol- amine 2.5 mg
Stief et al.[22]	Papaverine 30 mg/phentol- amine 1 mg
Wespes et al.[15]	Papaverine 60 mg

procedure. In the CIS test, a provocative injection of intracavernous vasoactive agents (usually 10 μg PGE₁) is combined with genital stimulation to produce erection. A patient with suspected venous leak achieves a full erection but is unable to sustain the erection for at least 5 min. When reviewing the results of the CIS test, we identified 25 patients with suspected venous leak (loss of rigidity at 5 min poststimulation). In 21 of these 25 patients (84%), moderate to severe venous leakage was documented on pharmacologic cavernosometry and cavernosography, and 4 (16%) evidenced no confirmation of leakage,[26] which was probably due to initial psychologic inhibition. This simple office examination provides a more physiologic assessment of the integrity of the venoocclusive mechanism.

THERAPY
Vacuum Therapy

Several vacuum constriction devices (VCD) are available commercially.[27,28] The standard VCD consists of a suction cylinder and pump to induce erection and a constricting band placed at the base of the penis to occlude venous return and maintain the erectionlike state after the suction device is removed. Initial models required both hands and a fair degree of manual dexterity for use. Newer models are single handed and contain built-in pumps in the vacuum cylinder or are motorized. Patient preference dictates the choice of device, as either model is satisfactory with proper education.[29] To prevent edema of the penis, the patient is advised to remove the constriction band within 30 min. Several studies have reported success after VCD use in a large number of patients. Ninety-two percent of 1517 patients responding to questionnaires achieved an erection or erectionlike state sufficient for intercourse, and 77% were able to have intercourse at least every 2 weeks.[30] Complications and minor discomforts[28,31] included petechiae (27%), ecchymosis (10%), initial penile pain (41%), ejaculatory difficulty (12%), dusky discoloration of the glans, penile numbness, and trapping of the ejaculate.

Medical Therapy

Intracavernous injection of pharmacologic agents also may be used therapeutically for those patients with mild to moderate venous leak. Papaverine, a vasodilator, and phentolamine, an alpha-blocker are commonly used. Prostaglandin E₁ may be used alone or in combination with papaverine and phentolamine. Response rates are reported to be near 80%. Simultaneous injection of intracavernous vasodilating drugs with use of a

VCD may help patients who cannot achieve adequate erection with either therapy alone.

Transluminal Venoablation

Percutaneous transluminal venoablation of abnormal venous leakage was first introduced by Courtheoux et al.[32] Twenty-six patients with venous leak were treated with implantation of 1.5 cm³ detachable balloons inflated by contrast and released to occlude abnormal venous leak. Initial results revealed improvement in sexual function in the majority, with absence of venous leak on follow-up cavernosography. However, the follow-up period for these patients was short, and no long-term results are available. Bookstein and Lurie reported their results with transluminal venoablation.[33] Embolization of abnormal venous drainage was performed with moderate success in 13 impotent patients. Subjective improvement was reported in 8 of the 13 patients, yet only 2 were considered cured and 9 of the 13 did not achieve an erection of sufficient rigidity to allow intercourse. With additional experience, Bookstein reports results comparable to those seen after penile vein ligation.[2] Schwartz et al. recently reported their results combining transluminal venoablation with the use of a venous sclerosant.[34] Best results were noted in a highly select subgroup of patients, namely, those with documented venoocclusive dysfunction in the presence of normal cavernous arteries and no glans or spongiosal leak, in whom an adequate technical procedure could be completed.

Surgery

Operative attempts to correct venous impotence began as early as 1908,[1] but it was only recently that a well designed operation based on a thorough understanding of the venoocclusive mechanism obtained from laboratory investigation was possible. As an understanding of the importance of the venoocclusive mechanism to the development of erection has been gained, the technique of penile vein ligation has been refined. The ability to eliminate patients with severe arterial disease by duplex ultrasonography and confirm the diagnosis in patients with venous leakage by cavernosometry and cavernosography should allow careful preselection of patients with pure venogenic impotence for surgical correction.

Given the difficulty in establishing the diagnosis of venogenic impotence and the technical challenge of the surgical procedure, it is not surprising that the operative results reported in the literature show great variability. Lewis et al. first presented their results of penile vein ligation in 1984[35] and have updated those results several times, most recently in 1990.[20] They report that of 77 patients who underwent penile vein ligation, 21 (27%) had an excellent result, 17 patients (22%) improved, and the rest were classified as failures. Average follow-up in these patients was 14 months. Lewis has defined an excellent result as the ability to obtain an erection postoperatively sufficient for vaginal intercourse and the patient's and his partner's satisfaction.[20,21] Improvement is defined as the ability to have intercourse but not complete satisfaction with the degree of tumescence with spontaneous erection after surgery. Lewis included in this group those patients with improved tumescence with intracavernous injection of vasoactive agents compared to preoperative responses. Knoll et al. reported on 41 patients with pure venogenic impotence who underwent penile vein ligation.[36] Resection of the dorsal vein alone was performed in 8 patients, and dorsal vein resection and cavernous vein ligation were performed in 33 patients. Follow-up ranged from 4 to 26 months, with an average of 18 months. These authors report a successful outcome in 22 of 41 patients (53%), with failure in 19 patients (47%). Rossman et al. report 16 patients who underwent vein ligation.[36a] Of the 16, 14 (89.5%) had a positive outcome initially, but 12 of the 14 patients deteriorated over time, for an overall long-term successful outcome of only 12.5%.

The European experience has been similar to that reported in the United States. Wespes and Schulman, in their initial report on 20 patients who underwent ligation of the deep dorsal vein for venous leakage, reported improvement in erection in 16 (80%).[37] They monitored corporal pressure intraoperatively and documented an increase in this pressure after vein ligation. Follow-up of this group of patients ranged from 3 to 24 months, with an average of 12 months. At the time of their report, they attributed their 4 failures to the coexistence of arterial inflow lesions. A later publication from these authors expanded their experience with 26 additional patients.[38] Fifteen of these patients (58%) had return of normal potency postoperatively. Of the 11 failures, 6 were noted to have converted from intracavernosal (ICI) nonresponders to ICI responders. Pfeiffer and Terhorst reported 32 patients who underwent venous ligation for venogenic impotence. Operative ligation of the plexus of Santorini was performed in 5 patients, with restoration of potency in 4.[39] Ligation of the deep dorsal vein was performed in 21 patients, with 15 reporting a successful outcome. An additional 6 patients underwent ligation of ectopic veins with dorsal vein ligation, and of these 4 were potent. Overall, these authors report that 23 of 32 patients (72%) experienced a positive outcome after vein ligation. All patients were followed for 6 to 12 months after operation. Treiber and Gilbert reported 116 patients who were operated for venogenic impotence.[40] They divided their patients into two groups; 54 patients had pure venous leakage, underwent penile vein ligation, and were followed for 12.4 months. Return of spontaneous erection occurred in 18 patients (33.3%), with an additional 16 patients (29.6%) converting from ICI nonresponders to ICI responders. A positive outcome then was achieved in 34 patients (62.9%). Treiber and Gilbert operated on 61 patients in their second group—those with venogenic impotence and a concomitant cause of erectile dysfunction. The length of follow-up was similar (13.3 months). Potency was restored in 10 of these patients (16.4%), and 23 patients converted to ICI responders. Overall, the positive outcome rate was 33 of 61 (54.1%). In this series, 9 of 11 patients who underwent separation of the corpora from the spongiosum for distal leakage between the two had a positive outcome, and of these, 4 had spontaneous erections and 5 required ICI therapy.

At our institutions, if the diagnosis of venous leakage is suspected by the CIS test and the patient has used vacuum or injection therapy and found them inadequate, we consider penile vein ligation. Duplex ultrasonography is performed to evaluate cavernous arterial function and previously published values are used to establish normal function.[41] Severe arterial insufficiency is a contraindication to penile vein ligation. Pharmacologic cavernosometry is performed preoperatively to confirm the diagnosis of venous leak and to identify the site of venous leakage. In our experience, the most important factors affecting surgical outcome in patients undergoing penile vein ligation for venogenic impotence are the findings on cavernosography.

At surgery, a 3-inch oblique inguinoscrotal incision is made 1 inch lateral to the root of the penis along the course of the spermatic cord. The last half of the incision is changed to a transverse direction across the midline when exposure of the corpus spongiosum is necessary. The suspensory ligaments are completely detached from the pubic bone. The superficial layer of Buck's fascia is incised to identify the deep dorsal vein and its branches. In approximately 70% of patients, there are more than one trunk of the deep dorsal vein. Each is identified and differentiated from the paired deep dorsal arteries and nerves that run just lateral to the veins. The lateral aspects of the penis are inspected along their entire length. Silk ties (4-0) and suture ligatures are used to ligate all the emissary and circumflex branches close to the tunica albuginea. A segment of deep dorsal vein from 1 cm proximal to the coronal sulcus to just under the lower margin of the pubic bone is dissected, ligated at both ends, and resected. Using a 5× power loupe magnification, careful dissection in the hilum of the penis is performed. The cavernous veins are usually multiple, each identified individually, and ligated. When a substantial crural leak also is seen on the cavernosogram, the crura are ligated. In a minority of patients, substantial cavernosal-to-spongiosal shunts may be visualized on cavernosography. In these patients, the spongiosum is carefully dissected off the cavernosa, and each individual venous communication is suture ligated as it is encountered.

At postoperative evaluation, patients are questioned about the quality and duration of their erections. Those who report normal erections with satisfactory intercourse undergo no further evaluation. Patients with residual erectile dysfunction, whether due to inadequate tumescence, insufficient rigidity, or short duration, undergo repeat CIS testing. Erectile responses are evaluated again, and the patients are offered adjunctive ICI therapy if they respond well and so desire. Patients with a full erection after stimulation that is maintained for more than 15 min are classified as improved, having converted from nonresponders to ICI to responders. Patients who do not respond to intracavernous injection or who decline repeat CIS testing are classified as operative failures. Repeat cavernosometry and cavernosography are reserved for those few patients desiring a second attempt at venous ligation.

We recently reviewed our treatment outcome after penile venous surgery. Ninety-six patients underwent vein ligation from January 1, 1987, to December 31, 1989. This period was chosen because the senior author (TFL) had modified the technique of penile vein ligation to include microscopic dissection of the penile hilum and ligation of the cavernous veins. Patients ranged in age from 17 to 72 years, with a mean age of 47 years. The combined ICI and self-stimulation test was performed on all patients. All of the patients showed either a poor response or the inability to maintain an erection.

Duplex ultrasonography was performed in all 96 patients, and data are available on 86 of these. Mean cavernous artery diameter was 0.05 cm bilaterally and increased to a mean of 0.08 bilaterally (60%) after injection. Mean peak flow velocity in the left cavernous artery was 33.4 cm/sec and 34.0 cm/sec in the right cavernous artery. Pharmacologic cavernosometry was performed on all patients. The initial intracorporal pressure ranged from 0 to 38 mm Hg 10 min after ICI, with a mean of 17 mm Hg. The maximal intracorporal infusion pressure ranged from 5 mm Hg to 200 mm Hg, with a mean of 74 mm Hg. Flow to maintain erection in those patients able to achieve an intracor-

poral pressure of greater than 80 mm Hg ranged from 15 ml/sec to 60 ml/sec, with a mean of 30 ml/sec, and the initial intracorporal pressure drop 30 sec after cessation of infusion ranged from 34 to 120 mm Hg, with an average of 62 mm Hg. Moderate leakage was documented in 62 patients (63.9%), and severe leakage was found in 34 patients (36.1%). Patients with severe venous leakage had a mean initial pressure of 13.8 mm Hg and a maximal intracorporal infusion pressure of 31.0 on the average. Flow to maintain erection and the maximal initial pressure decline could not be measured in these individuals. Review of cavernosography revealed leakage through deep dorsal vein and cavernous veins in all patients. In addition, the superficial system was visualized in 14 patients (14.5%), the deep system (crural veins) in 25 patients (26%), and the corpus spongiosum in 13 (13.5%).

All patients underwent ligation and excision of the deep dorsal veins, ligation of any superficial veins seen, dissection of the penile hilum with ligation of the cavernous veins, and crural plication as necessary. An additional 7 patients underwent separation of the cavernosa from the corpus spongiosum. No major complications occurred, and 11 patients suffered minor complications (Table 14–3).

Length of follow-up, measured in time from operation to last interview, is available on all 96 patients and ranges from 24 to 56 months. Normal erections were reported by 27 of 96 patients (28%), and 43 patients (45%) converted from ICI nonresponders to ICI responders. Failure of penile vein ligation to restore normal erection or to improve the patient's response to ICI was noted in 26 patients (27%). Most patients reported initial improvement in erectile function, but there was a steady decline in erectile capacity over time. Time to failure ranged from 6 weeks to 19 months. Time to failure in the 43 patients who responded to ICI injection after operation was 5.5 months, and the 27 patients who did not have normal erections postoperatively and who did not respond to ICI failed at 6.8 months on the average.

TABLE 14–3
Complications of Penile Venous Surgery

Complication	No.
Persistent paresthesias	5
Significant penile shortening	3
Hematoma requiring evacuation	1
Abscess	1
Loss of libido	1

In our series, all patients had a poor initial response to ICI when the CIS test was performed. With genital self-stimulation, that response improved, but in the absence of a properly functioning venoocclusive mechanism, the response could not be maintained. Failure to maintain erection after stimulation is suggestive of venous leakage, and we have demonstrated that 84% of these patients will have venous leakage at cavernosometry.[26] After penile vein ligation, even in those who fail to achieve erection spontaneously, the overall initial response to injection improved, and the drop in rigidity after stimulation was minimal. Those patients who fail to improve on repeat CIS testing can be presumed to have ongoing venous leakage. Overall, normal spontaneous erections were maintained in 28% of our patients. The degree of initial venous leakage, moderate or severe, also did not appear to influence final outcome.

The reasons for failure of penile vein ligation vary and include improper diagnosis, incomplete surgical resection of abnormal venous channels, the presence of an arteriogenic component, cavernosal pathology, and the formation of collateral vessels. In a retrospective review of 50 patients (25 successful and 25 failures) who had undergone penile venous surgery at our institution, the most important factors affecting surgical outcome were the findings on cavernosography and the consequent ease of identification and suture ligation of the abnormal leak. Those patients who leaked into unusual sites, such as the glans, corpus spongiosum, or crura, in combination with a large amount of drainage to the deep dorsal or cavernous vein had the highest rate of failure. If the venous leak could be easily identified on the cavernosogram and could be suture ligated at the tunica albuginea, success was more likely.

Unrecognized neurogenic dysfunction could lead to failure of sinusoidal relaxation at the cellular level. Both papaverine and PGE_1 activate erection through a mechanism possibly involving the cyclic AMP system. Failure of the primary erectile mechanism, mediated through nitric oxide cGMP, could account for the inability to have spontaneous erections satisfactory for intercourse that improves markedly when the secondary erectile mechanism is instituted by ICI.

Is spontaneous erection the primary outcome measurement of success after penile vein ligation? Or should we consider improved response to ICI a positive outcome? Taken together, a positive outcome occurred in 73% of our patients. Although many patients may not wish to perform ICI, the resultant erection is more natural than that of a penile prosthesis. Further, prosthetic erection may not lead the patient to sexual satisfaction despite a functional erectile capacity. Pederson et al. reported that 18% of men and 15% of their partners described themselves as moderately to extremely dissatisfied with sexual use of a penile prosthesis 4 years after implantation despite 88% satisfaction with the erection produced. Clearly, the results of penile vein ligation are far from satisfactory as the restoration of normal, spontaneous erection occurs in a minority of patients. However, natural erectile function, albeit with the need for adjunctive ICI, may produce a positive surgical outcome for many patients.

PERSPECTIVES

As our understanding of the physiology of erection and the pathophysiology of venoocclusive dysfunction increases, improved methods of treatment may become available. Taking a basic science discovery into the clinical realm, Stief et al. reported their preliminary results using the nitric oxide donor lindosimine (SIN-1) for ICI in impotent patients.[42] SIN-1 appears to be as effective as current intracavernous agents and may have a better safety profile in neurogenic patients. Preliminary animal studies of an implantable penile venous compression device also have shown promise.[43,44] New and emerging therapies should allow physicians to improve significantly the quality of life of patients suffering from cavernosal impotence due to corporal venoocclusive dysfunction.

REFERENCES

1. Lydston GF. The surgical treatment of impotency. Am J Clin Med 15:1571, 1908.
2. Bookstein JJ: Comment in Donatucci CF, Lue TF. Penile venous surgery: are we kidding ourselves? In: Lue TF, ed. World Book of Impotence. London: Smith-Gordon, 1992:221–227.
3. Breza J, Aboseif SR, Orvis BR, et al. Detailed anatomy of penile neurovascular structures: surgical significance. J Urol 141:437, 1989.
4. Fournier G Jr, Juenemann K-P, Lue TF, et al. Mechanism of venous occlusion during canine penile erection: an anatomic demonstration. J Urol 137:163, 1987.
5. Rajfer J, Aronson WJ, Bush PA, et al. Nitric oxide as a mediator of relaxation of the corpus cavernosum in response to nonadrenergic, noncholinergic neurotransmission. N Engl J Med 326:90, 1992.
6. Azadzoi KM, Kim N, Brown ML, et al. Endothelium-derived nitric oxide and cyclooxygenase products modulate corpus cavernosum smooth muscle tone. J Urol 147:220, 1992.
7. Tejada IS, Goldstein I, Azadzoi K, et al. Impaired neurogenic endothelium-mediated relaxation of penile smooth muscle from diabetic men with impotence. N Engl J Med 320:1025, 1989.
8. Christ G, Stone B, Melman A. Age-dependent alteration in the efficacy of phenylephrine-induced

contractions in vascular smooth muscle isolated from the corpus cavernosum of impotent men. Can J Physiol Pharmacol 69:909, 1991.

9. Kim SC, Oh MM. Norepinephrine involvement in response to intracorporeal injection of papaverine in psychogenic impotence. J Urol 147:1530, 1992.

10. Korenman SG, Morley JE, Mooradian AD, et al. Secondary hypogonadism in older men: its relation to impotence. J Clin Endocrinol Metab 71:963, 1990.

11. Johnson AR, Jarrow JP. Is routine endocrine testing of impotent men necessary? J Urol 147:1542, 1992.

12. Virag R, Spencer PP, Frydman D. Artificial erection in diagnosis and treatment of impotence. Urology 24:157, 1981.

13. Wespes E, Delcour C, Struyven J, et al. Cavernometry-cavernography: its role in organic impotence. Eur Urol 10:229, 1984.

14. Lue TF, Hricak H, Schmidt RA, et al. Functional evaluation of penile veins by cavernosography in papaverine-induced erection. J Urol 135:479, 1986.

15. Wespes E, Delcour C, Struyven J, et al. Pharmacocavernometry-cavernography in impotence. Br J Urol 58:429, 1986.

16. Goldstein I, Krane RJ, Greenfield AJ, et al. Vascular disease of the penis: impotence and priapism. In: Pollack HM, ed. Clinical Urography. Philadelphia: WB Saunders Co, 1990:2231–2252.

17. Bookstein JJ. Cavernosal venocclusive insufficiency in male impotence: evaluation of degree and location. Radiology 164:175, 1987.

18. Bookstein JJ, Fellmeth B, Moreland S, et al. Pharmacoangiographic assessment of the corpora cavernosa. Cardiovasc Intervent Radiol 11:218, 1988.

19. Bennett AH, Garofalo FA. Enhanced cavernometry: procedure for the diagnosis of venogenic impotence. Br J Urol 64:420, 1989.

20. Lewis RW. Venous ligation surgery for venous leakage. Int J Impot Res 2:1, 1990.

21. Lewis RW. Venous surgery for impotence. Urol Clin North Am 15:115, 1988.

22. Stief CG, Wetterauer U, Sommerkamp H. Intraindividual comparative study of dynamic and pharmacocavernography. Br J Urol 64:93, 1989.

23. Vickers MA, Benson C, Dluhy R, et al. The current cavernosometric criteria for corporovenous dysfunction are too strict. J Urol 147:614, 1992.

24. Peuch-Leo P, Chao S, Glina S, et al. Gravity cavernosometry—a simple diagnostic test for cavernosal incompetence. Br J Urol 65:391, 1990.

25. Meuleman EJH, Wijkstra H, Doesburg WH, et al. Comparison of the diagnostic value of pump and gravity cavernosometry in the evaluation of the cavernous veno-occlusive mechanism. J Urol 146:1266, 1991.

26. Donatucci CF, Lue TF. The combined intracavernous injection and stimulation test: diagnostic accuracy. J Urol 148:61, 1992.

27. Turner LA, Althof SE, Levine SB, et al. Treating erectile dysfunction with external vacuum devices: impact upon sexual, psychological and marital functioning. J Urol 144:79, 1990.

28. Witherington R. The Osbon Erecaid system in the management of erectile impotence. J Urol 33A:306, 1985.

29. Salvatore FT, Sharman GM, Hellstrom WJG. Vacuum constriction devices and the clinical urologist: an informed selection. Urology 38:323, 1991.

30. Witherington R. Vacuum constriction device for management of erectile impotence. J Urol 141:320, 1989.

31. Nadig PW, Ware JC, Blumoff R. Noninvasive device to produce and maintain an erection-like state. Urology 27:126, 1986.

32. Courtheoux P, Maiza D, Henriet JP, et al. Erectile dysfunction caused by venous leakage: treatment with detachable balloons and coils. Radiology 161:807, 1986.

33. Bookstein JJ, Lurie AL. Transluminal penile venoablation for impotence: a progress report. Cardiovasc Intervent Radiol 11:253, 1988.

34. Schwartz AN, Lowe M, Harley JD, et al. Preliminary report: penile vein occlusion therapy: selection criteria and methods of use for the transcatheter treatment of impotence caused by venous-sinusoidal incompetence. J Urol 148:815, 1992.

35. Lewis RW, Puyau FA, Kerstein MD, et al. Corpora cavernosa outflow as defined by dynamic cavernosography—implications in the evaluation and treatment of impotence. In: Virag R, Lappas HV, eds. First World Meeting on Impotence. Paris: Les Edition des CERI, 1984:172–178.

36. Knoll LD, Furlow WL, Benson RC. Penile venous surgery for the management of cavernosal venous leakage. Int J Impot Res 2:21, 1990.

36a. Rossman B, Mieza M, Melman A. Penile vein ligation for corporeal incompetence: an evaluation of short-term and long-term results. J Urol 144:679, 1990.

37. Wespes E, Schulman CC. Venous leakage: surgical treatment of a curable cause of impotence. J Urol 133:796, 1985.

38. Wespes E, Delcour C, Preserowitz L, et al. Impotence due to corporeal venoocclusive dysfunction: long-term follow-up of venous surgery. Eur Urol 21:115, 1992.

39. Pfeiffer G, Terhorst B. Chirurgische Therapie bei erektiler Impotenz vaskularer-venoser Genese. Urologe(A) 27:139, 1988.

40. Treiber U, Gilbert P. Venous surgery in erectile dysfunction: a critical report on 116 patients. Urology 34:22, 1989.

41. Lue TF, Mueller SC, Jow Y, et al. Functional evaluation of penile arteries with duplex ultrasound in vasodilator-induced erection. Urol Clin North Am 16:799, 1989.

42. Stief C, Holmquist F, Djamilian M, et al. Preliminary results with the nitric oxide donor linsidomine chlorhydrate in the treatment of human erectile dysfunction. J Urol 145:1437, 1992.

43. Paick JS, Marc B, Suh JK, et al. Implantable penile venous compression device: initial experience in the acute canine model. J Urol 148:188, 1992.

44. Knoll LD, Benson RC, Furlow WL. Inflatable cavernosal body device: feasibility and chronic safety study in the canine model. Int J Impot Res 4(Suppl. 2):A126, 1992.

CHAPTER 15

Vasculogenic Impotence Secondary to Atherosclerosis/Dysplasia

Ira D. Sharlip

Until the mid-1970s, erectile dysfunction was routinely attributed to abnormalities in testosterone metabolism or psychogenic causes. Little was known about the physiologic mechanism of erection, and even less was known about the physiology of erectile dysfunction. Probably because of liberalization of social attitudes toward sexuality and the development of effective therapy for impotence by penile prosthesis implantation, interest in erectile dysfunction began to escalate in the mid-1970s. Pioneer workers, such as R. Virag from Paris, V. Michal from Prague, the Ginestie team from Montpellier, A. Zorgniotti from New York, and others, began to focus attention on arterial insufficiency as the cause of erectile dysfunction. Since that time, indirect evidence has accumulated to suggest that arterial insufficiency of the corpus cavernosum is probably a common part of the pathophysiology of erectile impotence, in some cases as the sole cause and in other cases as a contributing factor.

Arterial insufficiency of the corpus cavernosum may be thought of as occurring in three different categories: arterial dysplasia, arteriosclerosis, and arterial spasm. Dysplasia is congenital and, therefore, is usually seen in men with a lifetime history of impotence. Its prevalence is rare. Arteriosclerotic impotence is common and develops in men who have a previous history of normal sexual function. Arterial spasm is probably common as well and may be seen in men of all ages. It is due to anxiety or to local irritation such as may occur with intraarterial injection of contrast agents. In our current state of diagnostic uncertainty, the true incidence of these various forms of arterial insufficiency is unknown.

Because both erectile dysfunction and arteriosclerosis are very common and increase in preva-lence with increasing age, it is tempting to think that arterial insufficiency of the corpus cavernosum is the pathophysiology that causes impotence in older men. Data now becoming available suggest that the prevalence of impotence is higher than previously suspected, especially in older men.[1] Important factors other than arterial insufficiency, however, such as smooth muscle myopathy, subtle neuropathy, and corporovenous insufficiency, may be involved as well in the pathophysiology of impotence. Improved diagnostic techniques are needed to clearly define the pathophysiology of age-related impotence.

The hemodynamics of impotence due to arterial insufficiency are conceptually simple. To create an erection, a combination of arterial dilation, venous constriction, and smooth muscle relaxation must occur simultaneously. A defect in any of these elements may be associated with impotence. If there is excellent venous constriction and smooth muscle relaxation, only severely reduced arterial flow would be expected to produce an inadequate erection. On the other hand, even if arterial flow were excellent, an adequate erection will not occur if there is poor smooth muscle relaxation or absent venous constriction. Various combinations of partially reduced arterial inflow, venous constriction, and smooth muscle relaxation may account for the erectile dysfunction that occurs in many men.

DIAGNOSIS

The prevalence of arterial insufficiency of the corpus cavernosum has not been clearly identified because standardized diagnostic methods with known normal parameters have not been studied until recently. In fact, some investigators have doubted that it was possible to diagnose vasculogenic impotence in any patient because of the absence of these standards for normal.

The earliest diagnostic techniques, which were based on Doppler measurements of penile blood pressure, such as the penile–brachial index (PBI), are now thought to be inaccurate and nearly useless. Penile arteriography was considered to be the gold standard for diagnosing arteriogenic impotence for a number of years, but it provides only anatomic information. It does not show whether an obstruction is functionally significant. Although some investigators continue to use penile arteriography as the basic diagnostic test for arteriogenic impotence, serious questions have been raised about its value for this purpose. Because most of the literature on this subject from the 1970s and early 1980s is based on diagnosis by PBI or penile arteriography or both, the literature from this period on penile revascularization cannot be rationally interpreted.

Currently, stimulation of erection by intracavernous injection of vasoactive drugs is the most commonly used diagnostic screening method for vasculogenic impotence, either arteriogenic or venogenic. An inadequate response to large doses of intracavernous vasoactive agents is generally thought to indicate that there is arterial or corporovenous insufficiency. However, increasing indirect evidence suggests that some, if not many, patients fail to respond to these injections because of inadequate smooth muscle relaxation caused by anxiety, thus introducing a group of false negative responders. Seftel et al. have suggested that a linear relationship between intracavernous pressure and flow-to-maintain pressure following intracavernous administration of papaverine and phentolamine shows that total relaxation of the smooth muscle has been achieved.[2] Validation of this concept remains to be proven by other investigators. If it is validated, false negative responses to intracavernous injection may be identified.

If a patient consistently fails to respond adequately to intracavernous stimulation, there are additional studies to support the diagnosis of vasculogenic impotence. These include duplex sonography of the central arteries of the corpus cavernosum, dynamic infusion cavernosometry (DICC), and penile arteriography. The accuracy and significance of these studies have not been proven. Researchers are beginning to define normal standards for these tests by studying normally potent men of various ages.

At the 1992 meeting of the International Society for Impotence Research (ISIR) in Milan, Pescatori et al. reported physiologic measurements of normal erections by DICC.[3] In 124 men who achieved a rigid and sustained erection following intracavernous injection of papaverine and phentolamine,

measurements showed equilibrium intracavernosal pressure of 82 mm Hg, flow-to-maintain corporal pressure of 1 to 2 ml/min, cavernosal artery systolic occlusion pressure of 105 mm Hg, brachial–cavernosal mean gradient of 33 to 34 mm Hg, and pressure decay over 30 sec of less than 30 mm Hg. This study seems to identify the hemodynamic characteristics of a normal erection by DICC, but it does not define limits of normal beyond which abnormal hemodynamic function of the corpus cavernosum may be diagnosed.

In 1993, Lee et al. reported penile blood flow parameters by duplex ultrasonography in normal men using intracavernous prostaglandin injection and visual sexual stimulation to induce erections.[4] These authors showed that a 70% or greater increase in cavernous artery diameter and a peak flow velocity greater than 30 cm/sec are normal under these circumstances. This study is compatible with the work of Lue (personal communication, 1992), the pioneer of duplex sonography for impotence evaluation, whose experience suggests that an increase in the cavernous artery diameter to more than 0.08 cm and a peak flow velocity of greater than 30 cm/sec are normal. The study of Lee et al. does define parameters that may be used to diagnose cavernous arterial dysfunction.

For penile arteriography, smooth-walled patent arteries in the entire arterial tree out to the distal dorsal penile artery and midcavernous artery are believed to be normal. However, no control study of penile arteriography in normally potent older men exists. It is entirely possible that normally potent older men have the same arteriographic abnormalities as do impotent older men. Until a control study of normal men is completed, the significance of penile arteriography for the diagnosis of arteriogenic impotence will remain in doubt.

The current limitations of diagnostic accuracy notwithstanding, to be considered as a candidate for penile revascularization, a patient should have a diagnosis of either pure arterial insufficiency or mixed arterial and corporovenous insufficiency. To make a diagnosis of pure arteriogenic impotence, there must be no evidence of corporovenous leakage. The method of identifying corporovenous leakage is covered in Chapter 14. It should be emphasized, however, that precise standards for patient selection for penile revascularization surgery do not exist.

NONSURGICAL TREATMENT

Several treatment methods have been developed over the past decade to deal with impotence due to a variety of causes. These include intracavernous injection of vasoactive drugs, external vacuum devices, and penile prostheses. Details of these approaches are covered in other chapters of this book. Each of these methods of treatment may be used for patients with vasculogenic impotence. Oral pharmacologic treatment with vasodilators and yohimbine has been tried, but there is no evidence that it is useful for patients with vasculogenic impotence.

Intracavernous injection of vasoactive drugs, such as papaverine, prostaglandin, and phentolamine, may be very effective for patients with vasculogenic impotence. It is generally thought that patients who have severe forms of vasculogenic impotence, either arteriogenic or venogenic, do not respond well to this method of therapy but that patients with mild or moderate forms of vasculogenic impotence may respond adequately. Because current methods of diagnosing vasculogenic impotence are uncertain, intracavernous pharmacotherapy is an option in virtually all impotent patients, even those who presumably have vasculogenic impotence. At the present time, it is difficult or impossible to predict which patients will respond adequately to this therapy, even if diagnostic physiologic tests suggest that there is advanced disease.

External vacuum devices are effective in approximately 75% of patients who use them regardless of the cause of reduced erections. They seem to work as well for patients with vasculogenic problems as they do for patients with other causes of impotence.

Penile prostheses remain another reliable and effective method of treatment for arteriogenic or venogenic impotence (Chapter 19).

PENILE REVASCULARIZATION BY ARTERIOARTERIAL PROCEDURES

Treatment for pure arteriogenic impotence may be attempted by neoarterialization of the penile arterial tree or by procedures that arterialize the dorsal penile vein system. In the neoarterialization (arterioarterial) procedures, a new source of arterial blood, usually the inferior epigastric artery, is anastomosed to the dorsal penile artery. This operation is performed for patients with pure arteriogenic impotence. Dorsal vein arterialization is applicable to both pure arteriogenic impotence and mixed arteriogenic with venogenic impotence. Dorsal vein arterialization is discussed in a later section.

To be considered a candidate for any form of penile vascular surgery, a patient should have an abnormal response to intracavernous pharmacodiagnosis, abnormal duplex sonography of the corpus cavernosum, or abnormal dynamic infusion cavernosometry and, if neoarterialization is to be done, abnormal penile arteriography. Penile arteriography is not a necessity before venous arterialization procedures. Endocrine and psychogenic factors

should be ruled out or treated before undertaking this surgery. It must be emphasized that it is not possible to draw definite conclusions about the efficacy of these operations from the current literature because almost all published studies are based on diagnostic techniques that have not been standardized and on follow-up methods that are not objective and not controlled. Postoperative success in most surgical series has been based predominantly on subjective patient reporting. Because patients are reluctant to have invasive studies postoperatively, very few studies report objective postoperative data, such as angiography or cavernosometry.

A variety of surgical techniques have been developed for neoarterialization of the penile artery. The first was a direct anastomosis of the inferior epigastric artery to the corpus cavernosum, now called the Michal I operation. This operation has been abandoned because of thrombosis of the artery at the anastomotic site in virtually all cases. Subsequently, the Michal II operation was developed. This operation consists of an end-to-side anastomosis of the inferior epigastric artery to the dorsal penile artery. The dorsal penile artery is exposed and isolated for a 2 to 3 cm segment at the base of the penis. The inferior epigastric artery is dissected from the external iliac artey to the umbilicus in its bed behind the rectus muscle. The small perforating muscular branches of the inferior epigastric artery must be secured meticulously to prevent inguinal and pararectal hematomas. The inferior epigastric artery is then transected at the umbilicus and transferred through a subcutaneous tunnel to the base of the penis, where it is microsurgically anastomosed with interrupted 10-0 nylon end-to-side to the dorsal penile artery.

In the 1970s, patients were selected for this operation by the finding of any abnormality on penile arteriography. More recently in the United States, selection of surgical candidates has been based on infusion cavernosometry or duplex ultrasonography plus angiographically demonstrated obstruction in the internal pudendal or common penile artery or both. This angiographic abnormality theoretically can be bypassed by an anastomosis from the inferior epigastric artery to the dorsal penile artery. In 1986, Michal et al. reported success with this operation in 44 of 73 cases (60%).[5] More recently, such investigators as Sarramon et al.[6] have reported similar success rates. These reports, however, contain the same diagnostic and follow-up limitations discussed previously and are, therefore, of uncertain significance.

Only a small amount of blood that engorges the corpora cavernosa during erection comes from the dorsal penile artery, and most of the filling comes from the cavernous artery. A theoretical objection to the Michal II operation is that the portion of blood that flows in the antegrade direction into the dorsal penile artey does not contribute significantly to filling of the corpora cavernosa. Consequently, retrograde revascularization of the dorsal penile artery was developed and first reported in 1984.[7] In this operation, an end-to-end anastomosis of the inferior epigastric artery to the dorsal penile artery is performed. The dorsal penile artery is divided at the base of the penis, the distal end is ligated, and the proximal end is used for the anastomosis. Theoretically, blood from the inferior epigastric artery will flow retrograde into the proximal dorsal penile artery and then into the cavernous artery, provided there is a more proximal focal obstruction of the internal pudendal or common penile artery.

The best candidates for this operation are patients with focal lesions of the internal pudendal or common penile artery and normal patency of the penile arterial tree distal to this. However, it is often difficult or impossible to prove distal patency by arteriography, especially if there is total occlusion of the internal pudendal artery. In general, patients with arteriosclerotic obstruction have diffuse arterial disease and, therefore, are not candidates for this operation. Most patients with focal arterial obstruction are young men with a history of severe abdominal/pelvic trauma, and therefore, the number of patients who are candidates for this operation is limited. I reported success with the retrograde revascularization approach in 4 of 5 patients with a history of severe pelvic trauma.[8] Carmignani et al. also reported good functional results in 4 of 5 patients.[9] Since some patients with arterial injury to the internal pudendal artery due to pelvic trauma also have traumatic injury to the adjacent cavernous nerve, undetectable neurogenic impotence may be present and limit the chances for good surgical results.

Levine and Goldstein have reported that arteriogenic impotence may result from injury to the common penile artery due to blunt perineal trauma, as well as from injury to the internal pudendal artery due to severe pelvic trauma.[10] Goldstein et al. reported in 1988 on the results of retrograde revascularization of the dorsal penile artery in 225 men. The pathogenesis of impotence was blunt perineal trauma in most of their patients, although in some, the history of perineal trauma was vague. The patients were selected by abnormal findings on DICC and arteriography. Since many of the operations were done bilaterally, the average length of surgery was 7 h. Surgical complications were rare and included an anastomotic rupture in 3 patients, pulmonary embolus in 2, and wound infection in 5 of 225 patients. They reported success in 37 of their last 50 evaluable patients (74%) in this series.[11] Fitch et al., using the same selection criteria and surgical technique, reported in 1991 that of 12 patients, 8 (67%) had an excellent result, 3 (25%) were improved, and only 1 (8%) failed.[12] However, other experts are uncertain about the validity of the postulated mechanism of injury to the common penile artery and about the accuracy of DICC and arteriography used in patient selection.[13] Application of the retrograde revascularization operation for impotence due to blunt perineal trauma, as opposed to pelvic trauma, remains controversial.

Austoni has suggested a further modification to neoarterialization of the penile artery by anastomosing branches of the inferior epigastric artery to both the distal and proximal divided ends of the dorsal penile arteries. He achieved functional success in 56% of 68 patients at 1 year following surgery.[14]

Several reports of direct anastomosis of the inferior epigastric artery to the cavernous artery have been published. In this operation, the inferior epigastric artery is dissected from its bed behind the rectus muscle, divided at the umbilicus, and transposed through a subcutaneous tunnel to the base of the penis. An opening is made in the tunica albuginea, and the cavernous artery is isolated in a nerve hook. An end-to-side anastomosis of the inferior epigastric artery to the cavernous artery is performed. The last report of this operation was published in 1989,[15] and no further reports, published or verbal, have appeared. The anastomosis is exceedingly delicate to perform, and it is likely that fibrosis develops at the site at which the inferior epigastric artery penetrates the tunica albuginea, resulting in arterial obstruction at this point. It is probable that this operation has been or will be abandoned for the management of arteriogenic impotence.

In 1987, Crespo et al. reported on interposition of a saphenous vein segment between the femoral artery and one or both of the dorsal penile arteries as well as one or both of the cavernous arteries. They reported cure in 107 patients (76.5%), improvement in 27 (10.5%), no change in 30 (11.7%), and worse function in 3 (1.1%) of 257 patients.[16] No further reports of their results have appeared.

There is general agreement that penile revascularization by arterioarterial procedures for those few patients with pure arteriogenic impotence caused by pelvic trauma, and possibly by perineal trauma, is reasonably successful and is, therefore, a possible option for clinical management. The role of these procedures for patients with arteriosclerotic arteriogenic impotence remains very uncertain despite the good success rates of 57% to 92% referenced here. Doubts exist about the reliability and reproducibility of these procedures because of the unstandardized diagnostic tests and unobjective and uncontrolled postoperative follow-up methods used for reporting.[17]

These doubts are supported by the possibility that a significant sham or placebo effect of this surgery exists. For example, Morales et al. studied the effect of oral yohimbine on impotent patients and found that 18% of patients treated by placebo alone were improved.[18] Michal has reported previously that many of his patients who were functionally successful after his Michal I operation actually had totally occluded anastomoses (personal communication, 1986). Sohn et al. recently reported a lack of correlation between subjective and objective responses to dorsal vein arterialization.[19] Savion et al. found that two thirds of impotent patients with no specific cause experienced improvement on a therapeutic regimen of oral yohimbine, thioridizine, and strychnine, all of which are probably ineffective drugs for the treatment of impotence.[20] Thus, it appears that the sham effect of any method of impotence treatment, including surgery, may be large.

Because of the doubts about the success of this surgery and because of the better reliability of other methods of impotence treatment, it is probably advisable to restrict penile revascularization procedures to medical centers with special interest and clincial expertise in this type of surgery.

PENILE REVASCULARIZATION BY ARTERIALIZATION OF THE DORSAL PENILE VEIN

Dorsal vein arterialization procedures usually are used for patients with mixed arteriogenic and venogenic pathophysiology. Some investigators use dorsal vein arterialization for patients with pure arteriogenic impotence, especially if there is diffuse arteriosclerotic pathology that cannot be bypassed by an arterioarterial anastomosis. This procedure has been used for pure venogenic impotence, though a penile vein resection/ligation operation alone is the more logical approach to this problem. Arterialization of the deep dorsal vein by anastomosis of the inferior epigastric artery to this vein was initially suggested by Virag. The anastomosis impedes venous outflow. At the same time, additional arterial blood may be supplied to the corpus cavernosum by retrograde flow from the inferior epigastric artery to the dorsal vein and then through the circumflex and emissary veins into the corpus cavernosum. A venocavernous window may be created to further increase backflow into the corpus cavernosum.

The surgical technique for this procedure requires isolation of the deep dorsal vein at the base of the penis. The inferior epigastric artery is isolated and transected at the umbilicus and then transposed to the base of the penis, where it is anastomosed to the dorsal vein. One of several variations in the management of the dorsal vein may be used (Table 15–1). The dorsal vein may be ligated proximal or distal (or both) to the site of the anastomosis. A venocavernous window may be added between the deep dorsal vein and the corpus cavernosum. In the United States, the most commonly performed of these procedures are the Virag 2 and Virag 5. In the Virag 2, the inferior epigastric artery is anastomosed to the deep dorsal vein without a venocavernous window. The deep dorsal vein is ligated proximally and may be ligated distally depending on pulsation in the glans following release of the clamps. The Virag 5 operation is identical, but in addition, a venocavernous window is created. Furlow has suggested a modification in which the vein is ligated proximally and distally without the construction of a venocavernous window. Lewis has suggested an end-to-end anastomosis of the inferior epigastric artery to the dorsal vein rather than an end-to-side anastomosis.[21] Success of the Virag procedure requires fracture of the valves in the deep dorsal vein with a valvulotomy. A serious complication of this procedure is glans hypervascularization, which can be prevented by distal ligation of the deep dorsal vein.

There is considerably more literature available

TABLE 15–1
Variations of Dorsal Vein Arterialization

Procedure	Method
Virag I	Inferior epigastric artery to deep dorsal vein end-to-side anastomosis, proximal vein open
Virag 2	Inferior epigastric artery to deep dorsal vein end-to-side anastomosis, proximal vein tied, distal vein may be tied
Virag 3	Saphenous vein graft to deep dorsal vein end-to-side anastomosis, proximal vein tied, distal vein may be tied
Virag 4	Virag 1 plus venocavernous shunt
Virag 5	Virag 2 plus venocavernous shunt
Virag 6	Virag 3 plus venocavernous shunt
Furlow-Fisher	Inferior epigastric artery to deep dorsal vein end-to-side anastomosis, proximal and distal veins tied
Lewis	Inferior epigastric artery to deep dorsal vein end-to-end anastomosis, proximal and distal veins tied

on the results of dorsal vein arterialization procedures than there is for arterioarterial methods of penile revascularization. Some of these reports are only in abstract form and, therefore, cannot be fully assessed. Other reports are updated series that probably contain some of the same patients reported in previous articles by the same authors. A literature review, excluding series that have been later updated, shows that the overall outcome of dorsal vein arterialization is successful (spontaneous erections without intracavernous injections) in 38% to 56% of patients and partially successful (erections with intracavernous injections) in another 14% to 30%. Together, success and partial success have varied from 60% to 81% of 290 cases in this literature review.[21-26] In addition to these published articles, five oral presentations dealing with dorsal vein arterialization were made at the ISIR meeting in 1992.[27-31] These showed success in 50% to 75% of 244 patients. Thus, a summary of both these published and oral reports reveals that in over 500 patients, dorsal vein arterialization procedures have produced good results in 50% to 81% of patients.

A variation of the technique of dorsal vein arterialization is Hauri's operation.[32] This consists of a side-to-side anastomosis of the dorsal penile artery and the dorsal penile vein with an end-to-side anastomosis of the inferior epigastric artery to the arteriovenous fistula created by the previous anastomosis. The theory of this operation is that the arteriovenous anastomosis provides rapid blood flow through the anastomosis of the inferior epigastric artery to the recipient vessels, thus reducing the chance for thrombotic occlusion of the anastomosis. Initially in 1986, Hauri reported success in 39 of 44 patients (89%).[32] At the ISIR meeting in 1992, Schraudenback et al. reported success with the Hauri operation in 28% of 105 patients, with an additional 33% showing partial success, as defined by conversion from nonresponding to responding to intracavernous injection of vasoactive drugs (8 to 46 months follow-up).[33] At the same meeting, Junemann et al., using a modified Hauri technique with three arteriovenous fistulas, reported resumption of spontaneous erections in 58% and intracavernous injection-aided erections in 26% of 40 patients with a 14-month follow-up.[34] Hemodynamic theory would suggest that once intracavernous pressure with sexual stimulation exceeds intravenous pressure, blood from the inferior epigastric artery will flow through the arteriovenous fistula and into the venous circulation rather than into the corpus cavernosum. Therefore, the mechanism by which the Hauri operation produces success is not understood. Because it is difficult to support the concept of an operative procedure that has no rational theoretical basis, this operation,

although popular in Europe, has not received worldwide application.

An overview of these multiple reports from many different medical centers throughout the world shows notable consistency, with approximately one half to three fourths of patients benefiting from the various types of dorsal vein arterialization. This consistency supports the argument that dorsal vein arterialization is effective treatment for impotence. However, there are strong arguments against dorsal vein arterialization. The arterial flow and pressure from the inferior epigastric artery are placed into the venous side of the circulation. Therefore, the new arterial circulation is not under the normal control mechanism of erectile physiology, which is located on the arterial side. In addition, selection of patients for dorsal vein arterialization has been based on unstandardized and uncontrolled diagnostic tests, and the methods for assessing postoperative results are, in general, subjective and uncontrolled.

Poor correlation between subjective and objective results of penile vascular surgery was shown in a recent study by Sohn et al.[35] They reported that no correlation could be found between postoperative patency of the inferior epigastric artery and the success of surgery following either Virag or Hauri operations. Of 65 patients, 50% reported subjective success. In 55%, a patent anastomosis was found by Doppler examination. No statistically significant relationship between subjective success and anastomotic patency was shown. Penile angiography was done on 38 patients postoperatively. Forty-seven percent of these patients were subjective responders, and 42% had angiographic bypass patency. Again, there was no statistically significant correlation between postoperative subjective success and angiographic patency. This study shows that many of the subjective responders did not have angiographic patency and many of the patients with angiographic patency were not subjective responders. Sohn et al. concluded that the mechanism of success for those patients who benefited subjectively from surgery could not be explained. The possibility of a significant placebo effect from penile revascularization was raised by these results.

Because of these uncertainties and doubts, the role of dorsal vein arterialization, like the role of arterioarterial forms of penile revascularization, remains unproven despite the apparently satisfactory results reported in the literature.

SUMMARY

Because of the flaws in diagnostic techniques and follow-up methods, the true incidence of success for penile revascularization operations is unknown. In the future, it will be necessary to find normal control standards for diagnostic methods by studying normally potent men at various ages by duplex sonography, DICC, and penile arteriography. It also will be necessary to have objective patient follow-up. Studies of the efficacy of penile vascular surgery need to be done in a prospective manner using preoperative and postoperative patient questionnaires, objective postoperative tests of hemodynamic and erectile function, and independent auditing by objective personnel. Only then will the value of penile revascularization for treatment of arteriogenic or mixed arteriogenic and venogenic impotence be known.

REFERENCES

1. Feldman H, Goldstein I, Hatzichristou DC, et al. Impotence and its medical and psychological correlates. Results of the Massachusetts male aging study. Int J Impot Res 4(s2): Abstract A17, 1992.
2. Seftel A, Saenz de Tejada I, Frohrid D, et al. Is it possible to achieve maximal smooth muscle relaxation during dynamic cavernosometry and thereby achieve standardization? J Urol 145:3434A, Abstract 521, 1991.
3. Pescatori ES, Nanburi S, Hatzichristou I, et al. Hemodynamic characteristics of rigid erection. Int J Impot Res 4(2): Abstract A51, 1992.
4. Lee B, Sikka SC, Randrup FR, et al. Standardization of penile blood flow parameters in normal men using intracavernous prostaglandin E1 and visual sexual stimulation. J Urol 149:49, 1993.
5. Michal V, Krysl I, Klika T, et al. Revascularization of the cavernous bodies. Presented at the Biennial Meeting of the International Society for Impotence Research, Prague, June 1986.
6. Sarramon JP, Rischmann P, Bertrand N, et al. Microsurgery reconstruction for pure arterial and mixed vascular impotence. Int J Impot Res 4(s2): Abstract P185, 1992.
7. Sharlip ID. Retrograde revascularization of the dorsal penile artery for arteriogenic erectile dysfunction. J Urol 131:232A, Abstract 513, 1984.
8. Sharlip ID. Role of vascular surgery in arteriogenic and combined arteriogenic and venogenic impotence. Semin Urol 8:129, 1990.
9. Carmignani G, Pirozzi F, Spano G. Cavernous artery revascularization in vasculogenic impotence: new simplified technique. Urology 30:23, 1987.
10. Levine FG, Goldstein I. Vascular reconstructive surgery in the management of erectile dysfunction. Int J Impot Res 2:59, 1990.
11. Goldstein I, Padma-Nathan H, Payton T, et al. Penile revascularization: 5 years experience in 225 patients. J Urol 139:298A, Abstract 542, 1988.
12. Fitch WF, Cookson MS, Phillips BL, et al. Analysis of penile revascularization results by arterial versus mixed arterial-venous etiology. J Urol 147:310A, Abstract 390, 1992.
13. Rajfer J. Comment: Dynamic infusion cavernosometry and cavernosography and the cavernosal artery system pressure gradient. In: Lue TF, ed. World Book of Impotence. London: Smith-Gordon/Nishimura, 1992:115.
14. Austoni R. Comment: arteriovenous surgeries. In: Lue TF, ed. World Book of Impotence. London: Smith-Gordon/Nishimura, 1992:217.
15. Konnak JW, Ohl DA. Microsurgical penile revascularization using the central corporal penile artery. J Urol 142:305, 1989.
16. Crespo EL, Bove D, Farrell C, et al. Microvascular surgery in vascular impotence: diagnosis, surgical technique, follow-up. Vasc Surg 21:277, 1987.
17. Sharlip ID. The incredible results of penile vascular surgery. Int J Impot Res 3:16, 1991.
18. Morales A, Condra MS, Owen JK, et al. Oral and transcutaneous pharmacologic agents in the treatment of impotence. Urol Clin North Am 15:87, 1988.
19. Sohn MH, Sikora RR, et al. Objective follow-up after penile revascularization. Int J Impot Res 4:73, 1992.
20. Savion M, Segenreich E, Kahan E, et al. Pharmacologic nonhormonal treatment of impotence. Urology 29:510, 1987.
21. Lewis RW. Arteriovenous surgeries: do they make sense? In: Lue TF, ed. World Book of Impotence. London: Smith-Gordon/Nishimura, 1992:199–205.
22. Belker AM, Bennett AH. Application of microsurgery in urology. Surg Clin North Am 68:1157, 1988.
23. Balko A, Malhotra CM, Wincze JP. Deep penile vein arterialization for arterial and venous impotence. Arch Surg 121:774, 1986.
24. Barada JH, Bennett AH. Penile revascularization: where do we stand? Int J Impot Res 2:79, 1990.
25. Furlow WL, Fisher J, Knoll LD. Current status of penile revascularization with deep dorsal vein arterialization experience of 95 patients. Int J Impot Res 2(s2):348, 1990.
26. Virag R, Bennett AH. Arterial and venous surgery for vasculogenic impotence: a combined French and American experience. It Arch Urol Nephr Androl 63:95, 1991.
27. Sarramon JP, Rischmann P, Malavaud B. Deep dorsal vein arterialization in arterial and venous vascular impotence. Int J Impot Res 4(s2): Abstract A136, 1992.
28. Sethis K, Pickard RS, Powell PH. Penile revascularization for arteriogenic impotence. Int J Impot Res 4(s2): Abstract 139, 1992.
29. Lizza E, Zorgniotti AW. Long-term results of penile revascularization. Int J Impot Res 4(s2): Abstract 141, 1992.
30. Furlow WL, Knoll LD, Benson RC. Deep dorsal vein arterialization: application of the Furlow-Fisher modification in 156 patients with vasculogenic impotence 1992. Int J Impot Res 4(s2): Abstract P187, 1992.
31. Constantinides C, Petraki C, Constantinides E, et al. The arterialization of deep dorsal vein (DDV) in the treatment of vascular impotence. Int J Impot Res 4(s2): Abstract P190, 1992.
32. Hauri D. A new operative technique in vasculogenic erectile impotence. World J Urol 4:237, 1986.

33. Schraudenback L, Klima M, Karft G, et al. Problems in penile revascularization using Hauri's technique: experience with 105 patients. Int J Impot Res 4(s2): Abstract A134, 1992.

34. Junemann KP, Schmidt P, Seemann O, et al. Modified microsurgical penile revascularization: two years experience in CCAT nonresponders. Int J Impot Res 4(s2): Abstract A135, 1992.

35. Sohn MH, Sikora RR, et al. Objective follow-up after penile revascularization. Int J Impot Res 4:73, 1992.

CHAPTER 16

Pelvic, Perineal, and Penile Trauma-Associated Arteriogenic Impotence: Pathophysiologic Mechanisms and the Role of Microvascular Arterial Bypass Surgery

Irwin Goldstein
Dimitrios G. Hatzichristou
Edoardo S. Pescatori

Alterations in the inflow and outflow of blood to and from the penis are the most frequent causes of organic impotence, resulting in cavernosal arterial insufficiency and corporal venoocclusive dysfunction, respectively.[1–4]

Cavernosal artery insufficiency, either atherosclerotic or traumatic in origin, can decrease the perfusion pressure and arterial inflow to the lacunar spaces.[5–7] It has been found that erectile dysfunction develops when arterial occlusive disease occludes more than 50% of the luminal diameter of the arterial supply to the penis.[7,8] The clinical consequences of the hemodynamic changes are lowered rigidity of the erect penis and prolonged time to maximum erection.[1]

Atherosclerotic vascular disease is the most common cause of cavernosal artery insufficiency.[1–3,5] This vascular disease induces diffuse hemodynamic lesions within the hypogastric-cavernous arterial bed and is associated with adverse affects in the corporal smooth muscle, lacunar space endothelium, and corporal microvasculature.[7,8] The main cause of cavernosal artery insufficiency in young patients without vascular risk factors is arterial disease associated with blunt trauma.[6] Blunt pelvic, perineal, and penile trauma have characteristic patterns of arteriographically demonstrated occlusive disease within the distal hypogastric-cavernous arterial bed consistent with the site of the traumatic injury.[6]

Young patients with cavernosal arterial insufficiency, an intact corporal venoocclusive mechanism, and a history of blunt pelvic, perineal, or penile trauma have been shown to be ideal candidates for penile microvascular bypass surgery.[9,10] The goal of penile microvascular arterial bypass surgery is similar to that of other arterial bypass procedures, that is, to provide an arterial pathway circumventing the arterial occlusive lesion. This bypass surgery aims to increase the arterial blood perfusion and inflow to the erectile tissue, thus enabling a more rigid, spontaneous penile erection. The motivation for this surgery is the desire by impotent patients, especially young men at the beginning of their sexual lives, to restore their impaired erectile function without the need for external or internal mechanical devices or intracavernosal injections of vasoactive agents.[10]

This chapter reviews pelvic, perineal, and penile trauma-associated impotence, the pathophysiology of each disorder, and their common treatment by microvascular arterial bypass surgery.

PATHOPHYSIOLOGY OF TRAUMA-ASSOCIATED VASCULOGENIC IMPOTENCE

It has been documented that arterial occlusive disease can be caused by blunt trauma to specific locations within the entire arterial system. Examples of site-specific arterial disease with their respective trauma include the occluded axillary artery from use of crutches, the occluded brachial artery from objects striking the antecubital fossa, the occluded common femoral artery from motorcycle accidents, and the occluded superficial palmar arch from repeated use of the hand as a hammer.[11] Blunt trauma has accounted for 5% to 41% of cases in studies on the etiology and incidence of civilian arterial injuries.[12-16] In this fashion, blunt pelvic, perineal, or penile trauma has caused occlusion of the arterial supply to the penis.[6]

Blunt Pelvic and Perineal Trauma and Arterial Occlusive Disease

Blunt pelvic trauma from pelvic fractures or crush injuries has been associated with a 23% to 80% incidence of impotence.[17-21] Sharlip reported on a case of impotence following multiple fractures of the pubic ring and urethral disruption in which the arteriogram revealed bilateral common penile and cavernosal arterial occlusions.[21] Blunt perineal trauma can also cause arteriogenic impotence, such as in cases of straddle injuries, kicks to or falls on the perineum.[22-25] Using penile Doppler ultrasonography, Kerstein et al. reported that 20 potent men, after sitting on an unpadded bicycle seat for 5 min, exhibited a decrease of normal penile blood pressure values to levels consistent with arterial vasculogenic impotence.[26] In a case of impotence following perineal trauma in a basketball game, St. Louis et al. documented arterial injuries consisting of bilateral total occlusion of the cavernosal and dorsal penile arteries.[25]

Levine et al. reviewed the findings of selective internal pudendal arteriograms in a group of impotent patients.[6] Twenty of these provided a history of blunt perineal trauma with immediate impotence, 7 had blunt pelvic trauma and immediate impotence, and 104 had either blunt trauma and delayed impotence or no history of blunt trauma. Those with impotence immediately following blunt pelvic trauma were found to have significantly dif-

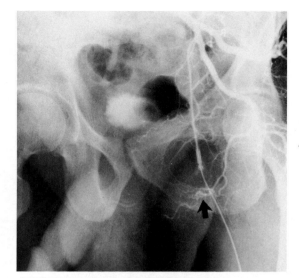

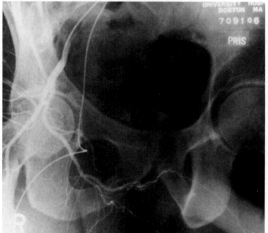

Figure 16–1. Selective internal pudendal arteriography of patients with (**A**) blunt pelvic trauma, illustrating arterial occlusion of the common penile artery as it crosses the ischiopubic ramus, and (**B**) blunt perineal trauma revealing proximal occlusion of the cavernosal artery.

ferent patterns of arteriographically demonstrated occlusive disease than patients who incurred blunt perineal trauma or patients without trauma and with vascular risk factors (Fig. 16–1). In the 7 patients with blunt pelvic trauma, there was a higher incidence (92%) of arterial lesions in the distal internal pudendal or common penile artery than in the 20 patients with blunt perineal trauma (35%). The incidence of a solitary arterial lesion in the cavernosal artery, without any proximal disease in the hypogastric-cavernous arterial bed, was significantly higher in patients with blunt perineal trauma (48%) than in patients with blunt pelvic trauma

(8%). The study confirmed that the arteriographic locations were related to the site of the blunt trauma. Blunt trauma without immediate impotence was also found to be a potential risk factor for later development of arterial vasculogenic impotence, and unrecognized or seemingly innocuous trauma was considered a potential factor in cases of idiopathic impotence. Patients without trauma and with vascular risk factors had a more diffuse pattern of arteriographically demonstrated arterial lesions, with a significantly higher incidence of arterial lesions in the aortoiliac system. This study suggested that the mechanism of arterial occlusion in atherosclerosis was more diffuse, consistent with a generalized systemic atherosclerotic process.

Blunt Penile Trauma and Arterial Occlusive Disease

The penis is vulnerable to blunt injury in the erect state.[27-32] High pressures within the corpora cavernosa during erection play the major role in such injuries.[32-34] Injury to the penis can occur during intercourse when the erect penis slips out of the vagina and is subsequently thrust against the partner's perineum or pubic bone, commonly with the partner in the superior position.[27] Penile injury also has been reported following accidents or self-inflicted abnormal bending of the penis during masturbation.[27-31] The classic injury is tunical rupture.[27,28,30] Intracavernosal bleeding may occur in conjunction with a tunical disruption or as an isolated event.[31]

In a recent study, Penson et al. reported on 19 patients with a history of impotence following blunt trauma to the erect penis during intercourse, during masturbation, or after an accident.[32] Corporal venoocclusive dysfunction was found in 84% and cavernosal artery insufficiency in 37% of the patients. A focal midshaft cavernosal artery occlusion was demonstrated in 28% of the patients, and a site-specific leak, consisting of abrupt filling of the dorsal vein or corpus spongiosum or both from a focal site on the penile shaft, was demonstrated in 79%.

Mechanism of Arterial Injury After Blunt Pelvic Trauma

The mechanisms of arterial injuries in the distal hypogastric-cavernous arterial bed after pelvic fractures have been proposed to be the same as those described for urethral injuries following similar trauma[17-21] (Fig. 16-2). The most common mechanism for urethral injury is an upward displacement of the symphysis causing rupture of the puboprostatic ligaments, stretching the urethra to the point of rupture at the urogenital diaphragm.[6] Such stretching in the area of the urogenital diaphragm could also lead to damage of the arteries that pierce and lie within it, that is, the common penile, cavernosal, and dorsal arteries. A second mechanism of urethral injury involves bilateral fractures of the superior and inferior pubic rami with posteroinferior displacement of the fractured segment. This causes a sudden retrocession of the urogenital diaphragm against the membranous urethra, with the diaphragm acting as a guillotine severing the urethra. This same guillotine action could sever the arteries that pierce the urogenital diaphragm. A

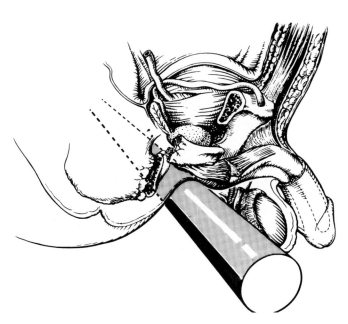

Figure 16–2. Mechanism of blunt pelvic trauma. The common penile artery bifurcates into the cavernosal and dorsal arteries just below the pubic symphysis. In blunt pelvic trauma from a fall onto a bar, the arteries may be crushed or injured between the object and the pubic bones. (From Goldstein I, Krane RJ. Diagnosis and therapy of erectile dysfunction. In: Walsh P, Retik A, Stamey TA, Vaughan DE Jr, eds. Campbell's Urology, 6th ed. WB Saunders Co, 1992; 3:3033.)

third mechanism of urethral injury, diastasis of the symphysis with rupture of one puboprostatic ligament, causes the urogenital diaphragm to be torn from its attachment to the contralateral pubic bone. This causes a shearing effect on the urethra as the urogenital diaphragm is pulled in the opposite direction. This shearing also could injure those arteries piercing the urogenital diaphragm. Finally, direct injury from a bony spicule may directly injure the urethra as well as an artery in close proximity. The internal pudendal and penile arteries lie in close apposition to the ischial and pubic rami.[6]

The cavernous nerves originate in the pelvis and course lateral to the urethra near the apex of the prostate before penetrating the urogenital diaphragm. Corporal innervation occurs at the penile hilum. Traumatic injury to the cavernous nerves may occur with bony, urethral, and crush injuries and may contribute to the otherwise vasculogenic-based traumatic erectile dysfunction.[32]

Mechanism of Arterial Injury After Blunt Perineal Trauma

The mechanism of the arterial injury after blunt perineal trauma can be explained by anatomic considerations.[6] The common penile artery lies medial to the inferior pubic ramus and bifurcates into the cavernosal and dorsal arteries just below the pubic symphysis. With such anatomic position, the arteries may be crushed between the object and the pubic bones. Such trauma has been reported to devitalize or sever the urethra.[17-25] Proximal arterial occlusive pathology in the internal pudendal artery is infrequent, as the more proximal internal pudendal artery would be protected from blunt perineal injury by virtue of its position superiorly and laterally in Alcock's canal.

Urethral injuries in impotent patients after perineal trauma are not usually present.[6] This may be explained by the fact that a blunt perineal injury of lesser severity may result in arterial rather than urethral injury. Arterial injury can result more readily, since the mechanism of arterial occlusive pathology depends on endothelial damage and not on severing of the artery. Alternatively, the main force of the blunt perineal trauma may be directed in a location more specifically related to the ischiopubic ramus and lateral to the urethra, thus causing arterial but avoiding urethral injury. It is also possible that other mechanisms interplay in blunt perineal trauma. The distal common penile and cavernosal arteries are both smaller and in closer proximity to the ischiopubic ramus, the rigid bony structure, than the proximal urethra. Such factors may allow clinically relevant arterial injury to occur independent of urethral injury.[6]

Is blunt perineal trauma a risk factor for arteriogenic impotence? A study showed that the pattern of arterial injury in patients who had previous perineal trauma and delayed impotence was similar to the pattern seen in patients with perineal trauma and immediate impotence.[6] Such observation may indicate that blunt perineal trauma, even if it does not result in immediate arterial occlusion, may still hasten its occurrence. The mechanism of such delayed arterial occlusive pathology is hypothesized to be intimal smooth muscle hyperplasia combined with fibrin, elastin, and lipid deposition secondary to increased endothelial and intimal permeability.[35,36] It may, therefore, be hypothesized that at the time of perineal trauma there is an injury to the artery not severe enough to cause an immediate arterial occlusion. The injury, however, may itself or in combination with other vascular risk factors progress to plaque formation, leading to an arteriographically demonstrated occlusion. Patterns of arterial injury after perineal trauma and immediate impotence were similar to the patterns of patients with no obvious perineal trauma and no vascular risk factors. This may suggest that the arterial lesions considered hemodynamically significant in blunt perineal trauma are not pathophysiologically related to the perineal trauma but are related to other unknown factors. Alternatively, it may be hypothesized that these men had perineal trauma in the past, perhaps during childhood, but it was not remembered. Bicycle accidents, falls or kicks to the perineum, or possibly several lesser incidents of repeated perineal trauma could conceivably have caused arterial endothelial damage to the hypogastric-cavernous beds and can be a factor inducing arterial occlusive lesions in such patients with idiopathic impotence.[6]

Mechanism of Arterial Injury After Trauma to the Erect Penis

In several organs, including the penis and the bladder, dramatic parallel increases in intraluminal pressure have been reported to induce dysfunction and rupture. This occurs when the organ is at or near maximum filling volume and is subjected to external loads capable of deforming the maximally stretched organ. For example, bladder rupture may occur when the full bladder is externally loaded by a force applied via blunt pelvic trauma. The marked elevation in intravesical pressure is equally directed toward all its surfaces. Wall rupture has been shown to occur at the weakest point.[32]

The normal structure of the tunica consists mainly of collagen, which, in the flaccid state, assumes an undulating pattern.[37] Elastic fibers are arranged longitudinally and connect to the wavelike pattern of collagen bundles. During erection, however, intracavernosal pressures approximate the systemic mean arterial blood pressure of 90 mm Hg, and there is a continuously distributed, cylindrical intracavernosal tissue stress state in both the axial and circumferential directions. The collagen and elastic fibers are stretched, with the wavelike pattern of the collagen assuming a more horizontal orientation. The tunica resists further expansion by the tunical tensile strength as well as by an intracavernous framework of fibrous columns that penetrate the corpora and attach to the intracavernosal vasculature.[38] Therefore, although the in vitro tensile strength of the isolated tunica albuginea is 600 to 750 mm Hg, the intracavernosal pressure necessary for in situ tunical disruption has been reported to be in excess of 1500 mm Hg.[37]

The tunica injury from blunt pelvic trauma may depend on several factors, including the final value of the intracavernosal pressure rise, the tensile strength of the tunica, and the contribution of tensile strength to the intact corpora from the fibrous columns. Using a typical patient data set, Penson et al. noted that a 60% diminution of circumference at the site of abrupt loading was calculated to in-duce a 15% increase in circumference in the non-loaded portion of the penile shaft and an elevated intracavernosal pressure exceeding 900 mm Hg[32] (Fig. 16–3). The authors proposed that the afore-mentioned hemodynamic abnormalities are caused by tunica and intracavernosal vasculature injuries induced by the marked short-term pressure increases, which approach or exceed the tunica tensile strength during acute abrupt loading of the erect penis.

The mechanism of site-specific injury of the cavernosal arteries after blunt trauma of the erect penis is unknown. In the human penis, the internal stress during erection is borne not only by the tunica albuginea but also by the intracavernous framework of fibromuscular columns that penetrate the corpora and attach to the intracavernosal vasculature.[38,39] Injury is hypothesized to result from short-term marked increases in intracavernosal pressures that approximate or exceed the tunica tensile strength. These supraphysiologic pressures result from re-distribution of corporal blood to nonloaded portions of the erect penile shaft. Such pressure elevations cause a spectrum of arterial injuries. It may include

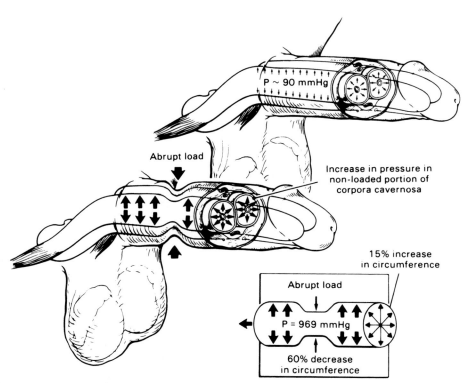

Figure 16–3. Biomechanical model showing the mechanism of blunt (compressive) trauma to the erect penis; 60% diminution of circumference at site of abrupt loading will result in 15% increase in circumference in the unloaded portion of the penile shaft and will increase intracavernosal pressure to 969 mm Hg. (From Penson DF, Seftel AD, Krane RJ, et al. The hemodynamic pathophysiology of impotence following blunt trauma to the erect penis. J Urol 148:1171, © by Williams & Wilkins, 1992.)

indirect trauma to the cavernosal arteries by means of a shearing action that might follow the excessive stresses on the fibrous columns, which attach to the tunica and to the intracavernosal neurovascular bundles. This shearing action may be the consequence of the corporal circumference increase in the nonloaded portion of the penile shaft.[38] Such a shearing action at excessive supraphysiologic pressures may result in focal bleeding or arterial occlusion or both.

PENILE MICROVASCULAR ARTERIAL BYPASS SURGERY

The main cause of cavernosal arterial insufficiency in young patients with impotence is blunt trauma-induced arterial occlusive pathology. Young patients with such arterial vasculogenic impotence and normal corporal venoocclusive function are considered to be the ideal candidates for microvascular arterial bypass surgery for impotence.

Microvascular arterial bypass surgery is the treatment option capable of restoring erectile function, impaired by arterial insufficiency, without the need for external or internal mechanical devices or pharmacotherapy.[10] Widely varying success rates following this procedure have led to concerns regarding selection criteria and technical aspects of the procedure.[1,9] The multiplicity of surgical approaches to penile arterial bypass surgery would suggest that no one procedure is effective in all instances. The major determinants of surgical outcome are surgical technique and selection criteria.[9,10,40,41] The lack of standardization of selection criteria in various institutions may be one factor responsible for the divergent outcomes of these procedures. Accurate and reproducible erectile hemodynamic testing is described though not used standardly. We review the literature and present our 11 year experience with patient selection, hemodynamic evaluation, and surgical technique.

Review of the Literature

The first vascular procedure in the penis, in a patient with priapism, was published by Gruber in 1972.[42] He performed one anastomosis of the inferior epigastric artery to the corpus cavernosum and a second anastomosis between the corpora cavernosa and the saphenous vein. A year later, Michal et al. published their results with vascular surgery in impotent patients.[43] In the first Michal procedure, the inferior epigastric artery was anastomosed to the corpora through a corporotomy. Most of the cases failed due to thrombosis of the anastomosis or the development of high-flow arterial priapism.[9] In 1977, the second Michal operation consisted of an anastomosis of the inferior epigastric artery end-to-side to the dorsal artery.[44] Michal et al. reported 60% success in 73 cases, and Sharlip[9] observed success in 3 of 7 cases.

McDougal and Jeffery modified this latter procedure using bilateral inferior epigastric arteries anastomosed end-to-side to both dorsal arteries.[45] Sharlip used an end-to-end anastomosis between the inferior epigastric artery and the dorsal artery, ligating the distal portion of the dorsal artery.[46] He reported improvement in 4 of 5 patients with a history of trauma, but in 5 patients with atherosclerotic disease, only 2 had minor improvement.[9] Similar success with this procedure was reported by Goldstein et al. (70% in 207 cases)[47] and Fitch (82% in 11 cases).[48] Recently, Cookson et al. reported on 50 cases, using both type of anastomoses, with a mean follow-up of 24 months.[49] They found 67% success in arteriogenic cases and 42% in mixed arteriogenic and venogenic. McGregor and Konnack proposed an anastomosis of the inferior epigastric artery to the cavernosal artery.[50] There was improvement in 1 of the 9 patients treated with this operation.[51] Crespo et al. suggested anastomosis of an autologous saphenous vein graft between the femoral artery and the dorsal or cavernosal artery.[52] Although the authors noticed 78% initial success, Sharlip, using the same procedure, reported only 1 success and 1 improvement in 8 cases.[9]

In 1980, Le Veen-Diaz reported arterialization of the deep dorsal vein for the first time as a treatment for impotence. He used a saphenous vein graft to anastomose the femoral artery to the deep dorsal vein.[53] Virag et al. popularized the use of the arterialized deep dorsal vein, describing five technical variations.[54–57] In a review, Virag and Bennett reported that 62% of 202 patients returned to a normal sexual life and 16% were improved with a mean follow-up 4.7 years.[56] Sohn et al. reported 80% success in 5 patients using either of the first two Virag operations.[58] Using the same techniques, Balko et al. reported a 64% improvement in 11 patients,[59] and Wagenknecht noticed that all 4 patients with a history of trauma but only 4 of 7 patients with atherosclerosis were cured.[60] A shunt between the corpora cavernosa and the arterialized deep dorsal vein has been used in conjunction with anastomosis of the inferior epigastric artery to the deep dorsal vein.[57] Virag and Bennett reported 38% success and 30% improvement in 100 patients,[56] Zorgnotti and Lizza observed 57% success and 29% improvement,[61] and Sharlip noted 1 success, 1 improvement, and 3 failures using this technique.[9]

In 1986, Hauri proposed an operation originally described by Dadrick for the lower extremities.[62] He created a fistula between the dorsal artery and the deep dorsal vein in a side-to-side fashion and then anastomosed the inferior epigastric artery end-to-side to the arteriovenous fistula. His success rate was 86%. Schramek et al. reported 77% cure or improvement,[63] and Sohn et al. documented a 71.4% success rate with a 1 to 1.5 year follow-up.[58] We recently described the use of two anastomoses of the inferior epigastric artery, the first in a side-to-side fashion with an isolated segment of the deep dorsal vein and the second end-to-end to the proximal dorsal artery, with a success rate of 68% and 24 months follow-up.[10,64]

In summary, short-term success with microvascular surgery varies from 38% to 86%. Further interpretation is difficult, as the selection criteria for success or improvement are varied. Moreover, long-term results are limited.

Patient Selection Criteria

Controversy exists in the literature concerning the selection criteria for penile microvascular arterial bypass surgery. We recently developed the Patient Profile-Oriented Algorithm to enable us to improve the selection of patients for this surgery.

Patient Profile-Oriented Algorithm
PATIENT PROFILE 1

Unless special concerns exist, the Patient Profile 1 consists of (1) those impotent patients with vascular risk factors, (2) those older patients (age > 55 years) who may or may not have documented vascular risk factors, and (3) those patients with documented neurogenic impotence. Epidemiologic and clinical data have shown that impotence determinants are associated with vascular risk factors (Chapter 1). These include hypertension, hyperlipidemia, cigarette smoking, diabetes mellitus, heart disease, pelvic radiation, chronic renal failure, and peripheral vascular disease.

Should impotent patients in Patient Profile 1 with systemic atherosclerotic disease or with arterial vascular risk factors be considered as candidates for microvascular arterial bypass surgery? Impotent patients with systemic atherosclerotic disease or with arterial vascular risk factors have been shown commonly to have corporal venoocclusive dysfunction. This hemodynamic abnormality is reflective of irreversible morphologic changes in the erectile tissue, possibly secondary to an excess of cross-linked collagen or to a dysfunctional endothelium.[1–3,5,8] Surgery for the treatment of corporal venoocclusive dysfunction has not had long-term success. Therefore, impotent patients in the Patient Profile 1 should not be considered good candidates for arterial bypass surgery. These impotent patients should undergo a sexual and medical history, phys-

ical examination, and psychologic consultation. There is generally no need for invasive erectile function testing in these patients.

PATIENT PROFILE 2

Patient Profile 2 consists of those young impotent patients without vascular risk factors or other health status concerns. Such young patients are often found to have site-specific arterial occlusive pathology in the distal internal pudendal, common penile, or cavernosal arteries in conjunction with a history of blunt pelvic or perineal trauma. These patients, who have arteriogenic impotence without concomitant corporal venoocclusive dysfunction or neurologic or endocrinologic factors, should consider microvascular arterial bypass surgery as a rational treatment option. These young patients, who are at the beginning of their personal lives and have potentially many years of sexuality ahead of them, will always desire the natural restoration of their erectile function without any mechanical or pharmacologic assistance.

Their history is characterized by a consistent reduction in the erectile rigidity during sexual activity. They have poorly spontaneous erections, often taking much effort and excessive time to achieve a poorly rigid erectile response. They often lose the partial erection during preparatory sexual stimulation before penetration or soon after penetration. They characteristically possess an ability to achieve a more rigid, long lasting erection on awakening in the morning.

Hemodynamic information is needed in those patients in Patient Profile 2, to obtain a more precise diagnosis of the etiology of their erectile insufficiency and thus facilitate selection of therapy.

Hemodynamic Criteria
Pharmacocavernosometry

During erection, the helicine arteries' resistant bed relaxes and systemic blood pressure is transmitted through the cavernosal arteries and the helicine arteries to the lacunar spaces. As a result, intracavernosal pressure approximates the systemic blood pressure. Systemic blood pressure value during penile hemodynamics testing is, therefore, the first critical consideration for any vascular testing of the erectile mechanism.[64]

Arterial inflow and venous outflow resistance, the two hemodynamic factors that determine erection, are associated with complete relaxation of the smooth muscle of the corpora cavernosa. Under such status of smooth muscle relaxation, hemodynamic testing is comparable and reproducible. Saenz de Tejada et al. studied the flow-to-maintain and venous outflow responses during pharmacocavernosometry in an animal model in the completely relaxed state (no added Ca^{2+} –papaverine combination) and in the fully contracted state (high K^+ –norepinephrine combination).[65] They found that in the presence of smooth muscle contraction, flow-to-maintain values were of a high magnitude and were nonlinear in their relationship to intracavernosal pressures. Venous outflow resistances, on the other hand, were of low magnitude and were nonconstant in their relationship to pressure. In the presence of smooth muscle relaxation, however, flow-to-maintain values were found to be of low magnitude and were linear with intracavernosal pressures, whereas venous outflow resistances were of high magnitude and were constant over the range of pressures studied. In a recent research study in humans, we also found low-magnitude flow-to-maintain values with a linear relationship to pressure over the pressure range studied. The same study showed that a positive response to the intracavernosal injection test does not rule out hemodynamic impairment, as arterial insufficiency has been well documented to exist in the presence of a positive test. Such data strongly imply that the state of smooth muscle tone should be known. For these reasons, hemodynamic information of the erectile mechanism obtained using intracavernosal injection testing cannot be reliable.

Using these research findings, a modified four-phase pharmacocavernosometry procedure has been proposed.[40] The advantage is that this pharmacocavernosometry procedure is the only available testing that evaluates both the arterial and the corporal venoocclusive function at the same time, under accurate assessment of the completeness of vasoactive agent-induced smooth muscle relaxation, with simultaneous recording of the systemic blood pressure.

Following intracavernosal administration of vasoactive agents, in phase 1, three parameters are documented: penile circumference, the steady-state intracavernosal equilibrium pressure achieved, and the time to achieve the steady-state equilibrium pressure. Organic vascular pathology is suspected when under conditions of complete smooth muscle relaxation, the intracavernosal pressure response is lower than the mean systemic arterial blood pressure.

During phase 2, assessment of (1) the corporal smooth muscle status and (2) the corporal venoocclusive function is possible by determining flow-to-maintain values at different intracavernosal pressures, typically chosen as 30, 60, 90, 120, and 150 mm Hg. A linear relationship between flow-to-maintain values and intracavernosal pressure values implies a constant venous outflow resistance and achievement of complete smooth muscle relaxation. If a nonlinear flow–pressure relationship is found, the study should be repeated with additional doses of vasoactive agents, as this pattern is characteristic of inadequate smooth muscle relaxation. Under such conditions of complete smooth muscle relaxation, normal venoocclusion is consistent with flow-to-maintain values of 3 ml/min or less.

Corporal venoocclusive function also may be studied by determining the capacitor function of energy storage capability of the erectile chambers. The capacitor function was estimated by recording intracavernosal pressure decay over time following termination of the infusion from a suprasystolic intracavernosal pressure. In clinical assessment, the intracavernosal pressure decay may be recorded from a suprasystolic pressure of 150 mm Hg over 30 sec. Normal corporal venoocclusive function has been found to be associated with an intracavernosal pressure decay less than 45 mm Hg in a period of 30 sec. This pump-independent test confirms the previous assessment of corporal venoocclusive dysfunction.

In phase 3, 10 mHz Doppler ultrasound is used to determine right and left cavernosal artery pulsatile flow. Arterial hemodynamics are assessed by recording the right and left cavernosal artery systolic pressures, as well as their gradients with the systemic systolic brachial arterial blood pressure. The advantage of this arterial function interpretation is that at this phase of the test, the corporal smooth muscle relaxation status is known. Patients who achieve an equilibrium pressure approximating the mean systemic arterial blood pressure have been found to have cavernosal artery systolic occlusion pressures approximating the brachial artery systolic occlusion pressures. Patients with arteriogenic impotence reveal cavernosal artery systolic occlusion pressures at least 35 mm Hg lower than the simultaneously determined brachial artery systolic occlusion pressure.

In phase 4, pharmacocavernosography is performed at a steady-state intracavernosal pressure of 90 mm Hg to confirm the findings of cavernosometry and to provide anatomic information of corporal venoocclusive dysfunction. Phase 4 need not be performed, at the discretion of the physician, if indices of corporal venoocclusive function are normal.

Further evaluation with selective internal pudendal pharmacoarteriography may be considered for those candidates for the microvascular penile arterial bypass procedure. Such patients have, on invasive hemodynamic testing, an abnormal equilibrium intracavernosal pressure, normal corporal venoocclusive function, and abnormal pressure gradients between brachial and cavernosal arteries systolic occlusion pressures. The anatomic pattern of arterial occlusive disease during subsequent pharamacoarteriography will lead the surgeon to select the appropriate microvascular surgical procedure.

Pharmacoarteriography

According to the anatomy, increased arterial blood flow to the lacunar spaces may be accomplished in several ways: (1) increasing the flow in the cavernosal arteries through their communications with the proximal dorsal arteries, and (2) increased inflow to the lacunar spaces may occur by arterialization of the deep dorsal vein, retrograde through the plexus of emissary and subtunical veins.

We recently described an anatomically oriented approach for penile microvascular arterial bypass surgery, based on the identification and the description of four common types of pharmacoarteriographic patterns of penile arterial occlusive disease[40,64] (Fig. 16–4). It should be noticed that each pattern has more than one selection option for the type of bypass. Based on the experience in other vascular beds, arterial grafts are superior to vein grafts in terms of longevity, and in situ vein grafts are preferable to reversed vein grafts.

FIRST PATTERN

This pattern involves bilateral occlusive lesions that are focal in nature and proximal to the cavernosal artery in the internal pudendal or common penile artery before the bifurcation to dorsal and cavernosal arteries. There are two pathways to increase the perfusion pressure and inflow to the cavernosal arteries: retrograde through the proximal dorsal arteries or through distal dorsal artery branches to the cavernosal artery. Patients with this pattern may be considered for one or two anastomoses of the inferior epigastric artery (one or two branches) to the proximal dorsal penile artery(ies) in an end-to-side or end-to-end fashion.

SECOND PATTERN

Arterial occlusive disease within both cavernosal and dorsal arteries is the characteristic of this pattern. Since there is no physiologic pathway available to increase the inflow to the corpora, a deep dorsal vein graft and its emissary and subtunical veins is used for this purpose. An anastomosis of the inferior epigastric artery end-to-side to an isolated deep dorsal vein segment is performed. The rationale of this bypass procedure is

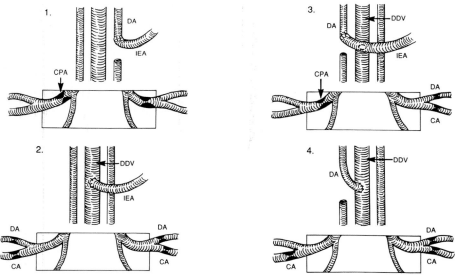

Figure 16–4. Arteriographic patterns and the associated types of bypass procedures. **Pattern 1,** bilateral arterial occlusive lesions that are focal in nature and proximal to the cavernosal artery (CA) before bifurcation to dorsal (DA) and cavernosal arteries. Anastomosis of the inferior epigastric artery (IEA) to the proximal dorsal penile artery. **Pattern 2,** arterial occlusive disease within both cavernosal arteries. Anastomosis of the inferior epigastric artery to an isolated deep dorsal vein segment (DDV). **Pattern 3,** arterial occlusive disease within the left cavernosal artery and within the right common penile artery (CPA). Anastomosis of the inferior epigastric artery to an isolated deep dorsal vein segment in a side-to-side fashion and to the proximal dorsal penile artery, end-to-end. **Pattern 4,** right cavernosal artery occlusion with an ipsilateral normal dorsal artery. Anastomosis of the dorsal artery to an isolated deep dorsal vein segment. (From Hatzichristou DG, Goldstein I. Penile microvascular arterial bypass surgery. Atlas Urol Clin North Am 1:XXX, 1993.)

based on the hypothesis that in the flaccid state, the normal high contractive tone of trabecular smooth muscle restricts retrograde flow, thus preventing high-flow priapism. During initiation of the erection, however, the trabecular smooth muscle relaxes and acts as a low-resistance pathway to the lacunar spaces. Although many investigators have failed to demonstrate arteriographic evidence of this retrograde arterial inflow, this operation has shown subjective success, based on postoperative patient questionnaire, as well as objective evidence of equilibrium pressures and time to equilibrium improvement, based on postoperative cavernosometric studies. Postoperative duplex ultrasonographic studies demonstrated a rapid increase of velocity and decrease of resistance index in the deep dorsal vein graft after intracavernosal admin-

istration of vasoactive agents (Fig. 16–5). In the presence of a activated venoocclusive mechanism, a small increase of about 15 ml in intracavernosal volume will dramatically increase rigidity.

THIRD PATTERN

This pattern may include unilateral cavernosal artery occlusion with an ipsilateral occluded dorsal artery (as in the second pattern) in conjunction with proximal contralateral arterial occlusive disease and a communication between the contralateral dorsal penile artery and the contralateral cavernosal artery (as in the first pattern). To increase perfusion pressure and inflow to the corpora using both available pathways, through the dorsal artery to the cavernosal artery and retrograde through the emissary veins off the deep dorsal vein graft, we use two

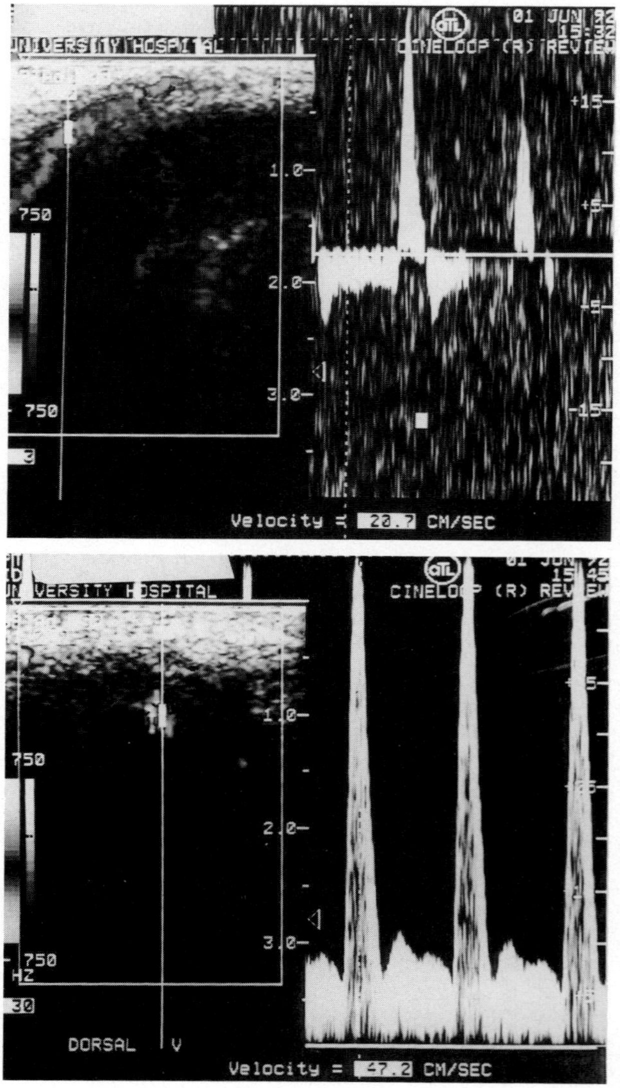

Figure 16–5. Postoperative (1 year) duplex ultrasound follow-up study of an arterialized deep dorsal vein graft, before **(A)** and after **(B)** intracavernosal injection of vasoactive agents. The velocity in the vein graft segment increased from 20.7 **(A)** to 47.2 cm/sec **(B)**.

anastomoses of the inferior epigastric artery: (1) to an isolated deep dorsal vein segment in a side-to-side fashion and (2) the protruding portion of the inferior epigastric artery to the dorsal penile artery in an end-to-end proximal or end-to-side fashion depending on the location of the dorsal artery to cavernosal artery communication.

FOURTH PATTERN

The fourth pattern consists of a bilateral cavernosal artery occlusion with an ipsilateral normal dorsal artery. To avoid an abdominal incision and the need to harvest the inferior epigastric artery, these patients could be treated as in pattern two, using this time the dorsal artery as neoarterial source.

VASCULAR AND MICROVASCULAR SURGICAL PRINCIPLES

The vascular principles used in microvascular arterial bypass surgery for impotence are similar to those vascular and microvascular principles used in arterial bypass procedures for occlusive disease in other vascular beds.[40,66,67] Long-term bypass patency is based on four microvascular principles: (1) prevention of ischemic, mechanical, or thermal injury to the vascular endothelium of the donor or recipient vascular structures, (2) transmission of systolic neoarterial inflow pressures and flow, (3) technically accurate arterial anastomoses, and (4) low recipient vascular outflow resistances.[64]

Recent studies at our institution have revealed results elucidating these vascular principles. The first study documents the role of prevention of endothelial injury during surgical preparation using technically sound no-touch techniques.[68] The second examined the quality of the donor and recipient vessels before the anastomoses.[69] The integrity of those vessels are of paramount concern, as the donor vessels provide transmission of the systemic blood pressure and the recipient vessels provide low resistance outflow runoff.

Vein grafts have been proposed as optimal conduits for small vessel arterial occlusive disease, since they possess native endothelium with intrinsic biologic properties that modulate the blood–graft interface and foster maintenance of vascular patency. In situ arterialization of the deep dorsal vein graft is a commonly performed procedure, especially in patients with bilateral cavernosal artery occlusions and absent dorsal–cavernosal arterial communications. Vein grafts however, used in coronary or peripheral artery bypass surgery have been reported to develop late occlusion on the basis of myointimal proliferative lesions in the arterialized vein wall.[70] Such lesions have been shown to be caused by injury to the vein graft endothelium. The

mechanism of endothelial injury in vein grafts remains controversial. Is the endothelial injury the result of ischemic, mechanical, or thermal insults during surgical preparation of the vein graft, or is the endothelial injury the consequence of exposure of the vein wall to arterial blood flow and pressures?

Histomorphometric tissue sections from the same deep dorsal vein before and 10 months after microvascular arterialization of an in situ deep dorsal vein graft were studied.[68] Extensive histomorphometric analysis revealed that the native architecture within the arterialized graft segment was preserved and that no myointimal proliferative lesions were noted 10 months later. This implied that exposure of the normal healthy deep dorsal vein bypass graft to systemic arterial blood pressures and flow for 10 months did not result in histologic alterations. Furthermore, iatrogenic ischemic, thermal, or mechanical trauma was not inflicted on the vein graft during surgery. Such observations strongly imply that the use of no-touch endothelium-preserving vascular techniques will improve long-term vascular patency. Such techniques already have yielded improved clinical results in other vascular beds.

The second study explored possible preexisting pathologic conditions of the donor and recipient vessels before anastomosis. Histomorphologic analyses revealed that preexisting atherosclerotic lesions existed in over 50% of the dorsal arteries studied.[69] Although present, such preexisting lesions rarely were identified in the inferior epigastric artery and the deep dorsal vein. Vascular risk factors did not per se predict the quality of the vessels.

These data reinforce the use of the inferior epigastric artery as the neoarterial pathway. In addition, they support the concept of using multiple blood supply to the corpora cavernosa.

SURGICAL TECHNIQUE

The goal of the procedure is to increase arterial perfusion pressure and inflow using the inferior epigastric artery as the donor artery and an in situ deep dorsal vein graft or the dorsal artery or both as recipients.[64] We briefly describe the surgical steps for a bypass procedure consistent with the third arteriographic pattern (Fig. 16–6).

Inguinal–Scrotal Incision

We use a curvilinear inguinal–scrotal skin incision, two fingerbreadths from the base of the penis, contralaterally from the best-quality inferior epigastric artery. The advantage of this incision is that it offers excellent proximal and distal exposure of the penile neurovascular bundle, and, particu-

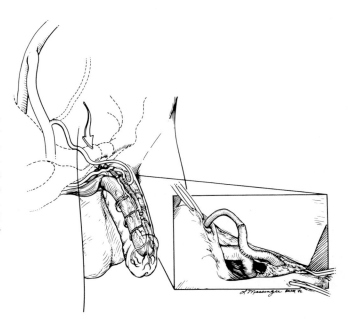

Figure 16–6. Anastomosis of the inferior epigastric artery to an isolated deep dorsal vein segment in a side-to-side fashion and to the proximal dorsal penile artery end-to-end or end-to-side depending on the location of the dorsal artery to cavernosal artery communication. The rationale of this modification is to increase perfusion pressure and inflow to the corpora using both available pathways, through the dorsal artery to the cavernosal artery and retrograde through the emissary veins off the deep dorsal vein graft.

larly, the proximal aspect of the deep dorsal vein may be easily exposed. It enables excellent exposure of the fundiform and suspensory ligaments so that they may be preserved. Furthermore, no subsequent scars will exist on the penile shaft or at the base of the penis.

Preservation of the Penile Ligaments

The two ligaments of the penis are preserved during dissection of the penis for two reasons: (1) they contain superficial cutaneous nerves important for sensation at the base of the penis, and (2) their integrity is important for the maintenance of postoperative penile length.

In Situ Preparation of the Isolated Deep Dorsal Vein Graft

Preparation of the deep dorsal vein for such arterial bypass surgery requires limited dissection. Ischemic, mechanical, and thermal trauma to the vein wall should be minimized by keeping the vein under maximal smooth muscle relaxation to decrease the endothelial damage. Inappropriate operating room and irrigating solution temperature can induce vasoconstriction, spasm, and possible endothelial cell damage.[71]

Irrigating Solution

Topical papaverine hydrochloride irrigation preserves vein and prevents spasm during vein graft preparation. For intraluminal irrigation, we use a dilute papaverine, heparin, and electrolytic solu-

tion to preserve endothelial and smooth muscle cell morphology.[72] This solution has been proposed to inhibit the early development of vein graft myointimal proliferative lesions during surgical preparation.

Avoiding Iatrogenic Trauma

Careful avoidance of mechanical twisting, stretching injury of the vessel, excessive dissection, or endothelial damage from high-pressure vascular occluding clamps is of critical concern. Thermal injury is avoided using a low-current microbipolar cautery set at the minimum level necessary for adequate coagulation. Care is taken not to injure any posterior emissary vein branches or the adjacent dorsal nerve. The vein is followed proximally under Buck's fascia, leaving the fundiform ligament intact. Exposure of the proximal deep dorsal vein ultimately is gained within the suspensory ligament. The vessel is ligated proximally under the pubic symphysis midway between the onset of the suspensory ligament and the urogenital diaphragm. At this proximal location, there are usually no emissary branches draining into the deep dorsal vein as the separate crural venous system drains the penile crurae. The isolated in situ vein graft segment is then prepared.

Vein Valves Ablation

This deep dorsal vein segment may have several valves within the lumen, which are often variable and unpredictable in number and location. Following the arterial anastomosis to the vein segment, it may be necessary to perform valve ablation maneuvers to achieve uniform arterial flow through the vein graft. Fewer than 10% of cases require this procedure in our experience. Valve ablation within the vein graft should be achieved with extreme caution to minimize mechanical trauma to the vein endothelium. A 2 mm Lemaitre valvulotome is, in our opinion, the most useful and safe instrument for this maneuver.

Abdominal Incision

A unilateral transverse abdominal incision provides excellent operative exposure of the inferior epigastric artery and heals with a better cosmetic scar than those observed with previously used paramedian skin incisions. The starting point of the incision is approximately five eighths of the total distance from the pubic bone to the umbilicus. It extends laterally along the skin lines of Langer to the lateral abdominal wall.

Harvesting of the Inferior Epigastric Artery

The rectus fascia is transected horizontally, and the rectus muscle is reflected medially to identify the inferior epigastric artery and its two accompanying veins. It is critical to harvest an inferior epigastric artery of appropriate length so that there will be no tension on any microvascular anastomosis. The vasa vasorum blood supply is preserved by dissecting the artery en bloc with its surrounding veins and fat.

Transfer of the Inferior Epigastric Artery

The internal ring is identified lateral to the origin of the inferior epigastric artery in the pelvis. Using blunt finger dissection through the inguinal canal, the finger is passed through the internal ring and through the external ring to the defect between the fundiform and suspensory ligaments at the base of the penis. A long, fine, right-angled vascular instrument is passed carefully from the fenestration between the fundiform and suspensory ligaments to the internal inguinal ring. The inferior epigastric vascular bundle is transferred to the base of the penis, and the abdominal incision may be closed in layers.

Microvascular Anastomoses

Exposure of a 1 cm segment of deep dorsal vein graft is made usually in the mid-third of the penile shaft, usually within the lower aspect of the fundiform ligament. The only location where the adventitia must be carefully removed is at the site of the vascular anastomosis to avoid causing subsequent thrombosis. Under microscopic control at $5\times$ to $10\times$ magnification, an oval section of the vein wall is excised with a curved microscissors, resulting in a 2 mm vertical venotomy. A similar sized vertical arteriotomy is made in the inferior epigastric artery for a side-to-side anastomosis. Typically 8-0 sutures are used to fashion an inferior epigastric artery anastomosis to the deep dorsal vein. Three interrupted sutures are placed into each side wall. Following release of the low-pressure angled temporary occluding vascular clamp on the inferior epigastric artery, the deep dorsal vein segment should reveal arterial pulsations along its length. Cannulation of the distal dorsal vein may be performed to identify postoperative oxygen tension and dorsal vein pressure changes. In our experience, the pressure in the deep dorsal vein graft approaches the systemic brachial arterial blood pressure. This pressure information provides evidence for the creation of a deep dorsal vein graft and not a low-pressure high-flow venous fistula.

A second anastomosis may be completed subsequently between the distal aspect of the inferior epigastric artery and the dorsal artery in an end-to-side or end-to-end fashion. The inferior epigastric artery and the dorsal artery are approximated, the arteriotomy in the dorsal artery is created, if needed, as previously described, and the anastomosis is created using interrupted 10-0 nylon sutures under $5\times$ to $10\times$ magnification. Closure of the inguinal–scrotal incision may begin in routine fashion.

RESULTS

Microvascular arterial bypass may fail due to inadequate arterial inflow, technical errors during the anastomosis, or poor arterial runoff due to preexisting vascular pathology, vein valves, or the development of myointimal proliferative lesions, especially within the deep dorsal vein grafts.[68] Failure also may result despite selection of those unique impotent patients with arterial insufficiency and normal corporal venoocclusive function. We have patients who denied postoperative improvement despite objective advantages in hemodynamic parameters by pharamacocavernosometry performed at 6 months to 3 years after surgery. Such patients may be unsatisfied secondary to unrealistic expectations of the surgery. Preoperative patient counseling, in addition to hemodynamic testing, hopefully will reflect in improved objective and subjective surgical treatment outcome.

Using the described anatomically oriented approach for arterial bypass surgery, we operated on 78 patients, aged 17 to 54 years (mean 38 years) following the described surgical principles.[64] Twenty-three patients underwent an anastomosis of the inferior epigastric artery to the proximal dorsal penile artery, 24 patients were treated with an anastomosis of the inferior epigastric artery to an isolated deep dorsal vein segment, 29 patients were treated with the modification that involves two anastomoses of the inferior epigastric artery, the first side-to-side to an isolated deep dorsal vein graft and the second end-to-end to the proximal dorsal artery, and 2 patients had an anastomosis of the normal dorsal artery to an isolated deep dorsal vein graft. With a mean follow-up of 21 months (range 14–37 months), 68% of our patients realized restoration of erectile potency as defined by a self-reported questionnaire.[64]

COMPLICATIONS

Complications include penile pain, diminished penile sensation, and altered penile length. Preservation of the two ligaments has resulted in a marked reduction of these complications in our patients.

Glans hyperemia is the most serious complication in cases of deep dorsal vein arterialization. Although the complication occurs immediately after the procedure, we have noticed this complication 10 months postoperatively following a zipper injury to the glans. In the 50 cases where we used a deep dorsal vein graft, there were 5 cases of glans hyperemia (10%).[64] Surgical exploration and ligation of distal branches of the deep dorsal vein graft is the first approach. In cases of persistent symptoms, embolization or ligation of the inferior epigastric artery is unavoidable.

CONCLUSIONS

Our experience with microvascular arterial bypass surgery for the treatment of arteriogenic impotence in over 400 cases has led us to identify three basic clinical principles.

1. STRICT SELECTION CRITERIA. Erectile hemodynamics differ from those of other vascular organs in that function is dependent not only on arterial inflow but also on the development of venous outflow resistance. The surgery should be restricted to those patients with arteriogenic impotence with normal corporal venoocclusion. In a recent clinical study considering failures after penile microvascular arterial bypass surgery, we found that patients with coexisting corporal venoocclusive dysfunction failed due to persistent venous leakage despite concomitant venous ligation surgery. This includes those young patients with site-specific arterial occlusive pathology following blunt pelvic or perineal trauma.

2. ANATOMICALLY ORIENTED ARTERIAL BYPASSES. Reconstruction should be based on the arteriographic pattern of arterial occlusive disease. There should not be one procedure universally applied.

3. ENDOTHELIUM-PRESERVING MICROVASCULAR TECHNIQUE. The surgical technique should consist of modern endothelium-sparing vascular and microvascular surgical principles similar to those applied for occlusive disease within other peripheral vascular beds.

To help patients with persistent impotence following blunt pelvic and perineal trauma achieve their goal, marked improvements in diagnosis and surgical technique, founded on objective hemodynamic testing and sound vascular and microvascular principles, have been made in the last decade. It is anticipated that the use of such principles will translate into improved long-term results of arterial reconstructive surgery for impotence.

REFERENCES

1. Krane RJ, Goldstein I, Saenz de Tejada I. Impotence. N Engl J Med 321:1648, 1989.
2. Virag R, Bouilly P, Frydaman D. Is impotence an arterial disorder? A study of arterial risk factors in 400 impotent men. Lancet 1:181, 1985.
3. Michal V. Arterial disease as a cause of impotence. Clin Endocrinol Metab 11:725, 1982.
4. Aboseif RS, Wetterauer U, Breza J, et al. The effect of venous incompetence and arterial insufficiency on erectile function: an animal model. J Urol 144:790, 1990.
5. Azadzoi KM, Goldstein I. Atherosclerosis-induced corporal leakage impotence. Surg Forum 38:647, 1987.
6. Levine FJ, Greenfield AJ, Goldstein I. Arteriographically determined occlusive disease within the hypogastric-cavernous bed in impotent patients following blunt perineal and pelvic trauma. J Urol 144:1147, 1990.
7. Rosen MP, Greenfield AJ, Walker TG, et al. Arteriogenic impotence: findings in 195 impotent men examined with selective internal pudendal angiography. Radiology 174:1043, 1990.
8. Azadzoi KM, Saenz de Tejada I. Hypercholesterolemia impairs endothelium-dependent relaxation of rabbit corpus cavernosum smooth muscle. J Urol 146:238, 1990.
9. Sharlip ID. The role of vascular surgery in arteriogenic and combined arteriogenic and venogenic impotence. Semin Urol 8:129, 1990.
10. Hatzichristou DG, Goldstein I. Arterial bypass surgery for impotence. Curr Opinion Urol 1:114, 1992.
11. Rich NM, Spencer FC. Vascular Trauma. Philadelphia: WB Saunders Co, 1978.
12. Moore CH, Wolma FJ, Brown RW, Derrick JR. Vascular trauma, a review of 250 cases. Am J Surg 122:576, 1971.
13. Ferguson IA Jr, Byrd WM, McAfee DK. Experi-

ences in the management of arterial injuries. Ann Surg 153:980, 1961.

14. Vollmar J. Surgical experience with 197 traumatic arterial lesions (1953–66). In: Hiertonn T, Rybeck B, eds. Traumatic Arterial Lesions. Stockholm: Forsvarets Forsningsanstalt, 1968.

15. Perry MO, Thal ER, Shires GT. Management of arterial injuries. Ann Surg 173:403, 1971.

16. Dillard BM, Nelson DL, Norman HG Jr. Review of 85 traumatic arterial injuries. Surgery 63:391, 1968.

17. Chambers HL, Balfour J. The incidence of impotence following pelvic fracture with associated urinary tract injury. J Urol 89:702, 1963.

18. Gibson J, Geoffrey R. Urological management and complications of fractured pelvis and ruptured urethra. J Urol 111:353, 1974.

19. King J. Impotence after fracture of the pelvis. J Bone Joint Surg 57:1107, 1975.

20. Cass AS, Godec CJ. Urethral injury due to external trauma. Urology 11:607, 1978.

21. Sharlip ID. Penile arteriography in impotence after pelvic trauma. J Urol 126:477, 1981.

22. Aboulker P, Benassayag E, Steg A. Les traumatismes du périnée par traction sur table orthopédique avec pelvi-support (3 observations). Rev Chir Orthop 60:165, 1974.

23. Schulak DJ, Bear TF, Summers JL. Transient impotence from positioning on the fracture table. J Trauma 20:420, 1980.

24. Simpson-Smith A. Traumatic rupture of the urethra, eight personal cases, with a review of 381 recorded ruptures. Br J Surg 24:309, 1936.

25. St. Louis EL, Jewett MAS, Gray RR, Grosman H. Basketball-related impotence. N Engl J Med 308:595, 1983.

26. Kerstein MD, Gould SA, French-Sherry E, Pirman C. Perineal trauma and vasculogenic impotence. J Urol 127:57, 1982.

27. Creecy AA, Beazlie FS Jr. Fracture of the penis: traumatic rupture of corpora cavernosa. J Urol 78:620, 1957.

28. Dever DP, Saraf PG, Catanese RP, et al. Penile fracture: operative management and cavernosography. Urology 22:394, 1983.

29. Kalash SS, Young JD Jr. Fracture of penis: controversy of surgical versus conservative treatment. Urology 24:21, 1984.

30. Godec CJ, Reiser R, Logush AZ. The erect penis: injury prone organ. J Trauma 28:124, 1988.

31. Grosman H, Gray RR, St. Louis EL, et al. The role of corpus cavernosography in the acute "fracture" of the penis. Radiology 144:787, 1982.

32. Penson DF, Seftel AD, Krane RJ, et al. The hemodynamic pathophysiology of impotence following blunt trauma to the erect penis. J Urol 148:1171, 1992.

33. Meehan JP, Goldstein AMB. High pressure within corpus cavernosum in man during erection. Urology, 21:385, 1983.

34. Purohit RC, Beckett SD. Penile pressures and muscle activity associated with erection and ejaculation in the dog. Am J Physiol 231:1343, 1976.

35. Moore S, Friedman RJ, Gent M. Resolution of lipid-containing atherosclerotic lesions induced by injury. Blood Vessels 14:192, 1977.

36. Ross R. The pathogenesis of atherosclerosis—an update. N Engl J Med 314:488, 1986.

37. Bitsch M, Kromann-Andersen B, Schou J, Sjøntoft E. The elasticity and the tensile strength of tunica albuginea of the corpora cavernosa. J Urol 143:642, 1990.

38. Goldstein AMB, Meehan JP, Padma-Nathan H. The microarchitecture of the intracavernosal smooth muscle and the cavernosal fibrous skeleton. J Urol 144:1144, 1990.

39. Frohib DA, Goldstein I, Payton TR, et al. Characterization of penile erectile states using external computer-based monitoring. J Biomech Eng 109:110, 1987.

40. Hatzichristou DG, Goldstein I. Penile arterial microvascular bypass surgery: indications and surgical considerations. Surg Annu 1993 (in press).

41. Sohn M, Sikora R, Bohndorf K, Deutz FJ. Selective microsurgery in arteriogenic erectile failure. World J Urol 8:104, 1990.

42. Gruber H. The treatment of priapsim: use of inferior epigastric artery: a case report. J Urol 108:882, 1972.

43. Michal V, Kramer R, Pospichal J, Hejhal L. Direct arterial anastomosis on corporal cavernosa penis in therapy of erectile impotence. Rozhl Chir 52:587, 1973.

44. Michal V, Kramar R, Pospichal J, Hejkal L. Arterial epigastricocavernous anastomosis for the treatment of sexual impotence. World J Surg 1:515, 1977.

45. McDougal WS, Jeffery RF. Microscopic penile revascularization. J Urol 129:517, 1983.

46. Sharlip I. Retrograde revascularization of the dorsal penile artery for arteriogenic erectile dysfunction. J Urol 131:232A, 1984.

47. Goldstein I, Levine F, Gasior B, et al. Role of vascular reconstructive surgery in impotence: a review of 335 patients over 7 years. J Urol 143:318A, 1990.

48. Fitch WP. Penile arterial revascularization. J Urol 139:402A, 1988.

49. Cookson MS, Phillips DL, Huff ME, Fitch WP III. Analysis of microsurgical penile revascularization results by etiology of impotence. J Urol 149:1308, 1993.

50. MacGregor RJ, Konnack JW. Treatment of vasculogenic erectile dysfunction by direct anastomosis of the inferior epigastric artery to the central artery to the corpus cavernosum. J Urol 127:136, 1982.

51. Konnack JW, Ohl DA. Microsurgical penile revascularization using the central corporal penile artery. J Urol 142:305, 1989.

52. Crespo E, Soltanik E, Bove D, et al. Treatment of vasculogenic sexual impotence by revascularizing cavernous and/or dorsal arteries using microvascular techniques. Urology 20:271, 1982.

53. Lewis RW. Arteriovenous surgeries: do they make any sense? In: Lue TF, ed. World Book of Impotence. London: Smith-Gordon 1992:199.

54. Virag R, Zwang G, Dermange H, Legman M. Vas-

culogenic impotence: a review of 92 cases with 54 surgical operations. Vasc Surg 15:9, 1981.

55. Bennett AH. Venous arterialization for erectile impotence. Urol Clin North Am 15:111, 1988.

56. Virag R, Bennett AH. Arterial and venous surgery for vasculogenic impotence: a combined French and American experience. Arch It Urol 63:95, 1991.

57. Barada JH, Bennett A. Penile revascularization: where do we stand? Int J Impot Res 2:79, 1990.

58. Sohn M, Sikora R, Bohndorf K, Deutz F-J. Selective microsurgery in arteriogenic erectile failure. World J Urol 8:104, 1990.

59. Balko A, Malhotra CM, Wincze JP, Susset JG. Deep penile vein arterialization for arterial and venous impotence. Arch Surg 121:774, 1986.

60. Wagenknecht LV. Microsurgical arterialization for vascular impotence. Microsurgery 9:258, 1988.

61. Zorgnotti AW, Lizza EF. Penile revascularization. In: Zorgnotti AW, Lizza EF, eds. Diagnosis and Management of Impotence. Toronto: BC Decker Inc, 1991.

62. Hauri D. A new operative technique in vasculogenic erectile impotence. World J Urol 4:237, 1986.

63. Schramek P, Engelmann U, Kaufmann F. Microsurgical arteriovenous revascularization in the treatment of vasculogenic impotence. J Urol 147:1028, 1992.

64. Hatzichristou DG, Goldstein I. Penile microvascular arterial bypass surgery. Atlas Urol Clin North Am 1:xx, 1993:

65. Saenz de Tejada I, Moroukian P, Tessier J, et al.

The trabecular smooth muscle modulates the capacitor function of the penis. Studies on a rabbit model. Am J Physiol 260 (Heart Circ Physiol):H1590, 1991.

66. Bergamini TM, Towne JB, Bandyc DF, et al. Experience with in situ saphenous vein bypasses during 1981 to 1989: determinant factors of long-term patency. J Vasc Surg 13:137, 1991.

67. Leather RP, Shah DM, Chang BB, Kaufman JL. Resurrection of the in situ saphenous vein bypass: 1000 cases later. Ann Surg 208:435, 1988.

68. Hatzichristou DG, Goldstein I, Kasznica J, Quist W. The native venous architecture is preserved in an "arterialized" deep dorsal vein graft for arteriogenic impotence: a case report. J Urol (in press).

69. Hatzichristou DG, Goldstein I, Quist W. Pre-existing vascular disease in donor and recipient vessels in microvascular arterial bypass surgery for impotence. Int J Impot Res 4:A137, 1992.

70. Clowes AW, Reidy MA. Prevention of stenosis after vascular reconstruction: pharmacologic control of intimal hyperplasia—a review. J Vasc Surg 6:885, 1991.

71. Leather RP, Shah DM. Experiences with in situ lower extremity saphenous vein bypass procedures. Surg Annu 20:257, 1988.

72. LoGerfo FW, Quist WC, Crawshaw HM, Haudenschild C. An improved technique for preservation of endothelial morphology in vein grafts. Surgery 90:1015, 1981.

CHAPTER 17

Vasoactive Pharmacotherapy

James H. Barada
Roger M. McKimmy

The treatment of erectile dysfunction has taken many paths over the last three decades. Oral therapy with a variety of agents has not proved satisfactory, so attention turned to the development of a mechanical substitute for the erection process in the form of penile prostheses. Despite tremendous advances in surgical technique and mechanical reliability, there has been resistance to widespread application of penile prostheses because of concerns over malfunction, infections, and the less than satisfying presence of a foreign device. The use of intracavernosal vasoactive therapy in the treatment of erectile dysfunction is the result of a fortuitous observation by Ronald Virag[1] in the course of a lower extremity vascular reconstruction procedure. Being a vascular surgeon, he recognized the utility of papaverine hydrochloride to attenuate vasospasm during small vessel vascular anastomoses.[2] The injection of 80 mg of papaverine into the hypogastric artery resulted in a rigid intraoperative erection. This observation was followed by direct intracavernosal injection in men with erectile dysfunction.

A year or so later, Brindley[3,4] performed intracavernosal self-injection of either phentolamine or phenoxybenzamine and then applied the findings of his pharmacologically induced erections to his patients. Thus, the era of intracavernosal vasoactive therapy for diagnosis and treatment of erectile dysfunction was ushered in. Since that time, there has been an explosion of laboratory and clinical research on various vasoactive agents and their combinations as well as diagnostic and treatment algorithms for their use.

The early enthusiasm for intracavernosal vasoactive therapy was quickly tempered by the realization that it did not prove to be a panacea for erectile dysfunction therapy and prolonged erection, priapism, or fibrosis could be sequelae of treatment.[5-7] Rather, it represents a viable treatment option for selected patients who must be educated in dosing, administration, and the potential for complications. There exists no ideal pharmacologic agent for on-demand treatment of erectile dysfunction. However, in many instances a carefully planned and implemented home pharmacologic erection program can achieve the goals of many patients, that is, a return to active and satisfactory sexual function in as natural a fashion as possible.

This chapter will review the clinical pharmacology of the various available intracavernosal vasoactive agents, their clinical utility, and treatment outcomes. A suggested method of patient selection and teaching for self-injection in the home setting and the treatment of potential complications are discussed.

PHARMACOLOGY OF INTRACAVERNOSAL AGENTS

In spite of a decade of intense vasoactive pharmacotherapy research, precise neurochemical events governing erection remain elusive. A number of putative nonadrenergic noncholinergic neurotransmitters have been isolated by immunohistochemical techniques from corporal tissue. Recently, the electrophysiology of corporal smooth muscle has been described,[8] clarifying the means by which very small volumes and doses of drugs can initiate and maintain the sequence of physiologic events culminating in an erection. Following is a brief discussion of the molecular physiology of penile erection, followed by monographs of agents known to induce pharmacologic erections.

Molecular Physiology of Erections

As discussed in earlier chapters, the key event in penile erection is relaxation of corporal smooth muscle. During periods of penile flaccidity, the corporal smooth muscle is in a state of tonic contraction maintained by an underlying sympathetic tone (adrenergic tone). As the smooth muscle relaxes, engorgement of the sinusoidal spaces with blood occurs, coinciding with an increase in penile arterial inflow in response to the simultaneous relaxation of arterial vascular smooth muscle. The emissary veins between the sinusoids and the tunica albuginea are compressed, retarding venous outflow from the corporal bodies. As inflow exceeds outflow, tumescence ensues. Continued stimulation further increases smooth muscle relaxation, and the increased turgor of the corporal tissue against the unyielding tunica albuginea increases intracavernosal pressure with a resultant rigid erection. Thus, an erection is a mechanical manifestation of a hemodynamic event.

At the cellular level, smooth muscle contraction is under the control of calcium ions and their action on regulatory proteins associated with thick myosin filaments called *light chains*. These are interspersed with actin filaments, which are anchored to dense bodies in a collagen matrix. As with skeletal muscle, the contractile cycle begins with charging of a myosin head to form a myosin-ATP intermediate, which then can bind with an actin filament to form an ATPase complex.[9] The ATPase complex rapidly splits ATP into ADP and inorganic phosphate. This energy-liberating step produces motion of the filaments relative to each other and, hence, contraction. The actin-myosin complex cannot dissociate to repeat the process until another ATP molecule binds with the myosin head. The activity of the ATPase formed by actin-myosin complexes is minimal until each of the light chains is phosphorylated, which is an ATP-dependent process. Once phosphorylated, the actin-myosin complex is free to hydrolyze additional ATP molecules for contraction. Myosin light chain kinase is the calcium-dependent enzyme responsible for light chain phosphorylation. Myosin light chain kinase can exist in active and inactive forms. Transition from inactive to active (calcium-sensitive) light chain kinase depends on the calcium-dependent regulatory protein, calmodulin.[10] When internal calcium concentrations fall during smooth muscle relaxation, light chain phosphorylation ceases. Phosphorylase enzyme acts to dephosphorylate the myosin chains, thus inactivating actin-myosin ATPase. During muscle contraction, the action of light chain kinase overwhelms that of phosphatase because increases in the free internal calcium concentration drive the phosphorylation of myosin light chain kinase.[11]

Smooth muscle may be made to contract by a variety of signals including nervous stimulation, hormones, physical distention, and a variety of drugs.[12] The action of any of these may be modified by a number of local factors. Neuromuscular junctions such as those in skeletal muscle are not found in smooth muscle. The autonomic nerve fibers innervating smooth muscle branch and ramify extensively near the outer sheet of muscle fibers, but never make direct contact with them. The terminal axons of these fibers have varicosities arrayed along their length, from which neurotransmitters are secreted.[13] These commonly act only on the outer sheet of muscle fibers to which they are exposed, and the underlying fibers then contract as the resulting action potential conducts through the muscle mass, either by subsequent diffusion of the neurotransmitter substance or by second messenger communication via gap junctions. Again, in contrast to the neuromuscular junction of skeletal muscle, which secretes only acetylcholine, the varicosities of smooth muscle may secrete either acetylcholine or norepinephrine according to the branch of the autonomic nervous system from which they originate.[12]

Ordinarily, acetylcholine serves to depolarize the smooth muscle cell membrane by opening voltage-dependent calcium channels. In human corporal smooth muscle, however, acetylcholine does not have a direct effect, but rather seems to exert a modulating effect on the action of other neurotransmitters.[14,15] This idea is supported by the observation that in vitro corporal smooth muscle treated with acetylcholine has equivocal relaxation responses.[16–18] It has long been known, however, that stimulation of preganglionic pelvic parasympathetic nerves can produce erections in animals.[19] Clearly, neurotransmitters other than acetylcholine are at work in producing erection and have come to be referred to collectively as nonadrenergic noncholinergic (NANC) substances. These include vasoactive intestinal polypeptide (VIP),[20–22] prostaglandins, endothelial-derived relaxation factor (EDRF) (now known to be nitric oxide [NO]),[23,24] neuropeptide Y,[25] peptide histidine methionine,[26] somatostatin,[27] and calcitonin gene-related peptide (CGRP).[28,29] The precise role of each in human erectile function remains to be clarified, but several have properties useful in the intracavernosal pharmacotherapy of erectile dysfunction.

Human erectile tissue has been shown to contain alpha-adrenergic receptors in a ratio of 9:1 to those of beta-adrenergic receptors.[30] The predominant receptor subtype is alpha$_1$, which has been shown to contract in response to catecholamines. The significance of these receptors lies in their coupling to membrane-bound adenylate cyclase or guanylate cyclase on the surface of most smooth muscle cells outside the genital system. Catecholamines classicly activate the cyclases, which then catalyze the formation of the second messenger cAMP. This begins a cascade terminating in the activation of phosphorylase,[31] which serves to dephosphorylate myosin light chains and thus relax smooth muscle.[11] In corporal smooth muscle, however, catecholamines induce smooth muscle contraction and detumescence.[32] In vitro preparations demonstrate that increased cyclic mononucleotide concentrations correspond to relaxation,[33] but adenylate cyclase activity in corporal smooth muscle appears to be coupled to transmitters or modulators other than catecholamines.

One such transmitter appears to be NO, originally described as EDRF. Release of NO from the sinusoidal endothelium of corporal tissue stimulates guanylate cyclase, leading to elevated intracellular concentrations of cGMP and smooth muscle relaxation.[34-36] In vitro preparations of human corporal tissue from diabetic patients with erectile dysfunction have displayed impaired endothelium-dependent relaxation,[37] and drugs supplying or liberating NO from endothelium in these patients are obviously of interest.

The intracellular concentrations of cAMP and cGMP have very important effects on smooth muscle contractility, chiefly by altering the degree of phosphorylation of several key enzymes that indirectly inhibits contraction.[11] For example, ATP-dependent pumps can drive calcium outside the cell or into the smooth muscle cell's rudimentary sarcoplasmic reticulum. This has the effect of lowering intracellular calcium concentrations and inhibiting contraction. The action of several of the drugs used in pharmacotherapy of erectile dysfunction can be explained by their effect on cyclic mononucleotide breakdown or production.

Left unexplained by our knowledge of corpus cavernosal anatomy and its sparse innervation is the fact that, for example, microgram quantities of prostaglandin E_1 (PGE_1) can promptly elicit an erection. The fact that simple drug diffusion cannot explain this observation led to the proposal of gap junctions between smooth muscle cells, serving to form a functional syncytium much the same way as they do in cardiac muscle.[38-41] These allow intercellular passage of ion flux and important second messenger molecules, including potassium, calcium, cAMP, and inositol triphosphate (ID3), which are believed to mediate calcium release from the sarcoplasmic reticulum of smooth muscle.[42] The actual number of cells acted upon directly by PGE_1 may in fact be quite low, but synchronous relaxation of all corporal smooth muscle may occur via gap junctions. It has been speculated that the previously described NANC transmitter substances are the true currency of coordinated corporal smooth muscle relaxation and erection.[20,21,28,32,43-46] Each may elicit its effects through passive diffusion and activity through gap junctions.

DRUGS USED IN INTRACAVERNOSAL THERAPY OF IMPOTENCE

For practical purposes, there are four drugs, or a combination thereof, currently used in intracavernosal pharmacotherapy of impotence. This may change with ongoing research investigating the role of NANC transmitters and intraurethral delivery systems. Additionally, a number of agents are being used in experimental investigations; for completeness they are considered here briefly as well.

Papaverine

Papaverine is a benzylisoquinoline alkaloid isolated from the opium poppy. It shares no pharmacologic properties with the opiate alkaloids, however, and derives its usefulness in medicine from its ability to relax smooth muscle, particulary vascular smooth muscle. Papaverine has long been employed in vascular surgery to prevent vasospasm, and it is this feature that led to the fortuitous discovery that it can produce a sustained erection in impotent men when injected into a corporal body. Papaverine's efficacy as a smooth muscle relaxant stems from several intracellular actions. First, it has an inhibitory effect on cyclic mononucleotide phosphodiesterases, leading to increased cAMP and cGMP concentrations.[47] Second, papaverine blocks voltage-dependent calcium channels, thus impairing calcium influx and downregulating myosin light chain kinase, and may impair calcium-activated potassium and chloride currents.[48,49] All of these actions relax smooth muscle, which has been demonstrated in the smooth muscle of the cavernous sinusoids as well as the vascular smooth muscle of the penile and helicine arteries.[50] Papaverine also has been shown to increase resistance to venous outflow from the penis, which probably results from corporovenous occlusion rather than from a contractile effect.[51]

Papaverine is one of few intracavernosal drugs for which pharmacokinetic data are available. It is metabolized extensively in the liver, and the plasma half-life is 1 to 2 hours.[52,53] Following intracavernosal injection, papaverine achieves peak serum concentrations in 10 to 30 minutes at approximately one fifth the concentration achieved with an intravenous injection of the same dose. The half-life of penile papaverine is much greater than that of the serum half-life, implying a deeper pharmacokinetic compartment when injected intracavernosally.

The toxicity of papaverine is limited to two effects: (1) a local corporal fibrosis believed to be related to the acidic pH (3 to 4) to which the solution is buffered[54] and (2) a hepatocellular toxicity manifested either as transient elevation of transaminases or, much less commonly, clinical hepatitis.[55]

Phentolamine

Phentolamine is a competitive, nonspecific alpha-adrenoceptor antagonist of the 2-substituted imidazoline class. In doses used intravenously in treatment of hypertension, its predominant mechanism of action, however, is a direct action on smooth muscle to cause relaxation.[55,56] The exact mechanism for this relaxation is not known, and which action predominates in doses used intracavernosally is also unknown. Intracavernous phentolamine as a single agent seldom produces a satisfactory erection, in contrast to the classic alpha-antagonist phenoxybenzamine.[57] Since phentolamine is both an alpha$_1$- and alpha$_2$-antagonist, it may be that the prejunctional alpha$_2$-blockade increases norepinephrine release from the presynaptic terminus, which would have the effect of competitively antagonizing the postjunctional alpha$_1$-blocking effect of the drug.

Phentolamine has been compared with papaverine regarding its effect on penile blood flow.[58] Both drugs decrease resistance to arterial inflow, but phentolamine does not increase resistance to venous outflow as papaverine does.

The plasma half-life of phentolamine is short (30 minutes) and is metabolized in the liver before excretion. Peak serum concentrations following intracavernosal administration occur in 20 to 30 minutes, then rapidly decline to unmeasurable levels.[53]

Intravenously administered phentolamine has been known to cause tachycardia and orthostatic hypotension. Cardiac arrhythmias and anginal pain may occur on rare occasion, and phentolamine also may cause gastrointestinal stimulation manifest as abdominal pain, nausea, vomiting, and diarrhea.[55] All of these effects are rarely, if ever, seen with intracavernosal administration.[59]

Prostaglandin E$_1$ (PGE$_1$, Alprostadil)

The prostaglandins, as a class of autocoids, are ubiquitous in the body. All are cyclic endoperoxides that are products of arachidonic acid metabolism, and an amazing variety of pharmacologic effects can be produced by slight variations in their structure. Different prostaglandins may have exactly opposite effects on the same tissue; such is the case for PGE$_1$, which is a potent smooth muscle relaxant, and PGF$_{2\alpha}$, a likewise potent smooth muscle contractant.[60] The exact mechanism by which this can be achieved is not known, but the fact that both of these substances, as well as thromboxane A$_2$, have been detected in human corporal tissue supports the contention that they function as NANC modulators of erectile function. They also may function as alpha-adrenergic blockers and may elevate intracellular levels of cGMP.[33,61]

The pharmacokinetics of the prostaglandins are not well characterized, but systemically administered PGE$_1$ is nearly completely cleared in a single pass through the pulmonary vascular bed.[62] There

is also evidence that PGE$_1$ is metabolized in the penis.[63] These two metabolic features may account for the fact that circulatory side effects and prolonged erections are seldom seen with intracavernosal PGE$_1$. The most bothersome side effect of PGE$_1$ is pain at the site of injection.[59]

Atropine

Atropine is a tropane alkaloid, the classic antimuscarinic anticholinergic drug that has received relatively recent interest in intracavernosal pharmacotherapy of erectile dysfunction.[64,65] In tissue concentrations in excess of those targeted for its anticholinergic effect, atropine is believed to stimulate release of EDRF (NO) from the sinusoidal endothelium of corporal tissue.

Systemic side effects of atropine would be expected to include tachycardia, xerostomia, drowsiness, mydriasis, and cycloplegia. These have not been observed in the limited number of clinical studies investigating intracavernosal atropine, and the pharmacokinetics of the drug following such therapy has not yet been described.

Phenoxybenzamine

Phenoxybenzamine, like phentolamine, is a nonspecific alpha-antagonist but differs from the latter in that it binds covalently with alpha-receptors, forming an irreversible or noncompetitive blockade.[55] It has been speculated that synthesis of new receptors is necessary to restore tissue responsiveness to alpha-agonists. Phenoxybenzamine also blocks receptors for acetylcholine, histamine, and serotonin (5-HT),[55] although the significance of this with regard to human erectile tissue is not known.

The metabolic fate of phenoxybenzamine is poorly understood. A haloalkylamine, it is very lipid soluble at physiologic pH, and it is known to accumulate in body fat. Phenoxybenzamine has a relatively long plasma half-life of at least 12 hours, which together with the noncompetitive nature of its alpha-blockade may explain both prolonged effects following systemic administration (in some cases lasting several days) and the relatively high incidence of prolonged erection following intracavernosal injection.[66]

The classic systemic adverse reaction to phenoxybenzamine is orthostatic hypotension, which may be associated with reflex tachycardia and possibly cardiac dysrhythmias. The lipid solubility of the drug allows penetration of the blood-brain barrier, and central nervous system effects such as hyperventilation, motor excitability, and nausea may be seen. Peripheral effects of alpha-blockade include nasal stuffiness, miosis, and inhibition of ejaculation.[55] Intracavernosal phenoxybenzamine produces pain at the site of injection, has a slow onset of action, and with repeated injections has a propensity to cause corporal fibrosis.[66] For all of these reasons, phenoxybenzamine has fallen into disfavor in clinical therapy of erectile dysfunction despite its undeniable efficacy.

Moxisylyte (Thymoxamine)

Moxisylyte is an alpha-adrenergic antagonist that attracted interest as an intracavernosal agent by virtue of its relatively selective action on alpha-receptors. It also may have antihistaminic properties and possesses a short duration of action (3 to 4 hours) following systemic administration. Moxisylyte has been shown in vitro to ameliorate the action of norepinephrine-contracted human corporal tissue[67] but is less potent than phentolamine in this regard. Not surprisingly, moxisylyte as a single agent has been shown to be less active than papaverine in inducing full erections.[68] Correspondingly, the incidence of prolonged erection and systemic side effects following intracavernosal injections is low, and investigators have stressed the advantage of safety with this agent.

Trazodone

Trazodone is a triazolopyridine derivative used orally as an antidepressant. A central inhibitor of 5-HT uptake and facilitator of brain dopamine turnover, it is generally classed with the tricyclic and tetracyclic antidepressants but is chemically unrelated and termed an *atypical* antidepressant, lacking the antimuscarinic properties of the former two groups.[69] In vitro experiments show that trazodone acts as an alpha-antagonist in human erectile tissue.[70] Numerous reports of increased erectile activity and even priapism associated with oral administration of the drug spurred interest in its use intracavernosally in treatment of impotence,[70] but the few investigations of this application have shown limited efficacy.[71]

VIP

VIP is a 28-amino-acid residue originally isolated from the small intestine and is a potent vasodilator, cardiac inotrope, bronchodilator, exocrine secretagogue, stimulant of gastrointestinal motility, and smooth muscle relaxant.[72] VIP has since been demonstrated throughout the CNS and in peripheral nerves[73] and is believed to be the nonadrenergic, noncholinergic neurotransmitter responsible for autonomic actions at a number of sites in the body, for example, the anticholinergic-resistant stimulation of salivary secretion. This

knowledge led to speculation that VIP may also be a key neurotransmitter involved in penile erection. In animal models, intracavernosal infusions of anti-VIP serum have abolished erections caused by electrical stimulation of pelvic nerves.[74] However, intracavernosal VIP even in high doses does not produce erection and is therefore unlikely to be the sole neurotransmitter in human penile erection.[75,76]

CGRP

CGRP is a 37-amino-acid residue and a potent vasodilator, which has been detected in blood vessels supplying the corporal bodies as well as in cavernosal smooth muscle. It has been shown to induce a dose-related increase in penile arterial inflow and cavernous smooth muscle relaxation.[28,77] In contrast to VIP, CGRP has been shown to be quite efficacious in producing erections, and combination therapy with PGE$_1$ has been effective in impotent men who are refractory to other combinations of drugs.[78] Systemic side effects consisting of facial flushing and hypotension have been observed with intracavernosal CGRP.

Linsidomine

Related to the antianginal drug molsidomine, linsidomine shares with atropine the property of releasing NO from endothelium, thus stimulating guanylate cyclase to generate intracellular cGMP.[79] This is likely responsible for linsidomine's action as a vasodilator. Linsidomine also has an inhibitory effect on platelet aggregation.[80] It is capable of producing a full erection when injected intracavernosally and has a short half-life of approximately 30 to 60 minutes. Linsidomine has not yet been studied extensively in controlled clinical trials, but recent studies have shown it to be markedly inferior to PGE$_1$ in efficacy.[81]

DRUGS USED IN TOPICAL THERAPY OF IMPOTENCE

Intracavernosal pharmacotherapy for impotence is invariably associated with a moderately high number of drop-outs from therapy, related in part to unwillingness to receive injections. This has led to interest in known topically active vasodilators in the treatment of impotence. Currently, two such agents have been investigated.

Nitroglycerin

In vitro studies have demonstrated the ability of both nitroglycerin and isosorbide to relax isolated human corporal smooth muscle. It is believed to act by stimulating guanylate cyclase.[82] Several trials investigating transcutaneous nitroglycerin administered via patches have shown activity in roughly one half of enrolled patients. Side effects of headache and hypotension occurred frequently (roughly 50%) in each group.[83,84]

Minoxidil

Minoxidil is a oral vasodilator used in the treatment of hypertension. Its activity is believed to stem from its ability to open ATP-dependent potassium channels, leading to hyperpolarization of the smooth muscle cell membrane and reduced sensitivity to contractile stimuli.[85] The oral preparation has a number of side effects, including hypertrichosis. Minoxidil is readily absorbed transcutaneously, a feature exploited in the topical preparation currently marketed for treatment of alopecia (Rogaine), and this preparation has been investigated in the treatment of impotence. Early double-blind trials show minoxidil to be superior to topical nitroglycerin or placebo in increasing penile rigidity when applied to the glans penis.[86]

CLINICAL STUDIES OF VASOACTIVE PHARMACOTHERAPY
Papaverine Monotherapy

Papaverine hydrochloride was the first of the intracavernous vasoactive agents to be used for the treatment of erectile dysfunction. This was a dramatic departure from the standard therapy of the day, penile prosthesis, and it sparked intensive research of the physiology and diagnostic evaluation of erectile dysfunction.

Virag's[1] original paper described bimonthly injection of 80 mg of papaverine followed by corporal infusion with heparin solution to maintain a rigid erection for 15 minutes. In 14 patients with presumed organic impotence, this therapy proved beneficial after two or more treatments in 9 (64%). Four of these patients returned to normal sexual activity without the need for further corporal infusion. This study was followed by a larger group of patients with organic impotence due to diabetes or arterial inflow disease based on radiographic studies.[87] Sixty-six percent of patients had return of functional erections and were satisfied. In a later report of 109 patients with psychogenic or neurogenic erectile dysfunction,[88] all patients were able to achieve an adequate erection. The average dose required was significantly less than the earlier organic impotence group (26 mg vs 60 mg).

The use of in-office vasoactive therapy did not prove to be as successful as initially hoped, that is, the intermittent stimulation therapy did not return the majority of patients to normal sexual function. The repeated office visits and patient inter-action may have served as a modified form of psychotherapy. Patients with organic impotence, although successfully able to achieve an erection with the in-office injection, were for the most part unable to return to successful intercourse without the aid of injections in the home setting. Thus, attention turned to the development of home pharmacologic erection programs to treat the majority of patients with erectile dysfunction.

Brindley[3] initially advocated phenoxybenzamine as a vasoactive intracavernosal injection agent but subsequently adopted papaverine as his primary drug for home therapy. In his initial report, 34 patients used papaverine injection for up to 2 years. Prolonged erection (greater than 12 hours) occurred in 12 patients (35%), the majority requiring pharmacologic reversal. Only one systemic reaction (trembling) to papaverine was reported (2.9%). Penile fibrosis at the injection site was identified in one patient (2.9%), who subsequently went on to prothesis implantation.

Gilbert and Gingell[89] reported on 194 men using papaverine alone with a minimum follow-up of 12 months (mean: 14 months). The cause of erectile dysfunction was primarily psychogenic. At follow-up, 59 men (30.4%) continued on therapy and were satisfied. Spontaneous return of erections was seen in 21 patients (10.8%) reflecting the high proportion of psychogenic patients. Prolonged erections occurred in 5 cases (2.6%), but corporal fibrosis was not observed.

Risk factors for prolonged erection (greater than 3 hours) following papaverine injection was examined by Lomas and Jarow.[90] Four hundred patients received a standard dose of papaverine (60 mg), which was reduced (15 mg) in spinal cord injury patients. Prolonged erection occurred in 67 patients (17%). Statistically significant risk factors were younger age, better quality of spontaneous erection, and neurogenic or psychogenic cause of erectile dysfunction. The presence of coronary artery disease or a vasculogenic cause of erectile dysfunction was associated with a statistically lower risk of prolonged erection.

The incidence of prolonged erection following the diagnostic and therapeutic use of papaverine as vasoactive pharmacotherapy is shown in Table 17–1. Difficulties in interpreting this data are encountered because of variations in the study population, dosage variability, and the differing duration of erection that comprises a prolonged or priapismic pharmacologic erection. Also contributing to the variability of results is the investigators' learning curve for judging papaverine dosing for the individual patient. Nonetheless, prolonged erection is recognized as a significant complication of papaverine monotherapy.

The same variability in reporting is also true for

TABLE 17–1
Reported Incidence of Papaverine-Induced Priapism

Reference	Papaverine Dose (mg)	No. of Patients	Incidence (%)
Brindley[3]	16–120	34	35.3
Lue et al.[99]	60	90	18.8
Lomas and Jarow[90]	30 or 15	400	17
Bodner et al.[164]	80	20	15.0
Cooper[161]	30–95	20	10
Pettirossi and Serenelli[165]	30–110	144	8.3
Postma et al.[166]	25–50	48	6.3
Gilbert and Gingell[89]	30–120	194	2.6
Lakin et al.[167]	30	8	0

determining the incidence of papaverine-induced corporal fibrosis. The pathophysiology of development of corporal fibrosis is not clearly understood; proposed mechanisms include microtrauma from needle injection, the low pH of the injection solution, or microprecipitation of papaverine at physiologic pH.[54,91] The presentation of fibrosis can be subtle, with changes apparent only on ultrasound examination of the corpora, or dramatic, with complete corporal fibrosis.[3,92–94] The incidence of fibrosis in clinical studies ranges from 1% to 33%.[3,93,95,96] It appears that the presence of fibrotic changes is both dose dependent and cumulative, although significant changes following limited injections coupled with prolonged erection has been reported.[97] When identified, the fibrotic changes usually result in the recommendation of discontinuing therapy, although significant penile curvature, except with concomitant Peyronie's disease, is not well documented. The natural course of the fibrosis upon withdrawal of injection therapy is also unknown; however, Sidi et al.[98] reported minimal histologic changes of corporal tissue at the time of prosthesis implantation for failure of vasoactive pharmacotherapy.

Systemic reactions to papaverine injection manifested as pallor, dizziness, facial flushing, and sweating have been reported with papaverine injection.[99–101] Tanaka[52] measured systemic papaverine levels following corporal injection and noted that patients who had a poor erectile response had statistically higher peripheral blood levels, suggesting corporovenous occlusive dysfunction. Wespes and Schulman[100] noted a systemic reaction in 6 out of 75 patients receiving 60 mg papaverine in the course of a diagnostic evaluation. The episodes were self-limiting and were managed by recumbency and lower-extremity elevation. All patients had severe venous leak on subsequent cavernosography.

Papaverine-Phentolamine Combination Pharmacotherapy

Papaverine as a single agent for vasoactive pharmacotherapy has a delayed onset of action, variability in its efficacy between doses, and significant risk of prolonged erection, systemic reaction, and delayed corporal fibrosis. Zorgniotti and Lafleur[57] combined papaverine with phentolamine in a ratio of 30 mg papaverine : .5 mg phentolamine in an effort to increase the safety profile of vasoactive pharmacotherapy. This dosage ratio has been extensively studied and is at present the most widely used vasoactive drug combination. The study's initial 250 patients were evaluated with a solution of 30 mg papaverine and 1 mg phentolamine. The mixture resulted in an erection satisfactory for intercourse in 72% of patients. Of these patients, 97% went on to self-injection with excellent response and a low drop-out rate. Prolonged erection occurred in four of the diagnostic injections (1.6%) but in only one patient on home therapy. Four of the 97 (4.1%) patients on home therapy developed fibrotic changes felt to be confined to the tunica albuginea, prompting discontinuation of therapy.[102]

A prospective double-blind placebo trial of papaverine-phentolamine vs saline injection by Gasser et al.[103] demonstrated the efficacy of this combination in men with organic erectile dysfunction. Twenty-four of 29 patients (83%) had a good erectile response to papaverine-phentolamine vs none in the saline group. One prolonged erection occurred (3.4%), resolving spontaneously.

Stief and Wetterauer[104] compared papaverine or phentolamine alone vs a papaverine-phentolamine combination in men with an organic cause of erectile dysfunction. The papaverine-phentolamine (15 mg/ml + .5 mg/ml [.5 to 3.0 ml]) combination was superior to papaverine (30 mg) or phentolamine (1.0 mg), with full erection occurring in 87% vs 40% (papaverine) and 7% (phentolamine).

The development of a home injection program using papaverine-phentolamine combination stresses the need for careful evaluation, meticulous teaching by the physician or nurse, and careful instructions for recognition and prompt treatment of complications.

In a follow-up study of 156 patients, Stief et al.[105] examined the efficacy and safety of papaverine-phentolamine combination therapy. Only 10 patients discontinued home therapy (6.4%). Satisfaction with this form of therapy was reported by 92.5% of the patients and 96.2% of the partners queried. Three patients (1.9%) had a prolonged erection, all of which followed a second injection after presumed failure of the initial injection. Three additional patients (1.9%) developed localized fibrosis at the injection site, all of which resolved by withholding injections for 8 weeks. No cavernosal fibrosis was present by clinical examination or cavernosal ultrasound.

Sidi et al.[106] retrospectively reviewed 239 patients using a papaverine-phentolamine combination for home injection therapy. They found that 78.2% were satisfied with the overall program, 75.3% with the degree of penile rigidity following injection, and 80% with the duration of erection. Most of the patients who continued to use self-injection were enthusiastic about the therapy and would continue as long as no complications occurred. The total drop-out rate was 25%, primarily due to tachyphylaxis, lack of spontaneity, inconvenience, and concern over long-term side effects.

Goldstein et al.[107] presented the early results of 300 patients who had a home pharmacologic erection. The solution used in their study contained 22.5 mg/ml papaverine and 1.25 mg/ml phentolamine, and patients were titrated to effect from .1 ml to 1.0 ml. More than two thirds of the patients had a vasculogenic cause of their erectile dysfunction, primarily corporovenous occlusive dysfunction. Of patients who completed 3 or more months of therapy, 79% continued to do so with satisfaction. The majority of patients discontinuing therapy elected no further treatment of their erectile dysfunction. Seven patients (2.3%) developed prolonged erections and were successfully treated with alpha-agonist therapy.

Less successful outcomes of papaverine-phentolamine combination pharmacotherapy was reported by Girdley et al.[108] in 78 patients. These patients used a drug dose of 30 mg/ml papaverine and 1.0 mg/ml phentolamine in volumes from .2 to 2.0 ml. Most patients (93.5%) reported at least one complication, primarily transient pain (78%), bruising (47%), or superficial/deep penile swelling (46%). Prolonged erection (>6 hours) occurred in 18 patients (23%). Induration and/or fibrosis was present in 13 patients (16%) and was more commonly seen in patients with a vasculogenic cause of erectile dysfunction. Most of these resolved with suspension of injections. Variability of erectile response was common: 49% of patients using a consistent dose experienced at least one episode of inadequate rigidity or duration of erection. Forty percent of patients were satisfied with the injection program, whereas 28% found the therapy unacceptable. Poor health of the patient or partner, or patient/partner dissatisfaction was cited as the primary reasons for drop-out. Less frequently, failure or variability of the erectile response or significant fibrosis prompted discontinuation of therapy.

Robinette and Moffat[109] used a papaverine-phentolamine combination (0.5 ml of papaverine 30 mg/ml and phentolamine 2.5 mg/ml) for diagnosis and home therapy in 101 patients with 2- to 12-month follow-up. Seventy-eight patients (77%) continued therapy, and all were reported to be satisfied or very satisfied with therapy. Prolonged erections occurred in seven patients (6.9%), three of which resolved spontaneously while two patients required a shunt procedure.

Nellans et al.[110] used papverine-phentolamine in 69 patients with various erectile dysfunction causes. A good response to injection was present in 67% of patients; failures were seen in the group with severe arterial disease or significant corporovenous occlusive dysfunction. Psychogenic or neurogenic causes of erectile dysfunction was present in 47% of patients. Forty-eight patients went on to a self-injection program, with good results reported by 74% of patients. Prolonged erection occurred in 6 patients (8.7%); one patient developed a localized fibrotic plaque (1.4%).

Special populations for which papaverine-phentolamine combinations have been successful include post–pelvic trauma patients,[111] psychogenic impotence patients,[112-114] spinal cord injury patients,[115-117] post–radical pelvic surgery patients,[118,119] and elderly patients.[120,121] In general, patients with psychogenic or neurogenic impotence have intact arterial inflow and competent veno-occlusive mechanisms and require reduced doses of vasoactive agents to achieve a satisfactory erection compared with patients with diabetic or vasculogenic causes of impotence. As expected, there is significant spontaneous return to natural erections in the psychogenic group. In patients who have had radical pelvic surgery, again a successful outcome can be achieved with low doses of papaverine-phentolamine combination.

The elderly patient represents a special challenge for institution of vasoactive pharmacotherapy. These patients tend to have a lower expectation of therapy and require special teaching because of decreased hand-eye coordination. Kerfoot and Carson[121] observed that the dose of papaverine-phentolamine required for adequate erectile response was higher in elderly men than that needed in a control group approximately 20 years younger in age; however, the incidence of prolonged erection and fibrosis was similar. Table 17–2 summarizes the incidence of prolonged erections and corporal fibrosis associated with papaverine-phentolamine combination therapy. The caveats of interpretation discussed in the papaverine section again apply.

PGE₁

The clinical use of PGE₁ began with the observation of Ishii et al.[122] that patients receiving intravenous PGE₁ for peripheral vascular disease had improvement in their erectile dysfunction. This finding prompted them to use an intracavernous injection of PGE₁ at the same dose (20 μg) as that used in intravenous therapy. The onset of action was rapid, within 2 to 3 minutes after injection. Full or partial erections were observed in 86% of 135 patients with all types of erectile dysfunction causes. Erection rates were lower in patients with previous pelvic fracture or diabetes mellitus. The duration of erection was 1 to 3 hours, and no patient had a prolonged pharmacologic erection requiring reversal. Dull penile pain following injection was present in "a limited number" of patients.

The diagnostic value of PGE₁ for erectile dysfunction as compared to papaverine was discussed by Buvat et al.[92] They found that 20 μg PGE₁ had a higher specificity for discriminating between psychogenic and organic impotence than did papaverine, but PGE₁ had a lower sensitivity. There was no clear correlation between PGE₁ testing and nocturnal penile tumescence monitoring. In 130 men tested with PGE₁, prolonged erection (greater than 4 hours) occurred in 3.8%. All of these resolved spontaneously. Painful injection and/or erection was seen in 47%. Forty-three percent of these patients had pain that was classified as moderate or severe. Systemic reactions of tachycardia, hypotension, or vasovagal response were present in 2.3% of patients. Their findings, compared with a personal series using 80 mg papaverine, showed that PGE₁ had an improved safety profile for prolonged erection or systemic reactions.

Chen et al.[123] found a statistical difference in onset and duration of erection comparing papaverine (60 mg) and PGE₁ (20 μg) in an office setting. A positive response was seen in 54% of the papaverine group and in 70% of the PGE₁ group. Papaverine had a more rapid onset of action; however, PGE₁ had a longer duration of erection. There was no difference in penile rigidity between the two groups. PGE₁ was superior in patients with a diabetic cause for their erectile dysfunction (60% vs 38%). Prolonged erection occurred in 2.9% of the papaverine group but in no patient injected with PGE₁. Penile pain following injection or with ensuing erection was present in 18% of the PGE₁ group vs 8.1% of the papaverine group. Systemic side effects of flushing or dizziness were present in 6% of the papaverine group but were not seen in the PGE₁ group. Their assessment was that PGE₁ was superior to papaverine for diagnostic use and potentially for therapy.

A single-blind crossover study comparing papaverine (18 mg) and PGE₁ (5 μg) 1 month apart by Earle et al.[124] demonstrated that PGE₁ resulted in a better erection as reported by one observer and the PGE₁ response was preferred by the patient. These results were statistically significant.

A double-blind comparison of 50 μg PGE₁ and papaverine-phentolamine (30 mg + 1.0 mg) in 25 patients was reported by Lee et al.[125] All patients had a response to injection, and in nine patients (36%) the PGE₁ was considered superior in rigidity and duration. No prolonged erections were seen in either group. Twenty patients (80%) receiving PGE₁ injections experienced pain on injection or erection. Four of these men felt the pain was severe enough to limit sexual activity. Reducing the concentration decreased the pain.

In the same study a second group of 8 men who

TABLE 17–2

Complications of Papaverine-Phentolamine Combination Therapy

Author	No. of Patients	Prolonged Erections (%)	Fibrosis (%)
Zorgniotti[102]	97	1.0	4.1
Stief and Wetterauer[105]	156	1.9	1.9
Goldstein et al.[107]	300	2.3	—
Girdley et al.[108]	78	23.1	16
Robinette and Moffat[109]	101	6.9	—
Nellans et al.[110]	69	8.7	1.4
Levine et al.[149]	111	1.8	—
Lakin et al.[167]	100	—	15

had a history of prolonged erection with papaverine or papaverine plus phentolamine received an escalating dose of PGE₁ (2.5–10 μg). All eight men responded to injection with erections lasting from 2.5 to 6 hours with spontaneous detumescence. This finding led the authors to suggest PGE₁ therapy for men who have had prolonged erections with vasoactive pharmacotherapy using papaverine or papaverine-phentolamine combinations.

Sarosdy et al.[126] compared 10 or 20 μg PGE₁ to 30 or 60 mg papaverine in 15 patients with erectile dysfunction. This double-blind prospective study revealed that all patients had a full or partial response to PGE₁ including two patients who did not respond to papaverine alone. No systemic side effects or prolonged erections occurred in either group. Although the study did not determine the optimum dose of PGE₁, it was proposed to use this PGE₁ therapy in patients failing papaverine therapy because of its differing mechanism or site of action on corporal smooth muscle relaxation.

In a prospective study of 119 consecutive patients Lui and Lin[127] compared a papaverine-phentolamine mixture (7.5–60 mg papaverine + .25–2.0 mg phentolamine) vs PGE₁ (10–20 μg). A good erectile response to papaverine and phentolamine was seen in 67.1% of 51 patients and 79.1% of 76 patients receiving PGE₁. Four patients in the papaverine-phentolamine group developed prolonged erections (5.3%), whereas none occurred in the PGE₁ group.

Stackl et al.[128] found PGE₁ to be useful as a diagnostic screening test and reported on 112 men entering a home pharmacologic erection program. There were no systemic complications, and no patient reported pain with erection. The required dose varied from 5 to 40 μg; a linear dose response for erection duration was observed. No patient required treatment for prolonged erection. At 4.5-month mean follow-up there were no cases of corporal nodules or fibrosis. The lack of systemic side effects was attributed to the local metabolism of PGE₁ and the rapid first-pass clearance in liver and lung tissue.[60,62]

PGE₁ therapy has been used in patients who failed to respond to office testing with papaverine or had limited success with home injection. Reiss[129] reported on 12 such patients, two of whom had a gradual loss of papaverine response over several months. A dose range of 5 to 20 μg of PGE₁ was used, and all 12 patients reported erections sufficient for intercourse. Seven of 12 patients, including the two papaverine tachyphylaxis failures, began a home injection program with good results. Only one patient reported transient pain with injection.

A double-blind crossover study comparing 60 mg papaverine and 20 μg PGE₁ in vasoculogenic impotence was done by Kattan et al.[130] Five patients were included who had previous diagnostic evaluation suggestive of vasculogenic impotence. All patients had failed previous papaverine injection. Failure to respond to either agent occurred in 52% of patients. Forty-six percent of patients responded to PGE₁ alone or both PGE₁ and papaverine, whereas only 14% responded to papaverine alone or both papaverine and PGE₁. This was statistically significant. There was no statistical difference in the occurrence of transient pain at the injection site, and no patient described pain with erection. Despite the low overall response rate in this selected group of patients, PGE₁ may be an effective agent for salvage in patients with moderate to severe vasculogenic impotence.

Ravnik-Oblak et al.[131] used PGE₁ as therapy for patients with erectile dysfunction due to diabetes mellitus. This patient population is known to have a blunted response to vasoactive injection.[37,132] Forty-one patients received 20 μg of PGE₁, and a response sufficient for intercourse was seen in 71%. These patients went on to home injection therapy with a follow-up ranging from 1 to 12 months. Erection duration ranged from 0.5 to 3 hours (average: 1.1 hour), and no patient had a prolonged erection. Of these patients 21% had mild pain during injection and/or erection, but no patient discontinued therapy for this reason. No fibrosis or nodules were seen at follow-up.

Beretta et al.[133] has used PGE₁ injection therapy in a home self-injection program in 30 patients who responded to 10 μg PGE₁ in an office setting. All patients reported satisfactory erections at up to 6 months follow-up without systemic side effects or prolonged erection. Only three patients had isolated penile hematoma following injection.

Schramek et al.[134] used PGE₁ for diagnosis and therapy in 149 men with erectile dysfunction. A vasculogenic cause was present in 72%, psychogenic in 17%, and neurogenic in 10%. A dose of 5 to 40 μg of PGE₁ was injected in the office with an overall response of erection sufficient for intercourse in 79%. Three patients had prolonged erection requiring treatment (2.0%). All three had a nonvasculogenic cause of impotence. Overall, 40% of patients reported tolerable or severe pain with injection and/or erection. Forty percent of these patients had severe penile discomfort. Again, this side effect was significantly greater in those patients with a nonvasculogenic cause. Corporovenous leak may result in decreased local concentration of PGE₁ and thus a lower incidence of pain. Eleven patients went on to home injection therapy with a mean follow-up of 7 months. Only one patient complained of tolerable pain with injection/erection. Six of seven patients had a good response to therapy. The remaining patient crossed over to papaverine-phentolamine because of inconsistent rigidity and had a good result. There was no reported prolonged erection or corporal fibrosis in this group of patients.

Mahmoud assessed the efficacy and safety of PGE_1 (20 μg) vs papaverine (30 mg) in a double-blind crossover study of 52 Egyptian patients. Overall, the positive response to PGE_1 was significantly greater than the response to papaverine (81% vs 63%). The latency period to full erection was shorter for papaverine, but the overall duration of erection was greater for PGE_1. There were no prolonged erections in either group, which included eight patients who had a previous prolonged erection with papaverine therapy. There was no significant difference in penile pain with injection and/or erection between the two groups. Mahmoud correctly points out that whereas PGE_1 appears to be a safe and effective agent for the diagnosis of erectile dysfunction and potentially for therapy, its use will be limited in developing countries because of its high cost and limited stability.

Gerber and Levine[135] reported on the largest group of patients on a PGE_1 home pharmacologic erection program. Seventy-two patients had a diagnostic evaluation and were candidates for home injection therapy. Thirty-seven patients (51%) failed to continue beyond the in-office dose titration/teaching period. Of the 35 patients (49%) who began therapy, 15 (43%) discontinued it during the follow-up period. This is a total drop-out rate of 72%. The most common reason for therapy drop-out was penile pain following injection (17%). There was no statistical difference among patients with vasculogenic vs nonvasculogenic causes of erectile dysfunction in regard to the presence of penile pain. Failure to achieve adequate erection with PGE_1 was a reason for drop-out in an additional 13% of patients. There were no instances of prolonged erection, significant hematoma, systemic reaction, or cavernosal fibrosis in the patients continuing on the PGE_1 pharmacologic erection program.

In summary, PGE_1 is an effective vasoactive agent for the diagnosis and treatment of erectile dysfunction. A specific advantage comparing PGE_1 with papaverine or papaverine-phentolamine combination therapy lies with its reliable dose-response effect. This results in a lower incidence of prolonged pharmacologic erection. The incidence of systemic side effects and delayed cavernosal fibrosis is significantly lower, perhaps because of its rapid local metabolism or its potential for membrane stabilization. On the negative side, PGE_1 is significantly more likely to result in pain with injection and/or erection, and in a number of patients this may lead to aversion for this form of therapy. Also its widespread acceptance may be limited by its high cost per dose and poor stability when not refrigerated when compared with papaverine-containing vasoactive agents.

Papaverine-Phentolamine-PGE_1 Combination Therapy

As shown above, the individual agents used in vasoactive pharmacotherapy of erectile dysfunction have limitations in their clinical success and potential for side effects. Papaverine as monotherapy has an unpredictable response with significant potential for prolonged erection and priapism. Chronic injection can result in cavernosal smooth muscle hypertrophy and fibrosis. Hepatic dysfunction is a reported side effect, although it may be more common in men with ongoing or past heavy alcohol use.[136] Phentolamine alone does not reliably produce an erection sufficient for intercourse.[104] In combination with papaverine, phentolamine decreases the latency between injection and erection and allows a reduction in the total papaverine dose, decreasing the incidence of prolonged erection and potentially the incidence of fibrosis. PGE_1 with its short half-life and dose-dependent duration of erection has an advantage over papaverine monotherapy or papaverine-phentolamine combination therapy, but significant pain with injection occurs in up to 40% of patients. In addition, PGE_1 is very expensive at the volumes required for clinical response. These shortcomings have prompted combination of all three agents for therapy. Because each agent acts on a specific site in the erection process through smooth muscle relaxation and arterial inflow, it is possible to take advantage of synergism at very low doses of each individual agent.

Bennett et al.[137] combined papaverine, phentolamine, and PGE_1 using the most expensive agent (PGE_1) as the base. The original formulation, which has been adopted by others, is shown in Table 17–3. Diagnostic evaluation of 116 patients was performed with the injection of the combination at a total volume of .25 ml containing a total of 4.4 mg papaverine, .15 mg phentolamine, and 1.5 μg PGE_1. A lower dose was used in patients with suspected psychogenic and neurogenic causes of dysfunction. Eighty-nine percent of the patients had a positive response and went on to home injection therapy. Overall, 78 patients (74%) were maintained at a volume of .25 ml per injection with a frequency of use averaging 3.1 times per month. Two episodes of prolonged erection requiring treatment were seen; both patients involved had psychogenic impotence. Two patients (1.9%) complained of pain at the injection site or with intercourse, prompting one to discontinue therapy. With an average follow-up of 12.7 months, no patient

TABLE 17–3
Formulation of Papaverine, Phentolamine, and Prostaglandin E₁ Solution

Vasoactive Agent	Dose (ml)
Papaverine HCL (30 mg/ml)	2.5
Phentolamine (5 mg/ml)	0.5
Prostaglandin E₁ (500 μg/ml)	0.05
0.9% Saline for injection	1.2
Total volume	4.25

From Bennett et al.: Improved vasoactive drug combination for pharmacological erection program. J Urol 146:1564, 1991, © American Urological Association, 1991.

had corporal fibrosis. In a later study, 110 patients with a minimum of 12-month and up to 28-month follow-up were contacted. Sixty-five continued injection therapy, and of these 89% were satisfied with the drug combination as a treatment option. Seven prolonged erections (greater than 3 hours) occurred (5.6%), but only one patient required intervention. No patient treated exclusively with this triple therapy developed fibrosis or nodules.[138]

Goldstein et al.[139] used a similar combination of papaverine, phentolamine, and PGE₁ in 32 patients who had failed previous pharmacotherapy with papaverine-phentolamine or PGE₁. Twenty patients (62%) were salvaged with the combination and had erections sufficient for satisfactory intercourse. Eight patients (25%) reported pain with injection, 6 of which were diabetic. No systemic side effects were seen, and no prolonged erections were encountered.

Hamid et al.[140] used Bennett's formulation in 100 consecutive patients with erectile dysfunction at a dose range of 0.05 to .35 ml. A positive response was seen in 88 patients, and only 5 patients complained of pain at the injection site. One patient required corporal aspiration for a prolonged (4-hour) erection.

McMahon,[141] in a randomized crossover study of 228 patients, compared the combination of papaverine, phentolamine, and PGE₁ to papaverine-phentolamine and PGE₁ alone. The dosage concentration for the triple therapy varied, but statistical significance in favor of triple therapy when compared with papaverine-phentolamine and PGE₁ was seen in men with severe arteriogenic or mild corporovenous occlusive disease. The incidence of prolonged erection was significantly lower in the triple therapy group than in the papaverine-phentolamine group (0.9% vs 7.3%) but was not statistically significant when compared with PGE₁ alone (1.3%).

Combination therapy has been used extensively by Virag, who continuously has changed his formula, adding new vasoactive agents and varying concentrations. Ceritine, a proprietary formulation, contains up to six vasoactive agents, several of which are unavailable in the United States. Virag's report indicates efficacy similar to that of triple therapy with a low incidence of fibrotic nodules and prolonged erections.[142] However, until this formulation is made more widely available, these results must be considered anecdotal.

In summary, a combination of papaverine, phentolamine, and PGE₁ has been used for the treatment of erectile dysfunction. The present literature, although limited, indicates that this vasoactive agent combination is equivalent to PGE₁ alone in efficacy with a lower cost and decreased incidence of painful erections. Further clinical evaluation is required to determine the long-term effects of therapy.

PATIENT SELECTION AND SELF-INJECTION EDUCATION

Intracavernosal pharmacotherapy should be presented to the patient as a treatment option based on the initial interview and physical examination. This discussion should be done in an unbiased manner, preferably using patient hand-outs or video presentations, which discuss the possible benefits and potential risks of each treatment modality available to the patient at the early stages of the diagnostic evaluation. The patient hand-out may double as an informed consent for vasoactive injection for diagnosis and potential therapy.

There are a few contraindications to vasoactive injection: penile fibrosis, coagulopathy, uncontrolled psychiatric disorders, or severe cardiovascular disease, which could be exacerbated by a complication of the injection.[143] Patients with chronic systemic illnesses should be followed in conjunction with their primary physician. Poor manual dexterity or morbid obesity, which could preclude self-injection, can be overcome by teaching an able and willing partner the technique of injection. If the patient and physician select intracavernosal therapy as a potential treatment option, then an office test injection of a selected agent is done. More important than the agent(s) selected is the environment in which the injection is made. A quiet and relaxed atmosphere is needed, free of extraneous personnel and equipment that can increase the anxiety of the patient who may already have significant adrenergic outflow. Since vasoactive pharmacotherapy relies on smooth muscle relaxation, a nervous patient will be less likely to respond to an office injection under stressful conditions. This may result in unnecessary testing and/or confusion regarding erectile dysfunction causes.

In addition, the patient will require additional dose titration to overcome this effect, with delay or refusal to enter a home injection program.

The dose of vasoactive agent(s) chosen for office testing is based on experience and the presumed cause of the erectile dysfunction. Patients suspected of having a significant psychogenic component, neurologic impairment in the absence of atherosclerotic risk factors, or known previous normal erections (as in the post–radical prostatectomy patient) are given a lower initial dose. The patient should already have read or been introduced to the technique of self-injection, and the physician should precisely follow each step of the injection sequence in a relaxed manner to reinforce patient understanding. Use of sterile technique for transfer of the medication to the injecting syringe and preparation of the penis for injection should be particularly stressed to reduce the small risk of infectious complications.

The intracavernosal injection is performed using a ½- to ⅝-inch 28- or 29-gauge needle. The smaller gauge needles decrease the amount of microtrauma to the tunica albuginea, a possible contributing factor to corporal nodules and fibrosis.[144] A 0.5 to 1.0 ml insulin syringe is used depending on the total volume of intracavernosal agent required. The patient is instructed to gently stretch the penis by grasping the glans penis with the nondominant hand. This exposes the base of the penis, and the underlying superficial veins become apparent. Generally, self-injection can be done in the sitting position, although patients with a large pannus may find it easier to inject in a semirecumbent position. After preparing the skin at the injection site with an alcohol pad, the injection syringe is held in the dominant hand as if holding a pencil or dart. The angle of injection is at the ten o'clock or two o'clock position to avoid injury to the dorsal penile or cavernosal vessels or intraurethral injection. Avoiding the superficial penile veins will decrease the complication of postinjection bruising or hematoma. With subsequent injections, the patient alternates sides as well as moving approximately 1 to 1.5 cm proximal and distal on the penile shaft. This provides multiple sites of injection, reducing microtrauma at any given point of the corpora. The needle is advanced in a smooth and continuous fashion through the skin, subcutaneous tissue, and tunica albuginea into the cavernosal body. Most patients are able to feel two distinct resistances, first at the skin level and then as the tunica albuginea is pierced. The contents of the syringe are gently and smoothly injected into the corporal body. Resistance to injection may indicate the needle tip is lying in the opposite wall of the tunica albuginea, and the needle should be withdrawn slightly. After injection, the needle and syringe are

removed in a rapid fashion, and pressure is applied to the injection site for 1 to 2 minutes. Patients receiving aspirin therapy or who have a history of easy bruising should maintain pressure for a longer period. Applying pressure should avoid the complication of subcutaneous or subfascial hematoma formation. Some patients may be apprehensive about self-injection because of poor dexterity or a fear of needles. These patients should be reassured that confidence will come with experience. Autoinjection devices have been developed that can increase the ease of injection in selected patients.[145–147]

After injection the patient remains or returns to a sitting position keeping the penis in a dependent position. The penis can be kneaded, to both distribute the medication and provide the benefit of self-stimulation to enhance its effect. Onset of erection depends on the agent used and the underlying cause of the erectile dysfunction. Patients with significant corporovenous occlusive dysfunction may benefit from standing after injection or using constricting bands to trap the vasoactive agents until a full erection is achieved.

After the office injection, further diagnostic tests may be performed that are appropriate to the specific suspected cause of dysfunction. The patient is observed for spontaneous detumescence. If the erection is rigid and persists for more than 2 hours without change, then the erection is reversed using an alpha-agonist. (See the section on management of prolonged pharmacologic erection.)

A medication dose is selected for the patient based upon the diagnostic evaluation and the results of the in-office vasoactive injection. The patient should understand that this is a "best-estimate" dose given the clinical findings, and further modifications may be needed. The dose used can be varied in an incremental fashion, higher or lower, depending upon his response in the home setting. The goal of vasoactive pharmacotherapy is to achieve an erection that lasts long enough for the patient to engage in satisfactory foreplay and sexual intercourse. The duration of erection needed to achieve this goal varies from patient to patient but need not exceed 1 hour. Factors affecting the amount of medication necessary for a successful clinical response vary with mood, alcohol consumption, and the amount of foreplay before and after injection. A dose that works well on one occasion may not be adequate on another. The patient is counseled not to double inject if an inadequate erection occurs but rather to adjust the dose on another occasion. If erections are inadequate on two consecutive attempts, despite an incremental escalation, he should return for further diagnostic evaluation, observation of technique, and dosage adjustment. It is reasonable to limit injections to two to three times per week, although over time patients will settle into a regular pattern of use.

We define a prolonged pharmacologic erection as that which is present for more than 4 hours or an erection of shorter duration that is painful. It is important that the patient be given a contact telephone number with the understanding that a call can be made at any hour of the day or night. A single 5 mg tablet of terbutaline can be dispensed to the patient to be taken in the event of a prolonged erection.[148] After terbutaline is taken, detumescence should occur within 1 hour; if it does not, the patient should go to the clinic or emergency department for immediate irrigation therapy. Whether terbutaline actually promotes detumescence is debatable. Its use does have the advantage of allowing the patient to self-intervene without contacting the physician and to "start the clock" leading to definitive detumescence therapy, if needed.

The follow-up of patients on vasoactive pharmacotherapy varies with the clinical situation. Home injection vasoactive pharmacotherapy can be divided into two periods: early and late. The early difficulties are primarily dose and technique related. If difficulties with bruising, urethral injection, inadequate rigidity, or marginally prolonged erections occur, the patient is seen again to reinforce the self-injection technique and to optimize dosing. Late follow-up is for penile surveillance to detect changes potentially resulting from chronic vasoactive pharmacotherapy, such as the development of corporal nodules or fibrosis, tachyphylaxis, and in the case of high-concentration papaverine compounds, abnormal liver enzyme elevation.[149,150]

The choice of intracavernosal pharmacotherapy for the treatment of erectile dysfunction places the patient in the situation of performing a minimally invasive drug injection procedure on an intermittent basis. For this reason, careful attention to detail on the part of the physician in the education of the patient is required. This approach should minimize patient frustration and decrease the probability of untoward side effects related to this therapy option.

Prolonged Pharmacologic Erection

The distinction between a prolonged pharmacologic erection and that of priapism is obscured. The hemodynamic changes seen in a rigid erection are low arterial inflow and minimal venous outflow.[151] With time there is a progressive decrease in penile blood oxygenation and pH because of reliance on anaerobic metabolism.[152] This further increases sinusoidal relaxation and blood trapping. An increasing cycle of sinusoidal epithelial edema and increased blood viscosity then results, with

corporal tissue damage. Pathologic ultrastructural changes have been identified within 12 hours after the onset of the rigid erection.[153] Prolonged pharmacologic erection is on the continuum of priapism, and if left untreated, the subsequent histologic fibrosis and lack of response to vasoactive agents are indistinguishable from classic priapism. Because the definitive diagnosis of the erectile dysfunction cause is as much a function of diagnostic experience as a reliance on objective testing, prolonged erections usually are seen during the diagnostic testing and early treatment phase. They are more common in men with psychogenic impotence or those on psychotropic agents for concomitant psychiatric disease. Papaverine monotherapy is more unpredictable than combination pharmacotherapy with occasional prolonged erections occurring at doses that were previously well tolerated.[154]

The prolonged erection/priapism complex is a true urologic emergency, but fortunately it can be readily reversed if treated within 4 to 6 hours. This again underscores the need for intense patient education and the willingness of the treating physician to be available at all times. If, during the course of a diagnostic evaluation that includes vasoactive injection, a rigid erection persists beyond 3 to 4 hours, then interventional detumescence should be performed using an alpha-agonist injection/irrigation protocol.

The alpha-agonists used for injection and/or irrigation and their properties are shown in Table 17–4. The most widely used agents are dilute solutions of phenylephrine or epinephrine. Norepinephrine and metaraminol have been associated with systemic toxicity, and deaths following metaraminol injection has been reported.[155-157] The choice of phenylephrine is due to its alpha$_1$ selective action and lack of beta$_1$ activity, although epinephrine's beta$_2$ activity theoretically may promote venous dilation, which improves outflow.[158] The penile skin is cleaned with a povidone-iodine (Betadine) solution and sterile drapes placed. A 19-gauge butterfly needle is placed for corporal irrigation therapy and connected to a three-way stopcock and the intravenous bag containing the prepared solution. This closed system lessens the possibility of infection or blood contamination. Aspiration/injection is continued until detumescence occurs. Pulse and blood pressure monitoring during irrigation therapy is suggested to identify systemic reactions.

After detumescence is achieved, the patient is observed for several hours to ensure success of the procedure. The cause of the prolonged erection is investigated, and the dose of vasoactive agent(s) is adjusted accordingly after several weeks of abstinence. One of the more likely reasons for a pro-

TABLE 17–4
Alpha-Adrenergic Agents for Corporal Irrigation

Drug	Adrenergic Activity	Preparation	Method of Use
Epinephrine [irrigation][158]	Alpha$_{1-2}$, beta$_{1-2}$	1 ml 1:1000 in 1000 ml saline	Aspirate 20 ml, inject 20 ml of solution, repeat q 5 min
Norepinephrine [irrigation][156]	Alpha$_{1-2}$, beta$_{1-2}$	1 ml 1:1000 in 1000 ml saline	Aspirate, inject 25 ml of solution
Phenylephrine [injection][168]	Alpha$_1$ Beta$_{1-2}$ at high doses	1 ml phenylephrine (10 mg/ml) and 9 ml saline	Inject 0.2–0.4 ml, repeat
Phenylephrine [irrigation][169]	Alpha$_1$ Beta$_{1-2}$ at high doses	1 ml phenylephrine (10 mg/ml) in 500 ml saline	Aspirate, irrigate with 10–15 ml of solution, repeat
Metaraminol [injection][170]	Indirect, nonspecific adrenergic agonist	10 mg/ml	0.3–2.0 ml, repeat at 1 hr

longed pharmacologic erection is double-dosing, which occurs when the patient injects the prescribed dose and an erection does not result. This may be due to technical factors permitting only partial injection or a potentially stressful circumstance. The patient then reinjects within a short interval and a prolonged erection ensues. This event is preventable through patient education and reinforcement of injection techniques.

Pharmacotherapy Drop-out

Therapy for erectile dysfunction is somewhat different than the treatment of other diseases in men. The disease process is not life threatening, and although commonly physical in origin, it can have a significant psychologic overlay for the patient and partner. The treatment of erectile dysfunction is elective, and the patient will have no physical sequelae by not initiating therapy or by discontinuing it once begun. Sexual activity, by its nature, is intermittent and generally involves a partner whose support is vital to the success of the therapy. The patient and partner must be sufficiently motivated to begin a therapy that may involve a period of frustration while the technique is mastered and dosing is adjusted. Given all of these factors, the patient has multiple opportunities to reject or discontinue therapy during the diagnostic/teaching phase, the early home phase, or later. This may result in a relatively high rate of patient drop-out when compared with that of therapy for other diseases, although it does not mean these patients will select penile prosthesis or vacuum devices as alternative therapy for their erectile dysfunction. Some patients also may suspend therapy for a major life event, returning to therapy upon resolution.

Unfortunately, while drop-out rates are reported in the literature for vasoactive pharmacotherapy, the reasons for discontinuing and subsequent alternate therapy are sketchy. Unexamined factors such as the office setting and personalities of the treating physicians and personnel may play a role unrelated to the vasoactive agent(s) used. Drop-out rates have ranged from none[128] to 47%,[159] with most reporting approximately 30% drop-out with at least a 6-month follow-up. In a report by Althof et al.,[160] 131 patients were evaluated for entry into a vasoactive pharmacotherapy program. A cumulative drop-out rate of 46% was observed. The phase of highest drop-out risk occurs in the diagnostic/teaching phase with patients who decline therapy accounting for approximately three quarters of the total drop-outs. The primary reasons stated were disagreement over the therapy selected and a fear of potential side effects (pain, prolonged erection, fibrosis). Once the patient enters home therapy, the drop-out rate falls off dramatically.[160] The primary reasons for late drop-out were loss of treatment effectiveness and the cost of treatment (medication, supplies, follow-up). Table 17–5 lists potential reasons for drop-out, some of which may occur in patients who can achieve a satisfactory erectile response to intracavernous pharmacotherapy.

Cooper[161] examined the reasons for drop-out in a small group of patients and found that drop-out patients were more likely to have a poor relationship with a sexual partner or that partner was not regularly available. In addition, all patients who discontinued therapy had a decline in libido during use.

Van Driel et al.[162] followed 152 patients who were considered candidates for intracavernous pharmacotherapy with papaverine or papaverine-

TABLE 17–5
Potential Reasons for Discontinuing Vasoactive Pharmacotherapy

Inadequate response to medication
Return of spontaneous erections
Fear of needles/injection
Concern over side effects
Dissatisfaction with artificial erection
Lack of spontaneity
Lack of partner support/satisfaction
Financial
Complications of therapy
   Pain following injection
   Prolonged erection
   Systemic reaction to injection
Significant life event
   Loss/death of partner
   Major illness/operation
   Social stressors (job loss/marital discord)

phentolamine. Fifty-three patients (34.8%) declined injection therapy for fear of injection, noncompliance, or side effects. The remaining 99 patients (65.2%) entered therapy. Seventy-six patients (77%) were able to attain a functional erection during the dose titration phase. Of these, 18 (29%) discontinued therapy early in the program, generally for reasons of fear of injection, episodes of prolonged erection, or inconsistency of erection rigidity. At the 2-year follow-up, an additional 32 patients (44%) had discontinued therapy, many for the reasons cited above, but additional patients experienced a return of normal erections or a loss of sexual interest. From the initial evaluation through to the follow-up, 82% (126 of 152 patients) are considered drop-outs or treatment failures by the criteria of intention to treat. This study indicates that despite the apparent utility of vasoactive pharmacotherapy in the treatment of erectile dysfunction, this treatment option will not be accepted initially or will be terminated early by many men.

To achieve the best outcome in erectile dysfunction therapy, one should not limit treatment to vasoactive pharmacotherapy alone and objectively should temper the patient's expectations of results. Patient concern over potential side effects should be addressed in an unbiased manner. Because these agents are not FDA approved, informed consent usually is involved. Informed consent, by its nature, tends to emphasize the potential deleterious effects of therapy at the cost of underemphasizing the potential benefits. Good technical teaching and a willingness to elucidate technique difficulties or observe injection technique periodically may decrease the incidence of improper injection and

failed responses. If appropriate, the patient should be able to adjust within specific bounds the total dose of medication injected to match the specific situation for which it is used.

One cannot emphasize enough the importance of involving the partner in the discussion of therapy alternatives and treatment goals. Interviewing and education of the partner can alleviate much of the stress that erectile dysfunction brings to a relationship, with the goal being an honest appraisal of the benefits and potential difficulties of therapy. There is also a role for sexual counseling for the patient and partner even if the cause is purely organic, because many men will have concomitant performance anxiety. Many relationships have erectile dysfunction only as a symptom of underlying marital discord due to other factors. Counseling by qualified personnel in certain circumstances can improve the outcome of vasoactive pharmacother-

TABLE 17–6
Guidelines for Reporting Techniques and Outcomes

Medication
   Preparation
   Dosage range
   Route/technique
Diagnostic modalities
Patient diagnosis
   Vasculogenic
      Arteriogenic
      Corporovenous occlusive dysfunction
   Neurogenic
   Diabetic
   Psychogenic
   Postoperative
   Mixed
   Unclassified
Complication rates
   Prolonged erection (definition)
   Corporal nodules/fibrosis
   Hematoma
   Liver dysfunction
   Pain
      Pain scale
   Systemic reactions
Outcome data
   Follow-up (mean, minimum, maximum)
      Return of spontaneous erections
   Rates of adequate rigidity/duration
   Rate of return to intercourse
   Injection frequency
   Patient satisfaction with therapy
   Partner satisfaction with therapy
   Drop-out rates and reasons

TABLE 17-7
Current Problems with Current Pharmacologic Agents

Agents are soluble in acid or alcohol only.
Pain is experienced with injection and/or erection.
Tachyphylaxis can develop.
Systemic effects can occur with injection.
Prolonged erection/priapism can occur.
Agents for treating prolonged erection can cause hypertension or arrhythmia.

Adapted from Lewis: Probl Urol 5:541, 1991.

apy and decrease the late drop-out rates of patients choosing this treatment option.

Vasoactive pharmacotherapy has gained widespread acceptance for the treatment of erectile dysfunction. Unfortunately, it is difficult to meaningfully compare different clinical studies because of the lack of consensus about diagnostics, technique, complications, and patient outcome. It is our suggestion that over time the use of vasoactive therapy has become relatively standardized enabling important outcomes to be measured consistently between different observers. Table 17-6 presents suggested guidelines for reporting techniques and outcomes that would permit different treatment modalities to be measured. The information contained within the body of a clinical report can be combined with other studies to produce meaningful statistical inference with a minimum of observer bias.

Vasoactive pharmacotherapy has traveled a somewhat tortuous path from an isolated case report to the development of large-scale pharmacologic erection programs. The ideal agent has not

TABLE 17-8
The Ideal Pharmacologic Agent

Can be given other than by injection
Consistent, predictable erections result
Dose-dependent erection
Low risk of prolonged erection
Specific for impotence-causing factor
Easily metabolized, preferably in cavernous tissue
Low toxicity/few side effects
Stable over time
Inexpensive

Adapted from Lewis: Probl Urol 5:541, 1991.

been identified, but active basic and clinical research of smooth muscle agents has produced promising leads. Tables 17-7 and 17-8 present the current problems associated with vasoactive pharmacotherapy and the characteristics of an ideal pharmacologic agent, respectively. Despite its shortcomings, vasoactive pharmacotherapy currently represents a viable treatment option in men with erectile dysfunction. Careful attention to diagnosis, teaching, and follow-up should facilitate patient acceptance and satisfaction with this form of therapy and minimize potential complications. Supervision of this form of therapy should be restricted to physicians who are familiar with the various vasoactive agents and combinations available and the diagnostic algorithm and who have the ability to treat potential complications aggressively.

REFERENCES

1. Virag R. Intracavernous injection of papaverine for erectile failure. Lancet 2:398, 1982.
2. Swartz WM, Brink RR, Buncke HJ. Prevention of thrombosis in arterial and venous microanastomosis by using topical agents. Plast Reconstr Surg 58:478, 1976.
3. Brindley GS. Maintenance treatment of erectile impotence by cavernosal unstriated muscle relaxant injection. Br J Psych 149:210, 1986.
4. Zorgniotti AW. Self Experimentation. Letter to the Editor. Lancet 336:1200, 1990.
5. Halsted DS, Weigel JW, Noble MJ, et al. Papaverine-induced priapism: two case reports. J Urol 137:292, 1986.
6. Larsen EH, Gasser TC, Bruskewitz RC. Fibrosis of the corpus cavernosum after intracavernous injection of phentolamine/papaverine. J Urol 137:292, 1987.
7. Fuchs ME, Brawer MK. Papaverine-induced fibrosis of the corpus cavernosum. J Urol 141:125, 1989.
8. Barr L, Burger W, Dewey M. Electrical transmission at the nexus between smooth muscle cells. J Gen Physiol 51:347, 1988.
9. Butler T, Siegman M. High-energy phosphate metabolism in vascular smooth muscle. Annu Rev Physiol 47:629, 1985.
10. Karum K, Stull J. Regulation of smooth muscle contractile elements by second messengers. Annu Rev Physiol 51:299, 1989.
11. Hartshorne D, Gorecka D. Biochemistry of the contractile proteins of smooth muscle. In: Handbook of Physiology. Baltimore: Williams & Wilkins, 1980; 2:83.
12. Guyton A. Textbook of Medical Physiology, 8th ed. Philadelphia: WB Saunders, 1991;1.
13. Morgan D, Proske U. Vertebrate smooth muscle: its structure, pattern of innervation, and mechanical properties. Physiol Rev 64:103, 1984.
14. Brindley GS. Pilot experiments on the actions of

drugs injected into the human corpus cavernosum penis. Br J Pharmacol 87:495, 1986.

15. Wagner G, Brindley G. The effect of atropine, alpha- and beta-blockers on human penile erection: a controlled pilot study. In: Vasculogenic Impotence. Proceedings of the First International Conference on Corpus Cavernosum Revascularization, Springfield, Mass, 1980:77–81.

16. Adaikan P, Karim S, Kottegoda S, et al. Cholinoceptors in the corpus cavernosum smooth muscle of the human penis. J Autonom Pharmacol 3:107, 1983.

17. Hedlund H, Andersson K. Comparison of the responses to drugs acting on adrenoreceptors and muscarinic receptors in human isolated corpus cavernosum and cavernous artery. J Autonom Pharmacol 5:81, 1985.

18. Benson G, McConnell J, Lipshultz L, et al. Neuromorphology and neuropharmacology of the human penis. J Clin Invest 65:506, 1980.

19. Eckhard C. Untersuchungen uber die erection des penis beim hunde: beitrage zur anatomie und physiologie., 1963.

20. Larsen J, Ottesen B, Fahrenkrug J, et al. Vasoactive intestinal polypeptide (VIP) in the male genitourinary tract. Invest Urol 19:211, 1981.

21. Polak J, Gu J, Mina S, et al. VIPergic nerves in the penis. Lancet 2:217, 1981.

22. Willis E, Ottesen B, Wagner B, et al. Vasoactive intestinal polypeptide as a putative neurotransmitter involved in penile erection. Life Sci 33:383, 1983.

23. Ignarro L, Buga G, Wood K, et al. Endothelium-derived relaxing factor produced and released from artery and vein is nitric oxide. Proc Natl Acad Sci 84:9265, 1987.

24. Palmer R, Ferrige A, Moncada S. Nitric oxide release accounts for the biological activity of endothelium-derived relaxing factor. Nature 327:524, 1987.

25. Weipes E, Schiffman S, Gilloteaux J, et al. Study of neuropeptide-Y containing nerve fibers in the human penis. Cell Tissue Res 254:69, 1988.

26. Yiangou Y, Christofides N, Gu J, et al. Peptide histidine methionine and the human genitalia. Neuropeptides 6:133, 1985.

27. Gu J, Polak J, Probert L, et al. Peptidergic innervation of the human male genital tract. J Urol 130:386, 1983.

28. Stief CG, Wetterauer U, Schaebsdau FH, et al. Calcitonin-gene-related peptide: a possible role in human penile erection and its therapeutic application in impotent patients. J Urol 146:1010, 1991.

29. Stief C, Benard F, Bosch R, et al. A possible role for calcitonin gene-related peptide in the regulation of the smooth muscle tone of the bladder and penis. J Urol 143:392, 1990.

30. Levin R, Wein A. Adrenergic alpha receptors outnumber beta receptors in human penile corpus cavernosum. Invest Urol 18:225, 1980.

31. Lehninger A. Principles of Biochemistry, 3rd ed. New York: Worth, 1982.

32. Christ GJ, Maayani S, Valcic M, et al. Pharma-cological studies of human erectile tissue: characteristics of spontaneous contractions and alterations in alpha-adrenoceptor responsiveness with age and disease in isolated tissues. Br J Pharmacol 101:375, 1990.

33. Bhargava G, Valcic M, Melman A. Human corpora cavernosa smooth muscle cells in culture: influence of catecholamines and prostaglandins on cAMP formation. Int J Impotence Res 2:35, 1990.

34. Moncada S, Palmer R, Higgs E. Nitric oxide: physiology, pathophysiology, and pharmacology. Pharmacol Rev 43:109, 1991.

35. Kim N, Azadzoi K, Goldstein I, et al. A nitric oxide–like factor mediates nonadrenergic noncholinergic neurogenic relaxation of penile corpus cavernosum smooth muscle. J Clin Invest 88:112, 1991.

36. Ignarro L, Bush P, Buga G, et al. Nitric oxide and cGMP formation upon electrical field stimulation cause relaxation of corpus cavernosum smooth muscle. Biochem Biophys Res Comm 170:843, 1980.

37. Saenz de Tejada I, Goldstein I, Azadzoi K, et al. Impaired neurogenic and endothelium-mediated relaxation of penile smooth muscle from diabetic men with impotence. N Engl J Med 320:1025, 1989.

38. Campos de Carvalho A, Moreno A, Christ G, et al. Gap junctions between human corpus cavernosum smooth muscle cells: identity of the connexin type and unitary conductance events. J Cell Biol 111:153A, 1990.

39. Moreno A, Campos de Carvalho A, Christ G, et al. Gap junctions between human corpus cavernosum smooth muscle cells in primary culture: electrophysiological and biochemical characteristics. Int J Impotence Res 2:55, 1990.

40. Christ G, Moreno A, Parker M, et al. Intercellular communication through gap junctions: a potential role in pharmacomechanical coupling and syncytial tissue contraction in vascular smooth muscle isolated from the human corpus cavernosum. Life Sci 49:PL, 1991.

41. Christ G, Moreno A, Melman A, et al. Gap junction-mediated intercellular diffusion of calcium in cultured human corporal smooth muscle cells. Amer J Physiol 263:C373, 1992.

42. Krall J, Fittinghoff M, Rajfer M. Characterization of cyclic nucleotide and inositol-sensitive calcium exchange activity of smooth muscle cells cultured from the human corpora cavernosa. Biol Reprod 39:913, 1987.

43. Melman A, Maayani S, Schwartzman M. Prostaglandin synthesis as a putative biochemical correlate of spontaneous myotonic oscillations in the isolated human penile erectile tissue. J Urol 135:361A, 1986.

44. Gu J, Polak J, Probert L, et al. Peptidergic innervation of the human male genital tract. J Urol 130:386, 1983.

45. Willis E, Ottesen B, Wagner G, et al. Vasoactive intestinal polypeptide as a putative neurotransmit-

ter involved with penile erection. Life Sci 33:383, 1983.

46. Steers W, McConnell J, Benson G. Anatomical localization and some pharmacological effects of vasoactive intestinal polypeptide in human and monkey corpus cavernosum. J Urol 132:1048, 1984.

47. Poch G, Kukovetz W. Papaverine-induced inhibition of phosphodiesterase activity in various mammalian tissues. Life Sci 10:133, 1971.

48. Brading A, Burdyga T, Scipnyuk Z. The effects of papaverine on the electrical activity of the guinea pig ureter. J Physiol 334:79, 1983.

49. Sungane N, Ugawa T, Uruno T, et al. Mechanism of relaxant action of papaverine. VI. Sodium ion dependence of its effects on 45-Ca-efflux in guinea pig taenea coli. JPN J Pharmacol 38:133, 1985.

50. Kirkeby H, Forman A, Andersson K. Comparison of the papaverine effects on isolated human penile circumflex veins and corpus cavernosum. Int J Impotence Res 2:49, 1990.

51. Delcour C, Wespes E, Vandenbosch G, et al. The effect of papaverine on arterial and venous hemodynamics of erection. J Urol 138:187, 1987.

52. Tanaka T. Papaverine hydrochloride in peripheral blood and the degree of penile erection. J Urol 143:1135, 1990.

53. Hakenberg O, Wetterauer U, Vandenbosch G, et al. Systemic pharmacokinetics of papaverine and phentolamine: comparison of intravenous and intracavernous application. Int J Impotence Res 2:247, 1990.

54. Seidmon EJ, Samaha AM Jr. The pH analysis of papaverine-phentolamine and prostaglandin E_1 for pharmacologic erection. J Urol 141:1458, 1989.

55. Needleman P, Corr P, Johnson E. Drugs used for the treatment of angina: organic nitrates, calcium channel blockers and beta-adrenergic antagonists. In: The Pharmacological Basis for Therapeutics, 7th ed. New York: Macmillan, 1985: 806–823.

56. Taylor S, Sutherland G, Mackenzie G, et al. The circulatory effect of intravenous phentolamine. Circulation 31:741, 1965.

57. Zorgniotti AW, Lefleur RS. Auto-injection of the corpus cavernosum with a vasoactive drug combination for vasculogenic impotence. J Urol 133:39, 1985.

58. Juenmann K, Lue T, Fournier J, et al. Hemodynamics of papaverine- and phentolamine-induced penile erection. J Urol 136:158, 1986.

59. Juenmann K, Atken P. Pharmacotherapy of erectile dysfunction: a review. Int J Impotence Res 1:71, 1989.

60. Hedlund H, Andersson KE. Contraction and relaxation induced by some prostanoids in isolated penile erectile tissue and cavernous artery. J Urol 134:1245, 1985.

61. von Heyden B, Donatucci C, Kaula N, et al. Intracavernous pharmacotherapy for impotence: selection of appropriate agent and dose. J Urol 149:1288, 1993.

62. Hamberg A, Samuelsson B. On the metabolism of prostaglandin E_1 and E_2 in man. J Biol Chem 246:6713, 1971.

63. Roy A, Adaikan P, Sen D, et al. Prostaglandin 15-hydroxydehydrogenase activity in human penile corpora cavernosa and its significance in prostaglandin-mediated penile erection. Br J Urol 64: 180, 1989.

64. Hall S, Honig S, Payton T, et al. Use of atropine sulfate in pharmacologic erections: initial experience with one-year follow-up in the United States. J Urol 147:265A, 1992.

65. Montorsi F, Guazzoni G, Bergamaschi F, et al. Four-drug intracavernous therapy for impotence due to corporal veno-occlusive dysfunction. J Urol 149:1291, 1993.

66. Brindley GS. Cavernosal alpha-blockade: a new technique for investigating and treating erectile impotence. Br J Psychiatry 143:332, 1983.

67. Imagawa A, Kimura K, Kawanishi Y, et al. Effect of moxisylyte hydrochloride on isolated human penile corpus cavernosum tissue. Life Sci 44:619, 1989.

68. Buvat J, Lemaire A, Buvat-Herbaut M, et al. Safety of intracavernous injections using an alpha-blocking agent. J Urol 141:1364, 1989.

69. Georgotas A, Forsell T, Mann J, et al. Trazodone hydrochloride: a wide spectrum antidepressant with a unique pharmacological profile. A review of its neurochemical effects, pharmacology, clinical efficacy, and toxicology. Pharmacotherapy 2:255, 1982.

70. Blanco R, Azadzoi K. Characterization of trazodone-associated priapism. J Urol 136:203A, 1987.

71. Azadzoi KM, Payton T, Krane RJ, et al: Effects of intracavernosal trazodone hydrochloride: animal and human studies. J Urol 144:1277, 1990.

72. Fahrenkrug J. VIP and autonomic neurotransmission. Pharmacol Ther 41:515, 1989.

73. Moncada S, Flower R, Vane J. Postaglandins, prostacyclin, thromboxane A_2 and leukotrienes. In: The Pharmacological Basis for Therapeutics, 7th ed. New York: Macmillan, 1985:823–830.

74. Aoki H, Matsuzaka J, Yeh K, et al. Studies on the role of VIP in penile erectile function. Int J Impotence Res 2:28, 1990.

75. Kiely EA, Bloom SR, Williams G. Penile response to intracavernosal vasoactive intestinal polypeptide alone and in combination with other vasoactive agents. Br J Urol 64:191, 1989.

76. Roy JB, Petrone RL, Said SI. A clinical trial of intracavernous vasoactive intestinal peptide to induce penile erection. J Urol 143:302, 1990.

77. Stief C, Benard F, Bosch R, et al. A possible role for calcitonin gene-related peptide in the regulation of the smooth muscle tone of the bladder and penis. J Urol 143:392, 1990.

78. Djamilian M, Stief C, Kuczyk M, et al. Follow-up results of a combination of calcitonin gene-related peptide and prostaglandin E_1 in the treatment of erectile dysfunction. J Urol 149:1296, 1993.

79. Stief C, Holmquist F, Allhoff E, et al. Preliminary report on the effect of nitric oxide donor SIN-1 on

human cavernous tissue in vivo. World J Urol 9:237, 1991.

80. Reden J. Moldisomine. Blood Vessels 27:282, 1990.

81. Porst H. Prostaglandin E₁ and the nitric oxide donor linsidomine for erectile failure: a diagnostic comparative study of 40 patients. J Urol 149:1280, 1993.

82. Heaton J. Synthetic vasodilators are effective, in vitro, in relaxing penile tissue from impotent men: the findings and their implications. Can J Physiol Pharmacol 67:78, 1989.

83. Owen JA, Saunders F, Harris C, et al. Topical nitroglycerin: a potential treatment for impotence. J Urol 141:546, 1989.

84. Claes H, Baert L. Transcutaneous nitroglycerin therapy in the treatment of impotence. Urol Int 44:309, 1989.

85. Edwards G, Weston A. Potassium channel openers and vascular smooth muscle relaxation. Pharmacol Ther 48:237, 1990.

86. Cavallini G. Minoxidil versus nitroglycerin: a prospective double-blind controlled trial in transcutaneous erection facilitation for organic impotence. J Urol 146:50, 1991.

87. Virag R, Frydman D, Legman M, et al. Intracavernous injection of papaverine as a diagnostic and therapeutic method in erectile failure. Angiology 35:79, 1984.

88. Virag R, Builly P, Daniel C, et al. Self intracavernous injection of vasoactive drugs for the treatment of psychogenic and neurologic impotence: late results in 109 patients. In: Proceedings of the Fifth Conference on Vasculogenic Impotence and Corpus Cavernosum Revascularization. Second World Meeting on Impotence. Prague: International Society for Impotence Research (ISIR), 11.1., 1986.

89. Gilbert HW, Gingell JC. The results of an intracorporeal papaverine clinic. Sex Marital Ther 6:49, 1991.

90. Lomas GM, Jarow JP. Risk factors for papaverine-induced priapism. J Urol 147:1280, 1992.

91. Aboseif M, Junemann KP, Luo JA, et al. Chronic papaverine treatment: the effect of repeated injections on the simian erectile response and penile tissue. J Urol 138:1263, 1987.

92. Buvat J, Lemaire A, Marcolin G, et al. Intracavernous injections on vasoactive drugs. J Urol 92:111, 1986.

93. Tullii RE, Degni M, Pinto AFC. Fibrosis of the cavernous bodies following intracavernous auto-injection of vasoactive drugs. Int J Impotence Res 1:49, 1989.

94. Desai KM, Gingell JC. Penile corporeal fibrosis complicating papaverine self-injection therapy for erectile impotence. Eur Urol 15:132, 1988.

95. Ruutu ML, Lindstrom BL, Virtanen JM, et al. Corporeal self-injection for erectile failure. Scand J Urol Nephrol 110(suppl):257, 1988.

96. Buvat J, Lemaire A, Marcolin G, et al. Intracavernous injection of papaverine (ICIP): assessment of its diagnostic and therapeutic value in 100 impotent patients. World J Urol 5:150, 1987.

97. Corriere JN Jr, Fishman IJ, Benson GS, et al. Development of fibrotic penile lesions secondary to the intracorporeal injection of vasoactive agents. J Urol 140:615, 1988.

98. Sidi AA, Brez HA, Bosch RJLH. The effect of intracavernous pharmacotherapy on human erectile tissue: a light microscopic analysis. Int J Impotence Res 1:27, 1989.

99. Lue TF, Hricak H, Marich KW, et al. Evaluation of arteriogenic impotence with intracorporeal injection of papaverine and duplex ultrasound scanner. Semin Urol 3:43, 1985.

100. Wespes E, Schulman CC. Systemic complication of intracavernous papaverine injection in patients with venous leakage. Urology 31:114, 1988.

101. Sidi AA, Chen KK. Clinical experience with vasoactive intracavernous pharmacotherapy for treatment of impotence. World J Urol 5:156, 1987.

102. Zorgniotti AW. Corpus cavernosum blockade for impotence: practical aspects and results in 250 cases. J Urol 135:306A, 1986.

103. Gasser TC, Roach RM, Larsen EH, et al. Intracavernous self-injection with phentolamine and papaverine for the treatment of impotence. J Urol 137:678, 1987.

104. Steif CG, Wetterauer U. Erectile responses to intracavernous papaverine and phentolamine: comparison of single and combined delivery. J Urol 140:1415, 1988.

105. Stief CG, Gall H, Scherb W, et al. Mid-term results of autoinjection therapy for erectile dysfunction. Urology 31:483, 1988.

106. Sidi AA, Reddy PK, Chen KK. Patient acceptance of and satisfaction with vasoactive intracavernous pharmacotherapy for impotence. J Urol 140:293, 1988.

107. Goldstein I, Payton T, Padma-Nathan H. Therapeutic roles of intracavernosal papaverine. Cardiovas Interventional Radiol 11:237, 1988.

108. Girdley FM, Bruskewitz RC, Feyzi J, et al. Intracavernous self-injection for impotence: a long-term therapeutic option? Experience in 78 patients. J Urol 140:972, 1988.

109. Robinette MA, Moffat MJ. Intracorporal injection of papaverine and phentolamine in the management of impotence. Br J Urol 58:692, 1986.

110. Nellans RE, Ellis LR, Kramer-Levien D. Pharmacological erection: diagnosis and treatment applications in 69 patients. J Urol 138:52, 1987.

111. Turini D, Barbanti G, Beneforti P, et al. Intracavernous therapy in impotence after pelvic trauma. A preliminary study. Eur Urol 12:413, 1986.

112. Dhabuwala CB, Kerkar P, Bhutwala A, et al. Intracavernous papaverine in the management of psychogenic impotence. Arch Androl 24:185, 1990.

113. Turner LA, Althof SE, Levine SB, et al. Self-injection of papaverine and phentolamine in the treatment of psychogenic impotence. J Sex Marital Ther 15:163, 1989.

114. Weiss JN, Ravalli R, Badlani GH. Intracavernous

pharmacotherapy in psychogenic impotence. Urology 37:441, 1991.

115. Wyndaele JJ, Meyer JM, Sy WA, et al. Intracavernous injection of vasoactive drugs, an alternative for treating impotence in spinal cord injury patients. Paraplegia 24:271, 1986.

116. Sidi AA, Cameron JS, Duffy LM, et al. Intracavernous drug-induced erections in the management of male erectile dysfunction: experience with 100 patients. J Urol 135:704, 1986.

117. Sidi AA, Cameron JS, Dykstra DD, et al. Vasoactive intracavernous pharmacotherapy for the treatment of erectile impotence in men with spinal cord injury. J Urol 138:539, 1987.

118. Dennis RL, McDougal WS. Pharmacological treatment of erectile dysfunction after radical prostatectomy. J Urol 139:775, 1988.

119. Al-Juburi AZ, O'Donnell PD. Penile self-injection for impotence in patients after radical cystectomy-ileal loop. Urology 30:29, 1987.

120. Richter S, Gross R, Nissenkorn I. Cavernous injection therapy for the treatment of erectile dysfunction in elderly men. Int J Impotence Res 2:43, 1990.

121. Kerfoot WW, Carson CC. Pharmacologically induced erections among geriatric men. J Urol 146:1022, 1991.

122. Ishii N, Watanabe H, Irisawa C, et al. Intracavernous injection of prostaglandin E_1 for the treatment of erectile impotence. J Urol 141:323, 1989.

123. Chen JK, Hwang TI, Yang C. Comparison of effects following intracorporeal injection of papaverine and prostaglandin E_1. Br J Urol 69:404, 1992.

124. Earle CM, Keogh EJ, Wisniewski ZS, et al. Prostaglandin E_1 therapy for impotence, comparison with papaverine. J Urol 143:57, 1990.

125. Lee LM, Stevenson RW, Szasz G. Prostaglandin E_1 versus phentolamine/papaverine for the treatment of erectile impotence: a double-blind comparison. J Urol 141:549, 1989.

126. Sarosdy MF, Hudnall CH, Erickson DR, et al. A prospective double-blind trial of intracorporeal papaverine versus prostaglandin E_1 in the treatment of impotence. J Urol 141:551, 1989.

127. Lui SM, Lin JS. Treatment of impotence: comparison between the efficacy and safety of intracavernous injection of papaverine plus phentolamine and prostaglandin E_1. Int J Impotence Res 2:147, 1990.

128. Stackl W, Hasun R, Marberger M. Intracavernous injection of prostaglandin E_1 in impotent men. J Urol 140:66, 1988.

129. Reiss H. Use of prostaglandin E_1 for papaverine-failed erections. Urology 33:15, 1989.

130. Kattan S, Collins JP, Mohr D. Double-blind, crossover study comparing prostaglandin E_1 and papaverine in patients with vasculogenic impotence. Urology 37:516, 1991.

131. Ravnik-Oblak M, Oblak C, Vodusek DB, et al. Intracavernous injection of PGE_1 in impotent diabetic men. Int J Impotence Res 2:143, 1990.

132. Blanco R, Saenz-de-Tejada I, Goldstein I, et al.

133. Dysfunctional penile cholinergic nerves in diabetic impotent men. J Urol 144:278, 1990.

133. Beretta G, Zanollo A, Ascani L, et al. Prostaglandin E_1 in the therapy of erectile deficiency. Acta Eur Fertil 20:305, 1989.

134. Schramek P, Dorninger R, Waldhauser M, et al. Prostaglandin E_1 in erectile dysfunction. Efficiency and incidence of priapism. Br J Urol 65:68, 1990.

135. Gerber GS, Levine LA. Pharmacological erection program using prostaglandin E_1. J Urol 146:786, 1991.

136. Lewis RW. The pharmacologic erection. Probl Urol 5:541, 1991.

137. Bennett AH, Carpenter AJ, Barada JH. Improved vasoactive drug combination for pharmacological erection program. J Urol 146:1564, 1991.

138. Barada JH, Bennett AH. A computerized database for outcome analysis in impotent patients treated with intracavernosal papaverine/phentoalmine/PGE_1. J Urol 145:232A, 1991.

139. Goldstein I, Borges FD, Fitch WP, et al. Rescuing the failed papaverine/phentolamine erection: a proposed synergistic action of papaverine, phentolamine, and PGE_1. J Urol 143:304A, 1990.

140. Hamid S, Dhabuwala CB, Pontes EJ. Combination intracavernous pharmacotherapy in the management of male erectile dysfunction. Int J Impotence Res 4:109, 1992.

141. McMahon CG. A comparison of the response to the intracavernosal injection of a combination of papaverine and phentolamine, prostaglandin PGE_1 and a combination of all three agents in the management of impotence. Int J Impotence Res 3:113, 1991.

142. Virag R, Shoukry K, Floresco J, et al. Intravenous self-injection of vasoactive drugs in the treatment of impotence: 8 year experience with 615 cases. J Urol 145:287, 1991.

143. Padma-Nathan H, Goldstein I, Payton T, et al. Intracavernosal pharmacotherapy: the pharmacologic erection program. World J Urol 5:160, 1987.

144. Seif SR, Brez HA, Bosch RLJH. Local and systemic effects of chronic intracavernous injection of papaverine, prostaglandin-E_1 and saline in primates. J Urol 142:403, 1990.

145. Kromann-Anderson B, Nielsen KK. Intracavernosal self-injection with injection pen. Int J Impotence Res 1:127, 1989.

146. Gilbert RW, Gingell JC. The autoinjector device: an aid to intracavernosal pharmacotherapy. Br J Urol 67:211, 1992.

147. Virag R, Shoukry K, Floresco J, et al. Intracavernous self-injection of vasoactive drugs in the treatment of impotence: 8-year experience with 615 cases. J Urol 145:287, 1991.

148. Shantha TR, Finnerty DP, Rodriquez AP. Treatment of persistent penile erection and priapism using terbutaline. J Urol 141:1427, 1989.

149. Levine SB, Althof SE, Turner LA, et al. Side effects of self-administration of intracavernous papaverine and phentolamine for the treatment of impotence. J Urol 141:54, 1989.

150. Turner LA, Althof SE, Levine SB, et al. Twelve-month comparison of two treatments for erectile dysfunction: self-injection vs. external vacuum devices. Urology 39:139, 1992.

151. Aboseif SR, Lue TF. Hemodynamics of penile erection. Urol Clin North Am 15:1, 1988.

152. Lue TF, Hellstrom WJG, McAninch JW, et al. Priapism: a refined approach to diagnosis and treatment. J Urol 136:104, 1986.

153. Spycher MA, Hauri D. The ultrastructure of erectile tissue in priapism. J Urol 135:142, 1986.

154. Slob AK, Rowland DL, Blom JH, et al. Psychologic factors affect erectile response to papaverine (letter). Urology 38:294, 1991.

155. Watters GR, Keogh EJ, Carati CJ, et al. Prolonged erections following intracorporeal injection of medications to overcome impotence. Br J Urol 62:173, 1988.

156. Carson CC III, Mino RD. Priapism associated with trazadone therapy. J Urol 139:369, 1988.

157. Stanners A, Colin-Jones D. Metaraminol for priapism (letter). Lancet 2:978, 1984.

158. Molina L, Bejany D, Lynne CM. Diluted epinephrine solution for the treatment of priapism. J Urol 141:1127, 1989.

159. Hollander JB, Gonzalez J, Norman T. Patient satisfaction with pharmacologic erection program. Urology 39:439, 1992.

160. Althof SE, Turner LA, Levine SB, et al. Why do so many people drop out from auto-injection therapy for impotence? J Sex Marital Ther 15:121, 1989.

161. Cooper AJ. Evaluation of intracorporeal papaverine in patients with psychogenic and organic impotence. Can J Psychiatry 36:574, 1991.

162. Van Driel MF, Mooibroek JJ, Van de Wiel HB, et al. Intracavernous pharmacotherapy: psychological, sexological and medical aspects. Int J Impotence Res 3:95, 1991.

163. Deleted.

164. Bodner DR, Lindan R, Leffler E, et al. The application of intracavernous injection of vasoactive medications for erection in men with spinal cord injury. J Urol 138:310, 1987.

165. Pettirossi O, Serenelli G. Intracavernous injection of papaverine, phentolamine and phenoxybenzamine. Acta Urol Belg 56:211, 1988.

166. Postma HJ, Steffens J, Steffens L. Experiences with a standardized diagnostic procedure on outpatient basis in 150 impotent males. Acta Urol Belg 56:220, 1988.

167. Lakin MM, Montague DK, VanderBrug-Medendorp S, et al. Intracavernous injection therapy: analysis of results and complications. J Urol 143:1138, 1990.

168. Barada JH, Bennett AH. Therapeutic penile detumescence by corporal irrigation. Contemp Urol 3:40, 1991.

169. Sidi AA. Vasoactive intracavernous pharmacotherapy. [Review]. Urol Clin North Am 15:95, 1988.

170. Brindley GS. New treatment for priapism. Lancet 2:220, 1984.

CHAPTER 18

Vacuum Therapy and Other Devices

Perry W. Nadig

The hope that some pill or external device could cause an erection is certainly as old as the problem of impotence, but although such a device was developed early in this century, it remained obscure for almost seven decades. In 1917, Doctor Otto Lederer, who described himself as a "subject of the Emperor of Austria" was granted a U.S. patent (number 1,225,341, May 8, 1917) for a "surgical device" through which

> by creating a vacuum, the blood is compelled to enter the cavernosum, whereby an erection is produced. By means of the ring remaining on the root of the penis, the erection is maintained for a considerable time after the sleeve has been removed, since owing to the existing compression, the blood can only flow back gradually.

Inventors in many countries have since patented numerous minor modifications, but Lederer's invention remains the prototype of today's vacuum constriction device (VCD).

The medical profession either ignored or was ignorant of the VCD until the first scientific report of its use was published in 1986.[1] Since that time, the VCD has gained popularity among physicians and patients and is now a widely prescribed treatment for impotence. About 40,000 VCDs were sold in the United States in 1991.

External devices are of three general types: (1) vacuum devices to cause penile rigidity, (2) constriction devices to maintain rigidity, and (3) a combination of the two, the VCD. A variant, the vacuum entrapment device (VE), does not rely on constriction to keep the penis hard but instead maintains the vacuum in a plastic sheath worn during intercourse.[2]

THE VACUUM CONSTRICTION DEVICE
Equipment and Technique

The VCD is simple. It consists of a vacuum chamber, a vacuum pump, and a constriction device that may be an elastic band, O-ring, or disc (Fig. 18–1). The vacuum chamber, made of transparent plastic, is of a length and diameter that will accommodate penises of various sizes and shapes. One end is open and must be of a size that allows the tumescent penis to fill it completely. Inside diameters of 4.14 cm, 4.45 cm, and 4.76 cm (1⅝, 1¾, and 1⅞ inches) are those most commonly required. If the opening is of optimum size, the expanded penis fills the proximal part of the cylinder, helping to seal the vacuum. If it is not large enough, the penis cannot expand completely and will not get rigid. If it is too large, the vacuum is difficult to maintain, and loose scrotal skin can be pulled into the cylinder to be trapped distal to the bands when they are applied.

Vacuum pressure must exceed 100 mm Hg. An early commercial version of the VCD used mouth suction, but most men prefer an electric or hand-operated mechanical pump. A safety valve to limit the maximum vacuum is essential, for as vacuum pressures increase, so does the incidence of ecchymosis and hematoma formation. Men taking aspirin or other anticoagulants are particularly vulnerable to this complication.

Water-soluble lubricant is applied generously to the penis, particularly at its base, where an airtight seal must form. The penis is placed in the chamber, and a vacuum is applied for 6 min (Fig. 18–2). Improved penile rigidity results from the technique of double pumping, i.e., applying the vacuum for 1 or 2 min, then relieving it momentarily and reapplying it for another 3 or 4 min.

To maintain rigidity when the vacuum is released, an elastic ring or band is used to constrict the base of the penis. This must be tight enough to maintain penile rigidity but not so tight that it injures the penis. The constricting device may be a simple rubber band, an O-ring, or a disc with a small opening in the center and may be placed about the base of the penis before or after penile rigidity has been induced by the vacuum. If a disc is used, it is applied before the vacuum, and the chamber then rests in contact with the disc rather than the body. Rubber bands or O-rings may be placed about the penis first but usually are mounted

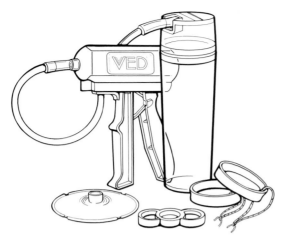

Figure 18–1. The VCD consists of a vacuum pump, a vacuum chamber, and constricting discs, bands, or O-rings. (From Nadig PW. World J Urol 8:114, 1990.)

on the open end of the vacuum cylinder, then pushed off to grip the base of the penis after it is rigid (Fig. 18–3). Constriction sufficient to maintain rigidity, by whatever method, can be maintained safely for 30 min.

Physiology

The evolution of the VCD was empirical. Few investigations of the underlying physiology have been published, but the general mechanism of action whereby the erectionlike state is produced by a vacuum and maintained by constriction has become clear.

The first description of the differences between the erectionlike state induced by the VCD and a normal erection appeared in 1986.[1] These differences include a decrease in penile arterial flow, decreased penile skin temperature, cyanosis and distention of veins of the penis, pivoting of the penis at the point of constriction, and increased penile circumference, presumably due to blood being trapped in all the tissues of the penis rather than only the corpora cavernosa.

These observations were followed by those of Marmar et al.,[3] who used penile plethysmography to obtain the pulse–volume tracings of 51 men impotent from a variety of causes before, during, and after use of a VCD. They found that during constriction, the pulse-volume tracing declined by 70% to 75% in all men and that within 60 sec after removal of the constricting bands, the tracings returned to the baseline level. Their studies confirmed earlier observations that arterial blood flow decreased but did not cease while constriction bands

were applied. Their findings suggested that the radial pressure produced by the constriction band exceeded the mean arterial blood pressure but did not exceed systolic blood pressure. They also confirmed increased penile circumference and lowered skin temperature while constriction was applied. Almost all of their subjects achieved penile rigidity adequate for vaginal penetration.

Do active mechanisms play any part in obtaining a vacuum-induced erectionlike state? Diederichs et al.[4] concluded that they do not and that the corporal distention that occurs is entirely passive. These investigators studied nine monkeys under anesthesia, measuring the cross-sectional area with a duplex scanner and recording intracavernous pressures. They found that cavernous cross-sectional area increased 50% after suction, compared to an 84% increase after papaverine injection. By contrast, the extratunical cross-sectional area increased 57% after suction but only 19% after papaverine. They also observed that intracavernous pressure after vacuum and constriction was equal to that after intracavernous injection of papaverine. Further, they demonstrated that partial constriction of the base of the penis, i.e., enough to block retrograde venous flow, applied before the vacuum did not alter the effect of the vacuum, and they concluded that arterial inflow caused the increased pe-

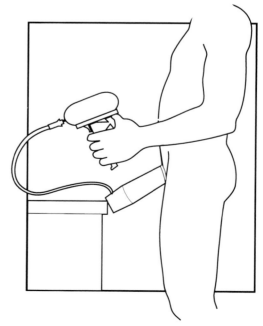

Figure 18–2. Applying the vaccum to the penis. Four to six minutes in the vacuum is needed for the penis to become rigid. The man should be sitting or standing. (From Nadig PW. World J Urol 8:114, 1990.)

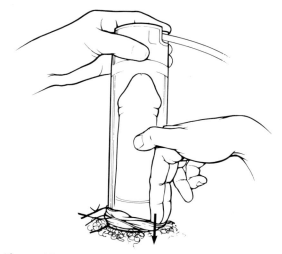

Figure 18–3. A constricting elastic band or an O-ring may be used to maintain rigidity. It is mounted on the open end of the cylinder and transferred to the base of the penis after the penis is rigid. (From Nadig PW. World J Urol 8:114, 1990.)

nile volume. Finally, they showed that tightening of the penile base alone does not readily change intracavernous pressure or induce tumescence.

Katz et al.[5] measured the xenon washout rate before, during application of vacuum, and after subsequent constriction of the base of the penis in 15 men, including 5 spinal cord-injury (SCI) patients, 5 older men with organic impotence, and 5 younger potent controls. They found that vacuum alone did not change the xenon washout measurements from flaccid state measurements among the three groups studied but that placement of a commercially available constriction band about the base of the penis decreased the washout significantly. They point out that venous outflow equals arterial inflow when a steady state exists and penile volume is constant. This implies that enough arterial inflow continues during constriction to replace the diminished amount of venous outflow.

Broderick et al.[6] used a duplex ultrasound with pulsed Doppler and color flow sonography to study the effect of vacuum and subsequent constriction on 5 organically impotent men. Two of the five subjects had failed to respond to intracavernous injection of papaverine 30 mg and phentolamine 0.5 mg, and two others had only transient rigidity with similar doses of these drugs. Cavernous arterial and cavernous body cross-sectional areas were measured before and after application of the VCD. Three patients also had measurements made after intracavernous injection of 20 μg of prostaglandin E_1 (PGE$_1$). Flow velocity studies were made. These investigators found that cavernous body cross-sectional area doubled after application of vacuum and subsequent constriction of the base of the penis, in contrast to a threefold increase after PGE$_1$. They also observed a transiently increased central cavernous arterial blood flow velocity immediately after application of the vacuum, but when constriction was applied, arterial flow became undetectable. They conclude that the erectile state maintained distal to the constricting band is low flow and relatively ischemic, thus confirming the observations of others.[1,3,5]

The mechanism by which an erectionlike state is produced by a vacuum and maintained by constriction appears to be as follows. (1) In a vacuum all tissues of the penis become engorged with blood, including the corpora cavernosa, which enlarge passively and not to the extent to which they enlarge after pharmacologically induced relaxation of the smooth muscle, (2) under vacuum the flow in the cavernous artery transiently increases, and (3) arterial flow then decreases markedly when constriction is applied but is sufficient to replace the small amount of venous blood that leaks past the constricting band. Although stasis of blood occurs and the penis is relatively ischemic while the constricting band is in place, the absence of reports of priapism or ischemic injury to the penis as a result of prolonged use implies that transient stasis and ischemia of this magnitude can be tolerated.

Complications

The majority of complications from the use of the VCD are minor and require no treatment. No serious injury has been reported. Petechiae often develop on the skin of the penis after use of the VCD, presumably as a result of capillary rupture. These are painless and disappear within 48 h. Ecchymoses can occur, particularly in men taking aspirin or other anticoagulant drugs, but have caused no problems. Men whose foreskin is tight risk developing paraphimosis when the penis becomes tumescent and should be circumcised before trying the VCD.[7]

Men with spinal cord injuries and other neurologic problems that impair sensation in the penis should use the VCD with caution. In particular, they should use only constriction devices obtained from a reputable manufacturer and should never exceed 30 min of constriction. Skin necrosis has been reported in a paraplegic man who used his VCD three times daily for three successive days.[8]

Men vary widely in their sensitivity to vacuum pressures. Some men have little or no discomfort with vacuums of as much as 600 mm Hg.[1] These men, as well as SCI patients, may repeatedly develop hematomas and ecchymoses of the penis if excessive vacuum pressure is applied.[9] Because negative pressure beyond 180 mm Hg is unnecessary and because unrestricted vacuums could harm some patients, a safety valve should be used to limit the maximum degree of vacuum. A VCD lacking a safety valve should not be used.

Patient Acceptance and Satisfaction

The VCD will cause penile rigidity sufficient for vaginal penetration for most men, regardless of the cause of impotence, including even those men with a malfunctioning penile prosthesis in place.[10] Only men with extensive scarring and deformity of the penis, such as that caused by an infected penile prosthesis, can be predicted to fail to obtain rigidity with the VCD.

Successful use of a VCD requires careful instruction. Patients who rely only on the manufacturer's printed or videotaped instructions are less likely to master the use of the VCD than those given a demonstration by a physician or experienced medical assistant.[11] Any man interested in trying the VCD should be given individual instruction on its use. About 80% of those men who obtain a VCD will continue to use it regularly. Men who discontinue regular use usually do so within the first 3 months.[10,12,13]

The great majority of men using the VCD report satisfaction with the rigidity, length and circumference, frequency of intercourse, and partner satisfaction. They also report improvement in their self-esteem and sense of well-being.

The most frequent complaint by men using VCD is the unnatural interruption of the act of lovemaking to use the VCD. Some complain of discomfort on ejaculation, but most do not describe this as objectionable. Other complaints include numbness of the penis, coldness of the penis, and difficulty in achieving orgasm.

Although sex involves two people and "sexual decisions are not solely a man's prerogative but should be looked upon as a couple's issue,"[14] most published studies have focused on the man's reaction to the restoration of his sexual function. Studies after implantation of a penile prosthesis show that the satisfaction of a man who has a prosthesis is markedly higher than that of his female partner. A critical assessment of the partner's views recently was published by Althof et al., who questioned the female partners of men using pharmacologic erection and vacuum constriction devices to learn the impact of these therapies on their psychologic and sexual functioning.[14] The subjects were 26 women whose partners were using self-injection and 21 whose partners were using the VCD. They were followed for 12 months. The women responded equally well to both treatments, experiencing significant increases in their level of

sexual satisfaction and arousal and frequency of intercourse and coital orgasm. They felt more at ease in their marital relationships, and they spontaneously commented on how relaxed, unhurried, assured, and enjoyable sex had become. Negative responses were the lack of spontaneity of both therapies, worry about side effects by the self-injection group, and annoyance at the coldness of the penis and the need for lubricant by the VCD group.

VCD Compared to Self-Injection

VCD has been compared directly with self-injection therapy using papaverine and phentolamine.[15] Patients using each type of treatment were followed for 12 months. Both treatment modalities caused a comparable improvement in the quality of erections, and frequency of intercourse and sexual satisfaction were comparably increased over pretreatment levels. The group using self-injection had a 59% dropout rate. Plaquelike nodules appeared in 26%. By contrast, the VCD group had only a 16% dropout rate, and the commonest side effect was blocked ejaculation. The authors concluded that fewer men are able to make use of the self-injection treatment, and the side effects are more worrisome.

Will the VCD make the penis as rigid as will pharmacologic erection? In monkeys, the intracavernous pressure can increase after suction to the same level as that seen after intracavernous papaverine injection.[4] Most VCD users agree. In response to a questionnaire returned after 2 months use of the VCD by 166 (72%) of 231 users,[12] 69.3% reported that they were very satisfied with the hardness of the erection produced by the VCD, 23.5% were somewhat satisfied, and 7.2% were dissatisfied. All of these men had individual hands-on instruction and demonstration of the VCD by a physician who stressed the importance of allowing the penis to be left in the vacuum for at least 6 min and who advised using the double-pumping technique described previously.

Use of the VCD in Conjunction with Injections and Prostheses

The VCD can enhance the effect of intracavernous injections in patients for whom the injections alone fail to induce penile rigidity adequate for vaginal penetration.[10,16] Lue states, "In patients with less than adequate response to repeated CIS (combined intracavernous and stimulation) tests, a vacuum constriction device is applied to see if the erection can be enhanced. If successful, a combination of VCD and injection therapy is recommended."[17] Smooth muscle relaxation caused by pharmacologic agents apparently augments the vacuum-induced tumescence. Ten or fifteen minutes should be allowed to pass from the time of injection before the vacuum is applied so as not to induce ecchymosis or hematoma as a result of blood leaking from the injection site.

Some patients who have had a penile prosthesis explanted can use the VCD successfully.[18,19] Some observed that use of the VCD compared favorably with the prosthesis. Even if a malfunctioning prosthesis is still in place, the VCD can be used to obtain rigidity or increase the girth of the penis.[10]

THE VACUUM ENTRAPMENT DEVICE

The VE uses a vacuum to draw blood into the penis, but the vacuum is sustained during use and constriction is unnecessary. The need for continuous vacuum necessitates the use of an individually fitted silicone sheath that conforms exactly to the shape of the tumescent penis and that is worn during intercourse. The penis is placed in the sheath, the vacuum is applied, the penis becomes tumescent, causing it to fill the sheath, and the vacuum is maintained.

The advantage of this system is that no constriction is required and penile arterial blood flow is not compromised.[5] The disadvantage is that the sheath must be worn during intercourse. The user may experience decreased sensitivity of the penis because of the required thickness of the material, and his sexual partner may experience discomfort, irritation, or trauma from the sheath.

Few reports of clinical experience with the VE have been published.[2,20–22] The largest of these,[20] which included 44 patients impotent from a variety of organic causes, reported that the VE was used successfully by 73%. Overall, 22% of the patients rated the erection obtained very good, 63% rated it satisfactory, and 16% rated it very poor. The vagina of the partner was reported traumatized by 2 patients, and the major complaint of the user was poor sensitivity due to the thickness of the device. The investigators also reported "many complaints" about improper sizing. Two of the reports, with a combined total of 30 patients, counted only 9 who continued to use the VE.[21,22] The fourth study was limited to patients with spinal cord injuries,[2] so that the question of decreased sensitivity could not be addressed.

CONSTRICTION BANDS

Constriction bands can be used by men who can achieve but not maintain an erection. No reports of the indications for or efficacy of this use have appeared in the peer-reviewed literature, but because constriction bands maintain the rigidity of a vacuum-induced erection, they should be expected to maintain a physiologically normal erection and can be recommended for trial by selected patients. Only elastic constriction bands offered by reputable manufacturers should be used. Men must not experiment with untested bands or rings, particularly rings made of metal or other inelastic materials.

CONCLUSIONS

External devices, especially the VCD, have proven safe, effective, and popular. Because of this, and because intracavernous injection of pharmacologic agents is also safe and effective, a new approach to the diagnosis and treatment of the impotent man has evolved. Elaborate and expensive testing of men who do not want surgery or who are not candidates for surgery is pointless and spendthrift. After a careful history, examination, and interview with the patient's sexual partner, the physician can, often without further testing, prescribe a reasonably priced and effective treatment that carries with it a minimum of risk.

REFERENCES

1. Nadig PW, Ware JC, Blumoff R. Noninvasive device to produce and maintain an erection-like state. Urology 27:126, 1986.
2. Zasler ND, Katz PG. Synergist erection system in the management of impotence secondary to spinal cord injury. Arch Phys Med Rehabil 70:712, 1989.
3. Marmar JL, DeBenedictis TJ, Praiss DE. Penile plethysmography on impotent men using vacuum constrictor devices. Urology 32:198, 1988.
4. Diederichs W, Kaula NF, Lue TF, et al. The effect of subatmospheric pressure on the simian penis. J Urol 142:1087, 1989.
5. Katz PG, Haden HT, Mulligan T, et al. The effect of vacuum devices on penile hemodynamics. J Urol 143:55, 1990.
6. Broderick GA, McGahan JP, Stone AR, et al. The hemodynamics of vacuum constriction erections: assessment by color Doppler ultrasound. J Urol 147:57, 1992.
7. Nadig PW. Six years experience with the vacuum constriction device. Int J Impot Res 1:55, 1989.
8. Meinhardt W, Kropman RF, Lycklama AAB, et al. Skin necrosis caused by use of negative pressure device for erectile impotence. J Urol 144:983, 1990.
9. Walden TB: Osbon Erec Aid (Letter). J Urol 136:689, 1986.
10. Sidi AA, Becher EF, Zhang G, et al. Patient acceptance of and satisfaction with an external negative pressure device for impotence. J Urol 144:1154, 1990.
11. Lewis JH, Sidi AA, Reddy PK. A way to help your patients who use vacuum devices. Contemp Urol 3:15, 1991.
12. Cookson MS, Nadig PW. Long-term results with the vacuum constriction device. J Urol 149:290, 1993.

13. Turner LA, Althof SE, Levine SB, et al. Treating erectile dysfunction with external vacuum devices: impact upon sexual, psychological and marital functioning. J Urol 144:79, 1990.

14. Althof SE, Turner LA, Levine SB, et al. Through the eyes of women: the sexual and psychological responses of women to their partner's treatment with self-injection or external vacuum therapy. J Urol 147:10024, 1992.

15. Turner LA, Bodner DR, Slthof SE, et al. Twelve-month comparison of two treatments for erectile dysfunction: self-injection versus external vacuum devices. Urology 38:139, 1992.

16. Marmar JL, DeBenedictis TJ, Praiss DE. The use of a vacuum constrictor device to augment a partial erection following an intracavernous injection. J Urol 140:975, 1988.

17. Lue TF. Patient's goal-directed impotence manage-ment. In: Crawford ED, ed. Urology Grand Rounds No. 29. Chicago: McCann Healthcare Advertising (Marion Laboratories, Inc.), 1989.

18. Moul JW, McLeod DG. Negative pressure devices in the explanted penile prosthesis population. J Urol 142:729, 1989.

19. Korenman SG, Viosca SP. Use of a vacuum tumescence device in the management of impotence in men with a history of penile implant or severe pelvic disease. J Am Geriatr Soc 40:61, 1992.

20. Al-Juburi AZ, O'Donnell PD. Synergist erection system: clinical experience. Urology 35:304, 1990.

21. Earle CM, Keogh EJ. Experience with the Synergist Erection System in the management of impotence. Int J Impot Res 3:33, 1991.

22. Asopa R, Williams G. Use of the Correctaid device in the management of impotence. Br J Urol 63:546, 1989.

CHAPTER 19

Penile Prostheses

Drogo K. Montague
Milton M. Lakin

HISTORICAL PERSPECTIVES

In an early attempt to manage erectile failure with a surgical implant, Bogoras in 1936 inserted a section of rib cartilage into a reconstructed penis.[1] Rib grafts, however, proved unsatisfactory because of protrusion, absorption, and infection. Goodwin and Scott in 1952 were the first to report the use of a synthetic acrylic prosthesis that they implanted beneath Buck's fascia in the shaft of the penis,[2,3] and similar rigid devices (Figs. 19–1 and 19–2) were implanted extracorporeally by others in the 1960s.[4–10]

Penile prosthetic surgery did not become popular, however, until the early 1970s, when Scott et al. introduced the first inflatable penile prosthesis[11] and Small et al. described paired, semirigid, intracorporeal sponge-filled silicone implants (Fig. 19–3).[12,13] In 1977, Finney introduced the Flexi-Rod prosthesis (Fig. 19–4), a semirigid rod implant with a softer hinged section beneath the pubis to provide better concealment and a trimmable proximal tail to reduce inventory requirements.[14,15] In 1980, Jonas and Jacobi introduced the first malleable device. This silicone penile implant (Fig. 19–5) had a twisted silver wire core that increased rigidity and allowed the prosthesis to be bent into either an upward or downward position.[16] Considerable experience with the Jonas prosthesis has been reported subsequently.[17–23] In the 1980s, two different one-piece hydraulic implants were introduced: Surgitek's Flexi-Flate prosthesis[24–26] (Fig. 19–6) and American Medical System's Hydroflex penile prosthesis[27–30] (Fig. 19–7). The AMS Hydroflex has been replaced by the AMS Dynaflex prosthesis, and Surgitek is no longer manufacturing or marketing penile prostheses. Before discontinuing activity in the prosthesis market, Surgitek also produced a two-piece hydraulic prosthesis, the Uniflate 1000.

IMPLANT TYPES

Penile implants can be divided into two general types, nonhydraulic and hydraulic. Nonhydraulic devices also are commonly referred to as semirigid rod prostheses, and hydraulic devices are often referred to as inflatable prostheses. The nonhydraulic penile prostheses currently marketed in the United States are listed in Table 19–1, and the hydraulic penile prostheses are listed in Table 19–2.

Nonhydraulic Prostheses
AMS Malleable 600

The AMS Malleable 600 prosthesis (Fig. 19–8) is a paired silicone device with a malleable core consisting of straight stainless steel wires twisted together and wrapped in a synthetic fabric. The prosthesis comes in three lengths (12 cm, 16 cm, and 20 cm), and 1 cm, 2 cm, and 3 cm rear tip extenders can be applied to adjust lengths between sizes. The diameter of this device is 13 mm; however, by removing a 1 mm outer silicone jacket with blunt scissors (Fig. 19–9), the device diameter can be changed to 11 mm. A smaller version of this device, the AMS Malleable 600M, has diameters of 11.5 mm and 9.5 mm, and comes in four lengths, 12 cm, 14 cm, 16 cm, and 18 cm. Experience with the AMS Malleable 600 device has been favorable,[31,32] and there have been no reports of mechanical failures.

DuraPhase (Dacomed)

The DuraPhase penile prosthesis[33,34] (Fig. 19–10) replaces the OmniPhase prosthesis,[35] an earlier device also marketed by Dacomed. The DuraPhase prosthesis consists of paired cylinders 13 cm in length and available in 10 mm and 12 mm diameters. Each cylinder contains 12 polysulfone segments that articulate with adjacent segments and are movable through an angle of approximately 17 degrees. A stainless steel cable runs through the center of each segment, and a spring on each end maintains constant tension between the segments. Each prosthetic cylinder is covered with polytetrafluoroethylene, and varying sized proximal and distal tips are attached to produce the proper length. This prosthesis design produces better device positionability than is possible with other implants. Early experience with this prosthesis has been encouraging.[36,37] However, in a multicenter

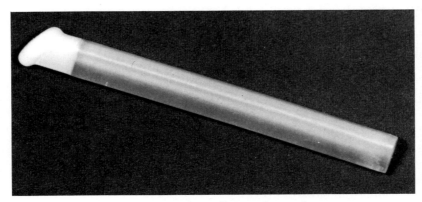

Figure 19–1. Lash-Loeffler penile prosthesis.

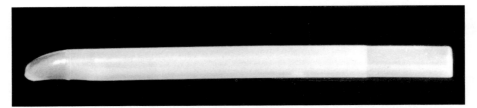

Figure 19–2. Pearman penile prosthesis.

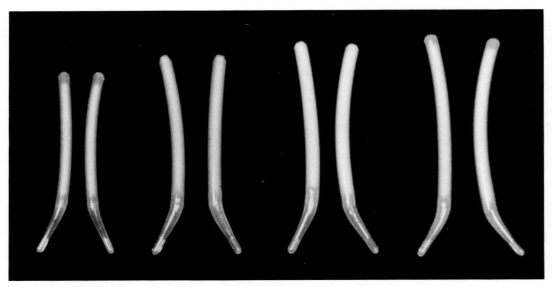

Figure 19–3. Small-Carrion penile prosthesis. (From Montague DK. Implant procedures for impotence. In: Stewart BH, ed. Operative Urology. Vol 2. © 1982, the Williams & Wilkins Co., Baltimore.)

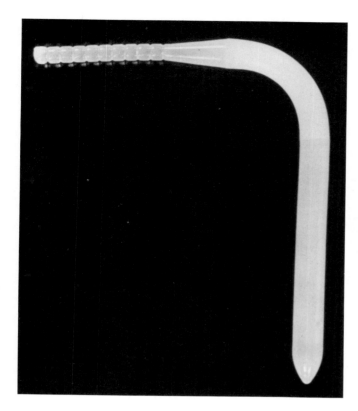

Figure 19–4. Finney Flexi-Rod prosthesis (one of a pair is shown). (From Montague DK. Implant procedures for impotence. In: Stewart BH, ed. Operative Urology, Vol 2. © 1982, the Williams & Wilkins Co., Baltimore.)

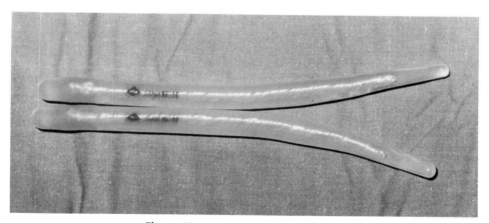

Figure 19–5. Jonas penile prosthesis.

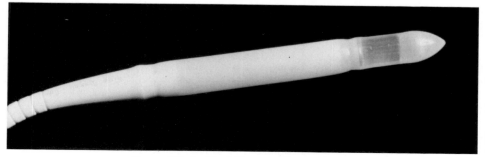

Figure 19–6. Flexi-Flate penile prosthesis.

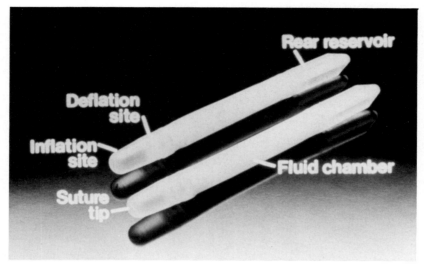

Figure 19–7. AMS Hydroflex penile prosthesis. (Courtesy of American Medical Systems, Inc., Minnetonka, Minn.)

TABLE 19–1
Nonhydraulic Penile Prostheses Marketed in the United States

Type	Name	Manufacturer	Cost
Malleable	AMS Malleable 600	AMS[a]	$1,295
Positionable	DuraPhase	Dacomed	$2,295
Positionable	Dura-II	Dacomed	Not available
Semirigid	Small-Carrion	Mentor	$950
Malleable	Mentor Malleable	Mentor	$1,450
Positionable	Acu-Form	Mentor	$1,695

[a]American Medical Systems.

TABLE 19–2
Hydraulic Penile Prostheses Manufactered in the United States

Type	Name	Manufacturer	Cost
One piece	AMS Dynaflex	AMS[a]	$3,570
Two piece	Mark II	Mentor	$3,750
Three piece	AMS 700CX	AMS	$3,595
Three piece	AMS Ultrex	AMS	$3,595
Three piece	AMS Ultrex Plus	AMS	$3,895
Three piece	Alpha I	Mentor	$3,550

[a]American Medical Systems.

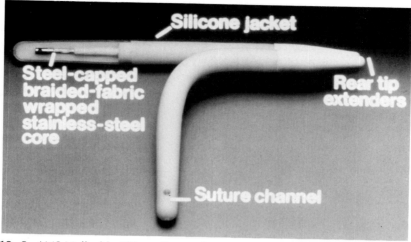

Figure 19–8. AMS Malleable 600 penile prosthesis. (Courtesy of American Medical Systems, Inc., Minnetonka, Minn.)

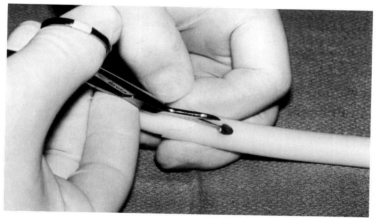

Figure 19–9. Blunt scissors are used to remove the outer jacket of an AMS Malleable prosthesis, changing its diameter from 13 mm to 11 mm. (From Montague DK. Penile prostheses. In: Montague DK, ed. Disorders of Male Sexual Function. Year Book Medical Publishers, Inc., 1988.)

study, 4 cable breaks occurred in 63 implant recipients.[38]

Dura-II (Dacomed)

The Dura-II prosthesis is a recently introduced, newly designed version of the DuraPhase device that reportedly extends cable life.

Small-Carrion (Mentor)

One of the earliest of the semirigid rod devices (Fig. 19–3), the Small-Carrion penile prosthesis, is still available through Mentor Corporation. This

prosthesis is available in three diameters, 9 mm, 11 mm, and 13 mm. The 9 mm device comes in five lengths, 12.0 cm, 13.3 cm, 14.5 cm, 15.8 cm, and 17.0 cm. The 11 mm device comes in six lengths, 12.0 cm, 13.3 cm, 14.5 cm, 15.8 cm, 17.0 cm, and 18.0 cm. The 13 mm device comes in five lengths, 17.0 cm, 18.0 cm, 19.0 cm, 20.0 cm, and 21.0 cm.

Mentor Malleable

The Mentor Malleable penile prosthesis[39] is shown in Figure 19–11. This prosthesis, which contains a coiled wire for malleability and en-

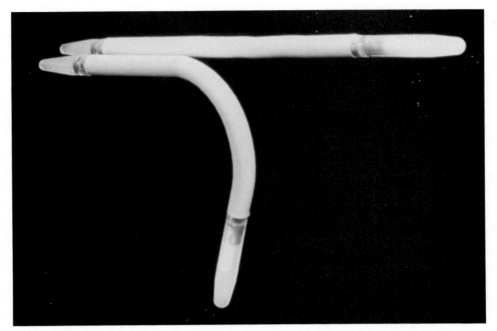

Figure 19–10. DuraPhase penile prosthesis. (Courtesy of Dacomed Corporation, Minneapolis, Minn.)

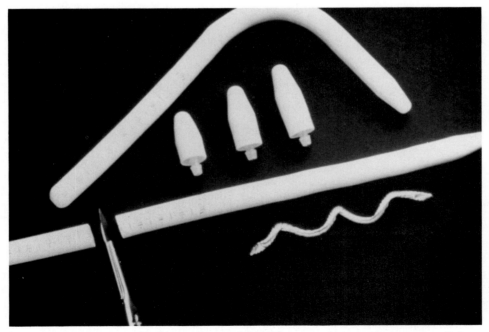

Figure 19–11. Mentor Malleable penile prosthesis. (Courtesy of Mentor Corporation, Goleta, Calif.)

hanced column strength, comes in three diameters: 9.5 mm, 11 mm, and 13 mm. Length adjustment is made by trimming the prosthesis at the desired centimeter mark and then applying either a standard, a +0.5 cm, or a +1 cm tail cap.

Acu-Form

The Mentor Acu-Form penile prosthesis (Fig. 19–12) is a semirigid rod prosthesis that contains no internal parts. Like the Mentor Malleable prosthesis, it is trimmable, comes in the same diameters, and has the same size tail caps.

Hydraulic Prostheses
One Piece

The AMS Dynaflex penile prosthesis (Fig. 19–13) is a paired, hydraulic device that is totally confined within the corpora cavernosa. The pump for this prosthesis is the distal portion of the device, and the reservoir is the proximal portion. Cycling the pump transfers fluid from the rear tip reservoir into a central nondistensible chamber. When the central chamber is full, further pumping does not produce expansion but does result in rigidity. The rigidity produced by the Dynaflex is comparable

to that produced by most semirigid rod prostheses. When prosthesis rigidity is no longer desired, the patient bends the penis over his thumb or a finger and maintains the penis in this flexed state for about 10 sec. When he releases the penis, fluid leaves the central chamber and returns to the rear tip reservoir. This results in a partial collapse of the central chamber, and the device loses a portion of its rigidity.

The Dynaflex prosthesis is supplied in two diameters: 11 mm and 13 mm. The 11 mm device comes in three lengths: 14 cm, 16 cm, and 18 cm. The 13 mm device comes in four lengths: 16 cm, 18 cm, 20 cm, and 22 cm. Adjustment between lengths is made by the addition of one or more snap-on rear tip extenders.

Two Piece

Mentor introduced a two-piece prosthesis in 1988.[40] This device, consisting of paired corporeal cylinders connected to a scrotal component that is both a pump and a fluid reservoir, was later named the Mentor G.F.S. inflatable prosthesis.[41] After connectors were eliminated from this device, it was renamed the Mark II inflatable penile prosthesis[42,43] (Fig. 19–14). This prosthesis is supplied in two

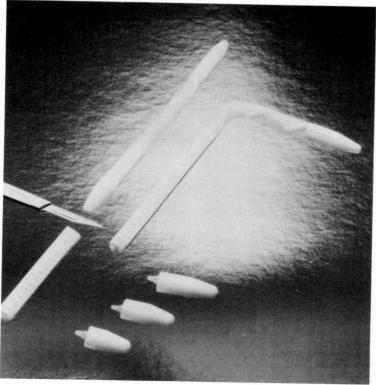

Figure 19–12. Acu-Form penile prosthesis. (Courtesy of Mentor Corporation, Goleta, Calif.)

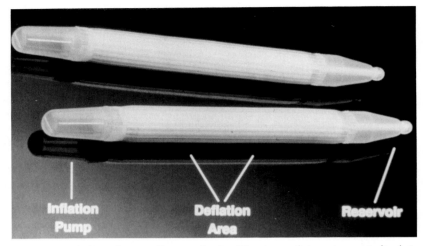

Figure 19–13. AMS Dynaflex penile prosthesis. (Courtesy of American Medical Systems, Inc., Minnetonka, Minn.)

versions, one with longer tubing for implantation via the infrapubic approach and one with shorter tubing for implantation via the scrotal approach. Each version comes with cylinders in six lengths: 12 cm, 14 cm, 16 cm, 18 cm, 20 cm, and 22 cm. Rear tip extenders are supplied to make length adjustments between cylinder sizes.

Three Piece

The Scott inflatable penile prosthesis manufactured by American Medical Systems is a three-piece device consisting of paired cylinders, a scrotal pump, and an abdominal fluid reservoir. After the initial report of Scott et al.,[11] numerous reports of clinical experience with this device followed.[44-67] These reports revealed initially high mechanical complication rates that became progressively lower as improvements both in prosthesis design and in implantation techniques occurred.

A major advancement in prosthesis design was the introduction of the triple-ply controlled expansion (CX) cylinder (Fig. 19–15). The outer layer of this cylinder is silicone, and this prevents tissue ingrowth into the device. The middle layer is a woven fabric that provides controlled cylinder girth expansion. The inner layer is a silicone tube into which fluid is pumped, causing it to expand against the controlled expansion middle layer. These cylinders have a diameter of 12 mm deflated and 18 mm inflated. With this new cylinder design, the symmetry of the erection is less dependent on penile tissue expansion characteristics than was the case with earlier cylinder designs. To date, no cylinder aneurysms have been reported, and the incidence of cylinder leaks with the CX cylinder has been very low.[50,68-70]

The AMS 700CX prosthesis comes with 12 cm, 15 cm, 18 cm, and 21 cm cylinders. Length adjustment between sizes is made by the addition of 1 cm, 2 cm, or 3 cm rear tip extenders. A 65 ml reservoir comes with this device. American Med-

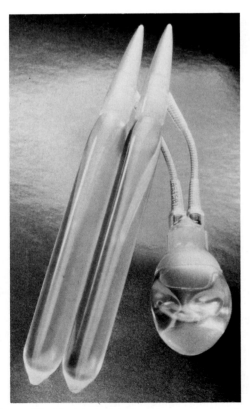

Figure 19–14. Mark II inflatable penile prosthesis. (Courtesy of Mentor Corporation, Goleta, Calif.)

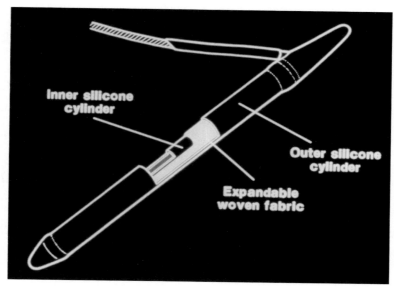

Figure 19–15. AMS controlled expansion (CX) cylinder. (Courtesy of American Medical Systems, Inc., Minnetonka, Minn.)

ical Systems also produces a smaller version of the AMS 700CX prosthesis: the AMS 700CXM device. This prosthesis comes with a smaller pump, a 50 ml reservoir, and four cylinders (12 cm, 14 cm, 16 cm, and 18 cm). These cylinders have a diameter of 9.5 mm when deflated and 14.2 mm when inflated.

The Ultrex cylinder is a modification of the CX cylinder. As in the CX cylinder, the middle fabric layer of the Ultrex cylinder also provides controlled girth expansion, allowing cylinder diameters to vary between 12 mm and 18 mm. Unlike the CX cylinder, however, the Ultrex cylinder also permits controlled length expansion, and the Ultrex cylinders are capable of expanding at least 20% in length. The AMS Ultrex penile prosthesis (Fig. 19–16) is the only prosthesis that provides penile length expansion. In a report concerning length expansion characteristics of this device, the intraoperative pubis to midglans length increase from deflated to inflated status varied between 1 cm and 4 cm, with a mean of 1.9 cm.[71]

The AMS Ultrex penile prosthesis comes with both 65 ml and 100 ml reservoirs. There are four cylinder lengths, 12 cm, 15 cm, 18 cm, and 21 cm. Length adjustment between sizes is made by the addition of 1 cm, 2 cm, or 3 cm rear tip extenders.

Recently, the AMS Ultrex Plus prosthesis was introduced. This prosthesis is supplied with a prefilled pump and prefilled cylinders connected directly to the pump. The reservoir, which is separate, is implanted empty and is filled by the surgeon after implantation. Thus, only one component

needs to be filled in the operating room, and only one tubing connection needs to be made. The AMS Ultrex Plus prosthesis is supplied both with long tubing between pump and cylinders (for infrapubic implantations) and with short tubing between the pump and cylinders (for penoscrotal implantations). Cylinder and reservoir sizes are the same as the AMS Ultrex prosthesis.

The Mentor inflatable penile prosthesis was introduced in 1983.[41,72–80] This three-piece hydraulic

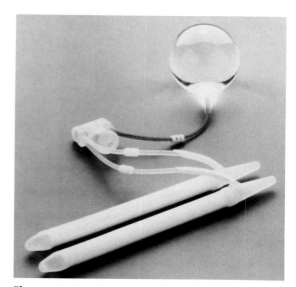

Figure 19–16. AMS 700 Ultrex penile prosthesis. (Courtesy of American Medical Systems, Inc., Minnetonka, Minn.)

prosthesis consists of an abdominal fluid reservoir, a scrotal pump, and paired cylinders made of bioflex, a polyurethane polymer. The current version of Mentor's three-piece prosthesis is the Alpha I inflatable penile prosthesis (Fig. 19–17), which has a pump preattached to the cylinders. This device comes with long tubing lengths for infrapubic implantations and shorter tubing lengths for scrotal implantations. Six cylinder lengths are supplied, 12 cm, 14 cm, 16 cm, 18 cm, 20 cm, and 22 cm. Length adjustment between sizes is made by the addition of 1 cm, 2 cm, or 3 cm rear tip extenders. Three reservoir sizes are available, 60 ml, 75 ml, and 100 ml.

PATIENT SELECTION

The ideal candidate for penile prosthesis implantation is the man with organic impotence who fails treatment by other means or finds them unacceptable and is a suitable surgical risk. Penile prostheses should not be implanted in men with situational, reversible, or temporary forms of erectile dysfunction. Men with psychogenic erectile dysfunction should be considered for penile pros-

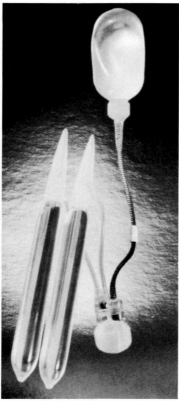

Figure 19–17. Alpha I inflatable penile prosthesis. (Courtesy of Mentor Corporation, Goleta, Calif.)

thesis implantation only if they have failed sex therapy and are recommended for a prosthesis by their therapist or if the therapist believes that sex therapy is not feasible for this individual or couple.

DEVICE SELECTION

Once the option of being implanted with a prosthesis has been selected, the different prostheses offered by the implanting surgeon should be discussed and contrasted with both the patient and, whenever possible, the partner. There is no single prosthesis that is best for every patient, and in addition to the factors subsequently discussed, the patient's or couple's own wishes should be factors in device selection.

If the patient wants a simple device that has the lowest possibility of subsequent mechanical failure and he is willing to accept the limitations inherent in a nonhydraulic prosthesis, a malleable or a positionable prosthesis should be considered. If, on the other hand, the patient wants either the most natural flaccidity or the most natural erection possible with today's devices, he should choose a three-piece hydraulic prosthesis. Other devices, such as one-piece and two-piece hydraulic devices, provide a compromise between nonhydraulic and three-piece hydraulic devices. When considering hydraulic penile prostheses, such factors as patient motivation, intelligence, manual dexterity, and strength should be considered to avoid implantation of a device that the patient will be unable to cycle. Costs can be an important factor in decision making, and this, of course, depends on the patient's insurance coverage and on his own financial resources. In general, the cost of a prosthesis is proportional to its design complexity, and the surgical implantation fee is usually dependent on device complexity as well.

Abnormalities of the corporeal tunica albuginea, such as fibrotic plaques or weakened areas, may complicate prosthesis implantation. Fibrosis of the cavernosal tissue also is often a problem in this regard. By using techniques, such as plaque incision or excision and corporeal augmentation procedures afforded by dacron or polytetrafluoroethylene patching, almost any type of prosthesis usually can be implanted.[81,82] However, nonhydraulic prostheses frequently can be implanted under these circumstances with little or no corporeal reconstruction, and this lessens the potential morbidity of the surgery. Abnormalities of the scrotum may influence decision making with regard to prostheses with scrotal components. Likewise, lower abdominal abnormalities may be factors in deciding about devices that have abdominal reservoirs.

SCI patients are at high risk for both infection and erosion.[83,84] Erosion in these patients occurs in part because of infection, and lack of sensation also contributes to the erosion problem. Hydraulic prostheses in SCI patients offer a reduced risk of erosion. Hydraulic prostheses often are considered advantageous in patients, such as those with a history of bladder tumor, who require periodic lower tract endoscopic procedures.

INFORMED CONSENT

Informed consent begins with telling the patient or couple that there are various treatment options for erectile dysfunction, including penile prosthesis implantation. Patients who are candidates for penile prosthesis implantation also are usually suitable candidates for treatment with a vacuum constriction device (VCD) or intracavernosal pharmacotherapy. Some may also be candidates for penile arterial or venous surgery.

Although some penile implantations are done under local anesthesia,[85] most continue to be done under general, spinal, or epidural anesthesia. The need for an anesthetic and the type of anesthetic to be used should be discussed. The operation is described in general to the patient or the couple.

Some implant procedures are done on an outpatient basis. When the procedure is done on an inpatient basis, the length of hospital stay is usually 1 or 2 nights. Patients should be aware that postoperative pain is significant and lasts about 4 to 6 weeks, although this is quite variable. Patients should plan to restrict strenuous physical activity for at least 4 weeks, and coitus usually is not advisable for at least 4 weeks.

Short-term complications, especially infection and erosion, should be discussed. The patient should be aware that infection and erosion usually require device removal. Less common short-term complications, such as device sizing or positioning problems, as well as device malfunction in the immediate postoperative period usually also require reoperation. The patient needs to be aware that implantation of a penile prosthesis does not ordinarily affect libido, orgasm, ejaculation, or genital sensation. However, a few implant recipients do experience either persistent pain or decreased penile sensation. This fortunately is rare and is often unexplainable.

It is very important that the potential implant recipient understand that the erection produced by a prosthesis always differs from a normal erection and that the appearance of the flaccid penis will be different to some degree as well. Of course, this departure from the normal state is variable, and this variability depends on the type of prosthesis chosen, differences in individual anatomy, and factors related to the healing process.

Infection and erosion need to be discussed also as possible long-term complications. Mechanical complications should be discussed. The patient needs to know that any type of penile prosthesis can fail mechanically and that the probability of device failure is usually proportional to device complexity. The potential implant recipient should be told that correction of device failure requires reoperation.

PREOPERATIVE PREPARATION

Preoperative preparation of the implant recipient is directed primarily at reducing the risk of infection. The penile prosthesis recipient should be free of urinary tract infection, and he should have no infections elsewhere in the body that might result in bacteria seeding during the healing phase. In addition, there should be no dermatitis, wounds, or other cutaneous lesions in the operative area. In diabetic implant recipients, good control of the diabetes mellitus may reduce the risk of infection.[86]

Broad-spectrum antibiotics providing gram-negative and gram-positive coverage are administered prophylactically. Frequently used agents are an aminoglycoside and vancomycin or an aminoglycoside and a cephalosporin. These antibiotics should be administered 1 h before the incision is made. They are usually continued for 24 to 48 h postoperatively.

Shaving of the operative area is done just before the operation. If shaving is done earlier, small cuts in the skin may become infected. After the patient is shaved, a 10 min skin preparation is performed. During the operation, traffic in the operating room should be limited. Alternatively, the Surgical Isolation Bubble System (Lonestar Medical Products, Houston, Texas) may be employed (Fig. 19–18).

SURGICAL APPROACHES

Implantation of a penile prosthesis can be performed through a variety of surgical approaches. However, those commonly used include only three, the infrapubic, subcoronal, and penoscrotal.

Infrapubic Approach

The primary advantage of the infrapubic approach is that it permits reservoir implantation under direct vision. Disadvantages include possible injury to the dorsal nerves of the penis, problems in extending corporeal exposure, and difficulty in scrotal pump fixation.

Subcoronal Approach

The subcoronal approach can be used only for nonhydraulic or one-piece hydraulic devices. The

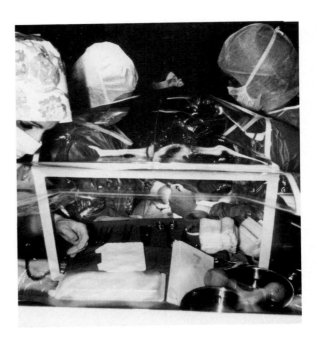

Figure 19–18. Surgical Isolation Bubble System. (Lonestar Medical Products, Houston, Tex.)

primary advantage of this approach is that it allows implantation of a prosthesis with minimal bending of the device. This is important with an implant, such as the DuraPhase, where excessive bending during implantation might weaken the cable. Disadvantages include prolonged sensitivity of the incision and possible difficulty in proximal crural dilatation from the distal corporotomy.

Penoscrotal Approach

Advantages of the penoscrotal approach, which was first used for semirigid rod implantation[87] and is now used for implantation of all types of penile prostheses, include optimal corporeal exposure, surgery away from the dorsal neurovascular bundle, and easy pump fixation in the scrotum. The disadvantage of this approach is that it requires blind reservoir placement for three-piece hydraulic devices.

IMPLANT TECHNIQUE: AMS DYNAFLEX PENILE PROSTHESIS
Position and Incision

The patient is in the supine position, and a 3 cm midline incision is made on the ventral surface of the penis starting at the penoscrotal junction. Dartos and Buck's fasciae are opened in line with the incision, and the urethra and both corpora cavernosa are exposed.

Corporeal Preparation

A 3 cm corporotomy is made, and stay sutures of 2-0 PDS (polydioxanone, Ethicon, Inc., Somerville, NJ) are placed (Fig. 19–19). The corpora are dilated with Hegar dilators beginning with 8 mm and proceeding to 15 mm proximally (Fig. 19–20) and distally (Fig. 19–21). A sizing instrument is used to obtain measurements from the proximal end of the corporotomy to the insertion of the crus onto the pelvic bone (Fig. 19–22) and from the distal end of the corporotomy to the distal end of the corpus cavernosum beneath the midglans penis (Fig. 19–23).

Prosthesis Selection

To determine the proper length for the prosthesis, the proximal and distal measurements are added together, and 1 cm is added to account for the corporotomy. Although the corporotomy is 3 cm long, only 1 cm is added because the actual internal length of the corpus cavernosum is about 2 cm less than the surface measurements. The AMS Dynaflex prosthesis comes in two diameters, 11 mm and 13 mm, and four lengths, 12 cm, 15 cm, 18 cm, and 21 cm. Length adjustment between sizes is made by the addition of one or more 0.5 cm snap-on rear tip extenders (Fig. 19–24). If corporeal dilatation to 15 mm was achieved, a 13 mm diameter implant is chosen. If corporeal dilatation to less than 15 mm was possible, an 11 mm diameter implant is chosen.

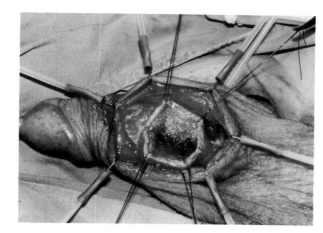

Figure 19-19. Three centimeter corporotomy with stay sutures.

Figure 19-20. Proximal corporeal (crural) dilatation.

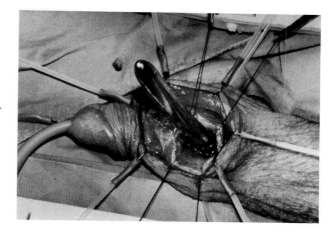

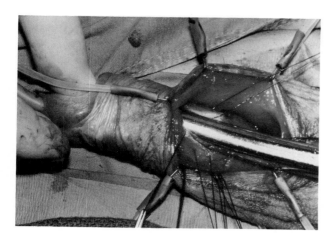

Figure 19-21. Distal corporeal dilatation.

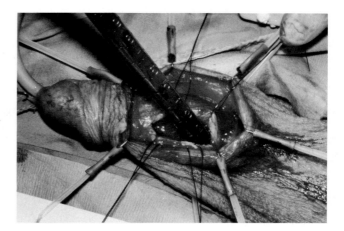

Figure 19–22. Proximal sizing.

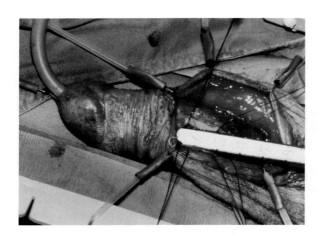

Figure 19–23. Distal sizing.

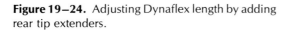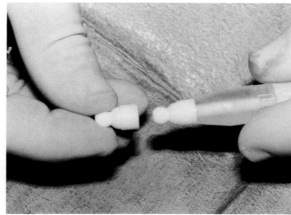

Figure 19–24. Adjusting Dynaflex length by adding rear tip extenders.

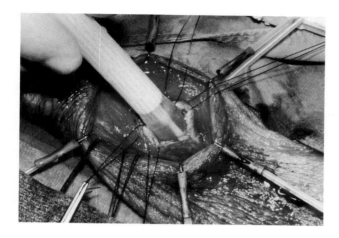

Figure 19–25. The inflated Dynaflex prosthesis is inserted proximally.

Prosthesis Implantation

The prosthesis, which has been prefilled with normal saline, is removed from its sterile foil wet pack, and if necessary rear tip extenders are added. The prosthesis is inflated to make it rigid, and it is inserted into the proximal corpus cavernosum (Fig. 19–25). The implant is then deflated (Fig. 19–26) and inserted into the distal corpus cavernosum (Fig. 19–27). The corporotomy is closed with a running horizontal mattress suture of 2-0 PDS (Fig. 19–28). Figure 19–29 shows a patient with an AMS Dynaflex deflated, and Figure 19–30 shows the same patient with the prosthesis inflated.

IMPLANT TECHNIQUE: AMA ULTREX PENILE PROSTHESIS
Position and Incision

The patient is placed in the supine position, a high transverse upper scrotal incision (Fig. 19–31) about 3 cm long is made, and dartos and Buck's fasciae are opened transversely. A 2 cm corporotomy is made, and 2-0 PDS stay sutures are placed (Fig. 19–32).

Corporeal Preparation

Dilatation is done with Hegar dilators, starting with a 8 mm dilator and proceeding to 13 mm distally (Fig. 19–33) and to 16 mm proximally (Fig. 19–34). A sizing instrument is used, and the total corporeal length is determined from each end of the corporotomy (Figs. 19–35 and 19–36). The corporotomy itself is not included in the measurement, since the sizing is done on the surface of the corpora and the actual internal corporeal length is shorter. To select the proper length cylinder for the Ultrex cylinder, 1 cm is subtracted from the total external corporeal measurement. This results in a cylinder selection that is somewhat shorter than the corpus cavernosum. This shorter cylinder fits well inside the corporeal body, and no bulging or buckling (which might result in early cylinder wear) occurs. Since the Ultrex cylinder can lengthen, a cylinder that is too long for the corpus cavernosum may, when inflated, cause an S-shaped penile deformity. With an Ultrex cylinder that is somewhat shorter than the corpus cavernosum, proper support of the glans penis can still be expected, since the cylinder lengthens with inflation.

Prosthesis Preparation

The correct length cylinders are obtained and then filled with normal saline. Since silicone is semipermeable, isotonic fluid must be used. The cylinders are filled but not distended. The pump is

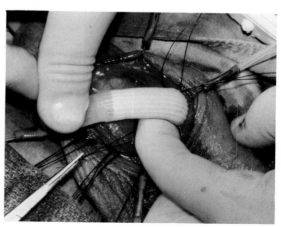

Figure 19–26. The Dynaflex device is deflated by bending it for 10 sec.

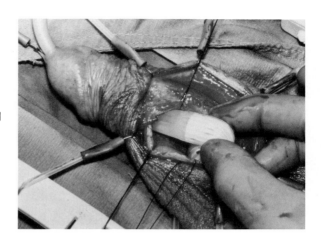

Figure 19–27. The deflated Dynaflex is inserted distally.

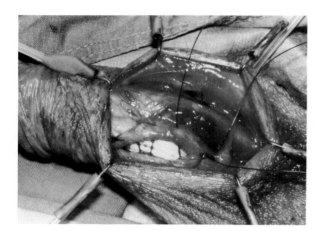

Figure 19–28. The corporotomy is closed with running 2-0 PDS suture.

Figure 19–29. A patient with a deflated AMS Dynaflex prosthesis.

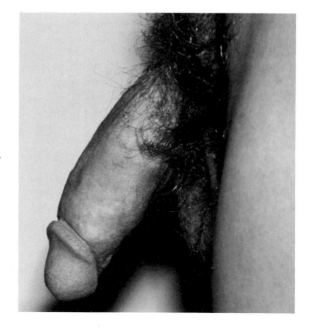

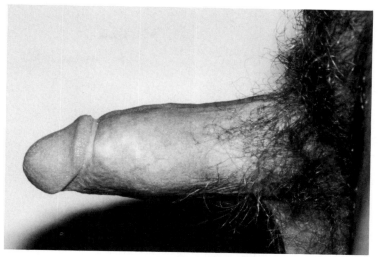

Figure 19–30. The patient in Figure 19–29 with his prosthesis inflated.

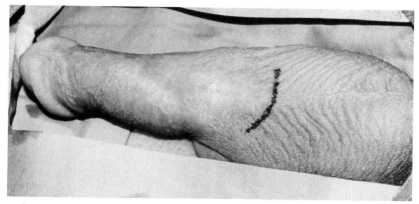

Figure 19–31. The 3 cm high transverse upper scrotal incision is marked.

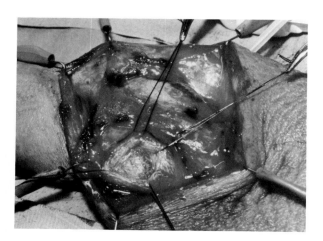

Figure 19–32. Two centimeter corporotomy with stay sutures.

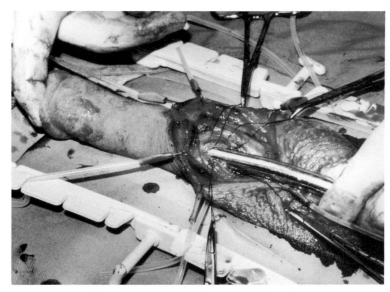

Figure 19–33. Distal corporeal dilatation.

Figure 19–34. Proximal corporeal (crural) dilatation.

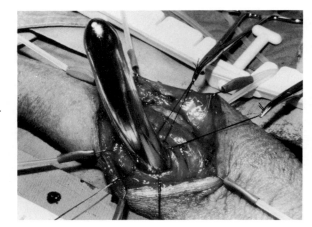

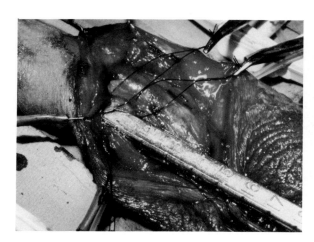

Figure 19–35. Distal sizing.

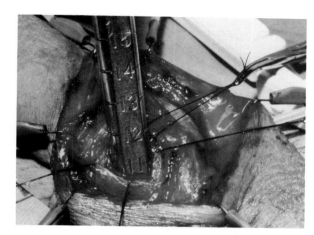

Figure 19–36. Proximal sizing.

filled by cycling the pump while the tubes are held under the surface of a basin of normal saline. The reservoir is filled with normal saline to displace the air, and the saline is then withdrawn, since the reservoir will be implanted empty.

Cylinder Implantation

A Furlow cylinder inserter (American Medical Systems, Minnetonka, MN) is used to pass a straight needle carrying a pulling suture through the inside tip of the corpus cavernosum out through the glans penis (Fig. 19–37). This suture, which passes through the tip of the cylinder, is used to

pull the cylinder into the distal corpus cavernosum (Fig. 19–38). If any rear tip extenders are needed, they are now applied (Fig. 19–39). A right angle clamp placed inside the proximal corpus cavernosum is used to create a stab incision approximately one half of the way between the corporotomy and the bone attachment of the crus (Fig. 19–40). A second right angle clamp is passed through this incision from the outside into the corpus cavernosum (Fig. 19–41), and this clamp is used to pull the cylinder tubing out through the stab incision (Figs. 19–42 and 19–43). Cylinder fit is checked, and the corporotomies are closed with running horizontal mattress sutures of 2-0 PDS

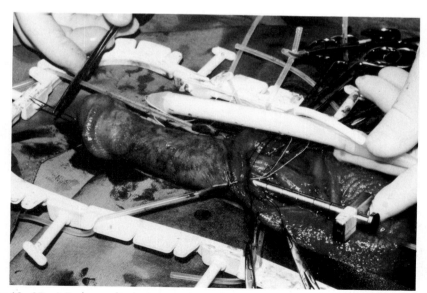

Figure 19–37. A Furlow cylinder inserter is used to pass a straight needle containing a pulling suture out through the tip of the corpus cavernosum and the overlying glans. (From Montague DK. Inflatable penile prostheses—AMS experience. In: Carson CC, ed. Prosthetics in Urology, Problems in Urology Series. JB Lippincott Co, [in press].)

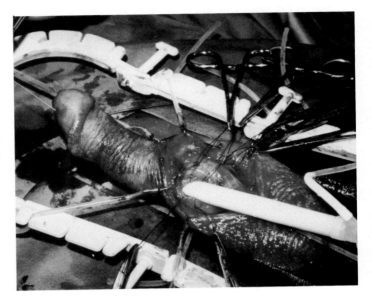

Figure 19–38. The pulling suture is used to pull the cylinder into the distal corpus cavernosum.

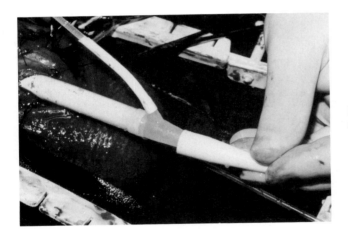

Figure 19–39. Rear tip extenders, if needed, are applied.

Figure 19–40. A right angle clamp creates a stab incision approximately halfway down the crus. (From Montague DK. Inflatable penile prostheses—AMS experience. In: Carson CC, ed. Prosthetics in Urology, Problems in Urology Series. JB Lippincott Co, [in press].)

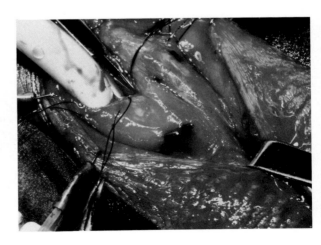

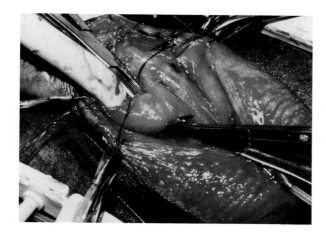

Figure 19–41. A second right angle clamp is passed through the stab incision into the corpus cavernosum.

(Fig. 19–44). The polytetrafluoroethylene covering around the cylinder tubing is removed (Fig. 19–45).

Pump Implantation

A small incision is made through dartos fascia in the septum of the scrotum. A long clamp is introduced through this incision and then spread to create a dartos pouch for the pump (Fig. 19–46). The pump is placed in this pouch so that the single tube going to the reservoir is located anteriorly. Placement of the pump in a septal location facilitates subsequent inflation of the prosthesis. The pump can be brought forward, allowing both testes to drop back. This provides ready exposure of both sides of the pump for device inflation (Fig. 19–47).

A right angled clamp is used to bring the pump tubing that goes to each cylinder out through the fascia that forms the back wall of the pouch (Fig. 19–48). Likewise, the pump tubing that goes to the reservoir is brought through the back wall of the pouch.

Pump–Cylinder Connections

The pump and cylinder tubing are irrigated with antibiotic solution to wash off any blood. Clean scissors are used to cut the tubing to appropriate lengths, making clean, right angled cuts. Each cylinder is connected to one of the cylinder tubes from the pump using straight connectors from the Quick Connect System (American Medical Systems). Connector rings are applied first to each of the tubes to be connected (Fig. 19–49). Each end of the tubing is inserted into a connector. Care should be taken to ensure that each tubing end is inserted completely into the connector up to the central stop (Fig. 19–50). After the closure tool (American

Medical Systems) is used to seat the connector rings (Fig. 19–51), the completed connection should be inspected to ascertain that both rings have been forced evenly and completely into each end of the connector. The Quick Connectors should be used only for initial implants or revisions where a connection is being made between two new components. If during a revision a connection is made to a component that was previously implanted, tie-on plastic connectors should be used. Quick Connectors may not be secure when they are used to connect tubing that has a lipid coating.

Reservoir Implantation

An 18F Foley catheter is inserted, and the bladder is completely emptied (Fig. 19–52). The surgeon introduces his or her index finger through the incision and then places it in the external inguinal ring. Long Metzenbaum scissors are used to per-

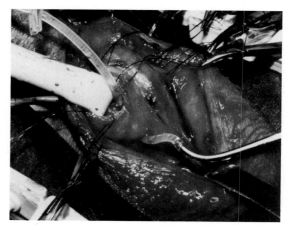

Figure 19–42. The second clamp is used to pull the cylinder tubing out.

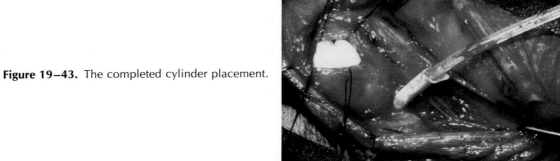

Figure 19–43. The completed cylinder placement.

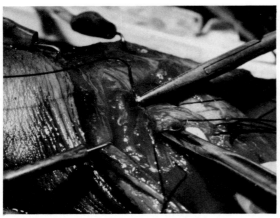

Figure 19–44. The corporotomy is closed with running 2-0 PDS suture.

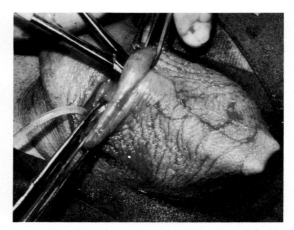

Figure 19–46. A long clamp creates a septal dartos pouch for the pump. (From Montague DK. Inflatable penile prostheses—AMS experience. In: Carson CC, ed. Prosthetics in Urology, Problems in Urology Series. JB Lippincott Co, [in press].)

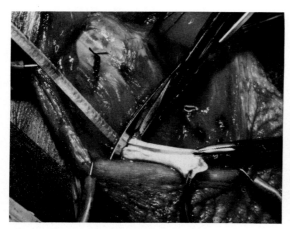

Figure 19–45. The polytetrafluoroethylene covering around the cylinder tubing is removed.

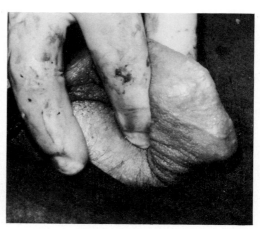

Figure 19–47. Septal placement of the pump allows it to be brought forward, creating ready access to both sides of the pump for inflation.

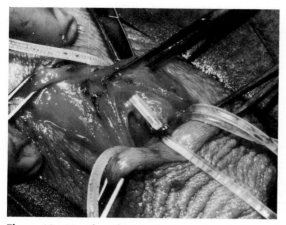

Figure 19–48. The tubing going to each cylinder and the reservoir is brought out through separate stab incisions in the back wall of the dartos pouch.

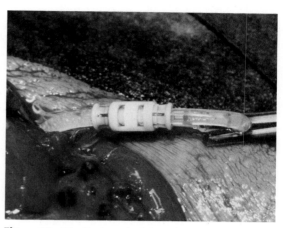

Figure 19–50. Each end of the tubing is inserted into the connector up to the central stop.

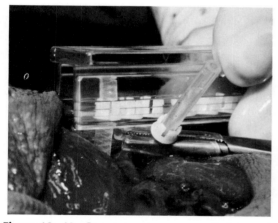

Figure 19–49. Connector rings are applied to each end of the tubing.

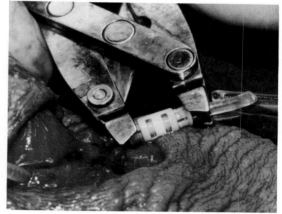

Figure 19–51. The closure tool is used to seat the connector rings, completing the connection. (From Montague DK. Inflatable penile prostheses—AMS experience. In: Carson CC, ed. Prosthetics in Urology, Problems in Urology Series. JB Lippincott Co, [in press].)

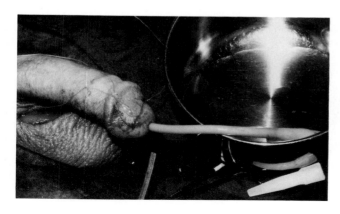

Figure 19–52. A catheter is inserted, and the bladder is emptied.

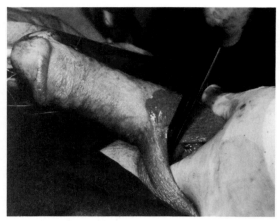

Figure 19–53. Long Metzenbaum scissors are used to perforate the transversalis fascia on the floor of the external inguinal ring. (From Montague DK. Inflatable penile prostheses—AMS experience. In: Carson CC, ed. Prosthetics in Urology, Problems in Urology Series. JB Lippincott Co, [in press].)

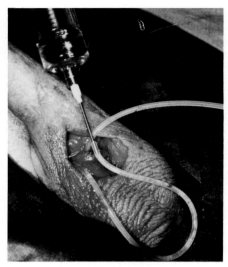

Figure 19–55. Saline is allowed to return to a glass syringe so that the fluid pressure in the reservoir will be zero.

forate the transversalis fascia in the floor of the ring (Fig. 19–53). The scissors are placed medial to the finger, and thus the cord structures, which are lateral to the finger, are protected. The scissors are spread and then withdrawn as the surgeon introduces his or her finger into the retropubic space. The surgeon should be able to feel the back of the symphysis pubis and the empty bladder. The inguinal reservoir introducer places the empty reservoir into the retropubic space (Fig. 19–54). The reservoir is filled with either 65 ml or 100 ml of normal saline, which is allowed to return to a glass syringe until the pressure in the reser-

voir is zero (Fig. 19–55). Generally 50 ml to 55 ml in a 65 ml reservoir and 85 ml to 90 ml in a 100 ml reservoir are the final zero pressure fluid volumes. A connection between the pump and the reservoir is made with a straight Quick Connector.

Hydraulic Dilatation and Intraoperative Testing

The prosthesis is fully inflated and deflated three times to stretch the corpora and to see that the prosthesis is functioning correctly. A cylinder sizing tool is used to determine the external pubis to midglans distance with the device both deflated (Fig. 19–56) and inflated (Fig. 19–57). Running 3-0 Dexon is used to close the dartos fascia over the pump. A second 3-0 Dexon suture is used to close dartos fascia transversely under the incision. The skin is closed with a running subcuticular 4-0 Vicryl suture. The prosthesis is left fully deflated, and to avoid chordee, the penis is kept up on the lower abdomen for the first 4 postoperative weeks.

Preventing Autoinflation

It has not been possible to incorporate a useful mechanism to prevent autoinflation in the prosthesis. Therefore, if the reservoir pressure is sufficiently high, fluid will flow from the reservoir through the pump and into the cylinders until cylinder pressure equals reservoir pressure. This results in partial erection, and this phenomenon is

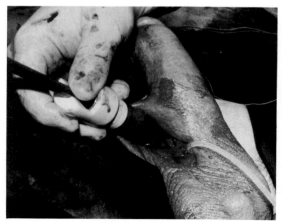

Figure 19–54. An empty reservoir is introduced into the retropubic space with the inguinal reservoir inserter.

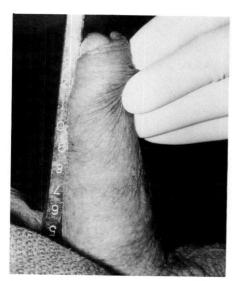

Figure 19–56. The pubis to midglans distance with the prosthesis deflated is 13 cm. (From Montague DK, Lakin MM. Early experience with the controlled girth and length expanding cylinder of the AMS Ultrex penile prosthesis. J Urol 148:1444–1446, © by Williams & Wilkins, 1992.)

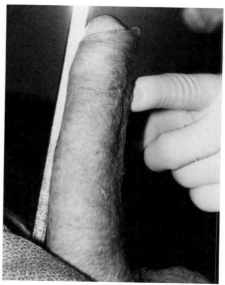

Figure 19–57. The pubis to midglans distance with the prosthesis inflated is 17 cm. (From Montague DK, Lakin MM. Early experience with the controlled girth and length expanding cylinder of the AMS Ultrex penile prosthesis. J Urol 148:1444–1446, © by Williams & Wilkins, 1992.)

known as autoinflation. The 65 ml and 100 ml reservoirs are designed to hold these amounts of fluid under zero pressure. However, this determination is made when the reservoirs are filled outside the body. As the reservoir expands with fluid in the body, it pushes against adjacent structures and the zero pressure state is reached sooner.

Two things should be done to avoid or minimize autoinflation. After the empty reservoir is implanted, it is filled with either 65 ml or 100 ml of normal saline. Fluid is allowed to escape from the reservoir tubing until the pressure is zero. The second step is to be sure that the cylinders are left deflated while healing takes place. It is not necessary to inflate the device early postoperatively. The first inflation can be done in 4 to 8 weeks, when the patient is relatively pain free. Although the body reacts to silicone by forming a fibrous pseudocapsule around it,[88] the energy generated by pumping will stretch the capsule that forms around the cylinders. On the other hand, deflation of the prosthesis takes place passively, and if the cylinders are left inflated while healing is taking place, the capsule that forms around the partially empty reservoir will prevent deflation at zero reservoir pressures. Figure 19–58 shows a man with his AMS Ultrex device deflated, and Figure 19–59 shows the same man with his prosthesis inflated.

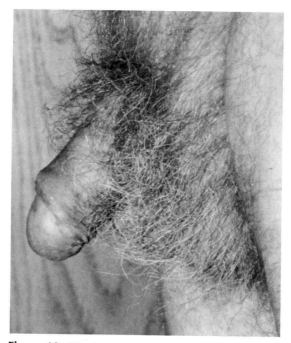

Figure 19–58. A patient with his AMS Ultrex deflated. (From Montague DK, Lakin MM. Early experience with the controlled girth and length expanding cylinder of the AMS Ultrex penile prosthesis. J Urol 148:1444–1446, © by Williams & Wilkins, 1992.)

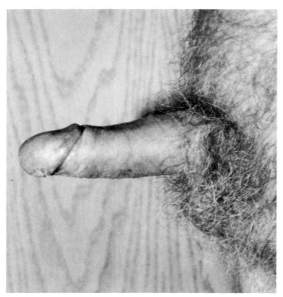

Figure 19–59. The patient in Figure 19–58 with his AMS Ultrex prosthesis inflated. The length increase in this patient was 2 cm. (From Montague DK, Lakin MM. Early experience with the controlled girth and length expanding cylinder of the AMS Ultrex penile prosthesis. J Urol 148:1444–1446, © by Williams & Wilkins, 1992.)

POSTOPERATIVE CARE

The Foley catheter is removed on the first postoperative day, and the patient is discharged on the second postoperative day. The patient is allowed to shower on the third postoperative day. One month after surgery, an attempt is made to inflate and deflate the prosthesis. If tenderness around the pump is still present, instruction on device inflation and deflation is delayed until 2 months after surgery. It is important to keep the cylinders fully deflated while healing is taking place to help prevent autoinflation, and the penis should be kept up on the lower abdomen to prevent ventral chordee.[89,90] Once the patient is able to learn how to cycle the prosthesis, he is instructed to inflate and deflate it fully twice daily for 4 weeks. Coitus can be attempted whenever the patient is pain free. The patient and his partner are instructed to use a water-soluble lubricant and to have adequate foreplay before vaginal intromission.

RESULTS
AMS Ultrex Prosthesis

We have implanted the AMS Ultrex prosthesis in 100 men. Follow-up is from 2 to 34 months (mean 14 months). One device was explanted at 3 weeks because of infection, and there were 2 me-

chanical failures, a reservoir leak and a pump leak. At the conclusion of each implant procedure, the pubis to midglans distance was measured with the cylinders deflated and then fully inflated. The increase in the pubis to midglans distance from the flaccid to the erect state in the first 50 patients is shown in Table 19–3.[71]

Experience with the Ultrex prosthesis obviously is still somewhat limited. However, some observations and projections can be made. Because of similarity in design, the mechanical reliability of this device will probably be similar to that of the AMS 700CX prosthesis. Because the Ultrex cylinders can lengthen, corporeal measurement and cylinder selection are no longer as critical as they once were. Indeed, implanters should implant a cylinder that is about 1 cm less than the total corporeal length. The patient can be told that his penis may lengthen with erection, but the amount of lengthening is variable and probably depends primarily on the elasticity of the patient's corpora. The Ultrex device is the only prosthesis that offers the advantage of cylinder and penile lengthening with inflation.

AMS 700CX Prosthesis

Longer experience is available with the AMS 700CX device, the prosthesis that preceded the AMS Ultrex. We have implanted the AMS 700CX prosthesis in 116 men. Follow-up is from 11 to 76 months (mean 48 months). There were 4 surgical complications resulting in device removal. One patient developed a periprosthetic infection and underwent prosthesis explantation at 7 months. Two patients who had previous penile prosthetic surgery developed urethral cylinder erosion, and 1 patient had reservoir erosion into the bladder. These patients all had their devices removed. There were 2 mechanical failures, a tubing leak, and a cylinder leak. The tubing leak occurred at 7 weeks, and this complication undoubtedly occurred because of tubing damage during closure. The only cylinder leak occurred at 4 years and 2 months. This experience compares favorably with other reports concerning this prosthesis.[68,70]

TABLE 19–3

Pubis to Midglans Penile Length Increase with Prosthesis Inflation

Increase (cm)	No. of patients
1	14
2	29
3	5

COMPLICATIONS

Most of the complications occurring during and after penile prosthesis implantation are listed in Table 19–4. The frequency of occurrence of many of these complications can be kept low by careful attention to detail and proper technique before, during, and after the operation. Nevertheless, the most careful surgeon will have some patients who experience these various complications, and the ability to recognize and manage these problems is essential.

Infection

Infection is probably the most significant complication of penile implant surgery.[91–97] Infection usually requires reoperation and frequently requires device removal. After an infected penile prosthesis is removed, cavernosal fibrosis occurs, making the penis smaller. Implantation of another prosthesis at a later date is not a significant problem with respect to pump or reservoir placement. However, implantation of new cylinders often is very difficult. The overall incidence of penile prosthesis infection has been estimated to be about 2%, with infection rates of 0.6% to 16.7% for nonhydraulic devices, 3.0% to 8.1% for one-piece hydraulic devices, and 0.8% to 8% for three-piece hydraulic devices.[94] Most periprosthetic infections are the direct result of the implant procedure. However, late hematogenous spread of infection from distant sources has been shown to occur.[91] Staphylococcal organisms are responsible for more than 50% of infections, with the rest usually caused by gram-negative bacteria.[92,93,98] Fungal infections,[99] gonococcal infections,[95] and Fournier's gangrene[100] are unusual infectious complications of penile prosthesis implantation. Penile necrosis occurs rarely following penile prosthesis implantation.[101–104]

This sometimes is caused by infection but also can be due to ischemia related to other factors. To help avoid penile necrosis after prosthesis implantation, pressure dressings on the penis either are not used or are applied with minimal compression of the penile tissues.

An early sign of infection is adherence of the skin and subcutaneous tissue to an underlying prosthesis component. This is seen most frequently in the scrotum, where the scrotal tissues become adherent to the pump. The tissue adherent to the pump gradually becomes thinner, and eventually pump erosion occurs (Fig. 19–60). Other signs of infection include persistent pain, swelling and erythema of tissue, fever, and purulent drainage.

Bacterial adherence to the prosthesis has been shown to be due to the ability of bacteria to produce an extracellular matrix or glycocalix composed of polysaccharides. This glycocalix acts as a physical barrier and impedes antibiotic and host defense mechanisms.[97] Superficial wound infections usually will respond to standard treatment, but deep infections in the periprosthetic space usually will not clear even with intensive antibiotic therapy. Because of adherence of bacteria to the prosthesis, when prosthesis explantation is required, it is important to remove all the prosthetic material. Standard treatment in the past has been to reimplant a new prosthesis at a later date. However, because of the difficulty with prosthesis implantation into fibrotic corpora, alternative methods of dealing with infection have been sought.

Furlow and Goldwasser introduced the concept of a salvage procedure for dealing with penile pros-

---

TABLE 19–4
Complications of Penile Prosthesis Implantation

Infection
Mechanical failures
Fibrosis
Autoinflation
Erosion
Sensory disturbances
Sizing errors
Ejaculatory incompetence
Insufficient rigidity
Phimosis, paraphimosis
Component displacement
Urinary retention

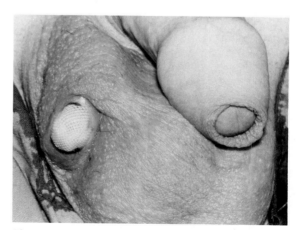

Figure 19–60. Pump erosion as a result of periprosthetic infection following implantation of an inflatable penile prosthesis. (From Montague DK. Penile prostheses. In: Montague DK, ed. Disorders of Male Sexual Function. Year Book Medical Publishers, Inc, 1988.)

thesis erosion. They were able to salvage successfully 16 of 22 cases of scrotal pump erosion, 8 of 8 cases of reservoir erosion, and 0 of 2 cases of cylinder erosion.[105] Because erosion is often associated with infection, salvage procedures are considered reasonable alternatives for dealing with infection. In a salvage procedure for infection, all prosthetic material is explanted, and cultures are taken. The operative field is irrigated with copious amounts of saline and antibiotic solution, and all new prosthetic material is implanted. Approximately 70% to 80% of these cases will heal successfully with no recurrent infection.

Fibrosis

Conditions associated with fibrosis are listed in Table 19–5. The most common cause of significant fibrosis is infection following previous penile prosthesis implantation. Fibrosis is usually severe following priapism and can lead to significant difficulties with prosthesis implantation.[106] Fortunately, priapism resulting in fibrosis is a rather uncommon occurrence. Fibrotic complications associated with intracavernous pharmacotherapy are common and consist of Peyronie's disease-like plaques and intracorporeal nodules.[107] Fortunately, the degree of fibrosis in men who have been on intracavernous pharmacotherapy rarely is severe, and prosthesis implantation usually is accomplished with only minimal difficulty.

Peyronie's disease causes fibrotic plaques that occur primarily on the surface of the corporeal bodies. Cavernosal smooth muscle is not usually affected, and the corpora are easy to dilate. If a malleable semirigid rod prosthesis is implanted, the penis often can be straightened by bending the prosthesis.[19] With an inflatable penile prosthesis and sometimes with nonmalleable semirigid rod devices, plaque excision, incision (Figs. 19–61 and 19–62), or a Nesbitt procedure may be necessary to correct penile curvature.[108–110]

Penile fibrosis can be expected in implant recipients who have one or more of the described conditions. However, idiopathic penile fibrosis

TABLE 19–5
Causes of Penile Fibrosis

Penile prosthesis infection
Priapism
Intracavernosal pharmacotherapy
Peyronie's disease
Idiopathic

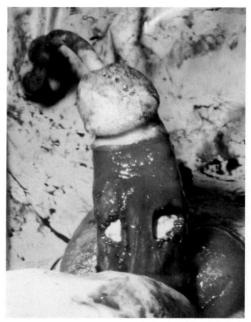

Figure 19–61. One transverse dorsal incision down to the cylinders has been made to correct dorsal curvature. (Note that the neurovascular bundle has been elevated.)

may be encountered unexpectedly during prosthesis implantation, and the surgeon should always be prepared to deal with this problem.

When the corporotomy is made for prosthesis implantation, the tunica albuginea and underlying cavernosal tissue, when normal, have a characteristic appearance (Fig. 19–63). The tunica has a uniform thickness of approximately 2 mm, and there is an abrupt transition between the tunica and the underlying erectile tissue, which is trabecular and beefy red in color. When cavernosal fibrosis is present, the erectile tissue is pale yellow, the trabecular appearance is lost, and the transition between the erectile tissue and the tunica albuginea is indistinct (Fig. 19–64).

If resistance to Hegar dilatation is encountered, force should not be used, as perforation is likely to occur. A Dilamezinsert instrument (Lone Star Medical Products, Inc., Houston, TX) (Fig. 19–65) may be used. This instrument has a sharper tip than a Hegar dilator, and it should be used with caution. Alternatively, long Metzenbaum scissors may be used (Fig. 19–66). Gently separating the tips of these scissors as they are advanced aids in their passage. As the scissors are withdrawn, the blades are more widely separated, and this procedure is repeated in three or four planes. After the Metzenbaum scissors are used in this fashion,

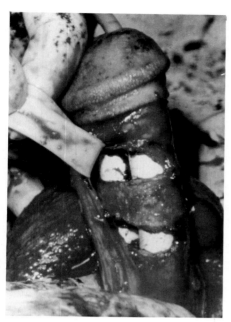

Figure 19–62. Two transverse incisions were required in this patient for complete penile straightening. (From Montague DK. Prosthesis insertion in the fibrotic penis. Urology Times 20:27, 1992.)

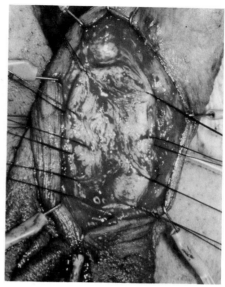

Figure 19–64. A patient with corporeal fibrosis. (From Montague DK. Penile prosthesis implantation in patients with corporeal fibrosis. In: McDougal WS, ed. Difficult Problems in Urologic Surgery. Year Book Medical Publishers, Inc, 1989.)

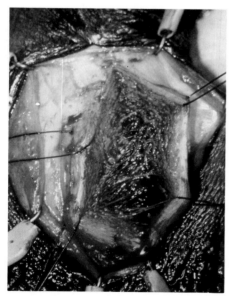

Figure 19–63. Normal tunica albuginea and erectile tissue. (From Montague DK. Penile prosthesis implantation in patients with corporeal fibrosis. In: McDougal WS, ed. Difficult Problems in Urologic Surgery. Year Book Medical Publishers, Inc, 1989.)

progressive dilatation with Hegar dilators usually is possible.

If these measures are not successful, the skin incision and the corporotomy should be extended. The penoscrotal incision has an advantage in this regard as it can be extended out to the frenulum if necessary for total distal corporeal exposure, and the resultant scar will be hidden when the patient stands. Proximal corporeal exposure can be obtained by retracting the scrotal contents (Fig. 19–67). If an infrapubic approach has been used, proximal corporeal exposure is limited and difficult, and distal corporeal exposure is usually obtained through a second circumcising, degloving incision.

Once an extended corporotomy has been made, a plane of dissection between the inner surface of the tunica albuginea and the fibrotic erectile tissue can be established under direct vision with sharp dissection (Fig. 19–68). This plane of dissection is extended until a fibrotic core of tissue can be removed (Fig. 19–69).[81,82] Finney has described another method of coring fibrotic tissue using sharpened hollow brass or stainless steel tubing.[111] After fibrotic tissue has been removed, a semirigid rod prosthesis can be placed into the corpus cavernosum (Fig. 19–70), or a hydraulic cylinder can be placed (Fig. 19–71). The tunica albuginea is then closed with running 2-0 polydioxanone suture. Sometimes, complete tunica closure is not possi-

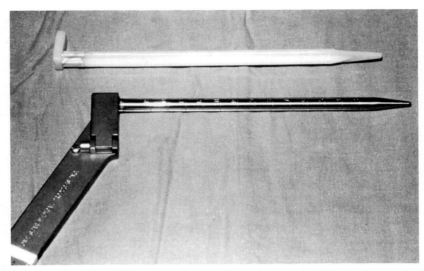

Figure 19–65. The Dilamezinsert instrument. (From Montague DK. Penile prosthesis implantation in patients with corporeal fibrosis. In: McDougal WS, ed. Difficult Problems in Urologic Surgery. Year Book Medical Publishers, Inc, 1989.)

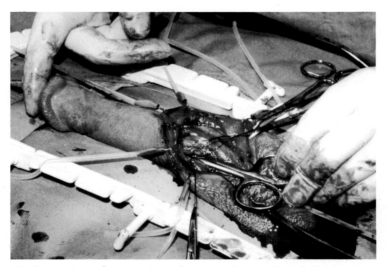

Figure 19–66. Long Metzenbaum scissor dissection frequently is helpful when cavernosal fibrosis is encountered.

ble, and the resultant defect can be covered with either dacron (Fig. 19–72) or polytetrafluoroethylene (Gore-Tex, Wakefield, Mass.) (Fig. 19–73). These patches of synthetic material must be sewn into place with nonabsorbable suture, such as 3-0 prolene.

Erosion

Factors associated with erosion are listed in Table 19–6. A common cause of erosion is tissue

injury during the implant procedure. If the urethra is entered, the implant procedure, at least on that side, should be abandoned. Lateral perforation of the tunica albuginea can still permit prosthesis implantation if another more medial plane for dilatation is established and the perforation is closed. If the crus is perforated during proximal corporeal dilatation, the crus usually can still be dilated adequately down to its bone attachment, and a rod prosthesis or hydraulic cylinder can be inserted, making certain that the proximal end of the pros-

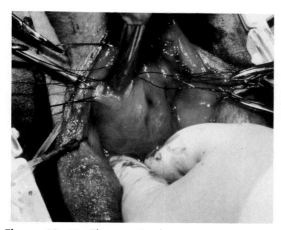

Figure 19–67. The proximal corpus cavernosum (crus) can be exposed by retracting the scrotal contents.

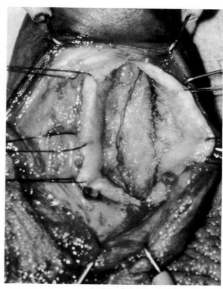

Figure 19–68. A plane of dissection between the fibrotic cavernosal tissue and the tunica albuginea can be established. (From Montague DK. Penile prosthesis implantation in patients with corporeal fibrosis. In: McDougal WS, ed. Difficult Problems in Urologic Surgery. Year Book Medical Publishers, Inc, 1989.)

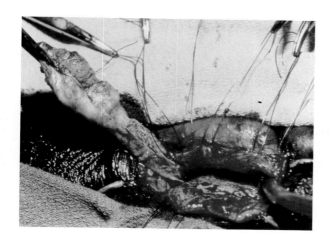

Figure 19–69. A core of fibrotic tissue is removed from the corpus cavernosum.

Figure 19–70. After making an extended corporotomy and resecting fibrotic cavernosal tissue, a malleable rod prosthesis is placed. (From Montague DK. Penile prosthesis implantation in patients with corporeal fibrosis. In: McDougal WS, ed. Difficult Problems in Urologic Surgery. Year Book Medical Publishers, Inc, 1989.)

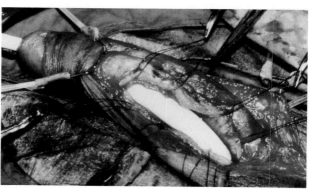

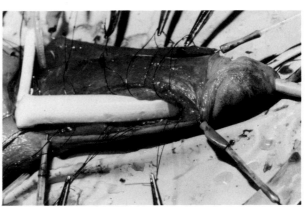

Figure 19–71. After making an extended corporotomy and resecting fibrotic cavernosal tissue, a penile cylinder is placed.

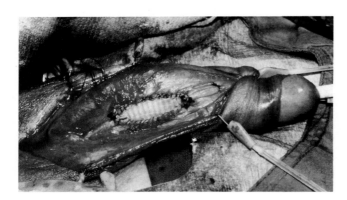

Figure 19–72. If the tunica albuginea cannot be closed primarily, the closure may be completed with a dacron patch.

thesis does not go out through the perforation. Alternatively, a dacron[112] or polytetrafluoroethylene[113] sock can be constructed to prevent prosthesis migration out into the perineum.

Infection is a common cause of erosion, and it is not always possible to tell whether erosion oc-

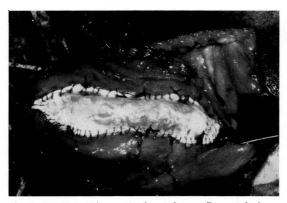

Figure 19–73. Alternatively, polytetrafluoroethylene (Gore-Tex) can be used as a patch for corporeal closure. (From Montague DK. Prosthesis insertion in the fibrotic penis. Urology Times 20:27, 1992.)

curred because of infection or other factors. This makes the true incidence of periprosthetic infection difficult to judge. As already discussed, erosion with or without infection requires device removal either with a salvage procedure[105] or reimplantation at a later date.[114]

Erosion can occur because of ischemia, which may be associated with many contributing factors (Table 19–6). The incidence of erosion is generally considered to be higher when a rod prosthesis is used than when a hydraulic device is implanted. This is particularly true if the prosthesis is too long to fit in the corpora without pressure. Absent sensation, usually associated with SCI, is a contributing factor to erosion. Radiation therapy, diabetes mellitus, and atherosclerosis are all factors that may contribute to erosion. Finally, ischemia, erosion, and gangrene (Fig. 19–74) may result from a pressure dressing or urethral catheter.[115]

After cystectomy the retropubic space is part of the abdominal cavity, and placement of a reservoir in a standard fashion results in an intraperitoneal reservoir placement. This has been associated with various complications, including small bowel obstruction,[116] erosion into an ileal conduit,[117] and erosion into small and large bowel (Fig. 19–75).[118]

TABLE 19–6
Factor Associated with Erosion

Operative injury
Ischemia
    Rod prostheses
    Oversized prostheses
    Lack of sensation
Infection
Radiation
Diabetes mellitus
Atherosclerosis
Pressure dressings
Urethral catheters

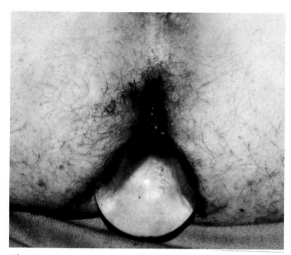

Figure 19–75. Erosion of an inflatable penile prosthesis reservoir into the rectum in a patient who had previously had a cystectomy.

If a three-piece hydraulic prosthesis is implanted in a patient who has had a cystectomy, extraperitoneal reservoir implantation through a separate incision can be performed.

Erosion of reservoirs into the bladder has been reported.[105,119,120] A salvage procedure is usually advisable in these cases. Scrotal pump erosion usually is a manifestation of infection, and either prosthesis removal with reimplantation at a later date or a salvage procedure should be done. Furlow and Goldwasser reported 22 salvage procedures for eroded pumps, with success in 16 cases.[105]

Sizing Errors

Inadequate distal dilation of the corpora and placement of a prosthesis that is too short will result in poor support of the glans penis (Fig. 19–76). This is commonly referred to as an SST deformity because of its resemblance to the supersonic transport aircraft. This is not only a cosmetic deformity but also a functional one, since poor glanular sup-

port usually causes pain during coitus. Treatment involves removal of the prosthesis. Long Metzenbaum scissors are inserted distally, and the fibrous capsule is perforated with the scissors. Hegar dilators are used to dilate the distal portion of the corpora. New measurements are taken, and a longer prosthesis is implanted. Alternatively, a dorsal subcoronal incision can be made, and subcutaneous horizontal mattress sutures can be placed, pulling the dorsal aspect of the glans back onto the distal

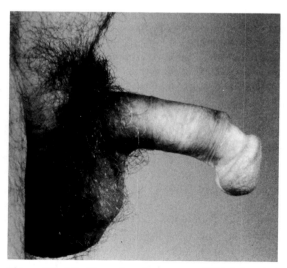

Figure 19–76. Poor glanular support (SST deformity) in a patient with a penile prosthesis that is too short. (From Montague DK. Penile prostheses. In: Montague DK, ed. Disorders of Male Sexual Function. Year Book Medical Publishers, Inc, 1988.)

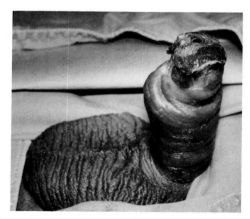

Figure 19–74. A patient with a semirigid rod penile prosthesis and dry gangrene of the glans penis.

penile shaft.[121] Care should be taken so these sutures do not injure the dorsal neurovascular structures or damage an underlying hydraulic device.

Placement of a hydraulic cylinder that is too long will result in buckling or folding of the cylinder, and this may result in early cylinder wear and fluid loss. With the AMX Ultrex cylinder where elongation takes place, a cylinder that is too long can result in an S-shaped deformity of the penis when the cylinders are inflated. For this reason, it is advisable to implant AMX Ultrex cylinders that are 1 cm shorter than usual. An SST deformity is unlikely, since these cylinders lengthen with inflation.

Implantation of a nonhydraulic or semirigid rod prosthesis may result in erosion. An early sign is persistent pain. Penile pain following prosthesis implantation generally persists for 1 to 2 months. Pain that lasts beyond this time may be caused by infection or a prosthesis that is too long. Treatment involves removal of the prosthesis, resizing of the corporeal bodies, and implantation of a shorter device.

Insufficient Rigidity

Penile prosthesis recipients frequently complain that their new erection is shorter than their natural erection used to be. This is a shortcoming inherent in prosthetic treatment of erectile dysfunction, and the length-elongating AMS Ultrex cylinders only partially correct this. Patients should be counseled preoperatively regarding the difference between natural and prosthetic erections. When an implant recipient complains of insufficient rigidity, his complaints may or may not be realistic, and the urologist should determine this by careful examination. Pressure on the glans penis toward the body is a good test of long axial rigidity. A one-piece or two-piece hydraulic prosthesis will provide sufficient rigidity for many men but often not enough for those with longer penises. When rigidity is insufficient, conversion to a three-piece inflatable prosthesis may be necessary. Men with semirigid rod prostheses may also have insufficient rigidity, and this is more likely if their penis is long or if they have a small-diameter or nonmalleable rod prosthesis. Again, conversion to another prosthesis may be necessary.

Component Displacement

The most common component displacement problem is upward pump migration. When the pump is low in the scrotum, the cosmetic appearance is better, and the pump is easier to cycle. Not only does upward pump migration affect the cos-metic appearance and make pumping more difficult, but also the pump may impinge on the base of the penis and interfere with complete vaginal intromission. Treatment is reoperation to move the pump to a lower location.

Distal cylinder crossover results in both distal cylinders being in the same corpus cavernosum. The cylinder that has crossed over pushes the other cylinder tip laterally, and this frequently results in pain. Treatment is removal of the cylinder that has crossed over, distal dilatation of that corpus cavernosum, and reimplantation of the same cylinder. This may occur also with nonhydraulic devices. Rarely, a reservoir may pop out through the transversalis fascia and appear as a bulge in the inguinal canal. This can be distinguished from a hernia by inflation of the prosthesis, which causes a bulge to disappear or become much smaller. Treatment is replacement of the prosthesis and repair of the fascial defect. This should be done through a separate inguinal incision.

Mechanical Failures

Mechanical failures of penile prostheses, although more common with hydraulic devices, also occur with nonhydraulic or semirigid rod prostheses. Breakage of strands in the silver wire core of the Jonas penile prosthesis,[18,21–23] fractures of the Small-Carrion and Finney Flexi-Rod devices,[122] and cable breakage of the OmniPhase[33,34] and DuraPhase[36,38] prostheses have been reported.

Early experience with the Scott-Bradley-Timm AMS inflatable penile prosthesis revealed mechanical failure rates ranging from 21% to 45%.[47,52,57,61,62] Four separate reports indicate significant improvement in mechanical reliability of the AMS 700 prosthesis compared to the pre-700 AMS models.[44,64,66,67] The current models of the AMS three-piece hydraulic prostheses (AMS 700CX, AMS Ultrex, and AMS Ultrex Plus) use triple-ply cylinders with input tubing protection, a sutureless connector system, kink-resistant tubing, and seamless reservoirs. Long-term experience with these new devices is not available, but preliminary reports[50,68,70] (see RESULTS) indicate that the mechanical reliability of these devices will be considerably better than the reliability of earlier models.

The Mentor three-piece hydraulic prosthesis was introduced in 1983. Initial reports indicated a 7.3% mechanical failure rate,[72,79] whereas a later report indicated a mechanical failure rate of 3%.[80] The primary difference between the current AMS and Mentor three-piece hydraulic devices is the cylinders. Mentor cylinders are constructed from polyurethane and, when deflated, produce palpable lateral folds at the base of the penis. This polyurethane material can be damaged by surgical cautery. The silicone cylinders of the AMS prostheses are not damaged by surgical cautery and have different expansion and contraction characteristics than the Mentor cylinders.

Autoinflation

Today's three-piece hydraulic devices do not contain a mechanism to prevent autoinflation. If pressure in the reservoir is high enough, fluid will be transferred from the reservoir through the pump into the cylinders until cylinder and reservoir pressures are equal. Autoinflation can be prevented or minimized by making sure that fluid pressure in the reservoir after implantation is zero and by maintaining the prosthesis in the deflated state during the healing process while a fibrous pseudocapsule is forming around the device. Finally, a reservoir in the prevesical space is less subject to increases in pressure due to physical stress than a reservoir implanted between the rectus muscle and the peritoneum. Treatment for autoinflation requires reoperation, at which time the noted principles are followed.

Sensory Disturbances

With the infrapubic and subcoronal surgical approaches for penile prosthesis implantation, injury to the dorsal nerves of the penis is possible. Even when these approaches are used, however, dorsal nerve injury is rare. With ventral (penoscrotal) approaches, dorsal nerve injury is not possible. Rarely, following penile prosthesis implantation with any of these approaches, the implant recipient complains of decreased sensation. An explanation for this usually is not evident unless dorsal nerve injury has occurred.

A somewhat more frequent but still rare problem is persistent pain following penile prosthesis implantation. Pain after prosthesis implantation generally persists for 1 to 2 months, although this is quite variable from patient to patient. Pain lasting more than 2 months may be the result of a nonhydraulic device that is too long or periprosthetic infection. Patients with sensory neuropathy associated with their primary disease (e.g., diabetes mellitus) often experience more severe and prolonged pain than other implant recipients. In addition, they often describe this pain as a burning sensation, which is a different pain description than that of other patients.

When persistent pain is the result of infection, clinical signs of infection eventually will develop. Treatment is directed toward the infection. Usually,

pain due to a sensory neuropathy will gradually resolve. Rarely, a prosthesis needs to be explanted because of pain.

Ejaculatory Incompetence

If the ability to have an orgasm (with or without ejaculation) is present before penile prosthesis implantation, it should still be present postoperatively. However, ejaculatory incompetence, a term used to describe the inability to reach orgasm, occasionally occurs after penile prosthesis implantation. In the early postoperative period when some discomfort is still present, this complaint is more common, and the problem usually resolves with further healing. It may, however, persist as a long-term problem, due at least in part to a difference between natural and prosthetic erections. A man without a prosthesis does not attempt coitus without being sexually aroused, since arousal is needed to obtain an erection. The implant recipient, on the other hand, can use his prosthesis for coitus without being sexually aroused. This results in less pleasure during coitus, and the threshold for orgasm might not be reached. When a couple is given permission to have coitus after prosthesis implantation, they are told to use a water-soluble lubricant and to use plenty of foreplay before vaginal intromission. Anxiety during initial coital attempts may impair vaginal lubrication. The lubricant can be discarded later if natural lubrication appears adequate. If a couple continues to have problems with coitus in spite of an absence of surgical or prosthetic problems, referral to a sex therapist is indicated.[123]

Phimosis, Paraphimosis

For every potential implant recipient, it is important to note whether he is circumcised or uncircumcised. Uncircumcised men should be examined to see if there are any abnormalities of the prepuce or glans penis. Early phimosis or mild balanitis may be an indication for circumcision either before or at the same time as prosthesis implantation. Postimplant problems with phimosis in uncircumcised men are unusual if their foreskins and glans are entirely normal. Paraphimosis is avoided, as in other situations, by keeping the foreskin pulled forward over the glans.

In patients with Peyronie's disease where a straightening procedure may be needed at the time of prosthesis implantation, this is usually done through a circumcising degloving approach. It is important to obtain permission from the uncircumcised man preoperatively for circumcision should this be necessary.

Urinary Retention

The voiding status of every implant recipient should be determined before implant. Men with significant bladder outlet obstruction should have a prostatectomy and wait for complete recovery before prosthesis implantation. If there is no significant history of voiding difficulty before implantation, urinary retention postoperatively is unusual.

SATISFACTION

Most satisfaction studies after penile prosthesis implantation have been retrospective. Some involve only the recipient,[124–126] whereas others involve both the recipient and his partner.[127–133] These studies indicate general reasonable levels of satisfaction postoperatively, although success rates in terms of satisfaction are not as high as success rates in terms of a good surgical result. Presumably, the patient (or couple) who is dissatisfied postoperatively yet has had a good surgical result did not have expectations met. Ideally, penile prosthesis implantation should include at least one preoperative counseling visit with a sex therapist and one or more visits as needed postoperatively. Unfortunately, the services of sex therapists often are not covered by third party payers.

SUMMARY

In spite of the development of alternative therapies for organic erectile dysfunction, such as vacuum constriction devices, intracavernous pharmacotherapy, and penile arterial and venous surgery, penile prosthesis implantation remains popular. The best devices approach the ideal in terms of providing penile flaccidity and erection that resembles that achieved naturally. Available devices also have acceptable mechanical reliability.

REFERENCES

1. Bogoras NA. Uber die volle plastiche Wiederherstellung eines rum koitus fahigen Penis (Peniplastica totalis). Zentralbl Chir 63:1271, 1936.
2. Goodwin WE, Scardino PL, Scott WW. Penile prosthesis for impotence: case report. J Urol 126:409, 1981.
3. Goodwin WE, Scott WW. Phalloplasty. J Urol 68:903, 1952.
4. Beheri GE. Beheri's operation for treatment of impotence—observations on 125 cases. Kasr el Aini J Surg 1:390, 1960.
5. Beheri GE. The problem of impotence solved by a new surgical operation. Kasr el Aini J Surg 1:50, 1960.
6. Beheri GE. Surgical treatment of impotence. Plast Reconstr Surg 38:92, 1966.
7. Lash H. Silicone implant for impotence. J Urol 100:709, 1968.
8. Loeffler RA, Sayegh ES. Perforated acrylic implants in management of organic impotence. J Urol 84:559, 1960.
9. Loeffler RA, Sayegh ES, Lash H. The artificial os penis. Plast Reconstr Surg 34:71, 1964.
10. Pearman RO. Treatment of organic impotence by implantation of a penile prosthesis. J Urol 97:716, 1967.
11. Scott FB, Bradley WE, Timm GW. Management of erectile impotence: use of implantable inflatable prosthesis. Urology 2:80, 1973.
12. Small MP. Small-Carrion penile prosthesis: a report on 160 cases and review of the literature. J Urol 119:365, 1978.
13. Small MP, Carrion HM, Gordon JA. Small-Carrion penile prosthesis: new implant for management of impotence. Urology 5:479, 1975.
14. Finney RP. New hinged silicone penile implant. J Urol 118:585, 1977.
15. Finney RP, Sharpe JR, Sadlowski RW. Finney hinged penile implant: experience with 100 cases. J Urol 124:205, 1980.
16. Jonas U, Jacobi GH. Silicone-silver penile prosthesis: description, operative approach and results. J Urol 123:865, 1980.
17. Benson RCJ, Barrett DM, Patterson DE. The Jonas prosthesis—technical considerations and results. J Urol 130:920, 1983.
18. Benson RCJ, Patterson DE, Barrett DM. Long-term results with the Jonas malleable penile prosthesis. J Urol 134:899, 1985.
19. Montague DK. Experience with the Jonas malleable penile prosthesis. Urology 23:83, 1984.
20. Pedersen B, Mieza M, Melman A. Instability and rotation of silver silicone penile prosthesis. Urology 31:116, 1988.
21. Tawil E, Hawatmeh IS, Apte S, et al. Multiple fractures of the silver wire strands as a complication of the silicone-silver wire prosthesis. J Urol 132:762, 1984.
22. Tawil EA, Gregory JG. Failure of the Jonas prosthesis. J Urol 135:702, 1986.
23. Walther M, Foster J. Complications of Jonas prosthesis. Urology 26:64, 1985.
24. Finney RP. Flexi-Flate penile prosthesis. Semin Urol 4:244, 1986.
25. Stanisic TH, Dean JC. The Flexi-Flate and Flexi-Flate II penile prosthesis. Urol Clin North Am 16:39, 1989.
26. Stanisic TH, Dean JC, Donovan JM, et al. Clinical experience with a self-contained inflatable penile implant: the Flexi-Flate. J Urol 139:947, 1988.
27. Fishman IJ. Experience with the Hydroflex penile prosthesis. Semin Urol 4:239, 1986.
28. Kabalin JN, Kessler R. Experience with the Hydroflex penile prosthesis. J Urol 141:58, 1989.
29. Mulcahy JJ. The Hydroflex self-contained inflatable penile prosthesis: experience with 100 patients. J Urol 140:1422, 1988.
30. Mulcahy JJ. The Hydroflex penile prosthesis. Urol Clin North Am 16:33, 1989.

31. Dorflinger T, Bruskewitz R. AMS malleable penile prosthesis. Urology 28:480, 1986.

32. Moul JW, McLeod DG. Experience with the AMS 600 malleable penile prosthesis. J Urol 135:929, 1986.

33. Huisman TK, Macintyre RC. Mechanical failure of Omniphase penile prosthesis. Urology 31:515, 1988.

34. Levinson K, Whitehead ED. Omniphase penile prosthesis: delayed bilateral central cable breakage. J Urol 141:618, 1989.

35. Mulcahy JJ. The OmniPhase and DuraPhase penile prostheses. Urol Clin North Am 16:25, 1989.

36. Hrebinko R, Bahnson RR, Schwentker FN, et al. Early experience with the Duraphase penile prosthesis. J Urol 143:60, 1990.

37. Thompson IM, Rodriguez FR, Zeidman EJ. Experience with Duraphase penile prosthesis: its use as replacement device. Urology 36:505, 1990.

38. Mulcahy JJ, Krane RJ, Lloyd LK, et al. Duraphase penile prosthesis—results of clinical trials in 63 patients. J Urol 143:518, 1990.

39. Nielson KT, Bruskewitz RC. Semirigid and malleable rod penile prostheses. Urol Clin North Am 16:13, 1989.

40. Fein RL. Clinical evaluation of inflatable penile prosthesis with combined pump-reservoir. Urology 32:311, 1988.

41. Merrill DC. Mentor inflatable penile prostheses. Urol Clin North Am 16:51, 1989.

42. Baum N, Suarez G, Mobley D. Use of infrapubic incision for insertion of Mentor Mark II inflatable penile prosthesis. Urology 39:436, 1992.

43. Fein RL. The G.F.S. Mark II inflatable penile prosthesis. J Urol 147:66, 1992.

44. Fallon B, Rosenberg S, Culp DA. Long-term follow-up in patients with an inflatable penile prosthesis. J Urol 132:270, 1984.

45. Fishman IJ, Scott FB, Light JK. Experience with inflatable penile prosthesis. Urology 23:86, 1984.

46. Furlow WL. The current status of the inflatable penile prosthesis in the management of impotence: Mayo Clinic experience updated. J Urol 119:363, 1978.

47. Furlow WL. Inflatable penile prosthesis: Mayo Clinic experience with 175 patients. Urology 13:166, 1979.

48. Furlow WL, Barrett DM. Inflatable penile prosthesis: new device design and patient–partner satisfaction. Urology 24:559, 1984.

49. Furlow WL, Goldwasser B, Gundian JC. Implantation of model AMS 700 penile prosthesis: long-term results. J Urol 139:741, 1988.

50. Furlow WL, Motley RC. The inflatable penile prosthesis: clinical experience with a new controlled expansion cylinder. J Urol 139:945, 1988.

51. Gregory JG, Purcell MH. Scott's inflatable penile prosthesis: evaluation of mechanical survival in the series 700 model. J Urol 137:676, 1987.

52. Kabalin JN, Kessler R. Five-year follow-up of the Scott inflatable penile prosthesis and comparison with semirigid penile prosthesis. J Urol 140:1428, 1988.

53. Kabalin JN, Kessler R. Penile prosthesis surgery: review of ten-year experience and examination of reoperations. Urology 33:17, 1989.

54. Kessler R. Surgical experience with the inflatable penile prosthesis. J Urol 124:611, 1980.

55. Kessler R. Complications of inflatable penile prosthesis. Urology 18:470, 1981.

56. Light JK, Scott FB. Management of neurogenic impotence with inflatable penile prosthesis. Urology 17:341, 1981.

57. Malloy TR, Wein AJ, Carpiniello VL. Further experience with the inflatable penile prosthesis. J Urol 122:478, 1979.

58. Malloy TR, Wein AJ, Carpiniello VL. Improved mechanical survival with revised model inflatable penile prosthesis using rear-tip extenders. J Urol 128:489, 1982.

59. Malloy TR, Wein AJ, Carpiniello VL. Revised surgical technique to improve survival of penile cylinders for the inflatable penile prosthesis. J Urol 130:1105, 1983.

60. Malloy TR, Wein AJ, Carpiniello VL. Reliability of AMS M700 inflatable penile prosthesis. Urology 28:385, 1986.

61. Merrill DC. Clinical experience with Scott inflatable penile prosthesis in 150 patients. Urology 22:371, 1983.

62. Montague DK. Experience with semirigid rod and inflatable penile prostheses. J Urol 129:967, 1983.

63. Montague DK, Hewitt CB, Stewart BH. Treatment of impotence with an inflatable penile prosthesis. Ohio State Med J 75:9, 1979.

64. Scarzella GI. Cylinder reliability of inflatable penile prosthesis: experience with distensible and nondistensible cylinders in 325 patients. Urology 31:486, 1988.

65. Scott FB, Byrd GJ, Karacan I, et al. Erectile impotence treated with an implantable, inflatable prosthesis. JAMA 241:2609, 1979.

66. Wilson SK, Wahman GE, Lange JL. Eleven years of experience with the inflatable penile prosthesis. J Urol 139:951, 1988.

67. Woodworth BE, Carson CC, Webster GD: Inflatable penile prosthesis: effect of device modification on functional longevity. Urology 38:533, 1991.

68. Knoll LD, Furlow WL, Motley RC. Clinical experience implanting an inflatable penile prosthesis with controlled-expansion cylinder. Urology 36:502, 1990.

69. Montague DK. Experience with the AMS 700CX penile prosthesis. Int J Impot Res 2:457, 1990.

70. Mulcahy JJ. Use of CX cylinders in association with AMS700 inflatable penile prosthesis. J Urol 140:1420, 1988.

71. Montague DK, Lakin MM. Early experience with the girth and length expanding cylinder of the AMS Ultrex penile prosthesis. J Urol 148:1444, 1992.

72. Brooks MB. 42 months of experience with the Mentor inflatable penile prosthesis. J Urol 139:48, 1988.

73. Engel RME, Smolev JK, Hackler R. Experience with the Mentor inflatable penile prosthesis. J Urol 135:1181, 1986.

74. Engel RME, Smolev JK, Hackler R. Mentor inflatable penile prosthesis. Urology 29:498, 1987.
75. Fein RL, Needell MH. Early problems encountered with the Mentor inflatable penile prosthesis. J Urol 134:62, 1985.
76. Fuerst DE, Bendo JJ. An unusual complication of the inflatable penile prosthesis. J Urol 136:913, 1986.
77. Hackler RH. Mentor inflatable penile prosthesis: a reliable mechanical device. Urology 28:489, 1986.
78. Merrill DC. Mentor inflatable penile prosthesis. Urology 22:504, 1983.
79. Merrill DC. Clinical experience with Mentor inflatable penile prosthesis in 206 patients. Urology 28:185, 1986.
80. Merrill DC. Clinical experience with the Mentor inflatable penile prosthesis in 301 patients. J Urol 140:1424, 1988.
81. Fishman IJ. Corporeal reconstruction procedures for complicated penile implants. Urol Clin North Am 16:73, 1989.
82. Montague DK. Penile prosthesis implantation in patients with corporeal fibrosis. In: McDougal WS. Difficult Problems in Urologic Surgery. Chicago: Year Book Medical Publishers, 1989.
83. Golji H. Experience with penile prosthesis in spinal cord injury patients. J Urol 121:288, 1979.
84. Rossier AB, Fam BA. Indications and results of semirigid penile prostheses in spinal cord injury patients: long-term follow-up. J Urol 131:59, 1984.
85. Kaufman JJ. Penile prosthetic surgery under local anesthesia. J Urol 128:1190, 1982.
86. Bishop JR, Moul JW, Sihelnik SA, et al. Use of glycosylated hemoglobin to identify diabetics at high risk for penile periprosthetic infections. J Urol 147:386, 1992.
87. Barry JM, Seifert A. Penoscrotal approach for placement of paired penile implants for impotence. J Urol 122:325, 1979.
88. Habal MB. The biologic basis for the clinical application of the silicones. Arch Surg 119:843, 1984.
89. Baum N, Scott FB, Suarez G. Iatrogenic chordee following insertion of inflatable penile prosthesis. Urology 32:442, 1988.
90. Mulcahy JJ, Rowland RG. Tunica wedge excision to correct penile curvature associated with the inflatable penile prosthesis. J Urol 138:63, 1987.
91. Carson CC, Robertson CN. Late hematogenous infection of penile prostheses. J Urol 139:50, 1988.
92. Kabalin JN, Kessler R. Infectious complications of penile prosthesis surgery. J Urol 139:953, 1988.
93. Montague DK. Periprosthetic infections. J Urol 138:68, 1987.
94. Moul JW, Carson CC. Infectious complications of penile prostheses. Infections Urol, p 97, 1989.
95. Nelson RP, Gregory JC. Gonococcal infections of penile prostheses. Urology 31:391, 1988.
96. Radomski SB, Herschorn S. Risk factors associated with penile prosthesis infection. J Urol 147:383, 1992.
97. Thomalla JV, Thompson ST, Rowland RG, et al. Infectious complications of penile prosthetic implants. J Urol 138:65, 1987.
98. Persky L, Luria S, Porter A, et al. *Staphylococcus epidermidis* in diabetic urological patient. J Urol 136:466, 1986.
99. Peppas DS, Moul JW, McLeod DG. *Candida albicans* corpora abscess following penile prosthesis placement. J Urol 140:1541, 1988.
100. Walther PJ, Andriani RT, Maggio MI, et al. Fournier's gangrene: a complication of penile prosthesis implantation in a renal transplant patient. J Urol 137:299, 1987.
101. Bour J, Steingardt G. Penile necrosis in patients with diabetes mellitus and end-stage renal disease. J Urol 132:560, 1984.
102. McClellan DS, Masih BK. Gangrene of the penis as a complication of penile prosthesis. J Urol 133:862, 1985.
103. McDowell GC, Hayden LJ, Wise HAI. Penile necrosis secondary to an indwelling Foley catheter. J Urol 138:1243, 1987.
104. Shelling RH, Maxted WC. Major complications of silicone penile prostheses: predisposing clinical situations. Urology 15:131, 1980.
105. Furlow WL, Goldwasser B. Salvage of the eroded inflatable penile prosthesis: a new concept. J Urol 138:312, 1987.
106. Bertram RA, Carson CCI, Webster GD. Implantation of penile prostheses in patients impotent after priapism. Urology 26:325, 1985.
107. Lakin MM, Montague DK, Mendendorp SV, et al. Intracavernous injection therapy: analysis of results and complications. J Urol 143:1138, 1990.
108. Eigner EB, Kabalin JN, Kessler R. Penile implants in the treatment of Peyronie's disease. J Urol 145:69, 1991.
109. Knoll LD, Furlow WL, Benson RC Jr. Management of Peyronie disease by implantation of inflatable penile prosthesis. Urology 34:406, 1990.
110. Subrini L. Surgical treatment of Peyronie's disease using penile implants: survey of 69 patients. J Urol 132:47, 1984.
111. Finney RP. Coring fibrotic corpora for penile implants. Urology 24:73, 1984.
112. Fritzler M, Flores-Sandoval FN, Light JK. Dacron "sock" repair for proximal corporeal perforation. Urology 28:524–526, 1986.
113. Mulcahy JJ. A technique of maintaining penile prosthesis position to prevent proximal migration. J Urol 137:294–296, 1987.
114. Gasser TC, Larsen EH, Bruskewitz RG. Penile prosthesis reimplantation. J Urol 137:46, 1987.
115. Steidle CP, Mulcahy JJ. Erosion of penile prostheses: a complication of urethral catheterization. J Urol 142:736, 1989.
116. Nelson RPJ. Small bowel obstruction secondary to migration of an inflatable penile prosthesis reservoir: recognition and prevention. J Urol 139:1053, 1988.
117. Godiwalla SY, Beres J, Jacobs SC. Erosion of an inflatable penile prosthesis reservoir into an ileal conduit. J Urol 137:297, 1987.
118. Singh I, Godec CJ. Asynchronous erosion of in

flatable penile prosthesis into small and large bowel. J Urol 147:709, 1992.

119. Dupont MC, Hochman HI. Erosion of an inflatable penile prosthesis reservoir into the bladder, presenting as bladder calculi. J Urol 139:367, 1988.

120. Fitch WPI, Roddy T. Erosion of inflatable penile prosthesis reservoir into bladder. J Urol 136:1080, 1986.

121. Ball TPJ. Surgical repair of penile "SST" deformity. Urology 15:603, 1980.

122. Agatstein EH, Farrer JH, Raz S. Fracture of semi-rigid penile prosthesis: a rare complication. J Urol 135:376, 1986.

123. Schover LR. Sex therapy for the penile prosthesis recipient. Urol Clin North Am 16:91, 1989.

124. Berg R, Mindus P, Berg G, et al. Penile implants in erectile impotence: outcome and prognostic indicators. Scand J Urol Nephrol 18:1983.

125. Beutler LE, Scott FB, Rogers RRJ, et al. Inflatable and noninflatable penile prostheses: comparative follow-up evaluation. Urology 27:136, 1986.

126. Hollander JB, Diokno AC. Success with penile prosthesis from patient's viewpoint. Urology 23:141, 1984.

127. Beutler LE, Scott FB, Karacan I, et al. Women's satisfaction with partners' penile implant. Urology 24:552, 1984.

128. Blake DJ, McCartney C, Fried FA, et al. Psychiatric assessment of penile implant recipient. Urology 21:252, 1983.

129. Gerstenberger DL, Osborne D, Furlow WL. Inflatable penile prosthesis: follow-up study of patient–partner satisfaction. Urology 14:583, 1979.

130. Krauss DJ, Lantinga LJ, Carey MP, et al. Use of the malleable penile prosthesis in the treatment of erectile dysfunction: a prospective study of postoperative adjustment. J Urol 142:988, 1989.

131. McLaren RH, Barrett DM. Patient and partner satisfaction with the AMS 700 penile prosthesis. J Urol 147:62, 1992.

132. Pedersen B, Tiefer L, Ruiz M, et al. Evaluation of patients and partners 1 to 4 years after penile prosthesis surgery. J Urol 139:956, 1988.

133. Schlamowitz KE, Beutler LE, Scott FB, et al. Reactions to the implantation of an inflatable penile prosthesis among psychogenically and organically impotent men. J Urol 129:295, 1983.

National Institutes of Health Consensus Development Conference Statement: Impotence

December 7–9, 1992*

INTRODUCTION

The term "impotence," as it has been applied to the title of this conference, has traditionally been used to signify the inability of the male to attain and maintain erection of the penis sufficient to permit satisfactory sexual intercourse. However, this use has often led to confusing and uninterpretable results in both clinical and basic science investigations. This, together with its pejorative implications, suggests that the more precise term "erectile dysfunction" be used instead to signify an inability of the male to achieve an erect penis as part of the overall multifaceted process of male sexual function. This process comprises a variety of physical aspects with important psychological and behavioral overtones. In an effort to be precise in the analysis of the material discussed at this conference, this consensus report addresses issues of male erectile dysfunction as implied by use of the term "impotence" in the reports that have been presented. However, it should be recognized that desire, orgasmic capacity, and ejaculatory capacity may be intact even in the presence of erectile dysfunction or may be deficient to some extent and contribute to the sense of inadequate sexual function.

Erectile dysfunction affects millions of men. Although for some men erectile function may not be the best or most important measure of sexual satisfaction, for many men erectile dysfunction creates mental stress that affects their interactions with family and associates. Many advances have occurred in both diagnosis and treatment of erectile dysfunction. However, its various aspects remain poorly understood by the general population and by most health care professionals. Lack of a simple definition, failure to delineate precisely the problem being assessed, and the absence of guidelines and parameters to determine assessment and treatment outcome and long-term results, have contributed to this state of affairs by producing misunderstanding, confusion, and ongoing concern. That

---

*Consensus Development Conferences are convened to evaluate available scientific information and to resolve safety and efficacy issues related to a biomedical technology. The resultant NIH consensus statements are intended to advance understanding of the technology or issue in question and to be useful to health professionals and the public.

NIH consensus statements are prepared by a nonadvocate, non-Federal panel of experts, based on (1) presentations by investigators working in areas relevant to the consensus questions during a 2-day public session; (2) questions and statements from conference attendees during open discussion periods that are part of the public session; and (3) closed deliberations by the panel during the remainder of the second day and morning of the third. This statement is an independent report of the panel and is not a policy statement of the NIH or the Federal Government.

Copies of this statement and bibliographies prepared by the National Library of Medicine are available from the Office of Medical Applications of Research, National Institutes of Health, Federal Building, Room 618, Bethesda, MD 20892.

For making bibliographic reference to the consensus statement from this conference, it is recommended that the following format be used, with or without source abbreviations, but without authorship attribution:

Impotence. NIH Consens Statement 1992 Dec 7–9;10(4):1–31.

results have not been communicated effectively to the public has compounded this situation.

Cause-specific assessment and treatment of male sexual dysfunction will require recognition by the public and the medical community that erectile dysfunction is a part of overall male sexual dysfunction. The multifactorial nature of erectile dysfunction, comprising both organic and psychologic aspects, may often require a multidisciplinary approach to its assessment and treatment. This consensus report addresses these issues, not only as isolated health problems but also in the context of societal and individual perceptions and expectations.

Erectile dysfunction is often assumed to be a natural concomitant of the aging process to be tolerated along with other conditions associated with aging. This assumption may not be entirely correct. For the elderly and for others, erectile dysfunction may occur as a consequence of specific illnesses or of medical treatment for certain illnesses, resulting in fear, loss of image and self-confidence, and depression.

For example, many men with diabetes mellitus may develop erectile dyfunction during their young and middle adult years. Physicians, diabetes educators, and patients and their families are sometimes unaware of this potential complication. Whatever the causal factors, discomfort of patients and health care providers in discussing sexual issues becomes a roadblock to pursuing treatment.

Erectile dysfunction can be effectively treated with a variety of methods. Many patients and health care providers are unaware of these treatments, and the dysfunction thus often remains untreated, compounded by its psychological impact. Concurrent with the increase in the availability of effective treatment methods has been increased availability of new diagnostic procedures that may help in the selection of an effective, cause-specific treatment. This conference was designed to explore these issues and to define the state of their art.

To examine what is known about the demographics, etiology, risk factors, pathophysiology, diagnostic assessment, treatments (both generic and cause-specific), and the understanding of their consequences by the public and the medical community, the National Institute of Diabetes and Digestive and Kidney Diseases and the Office of Medical Applications of Research of the National Institutes of Health, in conjunction with the National Institute of Neurological Disorders and Stroke and the National Institute on Aging, convened a consensus development conference on male impotence on December 7–9, 1992. After 1-½ days of presentations by experts in the relevant fields involved with male sexual dysfunction and erectile impotence or dysfunction, a consensus panel comprised of representatives from urology, geriatrics, medicine, endocrinology, psychiatry, psychology, nursing, epidemiology, biostatistics, basic sciences, and the public considered the evidence and developed answers to the following questions.

1. WHAT ARE THE PREVALENCE AND CLINICAL, PSYCHOLOGICAL, AND SOCIAL IMPACT OF IMPOTENCE (CULTURAL, GEOGRAPHICAL, NATIONAL, ETHNIC, RACIAL, MALE/FEMALE PERCEPTIONS AND INFLUENCES)?
Prevalence and Association with Age

Estimates of the prevalence of impotence depend on the definition employed for this condition. For the purposes of this consensus development conference statement, impotence is defined as male erectile dysfunction, that is, the inability to achieve or maintain an erection sufficient for satisfactory sexual performance. Erectile performance has been characterized by the degree of dysfunction, and estimates of prevalence (the number of men with the condition) will vary depending upon the definition of erectile dysfunction used.

Appallingly little is known about the prevalence of erectile dysfunction in the United States and how this prevalence varies according to individual characteristics (age, race, ethnicity, socioeconomic status, and concomitant diseases and conditions). Data on erectile dysfunction available from the 1940's applied to the present U.S. male population produce an estimate of erectile dysfunction prevalence of 7 million. More recent estimates suggest that the number of U.S. men with erectile dysfunction may more likely be near 10-20 million. Inclusion of individuals with partial erectile dysfunction increases the estimate to about 30 million. The majority of these individuals will be older than 65 years of age. The prevalence of erectile dysfunction has been found to be associated with age. A prevalence of about 5% is observed at age 40, increasing to 15-25% at age 65 and older. One-third of older men receiving medical care at a Department of Veterans' Affairs ambulatory clinic admitted to problems with erectile function.

Causes contributing to erectile dysfunction can be broadly classified into two categories: organic and psychologic. In reality, while the majority of patients with erectile dysfunction are thought to demonstrate an organic component, psychological aspects of self-confidence, anxiety, and partner communication and conflict are often important contributing factors.

The 1985 National Ambulatory Medical Care

Survey indicated that there were about 525,000 visits for erectile dysfunction, accounting for 0.2% of all male ambulatory care visits. Estimates of visits per 1,000 population increased from about 1.5 for the age group 25-34 to 15.0 for those age 65 and above. The 1985 National Hospital Discharge Survey estimated that more than 30,000 hospital admissions were for erectile dysfunction.

Clinical, Psychological and Social Impact
GEOGRAPHIC, RACIAL, ETHNIC, SOCIOECONOMIC, AND CULTURAL VARIATION IN ERECTILE DYSFUNCTION

Very little is known about how erectile dysfunction prevalence varies across geographic, racial, ethnic, socioeconomic, and cultural groups. Anecdotal evidence points to the existence of racial, ethnic, and other cultural diversity in the perceptions and expectation levels for satisfactory sexual functioning. These differences would be expected to be reflected in these groups' reaction to erectile dysfunction, although few data on this issue appear to exist.

One report from a recent community survey concluded that erectile failure was the leading complaint of males attending sex therapy clinics. Other studies have shown that erectile disorders are the primary concern of sex therapy patients in treatment. This is consistent with the view that erectile dysfunction may be associated with depression, loss of self-esteem, poor self-image, increased anxiety or tension with one's sexual partner, and/or fear and anxiety associated with contracting sexually transmitted diseases, including AIDS.

MALE/FEMALE PERCEPTIONS AND INFLUENCES

The diagnosis of erectile dysfunction may be understood as the presence of a condition limiting choices for sexual interaction and possibly limiting opportunity for sexual satisfaction. The impact of this condition depends very much on the dynamics of the relationship of the individual and his sexual partner and their expectation of performance. When changes in sexual function are perceived by the individual and his partner as a natural consequence of the aging process, they may modify their sexual behavior to accommodate the condition and maintain sexual satisfaction. Increasingly, men do not perceive erectile dysfunction as a normal part of aging and seek to identify means by which they may return to their previous level and range of sexual activities. Such levels and expectations and desires for future sexual interactions are important

aspects of the evaluation of patients presenting with a chief complaint of erectile dysfunction.

In men of all ages, erectile failure may diminish willingness to initiate sexual relationships because of fear of inadequate sexual performance or rejection. Because males, especially older males, are particularly sensitive to the social support of intimate relationships, withdrawal from these relationships because of such fears may have a negative effect on their overall health.

2. WHAT ARE THE RISK FACTORS CONTRIBUTING TO IMPOTENCE? CAN THESE BE UTILIZED IN PREVENTING DEVELOPMENT OF IMPOTENCE?
Physiology of Erection

The male erectile response is a vascular event initiated by neuronal action and maintained by a complex interplay between vascular and neurological events. In its most common form, it is initiated by a central nervous system event that integrates psychogenic stimuli (perception, desire, etc.) and controls the sympathetic and parasympathetic innervation of the penis. Sensory stimuli from the penis are important in continuing this process and in initiating a reflex arc that may cause erection under proper circumstances and may help to maintain erection during sexual activity.

Parasympathetic input allows erection by relaxation of trabecular smooth muscle and dilation of the helicine arteries of the penis. This leads to expansion of the lacunar spaces and entrapment of blood by compressing venules against the tunica albuginea, a process referred to as the corporal veno-occlusive mechanism. The tunica albuginea must have sufficient stiffness to compress the venules penetrating it in order to block venous outflow for sufficient tumescence and rigidity to occur.

Acetylcholine released by the parasympathetic nerves is thought to act primarily on endothelial cells to release a second nonadrenergic-noncholinergic carrier of the signal that relaxes the trabecular smooth muscle. Nitric oxide released by the endothelial cells, and possibly also of neural origin, is currently thought to be the leading of several candidates as this nonadrenergic-noncholinergic transmitter; but this has not yet been conclusively demonstrated to the exclusion of other potentially important substances (e.g., vasoactive intestinal polypeptide). Its relaxing effect on the trabecular smooth muscle may be mediated through its stimulation of guanylate cyclase and the production of cyclic guanosine monophosphate (cGMP), which would then function as a second messenger in this system.

Constriction of the trabecular smooth muscle and helicine arteries induced by sympathetic innervation makes the penis flaccid, with blood pressure in the cavernosal sinuses of the penis near venous pressure. Acetylcholine is thought to decrease sympathetic tone. This may be important in a permissive sense for adequate trabecular smooth muscle relaxation and consequent effective action of other mediators in achieving sufficient inflow of blood into the lacunar spaces. When the trabecular smooth muscle relaxes and helicine arteries dilate in response to parasympathetic stimulation and decreased sympathetic tone, increased blood flow fills the cavernous spaces, increasing the pressure within these spaces so that the penis becomes erect. As the venules are compressed against the tunica albuginea, penile pressure approaches arterial pressure, causing rigidity. Once this state is achieved, arterial inflow is reduced to a level that matches venous outflow.

Erectile Dysfunction

Because adequate arterial supply is critical for erection, any disorder that impairs blood flow may be implicated in the etiology of erectile failure. Most of the medical disorders associated with erectile dysfunction appear to affect the arterial system. Some disorders may interfere with the corporal veno-occlusive mechanism and result in failure to trap blood within the penis, or produce leakage such that an erection cannot be maintained or is easily lost.

Damage to the autonomic pathways innervating the penis may eliminate "psychogenic" erection initiated by the central nervous system. Lesions of the somatic nervous pathways may impair reflexogenic erections and may interrupt tactile sensation needed to maintain psychogenic erections. Spinal cord lesions may produce varying degrees of erectile failure depending on the location and completeness of the lesions. Not only do traumatic lesions affect erectile ability, but disorders leading to peripheral neuropathy may impair neuronal innervation of the penis or of the sensory afferents. The endocrine system itself, particularly the production of androgens, appears to play a role in regulating sexual interest, and may also play a role in erectile function.

Psychological processes such as depression, anxiety, and relationship problems can impair erectile functioning by reducing erotic focus or otherwise reducing awareness of sensory experience. This may lead to inability to initiate or maintain an erection. Etiologic factors for erectile disorders may be categorized as neurogenic, vasculogenic, or psychogenic, but they most commonly appear to derive from problems in all three areas acting in concert.

Risk Factors

Little is known about the natural history of erectile dysfunction. This includes information on the age of onset, incidence rates stratified by age, progression of the condition, and frequency of spontaneous recovery. There also are very limited data on associated morbidity and functional impairment. To date, the data are predominantly available for whites, with other racial and ethnic populations being represented only in smaller numbers that do not permit analysis of these issues as a function of race or ethnicity.

Erectile dysfunction is clearly a symptom of many conditions, and certain risk factors have been identified, some of which may be amenable to prevention strategies. Diabetes mellitus, hypogonadism in association with a number of endocrinologic conditions, hypertension, vascular disease, high levels of blood cholesterol, low levels of high density lipoprotein, drugs, neurogenic disorders, Peyronie's disease, priapism, depression, alcohol ingestion, lack of sexual knowledge, poor sexual techniques, inadequate interpersonal relationships or their deterioration, and many chronic diseases, especially renal failure and dialysis, have been demonstrated as risk factors. Vascular surgery is also often a risk factor. Age appears to be a strong indirect risk factor in that it is associated with an increased likelihood of direct risk factors. Other factors require more extensive study. Smoking has an adverse effect on erectile function by accentuating the effects of other risk factors such as vascular disease or hypertension. To date, vasectomy has not been associated with an increased risk of erectile dysfunction other than causing an occasional psychological reaction that could then have a psychogenic influence. Accurate risk factor identification and characterization are essential for concerted efforts at prevention of erectile dysfunction.

Prevention

Although erectile dysfunction increases progressively with age, it is not an inevitable consequence of aging. Knowledge of the risk factors can guide prevention strategies. Specific antihypertensive, antidepressant, and antipsychotic drugs can be chosen to lessen the risk of erectile failure. Published lists of prescription drugs that may impair erectile functioning often are based on reports implicating a drug without systematic study. Such studies are needed to confirm the validity of these suggested associations. In the individual patient, the physician can modify the regimen in an effort to resolve the erectile problem.

It is important that physicians and other health care providers treating patients for chronic conditions periodically inquire into the sexual functioning of their patients and be prepared to offer counsel for those who experience erectile difficulties. Lack of sexual knowledge and anxiety about sexual performance are common contributing factors to erectile dysfunction. Education and reassurance may be helpful in preventing the cascade into serious erectile failure in individuals who experience minor erectile difficulty due to medications or common changes in erectile functioning associated with chronic illnesses or with aging.

3. WHAT DIAGNOSTIC INFORMATION SHOULD BE OBTAINED IN ASSESSMENT OF THE IMPOTENT PATIENT? WHAT CRITERIA SHOULD BE EMPLOYED TO DETERMINE WHICH TESTS ARE INDICATED FOR A PARTICULAR PATIENT?

The appropriate evaluation of all men with erectile dysfunction should include a medical and detailed sexual history (including practices and techniques), a physical examination, a psychosocial evaluation, and basic laboratory studies. When available, a multidisciplinary approach to this evaluation may be desirable. In selected patients, further physiologic or invasive studies may be indicated. A sensitive sexual history, including expectations and motivations, should be obtained from the patient (and sexual partner whenever possible) in an interview conducted by an interested physician or another specially trained professional. A written patient questionnaire may be helpful, but is not a substitute for the interview. The sexual history is needed to accurately define the patient's specific complaint and to distinguish between true erectile dysfunction, changes in sexual desire, and orgasmic or ejaculatory disturbances. The patient should be asked specifically about perceptions of his erectile dysfunction, including the nature of onset, frequency, quality, duration of erections, the presence of nocturnal or morning erections, and his ability to achieve sexual satisfaction. Psychosocial factors related to erectile dysfunction should be probed, including specific situational circumstances, performance anxiety, the nature of sexual relationships, details of current sexual techniques, expectations, motivation for treatment, and the presence of specific discord within the patient's relationship with his sexual partner. The sexual partner's own expectations and perceptions should

also be sought since they may have important bearing on diagnosis and treatment recommendations.

The general medical history is important in identifying specific risk factors that may account for or contribute to the patient's erectile dysfunction. These include vascular risk factors such as hypertension, diabetes, smoking, coronary artery disease, peripheral vascular disorders, pelvic trauma or surgery, and blood lipid abnormalities. Decreased sexual desire or history suggesting a hypogonadal state could indicate a primary endocrine disorder. Neurologic causes may include a history of diabetes mellitus or alcoholism with associated peripheral neuropathy. Neurologic disorders such as multiple sclerosis, spinal injury, or cerebrovascular accidents are often obvious or well defined prior to presentation. It is essential to obtain a detailed medication and illicit drug history since an estimated 25% of cases of erectile dysfunction may be attributable to medications for other conditions. Past medical history can reveal important causes of erectile dysfunction, including radical pelvic surgery, radiation therapy, Peyronie's disease, penile or pelvic trauma, prostatitis, priapism, or voiding dysfunction. Information regarding prior evaluation or treatment for "impotence" should be obtained. A detailed sexual history, including current sexual techniques, is important in the general history obtained. It is also important to determine if there have been previous psychiatric illnesses such as depression or neuroses.

Physical examination should include the assessment of male secondary sex characteristics, femoral and lower extremity pulses, and a focused neurologic examination including perianal sensation, anal sphincter tone, and bulbocavernosus reflex. More extensive neurologic tests, including dorsal nerve conduction latencies, evoked potential measurements, and corpora cavernosal electromyography lack normative (control) data and appear at this time to be of limited clinical value. Examination of the genitalia includes evaluation of testis size and consistency, palpation of the shaft of the penis to determine the presence of Peyronie's plaques, and a digital rectal examination of the prostate with assessment of anal sphincter tone.

Endocrine evaluation consisting of a morning serum testosterone is generally indicated. Measurement of serum prolactin may be indicated. A low testosterone level merits repeat measurement together with assessment of luteinizing hormone (LH), follicle-stimulating hormone (FSH), and prolactin levels. Other tests may be helpful in excluding unrecognized systemic disease and include a complete blood count, urinalysis, creatinine, lipid profile, fasting blood sugar, and thyroid function studies.

Although not indicated for routine use, nocturnal penile tumescence (NPT) testing may be useful in the patient who reports a complete absence of erections (exclusive of nocturnal "sleep" erections) or when a primary psychogenic etiology is suspected. Such testing should be performed by those with expertise and knowledge of its interpretation, pitfalls, and usefulness. Various methods and devices are available for the evaluation of nocturnal penile tumescence, but their clinical usefulness is restricted by limitations of diagnostic accuracy and availability of normative data. Further study results regarding standardization of NPT testing and its general applicability is indicated.

After the history, physical examination, and laboratory testing, a clinical impression can be obtained of a primarily psychogenic, organic, or mixed etiology for erectile dysfunction. Patients with primary or associated psychogenic factors may be offered further psychologic evaluation, and patients with endocrine abnormalities may be referred to an endocrinologist to evaluate the possibility of a pituitary lesion or hypogonadism. Unless previously diagnosed, suspicion of neurologic deficit may be further assessed by complete neurologic evaluation. No further diagnostic tests appear necessary for those patients who favor noninvasive treatment (e.g., vacuum constrictive devices or pharmacologic injection therapy). Patients who do not respond satisfactorily to these noninvasive treatments may be candidates for penile implant surgery or further diagnostic testing for possible additional invasive therapies.

A rigid or nearly rigid erectile response to intracavernous injection of pharmacologic test doses of a vasodilating agent (see below) indicates adequate arterial and veno-occlusive function. This suggests that the patient may be a suitable candidate for a trial of penile injection therapy. Genital stimulation may be of use in increasing the erectile response in this setting. This diagnostic technique also may be used to differentiate a vascular from a primarily neuropathic or psychogenic etiology. Patients who have an inadequate response to intracavernous pharmacologic injection may be candidates for further vascular testing. It should be recognized, however, that failure to respond adequately may not indicate vascular insufficiency but can be caused by patient anxiety or discomfort. The number of patients who may benefit from more extensive vascular testing is small, but includes young men with a history of significant perineal or pelvic trauma, who may have anatomic arterial blockage (either alone or with neurologic deficit) to account for erectile dysfunction.

Studies to further define vasculogenic disorders include pharmacologic duplex grey scale/color ultrasonography, pharmacologic dynamic infusion cavernosometry/cavernosography, and pharmacologic pelvic/penile angiography. Cavernosometry, duplex ultrasonography, and angiography performed either alone or in conjunction with intracavernous pharmacologic injection of vasodilator agents rely on complete arterial and cavernosal smooth muscle relaxation to evaluate arterial and veno-occlusive function. The clinical effectiveness of these invasive studies is severely limited by several factors, including the lack of normative data, operator dependence, variable interpretation of results, and poor predictability of therapeutic outcomes of arterial and venous surgery. At the present time these studies might best be done in referral centers with specific expertise and interest in investigation of the vascular aspects of erectile dysfunction. Further clinical research is necessary to standardize methodology and interpretation, to obtain control data on normals (as stratified according to age), and to define what constitutes normal in order to assess the value of these tests in their diagnostic accuracy and in their ability to predict treatment outcome in men with erectile dysfunction.

4. WHAT ARE THE EFFICACIES AND RISKS OF BEHAVIORAL, PHARMACOLOGICAL, SURGICAL, AND OTHER TREATMENTS FOR IMPOTENCE? WHAT SEQUENCES AND/OR COMBINATION OF THESE INTERVENTIONS ARE APPROPRIATE? WHAT MANAGEMENT TECHNIQUES ARE APPROPRIATE WHEN TREATMENT IS NOT EFFECTIVE OR INDICATED?
General Considerations

Because of the difficulty in defining the clinical entity of erectile dysfunction, there have been a variety of entry criteria for patients in therapeutic trials. Similarly, the ability to assess efficacy of therapeutic interventions is impaired by the lack of clear and quantifiable criteria of erectile dysfunction. General considerations for treatment follow:

- Psychotherapy and/or behavioral therapy may be useful for some patients with erectile dysfunction without obvious organic cause, and for their partners. These may also be used as an adjunct to other therapies directed at the treatment of organic erectile dysfunction. Outcome data from such therapy, however, have not been well-documented or quantified, and additional studies along these lines are indicated.

- Efficacy of therapy may be best achieved by inclusion of both partners in treatment plans.
- Treatment should be individualized to the patient's desires and expectations.
- Even though there are several effective treatments currently available, long-term efficacy is in general relatively low. Moreover, there is a high rate of voluntary cessation of treatment for all currently popular forms of therapy for erectile dysfunction. Better understanding of the reasons for each of these phenomena is needed.

Psychotherapy and Behavioral Therapy

Psychosocial factors are important in all forms of erectile dysfunction. Careful attention to these issues and attempts to relieve sexual anxieties should be a part of the therapeutic intervention for all patients with erectile dysfunction. Psychotherapy and/or behavioral therapy alone may be helpful for some patients in whom no organic cause of erectile dysfunction is detected. Patients who refuse medical and surgical interventions also may be helped by such counseling. After appropriate evaluation to detect and treat coexistent problems such as issues related to the loss of a partner, dysfunctional relationships, psychotic disorders, or alcohol and drug abuse, psychological treatment focuses on decreasing performance anxiety and distractions and on increasing a couple's intimacy and ability to communicate about sex. Education concerning the factors that create normal sexual response and erectile dysfunction can help a couple cope with sexual difficulties. Working with the sexual partner is useful in improving the outcome of therapy. Psychotherapy and behavioral therapy have been reported to relieve depression and anxiety as well as to improve sexual function. However, outcome data of psychological and behavioral therapy have not been quantified, and evaluation of the success of specific techniques used in these treatments is poorly documented. Studies to validate their efficacy are therefore strongly indicated.

Medical Therapy

An initial approach to medical therapy should consider reversible medical problems that may contribute to erectile dysfunction. Included in this should be assessment of the possibility of medication-induced erectile dysfunction with consideration for reduction of polypharmacy and/or substitution of medications with lower probability of inducing erectile dysfunction.

For some patients with an established diagnosis of testicular failure (hypogonadism), androgen replacement therapy may sometimes be effective in improving erectile dysfunction. A trial of androgen replacement may be worthwhile in men with low serum testosterone levels if there are no other contraindications. In contrast, for men who have normal testosterone levels, androgen therapy is inappropriate and may carry significant health risks, especially in the situation of unrecognized prostate cancer. If androgen therapy is indicated, it should be given in the form of intramuscular injections of testosterone enanthate or cipionate. Oral androgens, as currently available, are not indicated. For men with hyperprolactinemia, bromocriptine therapy often is effective in normalizing the prolactin level and improving sexual function. A wide variety of other substances taken either orally or topically have been suggested to be effective in treating erectile dysfunction. Most of these have not been subjected to rigorous clinical studies and are not approved for this use by the Food and Drug Administration (FDA). Their use should therefore be discouraged until further evidence in support of their efficacy and indicative of their safety is available.

Intracavernosal Injection Therapy

Injection of vasodilator substances into the corpora of the penis has provided a new therapeutic technique for a variety of causes of erectile dysfunction. The most effective and well-studied agents are papaverine, phentolamine, and prostaglandin E_1. These have been used either singly or in combination. Use of these agents occasionally causes priapism (inappropriately persistent erections). This appears to have been seen most commonly with papaverine. Priapism is treated with adrenergic agents, which can cause life-threatening hypertension in patients receiving monoamine oxidase inhibitors. Use of the penile vasodilators also can be problematic in patients who cannot tolerate transient hypotension, those with severe psychiatric disease, those with poor manual dexterity, those with poor vision, and those receiving anticoagulant therapy. Liver function tests should be obtained in those being treated with papaverine alone. Prostaglandin E_1 can be used together with papaverine and phentolamine to decrease the incidence of side effects such as pain, penile corporal fibrosis, fibrotic nodules, hypotension, and priapism. Further study of the efficacy of multitherapy versus monotherapy and of the relative complications and safety of each approach is indicated. Although these agents have not received FDA approval for this indication, they are in widespread clinical use. Patients treated with these agents should give full informed consent. There is a high rate of patient dropout, often early in the treatment. Whether this is related to side effects, lack of spontaneity in sexual relations, or general loss of interest is unclear. Patient education and follow-up support might improve compliance and lessen the dropout rate. However, the reasons for the high dropout rate need to be determined and quantified.

Vacuum Constrictive Devices

Vacuum constriction devices may be effective at generating and maintaining erections in many patients with erectile dysfunction and these appear to have a low incidence of side effects. As with intracavernosal injection therapy, there is a significant rate of patient dropout with these devices, and the reasons for this phenomenon are unclear. The devices are difficult for some patients to use, and this is especially so in those with impaired manual dexterity. Also, these devices may impair ejaculation, which can then cause some discomfort. Patients and their partners sometimes are bothered by the lack of spontaneity in sexual relations that may occur with this procedure. The patient is sometimes also bothered by the general discomfort that can occur while using these devices. Partner involvement in training with these devices may be important for successful outcome, especially in regard to establishing a mutually satisfying level of sexual activity.

Vascular Surgery

Surgery of the penile venous system, generally involving venous ligation, has been reported to be effective in patients who have been demonstrated to have venous leakage. However, the tests necessary to establish this diagnosis have been incompletely validated; therefore, it is difficult to select patients who will have a predictably good outcome. Moreover, decreased effectiveness of this approach has been reported as longer term follow-ups have been obtained. This has tempered enthusiasm for these procedures, which are probably therefore best done in an investigational setting in medical centers by surgeons experienced in these procedures and their evaluation.

Arterial revascularization procedures have a very limited role (e.g., in congenital or traumatic vascular abnormality) and probably should be restricted to the clinical investigation setting in medical centers with experienced personnel. All patients who are considered for vasular surgical therapy need to have appropriate preoperative evaluation, which may include dynamic infusion pharmaco-cavernosometry and cavernosography (DICC), duplex ultrasonography, and possibly arteriography. The indications for and interpretations of these diagnostic procedures are incompletely

standardized; therefore, difficulties persist with using these techniques to predict and assess the success of surgical therapy, and further investigation to clarify their value and role in this regard is indicated.

Penile Prostheses

Three forms of penile prostheses are available for patients who fail with or refuse other forms of therapy: semirigid, malleable, and inflatable. The effectiveness, complications, and acceptability vary among the three types of prostheses, with the main problems being mechanical failure, infection, and erosions. Silicone particle shedding has been reported, including migration to regional lymph nodes; however, no clinically identifiable problems have been reported as a result of the silicone particles. There is a risk of the need for reoperation with all devices. Although the inflatable prostheses may yield a more physiologically natural appearance, they have had a higher rate of failure requiring reoperation. Men with diabetes mellitus, spinal cord injuries, or urinary tract infections have an increased risk of prosthesis-associated infection. This form of treatment may not be appropriate in patients with severe penile corporal fibrosis or severe medical illness. Circumcision may be required for patients with phimosis and balanitis.

Staging of Treatment

The patient and partner must be well informed about all therapeutic options including their effectiveness, possible complications, and costs. As a general rule, the least invasive or dangerous procedures should be tried first. Psychotherapy and behavioral treatments and sexual counseling alone or in conjunction with other treatments may be used in all patients with erectile dysfunction who are willing to use this form of treatment. In patients in whom psychogenic erectile dysfunction is suspected, sexual counseling should be offered first. Invasive therapy should not be the primary treatment of choice. If history, physical, and screening endocrine evaluations are normal and nonpsychogenic erectile dysfunction is suspected, either vacuum devices or intracavernosal injection therapy can be offered after discussion with the patient and his partner. These latter two therapies may also be useful when combined with psychotherapy in those with psychogenic erectile dysfunction in whom psychotherapy alone has failed. Since further diagnostic testing does not reliably establish specific diagnoses or predict outcomes of therapy, vacuum devices or intracavernosal injections often are applied to a broad spectrum of etiologies of male erectile dysfunction.

The motivation and expectations of the patient and his partner and education of both are critical in determining which therapy is chosen and in optimizing its outcome. If single therapy is ineffective, combining two or more forms of therapy may be useful. Penile prostheses should be placed only after patients have been carefully screened and informed. Vascular surgery should be undertaken only in the setting of clinical investigation and extensive clinical experience. With any form of therapy for erectile dysfunction, long-term follow-up by health professionals is required to assist the patient and his partner with adjustment to the therapeutic intervention. This is particularly true for intracavernosal injection and vacuum constriction therapies. Follow-up should include continued patient education and support in therapy, careful determination of reasons for cessation of therapy if this occurs, and provision of other options if earlier therapies are unsuccessful.

5. WHAT STRATEGIES ARE EFFECTIVE IN IMPROVING PUBLIC AND PROFESSIONAL KNOWLEDGE ABOUT IMPOTENCE?

Despite the accumulation of a substantial body of scientific information about erectile dysfunction, large segments of the public—as well as the health professions—remain relatively uninformed, or—even worse—misinformed, about much of what is known. This lack of information, added to a pervasive reluctance of physicians to deal candidly with sexual matters, has resulted in patients being denied the benefits of treatment for their sexual concerns. Although they might wish doctors would ask them questions about their sexual lives, patients, for their part, are too often inhibited from initiating such discussions themselves. Improving both public and professional knowledge about erectile dysfunction will serve to remove those barriers and will foster more open communication and more effective treatment of this condition.

Strategies for Improving Public Knowledge

To a significant degree, the public, particularly older men, is conditioned to accept erectile dysfunction as a condition of progressive aging for which little can be done. In addition, there is considerable inaccurate public information regarding sexual function and dysfunction. Often, this is in the form of advertisements in which enticing promises are made, and patients then become even more demoralized when promised benefits fail to materialize. Accurate information on sexual function

and the management of dysfunction must be provided to affected men and their partners. They also must be encouraged to seek professional help, and providers must be aware of the embarrassment and/or discouragement that may often be reasons why men with erectile dysfunction avoid seeking appropriate treatment.

To reach the largest audience, communications strategies should include informative and accurate newspaper and magazine articles, radio and television programs, as well as special educational programs in senior centers. Resources for accurate information regarding diagnosis and treatment options also should include doctors' offices, unions, fraternal and service groups, voluntary health organizations, state and local health departments, and appropriate advocacy groups. Additionally, since sex education courses in schools uniformly address erectile function, the concept of erectile dysfunction can easily be communicated in these forums as well.

Strategies for Improving Professional Knowledge

1. Provide wide distribution of this statement to physicians and other health professionals whose work involves patient contact.
2. Define a balance between what specific information is needed by the medical and general public and what is available, and identify what treatments are available.
3. Promote the introduction of courses in human sexuality into the curricula of graduate schools for all health care professionals. As sexual well-being is an integral part of general health, emphasis should be placed on the importance of obtaining a detailed sexual history as part of every medical history.
4. Encourage the inclusion of sessions on diagnosis and management of erectile dysfunction in continuing medical education courses.
5. Emphasize the desirability for an interdisciplinary approach to the diagnosis and treatment of erectile dysfunction. An integrated medical and psychosocial effort with continuing contact with the patient and partner may enhance their motivation and compliance with treatment during the period of sexual rehabilitation.
6. Encourage the inclusion of presentations on erectile dysfunction at scientific meetings of appropriate medical specialty associations, state and local medical societies, and similar organizations of other health professions.
7. Distribute scientific information on erectile dysfunction to the news media (print, radio, and television) to support their efforts to disseminate accurate information on this subject and to

counteract misleading news reports and false advertising claims.

8. Promote public service announcements, lectures, and panel discussions on both commercial and public radio and television on the subject of erectile dysfunction.

6. WHAT ARE THE NEEDS FOR FUTURE RESEARCH?

This consensus development conference on male erectile dysfunction has provided an overview of current knowledge on the prevalence, etiology, pathophysiology, diagnosis, and management of this condition. The growing individual and societal awareness and open acknowledgment of the problem have led to increased interest and resultant explosion of knowledge in each of these areas. Research on this condition has produced many controversies, which also were expressed at this conference. Numerous questions were identified that may serve as foci for future research directions. These will depend on the development of precise agreement among investigators and clinicians in this field on the definition of what constitutes erectile dysfunction, and what factors in its multifaceted nature contribute to its expression. In addition, further investigation of these issues will require collaborative efforts of basic science investigators and clinicians from the spectrum of relevant disciplines and the rigorous application of appropriate research principles in designing studies to obtain further knowledge and to promote understanding of the various aspects of this condition.

The needs and directions for future research can be considered as follows:

- Development of a symptom score sheet to aid in the standardization of patient assessment and treatment outcome.
- Development of a staging system that may permit quantitative and qualitative classification of erectile dysfunction.
- Studies on perceptions and expectations associated with racial, cultural, ethnic, and societal influences on what constitutes normal male erectile function and how these same factors may be responsible for the development and/or perception of male erectile dysfunction.
- Studies to define and characterize what is normal erectile function, possibly as stratified by age.
- Additional basic research on the physiological and biochemical mechanisms that may underlie the etiology, pathogenesis, and response to treatment of the various forms of erectile dysfunction.
- Epidemiological studies directed at the prevalence of male erectile dysfunction and its medical and psychological correlates, particularly in the context of possible racial, ethnic, socioeconomic, and cultural variability.
- Additional studies of the mechanisms by which risk factors may produce erectile dysfunction.
- Studies of strategies to prevent male erectile dysfunction.
- Randomized clinical trials assessing the effectiveness of specific behavioral, mechanical, pharmacologic, and surgical treatments, either alone or in combination.
- Studies on the specific effects of hormones (especially androgens) on male sexual function; determination of the frequency of endocrine causes of erectile dysfunction (e.g., hypogonadism and hyperprolactinemia) and the rates of success of appropriate hormonal therapy.
- Longitudinal studies in well-specified populations; evaluation of alternative approaches for the systematic assessment of men with erectile dysfunction; cost-effectiveness studies of diagnostic and therapeutic approaches; formal outcomes research of the various approaches to the assessment and treatment of this condition.
- Social/psychological studies of the impact of erectile dysfunction on subjects, their partners, and their interactions, and factors associated with seeking care.
- Development of new therapies, including pharmacologic agents, and with emphasis on oral agents, that may address the cause of male erectile dysfunction with greater specificity.
- Long-term follow-up studies to assess treatment effects, patient compliance, and late adverse effects.
- Studies to characterize the significance of erectile function and dysfunction in women.

CONCLUSIONS

- The term "erectile dysfunction" should replace the term "impotence" to characterize the inability to attain and/or maintain penile erection sufficient for satisfactory sexual performance.
- The likelihood of erectile dysfunction increases progressively with age but is not an inevitable consequence of aging. Other age-related conditions increase the likelihood of its occurrence.
- Erectile dysfunction may be a consequence of medications taken for other problems or a result of drug abuse.
- Embarrassment of patients and the reluctance

of both patients and health care providers to discuss sexual matters candidly contribute to underdiagnosis of erectile dysfunction.

- Contrary to present public and professional opinion, many cases of erectile dysfunction can be successfully managed with appropriately selected therapy.
- Men with erectile dysfunction require diagnostic evaluations and treatments specific and responsive to their circumstances. Patient compliance as well as patient and partner desires and expectations are important considerations in the choice of a particular treatment approach. A multidisciplinary approach may be of great benefit in defining the problem and arriving at a solution.
- The development of methods to quantify the degree of erectile dysfunction objectively would be extremely useful in the assessment both of the problem and of treatment outcomes.
- Education of physicians and other health professionals in aspects of human sexuality is currently inadequate, and curriculum development is urgently needed.
- Education of the public on aspects of sexual dysfunction and the availability of successful treatments is essential; media involvement in this effort is an important component. This should be combined with information designed to expose "quack remedies" and protect men and their partners from economic and emotional losses.
- Important information on many aspects of erectile dysfunction is lacking; major research efforts are essential to the improvement of our understanding of the appropriate diagnostic assessments and treatments of this condition.
- Erectile dysfunction is an important public health problem deserving of increased support for basic science investigation and applied research.

CONSENSUS DEVELOPMENT PANEL

Michael J. Droller, M.D.
Panel and Conference Chairperson
Professor and Chairman, Department of Urology
The Mount Sinai Medical Center
New York, New York

James R. Anderson, Ph.D.
Professor and Chair
Department of Preventive and Societal Medicine
University of Nebraska Medical Center
Omaha, Nebraska

John C. Beck, M.D.
Director
Professor of Medicine-Geriatrics
Multicampus Program of Geriatric Medicine and Gerontology
UCLA School of Medicine
Los Angeles, California

William J. Bremner, M.D., Ph.D.
Chief of Medicine
Seattle Veterans' Affairs Medical Center
Professor and Vice-Chairman of Medicine
University of Washington
Seattle, Washington

Kurt Evans, M.D.
Chief
Department of Urology
Kaiser Permanente
Dallas, Texas

Mikel Gray, Ph.D., CURN
Clinical Uro Dynamics
Adjunct Professor
Georgia State University School of Nursing
Alpharetta, Georgia

Arthur H. Keeney, III
Executive Director
American Foundation for Urologic Disease
Baltimore, Maryland

Philip J. Lanzisera, Ph.D.
Director of Psychology Internship Program
Department of Psychiatry
Henry Ford Health Sciences Center
Detroit, Michigan

Winston C. Liao, Ph.D.
Associate Program Director
Center for Epidemiologic and Medical Studies
Research Triangle Institute
Research Triangle Park, North Carolina

David W. Richardson, M.D.
Professor of Medicine
Department of Cardiology
Medical College of Virginia
Richmond, Virginia

Thomas J. Rohner, Jr., M.D.
Professor of Surgery (Urology)
Chief Division of Urology
Pennsylvania State University College of Medicine
Milton S. Hershey Medical Center
Hershey, Pennsylvania

Linda D. Shortliffe, M.D.
Associate Professor
Chief, Pediatric Urology
Department of Urology
Packard Children's Hospital at Stanford
Stanford University Medical School
Stanford, California

William R. Turner, M.D.
Professor and Chairman
Department of Urology
Medical University of South Carolina Charleston
Charleston, South Carolina

Arthur Zitrin, M.D.
Professor of Psychiatry
Associate Dean
New York University School of Medicine
New York, New York

SPEAKERS

Stanley E. Althof, Ph.D.
Choosing Among Contemporary Alternatives: Self-Injection Versus Vacuum Pump Therapy

Alan H. Bennett, M.D.
When to Perform Venous Studies in the Impotent Patient

Gregory Broderick, M.D.
Drug-Induced Male Sexual Dysfunction

Irwin Goldstein, M.D.
The Effect of Age-Related Diseases on the Development of Impotence
The Venous System in the Diagnosis of Erectile Impotence
Intracavernosal Therapy for Erectile Impotence

Helen Singer Kaplan, Ph.D.
The Psychological Evaluation of the Impotent Male

Stanley G. Korenman, M.D.
The Relationship Between Impotence and Aging

Ronald W. Lewis, M.D.
Penile Prosthesis

Tom F. Lue, M.D.
Anatomy and Physiology of Normal and Abnormal Erection
The Diagnosis of Arterial-Related Impotence Peyronie's Disease

William H. Masters, M.D.
Introduction: A History of the Diagnosis and Treatment of Impotence

John B. McKinlay, Ph.D.
The Prevalence and Demographics of Impotence

Arnold Melman, M.D.
The Argument Against the Utilization of Arterial Studies in the Diagnosis of Impotence

Drogo K. Montague, M.D.
General Diagnostic Procedures Employed in the Diagnosis of Erectile Impotence

Alvaro Morales, M.D., F.R.C.S.(C)
Hormonal Studies in the Evaluation of the Impotent Man
The Medical Management of Impotence

David Osborne, Ph.D.
Behavioral Intervention in the Treatment of Erectile Impotence

Jacob Rajfer, M.D.
Nitric Oxide and Erections

John Rowe, M.D.
The Prevention of Erectile Impotence—The Need for Education

Iñigo Saenz de Tejada, M.D.
Vascular Physiology of Erection

Michael H.H. Sohn, M.D.
Vascular Procedures for the Treatment of Erectile Impotence

William D. Steers, M.D.
Neurophysiology of Penile Erection

Leonore Tiefer, Ph.D.
Nomenclature

Gorm Wagner, M.D., Ph.D.
Partner Issues in Diagnosis and Treatment
Neurologic Evaluation of the Impotent Male

PLANNING COMMITTEE

Leroy M. Nyberg, Ph.D., M.D.
Planning Committee Chairperson
Director
Urology Program
Division of Kidney, Urologic, and Hematologic Diseases
National Institute of Diabetes and Digestive and Kidney Diseases
National Institutes of Health
Bethesda, Maryland

Alan H. Bennett, M.D.
Professor of Surgery
Head, Division of Urological Surgery
Albany Medical Center Hospital and Albany Medical College
Albany, New York

Benjamin T. Burton, Ph.D.
Associate Director for Disease Prevention and Technology Transfer
National Institute of Diabetes and Digestive and Kidney Diseases
National Institutes of Health
Bethesda, Maryland

Michael J. Droller, M.D.
Conference and Panel Chairperson
Professor and Chairman
Department of Urology
Mount Sinai Medical Center
New York, New York

Jerry M. Elliott
Program Analyst
Office of Medical Applications of Research
National Institutes of Health
Bethesda, Maryland

John H. Ferguson, M.D.
Director
Office of Medical Applications of Research
National Institutes of Health
Bethesda, Maryland

Willis R. Foster, M.D.
Senior Staff Physician
Office of Disease Prevention and Technology Transfer
National Institute of Diabetes and Digestive and Kidney Diseases
National Institutes of Health
Bethesda, Maryland

Jean Fourcroy, M.D.
Medical Officer
Division of Metabolism and Endocrinology Drug Products
Center for Drug Evaluation and Research
Food and Drug Administration
Rockville, Maryland

Irwin Goldstein, M.D.
Professor of Urology
Department of Urology
Boston University School of Medicine
Boston, Massachusetts

William H. Hall
Director of Communications
Office of Medical Applications of Research
National Institutes of Health
Bethesda, Maryland

F. Terry Hambrecht, M.D.
Head
Neural Prosthesis Program
Division of Fundamental Neurosciences
National Institute of Neurological Disorders and Stroke
National Institutes of Health
Bethesda, Maryland

Mary M. Harris
Writer/Editor
Office of Health Research Reports
National Institute of Diabetes and Digestive and Kidney
   Diseases
National Institutes of Health
Bethesda, Maryland

Stuart S. Howards, M.D.
Professor of Urology
Department of Urology
University of Virginia Hospital
Charlottesville, Virginia

Mark D. Kramer
Chief
Urology and Lithotripsy Devices Branch
Food and Drug Administration
Rockville, Maryland

Tom F. Lue, M.D.
Professor
Department of Urology
University of California at San Francisco
San Francisco, California

William H. Masters, M.D.
Masters & Johnson Institute
St. Louis, Missouri

Arnold Melman, M.D.
Professor and Chairman
Department of Urology
Albert Einstein College of Medicine
Montefiore Medical Center
Bronx, New York

Stanley L. Slater, M.D.
Acting Deputy Associate Director for Geriatrics
National Institute on Aging
National Institutes of Health
Bethesda, Maryland

Donna L. Vogel, M.D., Ph.D.
Head, Reproductive Medicine Unit
Reproductive Sciences Branch
National Institute of Child Health and Human Development
National Institutes of Health
Bethesda, Maryland

CONFERENCE SPONSORS

National Institute of Diabetes and Digestive and Kidney Diseases
Phillip Gorden, M.D.
Director

Office of Medical Applications of Research, NIH
John H. Ferguson, M.D.
Director

Index

Note: Page numbers in *italics* refer to illustrations; page numbers followed by t refer to tables.

309

ISBN 0-7216-3768-X

90038